TWO DISCOURSES
concerning
THE SOUL OF BRUTES

HISTORY OF PSYCHOLOGY SERIES
General Introduction

The historically interesting works reprinted in this series helped to prepare the way for the science of psychology. Most of these books are long forgotten, but their relevance to the field is unmistakable. Many of the writings on mental and moral philosophy, published before the dawn of scientific procedures, have much to commend them to present-day scholars. These books serve as groundwork for a fuller account of the background from which the field emerged, and they should be attractive to students who seek in the past for hints of the future direction that certain types of research can take. Each work will have an Introduction stating the provenance and significance of the book and will add appropriate biographical information.

Robert I. Watson
General Editor
University of New Hampshire

TWO DISCOURSES

CONCERNING

The Soul of Brutes,

Which is that of the

Vital and Sensitive of Man.

BY

Thomas Willis

A FACSIMILE REPRODUCTION
OF THE TRANSLATION BY S. PORDAGE, 1683,
WITH AN INTRODUCTION

BY

Solomon Diamond

GAINESVILLE, FLORIDA
SCHOLARS' FACSIMILES & REPRINTS
1971

SCHOLARS' FACSIMILES & REPRINTS

1605 N.W. 14TH AVENUE

GAINESVILLE, FLORIDA 32601 U.S.A.

HARRY R. WARFEL, GENERAL EDITOR

REPRODUCED FROM A COPY
OWNED BY SOLOMON DIAMOND

L. C. CATALOG CARD NUMBER: 72-161936

ISBN 0-8201-1096-5

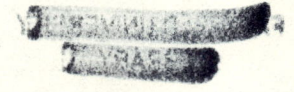

Manufactured in the U.S.A.

INTRODUCTION

Thomas Willis was born in 1621, lived in his boyhood near Oxford, enlisted there as a royalist soldier in his student years, was rewarded after the Restoration by appointment to the Sedleian chair of natural philosophy (made vacant by the ousting of an incumbent with wrong affiliations), and was active at Oxford until 1666. In that year he moved to London, where he enjoyed a prosperous practice until pneumonia caused his untimely death in 1675. Of his two chief works, one, the *Cerebri anatome* (1664), is the product of his Oxford years, and smells one may say of the "Anatomical Court" where he had "slain whole Hecatombs almost of all animals;" the other (*De anima brutorum,* 1672, presently before us in a reproduction of its first English edition) issues from the consulting room of a practising physician who writes chiefly from the points of view of the clinician and the humanist scholar. It fulfills, however, the promise given in the Conclusion to the earlier work, that "for the Crown of the Work, a certain Theory of the Soul of Brutes should be added. . . . Truly it is but just and equal, that we enter upon this Discourse of the Soul, and that other task of *Pathologie,* to wit, that the Asperities and hard sence of our already instituted Anatomy may be sweetned with those kind of more pleasant Speculations, as it were cloathing the Skeleton with flesh."

The reader who wishes to learn more about the biographic circumstances of Willis's life, his associations, and his lesser writings, may turn to the excellent volume of introductory materials which accompanies the recent reproduction of Samuel Pordage's English translation of the *Cerebri anatome*. (*The Anatomy of the Brain and Nerves*, ed. by Wm. Feindel. 2 vols. Montreal: McGill University Press, 1965.) There is also a fine monograph by Hansruedi Isler: *Thomas Willis . . . Doctor and Scientist* (Hafner, 1968). This introduction has a more narrow scope.

Willis is remembered chiefly as an anatomist who immeasurably advanced the study of the brain and nervous system. But his anatomy is always relevant to function. The "circle of Willis" is an anatomical designation, but its discovery resulted from the investigation of the circulation of blood through the brain using the new technique of injecting "inky liquor" into the carotid artery. This appreciation of the importance of blood supply to the brain leads on to the view which Horwicz (*Analyse des Denkens*, 1875) expressed 200 years later in the phrase, startling even to his contemporaries, "ohne Blut kein Gedanke." It also foreshadows our present awareness of the critical importance of uninterrupted blood supply not merely for the present functioning but for the maintenance of the brain.

Another illustration: Willis's careful charting of the cranial and spinal nerves (which led him to coin the term neurology—that subsequently acquired much broader meaning—to designate this branch of his anatomical labors) was similarly motivated by interest in function, "because without the perfect knowledge of the Nerves the Doctrine of the Brain and its Appendix would be left wholly lame and imperfect." In this respect he is the precursor of Charles Bell, who only echoed Willis in stating that "to arrive at any understanding of the internal parts of the cerebrum, we must keep in view the relations of the nerves, and must class and distinguish the nerves, and follow them into its substance [*Idea for a New Anatomy of the Brain*, 1811, p. 28]."

Although Willis likened the *Anatomy* to a foundation upon which the present work would be erected as a superstructure, it is by no means necessary to read one before the

INTRODUCTION

other. It may, however, be of value to have a summary statement of Willis's neurophysiological theories, and we can conceive of no better way of doing this than to borrow it from George Prochaska, the Czech physiologist whose *Dissertation on the Functions of the Nervous System* (1784, English translation 1851) showed the influence of Willis (as its translator, Thomas Laycock, points out) in distinguishing between a "soul-sensorium" seated in the brain and a "corporeal sensorium" seated in brain, spinal cord, and nerves. Prochaska wrote:

"Thomas Willis, a celebrated member of the chemical sect, advanced, with some ingenuity, many new hypotheses as to the uses of the nervous system. ... His own peculiar doctrines chiefly are: that the cerebrum subserves to the animal functions and the voluntary motions, the cerebellum to the involuntary; that a perception of all the sensations takes place in the ascending fibres of the corpora striata, and that through the descending, voluntary movements are excited; that the understanding is seated in the corpus callosum, and memory in the convolutions, which are its storehouses; that the animal spirits are generated in the cortex of the cerebrum and cerebellum from the arterial blood; that they collect in the medulla, are variously distributed and arranged to excite the animal actions, and distil through the fornix as through a pelican: that the animal spirits secreted in the cerebellum are ever flowing, equably and continuously, into the nerves which regulate involuntary movements; but those of the cerebrum tumultuously and irregularly, according as the animal actions are vehemently performed or quiescent. To excite sensation, the spirits flow along the nerves to the brain. He distinguishes between a thick nervous fluid, suitable to nutrition, and the extremely volatile animal spirits, subservient to sensation and movement, and commingled in the preceding as their vehicle. He maintains, that there are two souls in man, the one rational, the other corporeal; the latter alone is given to brutes. ... He explains the unity of the nerves by their communications and connections with each other, or their anastomoses, as anatomists term them: and he also explains, that the union of the cerebrum and cerebellum is attained by the tubercula quadrigemina, or nates and testes. As to the loops of nerves with which the arteries here and there are encircled, he states their use to be, to relax or close the arteries, and thus during various emotions of the mind to admit the blood in greater or less quantity to certain parts. He decided that the pineal gland is not the seat of the soul, but a lymphatic gland, having no relation with the substance of the brain, which absorbs lymph, and carries it off again through other vessels, and keeps the plexus choroides expanded [1851, p. 375-376]."

The modern reader will not fail to be impressed by one aspect of Willis's work which Prochaska omitted to mention: his great contribution in founding comparative neuroanatomy.

Quite another face of Willis, which appears in the second of these *Two dissertations,* is that of the practitioner dealing with "diseases which affect . . . the brain and nervous stock." The views of Willis were quite influential in this area, too. Zilboorg (*History of Medical Psychology,* 1941), who is hostile to every attempt to give mental illness an organic basis, looks upon Willis as a *bête noire* "whose psychological acumen lagged behind his other scientific achievements," and as one who helped lay "the foundations of a psychiatry without psychology which took root in medical science and which, while rendering inestimable service to neuroanatomy, neurophysiology, and neuropathology, almost totally discarded the study of the very psychological phenomena which these men seem to have set out to study." For Zilboorg, the baleful influence of Willis is symbolized by the persistence of the term "neurologist" as a synonym for "psychiatrist."

This condemnation seems unfair, for in fact Willis (in his preface) declares "some to be rather sick in Soul; yea first, and chiefly than in Body; otherways than the Schools of Physicians, which refer the primary seats of all Diseases, into solid Parts, Humors, and Vital Spirits, or innate Heat." However, he views these sicknesses as affections of a corporeal soul, which has "not only Extension, but Members, and as it were Organical Parts, yea Peculiar Diseases." Hunter and Macalpine (*Three Hundred Years of Psychiatry*, 1964) point out in a more balanced appraisal that it was Willis who "convincingly vindicated the uterus and the humours from causing hysteria." Also, "he attributed 'melancholy' or affective psychosis to 'passions of the heart'; and 'madness' or psychosis accompanied by thought disorder, delusions or hallucination—that is schizophrenia—to 'vice or fault of the Brain'. He recognised the difference between the symptoms of gross brain disease and those of mental illness by postulating a disturbance of the brain and nerves in terms of disordered 'Animal Spirits'. For this reason he is often credited with having first equated mind disease with brain disease."

Even if Willis had not left so deep a mark on what we may call the "two neurologies," neuroanatomy and psychiatry, his work would still have special appeal to psychologists because it represents the highest point reached by the psychology of Renaissance medicine, in which the Galenic tradition is still strong, though no longer blindly followed. His discussions of animal instinct, animal learning, human passions, and "stupidity, or foolishness" seem to this reader to be particularly rewarding. No doubt, however, each reader will find his own favorite topics. The book is, besides, a literary treat, even in translation. Soury (*Le systéme nerveux centrale*, 1899) declared that Willis's "great imagination, brilliance of language [in the Latin original!], and profundity of thought remind us of Shakespeare."

With this work, Willis closed an epoch in the history of psychology. Among those who listened to his lectures at Oxford was John Locke, who, though probably departing little in his beliefs from any of the specific teachings of Willis, chose in his *Essay concerning Human Understanding*

(1690) not to "meddle with the physical considerations of mind." The imaginations of the generation after Willis were captivated by the achievements of Newton and soon, under the banner of "empiricism," a thoroughly rationalistic psychology would hold sway, and metaphysical speculations would replace physiological hypotheses. Not before the time of Cabanis (*Rapports du physique et du moral de l'homme,* 1802) would there be another work to stand beside this, as a comprehensive effort to deal with the full range of behavior in terms of the most advanced contemporary knowledge of the nervous system.

SOLOMON DIAMOND

California State College
Los Angeles

TWO DISCOURSES

CONCERNING

The Soul of Brutes,

Which is that of the

Vital and Senſitive of Man.

The Firſt is PHYSIOLOGICAL, ſhewing the NATURE, PARTS, POWERS, and AFFECTIONS of the ſame.

The Other is PATHOLOGICAL, which unfolds the DISEASES which Affect it and its Primary Seat; to wit, The BRAIN and NERVOUS STOCK, And Treats of their CURES: With Copper Cuts.

By *THOMAS WILLIS* Doctor in PHYSICK, Profeſſor of Natural Philoſophy in *OXFORD*, and alſo one of the Royal Society, and of the renowned College of Phyſicians in *LONDON*.

Engliſhed
By *S. PORDAGE*, Student in PHYSICK.

LONDON,

Printed for *Thomas Dring* at the *Harrow* near *Chancery-Lane* End in *Fleet-ſtreet*, *Ch. Harper* at the *Flower-de-Luce* againſt St. *Dunſtan*'s Church in *Fleet-ſtreet*, and *John Leigh* at *Stationers-Hall*. 1683.

To the most Reverend Father in God

GILBERT

(By Divine Providence)

Arch-Bishop of Canterbury,

Primate and Metropolitan of all *ENGLAND*, and one of the Privy Council to His Sacred Majesty *CHARLES* the Second, King of *Great Britain, France*, and *Ireland*, &c.

Most Renowned Prelate,

IN *that I still become troublesom to your greater Cares, by this Kind of often repeated Duty, I must also repeat my former Excuse. For that these my VVritings, with those formerly Published, for the most part consist of those things which I have delivered in my Academical Readings, by a necessitated Duty belong to you, for that I received them from your Favours; and indeed, neither these had ever seen the Light, nor perhaps my self had ever been in the number of Authors, unless I had been made at first your* Sidlie *Professor at* Oxford; *yours I say, both for the ancient Honour with which you had advanced me, and also for the more fresh magnificent Liberality, which has obliged the whole* Academy, *and all its Gowned Company. All the Schools partake of what is imputed to your* Theatre; *and moreover all the Professors, whil'st every one of their private Patrons are acknowledged,Celebrate* Sheldon; *who exceeds, by your gifts that of other Mecænatuses, and Crowns the whole.*

But as these Disquisitions are indebted to your Munificence, so they require your Patronage, and we offer them not more in Duty to your Grace, than for the Cause of your

A 2 *Tutelage.*

The Epistle Dedicatory.

Tutelage. Concerning the Soul, I have enter'd upon a great and difficult thing, and full of hazard; where we may equally fear the Censures of the Church, as the Schools. For that I assert a Man (as the Mad-man in the Gospel possess't with a Legion) to be indued with many distinct Souls, and design sometimes a legitimate Subordination of them, and sometimes wicked Combinations, troublesom Contests, and more than Civil Wars; yea, and in that I importunately describe, the Manners and Affections, the Mutual Exaltations, Dejections, and Productions of either, and their state after Separation: These, I say, some not only Philosophers, but Theologists perhaps may find fault with. And altho I have a place of Safety, in that the Arguments and Reasons fight on my Side, and that I have got the Suffrages of the ancient Philosophers, and the holy Fathers (and especially of St. Hierome *and* Augustine, *and among the Moderns of* Gassendus *and our* Hammond*) yet suffer your Grace for my greater Safety, to extend your help to me, and grant that I may profess in the Entrance to this Discourse, that I am*

Your Graces

Most humble and devoted Servant

Tho. Willis.

To the Most LEARNED and WORSHIPFUL

By me ever Respected

The Vice-Chancellor, Doctors, *and* Masters, *who diligently Profess, greatly Adorn, and happily Promote good Letters in the most Famous University of* Oxford, *Health.*

Excuse me, Learned Men, if you, who were once my Auditors, I now desire to be my Readers, and you whom I ever found Propitious and Favourable, that I therefore wish you may be my Judges and Patrons. Your singular Humanity hath formerly enflamed my Industry, in this Physiological Undertaking, and given me Life and Strength; so that if that any thing of Praise be due to me, it ought to be imputed and referred to you. I know indeed how great difference there is, betwixt the flying words of Speakers, and those impress'd upon lasting Papers; but it seems of great Authority, that they have not been displeasing to your most Curious Judgments, in their utterance, and I hope they may now pass any Examen, having already passed your Critical Ears. It therefore belongs to you to defend, if not these my Endeavours, yet at least your own Judgments; and if perchance, the litterate *Thrasoe's* of this Age, who are wholly ignorant in Philosophy, every where wandring about, attempt to overthrow me with their Clamors, which is their chief Eloquence, to oppose your Authority against them, by which, if they are not put to Silence, it will be however an high Confidence and inviolable Security to

Honored Sirs,

the Admirer of you all,

THO. WILLIS.

THE PREFACE TO THE READER.

Courteous Reader.

I Have here given you what I had long promised, the Pathology of the Brain and Nervous Stock, and with it the previous Physical Meditations of the Soul of the Brutes, which is that inferior one of Man. This difficult task, when at first denied leisure and retirement, it could not be performed; after the Death of my Dear Wife, being lonely, with frequent and unseasonable Studies, that I might the less think on my Grief, I have at last finished this, according to my slender Capacity. But indeed in these Disquisitions (which the Anatomy of the Brain, and its Appendixes, hath lately and more exactly shown) as we have enter'd into a by-way, and not before trodden, there was a necessity to lead thee, thorow some sharp and stony ways, beset with bushes and thorns, which might offend thee. And indeed I know not, whether it will be pleasing to all, that instituting the something Paradoxical Doctrine of the Animal Soul, that I should assign to that Soul, by which the Brutes as well as Men live, feel, move, not only Extension, but Members, and as it were Organical Parts, yea peculiar Diseases, and proper means or methods of Curing them; and that moreover, I should form this, which is meerly Vital, and different from the Rational, and subordinate to it, and so Man, a Two-soul'd Animal, and as it were a manifold Geryon.

That I may remove out of the way these little rubs, I do not at all doubt to overcome them, and evince the Corporeity of the Soul, by Reasons not to be contemned, and also by the full suffrage, both of the Ancients and the Moderns; and besides, that it is Bipart or Twofold, I have already, in another place, by a necessary Consequence deduced, from the Life of the Blood, as it were a flame, and from the existency of the Animal Spirits, and as it were lucid or ætherial Hypostasis, asserted and proved. For granting to the Soul, one Vital Portion living in the Blood, to be a certain inkindling of it, and another Sensitive, to be only an heap of Animal Spirits every where diffused thorow the Brain and Nervous Stock; it follows from hence, that Brutes have a Soul Co-extended to the whole Body, and Parts not only many and distinct, but after a manner dissimilar. But that some object, that the Soul of the Beast, because it perceives, or knows that it feels, to be immaterial, for that Matter seems to be incapable of Perception, that indeed, had been likely, if that Perception should pass beyond the limits of Material things; or higher, than what inspires them, which things are usually attributed to Natural Instinct, or Idiocrasie or peculiar Temperaments, that I may omit Sympathies and Antipathies. But who should be the Betrother? I profess the great God, as the only Work-man, so also as the first Mover, and auspiciously present, every where, was he not able to impress strength, Powers, and Faculties to Matter, fitted to the offices of a Sensitive Life? The Pen in the hand of the Writer, Disputes, Intreats, gives Relations of Things, and is in the midst between things past and things to come; and why should we not believe that greater things than any of these, may be done, when the Skill

of

of the Deity is present? Lastly, If any one shall affirm, that most subtile Substance, and wholly Etherial, which serves for the Vital Oeconomy or Government to be immaterial, for that it enters upon the sluggish Disposition of inanimate Bodies, let him remember to be indulgent to me, if by chance I call it material, for that it subsists very much below the Prerogatives of Reason.

But I shall not stand upon these things, for truly I have prepared a far othergates defence; to wit, I speak not from the Tripos like an Oracle, nor from the Chair, but as one of a low form: I play not the Prophet, or Dictator, but the Philosopher, neither do I plant an Opinion, but propose an Hypothesis, and open my Judgment. Geometry has its Demonstrations in it self; we are Skill'd in that part of Philosophy, where it aboundantly suffices to have brought Logical Proofs: Surely he only certainly pronounces, who professes his Errors, and whilst he Philosophizes about Man, remembers himself that he is a Man.

But that according to the Adage, that I should declare some to be rather sick in Soul, yea first, and chiefly than in Body; otherways than the Schools of Physicians, which refer the Primary Seats of all Diseases, into solid Parts, Humors, and Vital Spirits, or innate Heat: I say from our Hypothesis, to wit, that this Soul hath a material Subsistence, extended equally with the Body, and peculiar Parts, Powers, and Affections; may be concluded, that it is found obnoxious also to preternatural Diseases, and not seldom wants Medical help.

Moreover, That the Corporeal Soul doth extend its Sicknesses, not only to the Body, but to the Mind or rational Soul, which is of an higher linage, and that it often-times involves it with its failings and faults, I think is clear enough in our Pathology or Method of Curing. Further, for the proving these two distinct Souls, to be together and subordinately in Man, as much as Authority and the force of Reasons can, I think is there proved; which Opinion is so far from that I need to fear it should be censured for Pernicious or Heretical; that on the contrary, we hope it is altogether Orthodox, and appears agreeable to a good Life, and Pious Institution: from hence the Wars and Strivings between our two Appetites, or between the Flesh and Spirit, both Morally and Theologically inculcated to us, are also Physically understood; for that, I see and approve the better things, and follow the worser; and this, The Flesh lusts against the Spirit, and the Spirit against the Flesh. So generally comes to pass in us, for as much as the Corporeal Soul adhering to the Flesh, inclines Man to Sensual Pleasures, whil'st in the mean time, the Rational Soul, being help'd by Ethical Rules, or Divine favour, invites it to good Manners, and the works of Piety. Further, from hence, the chief Argument is brought against Epicurism, and Atheism, for that it is moved by the force of Reasons, our Sensitive Soul even as that of the Brutes, miscarrying, the other perpetually survives; for truly being perswaded of an after and Eternal State, why doth it not make it its whole business, that it may live more happily in it, or at least not miserably?

But also, that it may be objected, that there cannot be therefore two Souls in Man, because many forms cannot actuate at once the same Matter; It may be answer'd; that the Supream form of the same Subject, doth sometimes subordinately include many others, but specifies it only a Compound. Also, the Corporeal Soul being subordinate to the Rational, subsists immediately in the Humane Body, and this Superior is in the same, that mediating. It would be a much more difficult solution of this hard Business, if the Inferior Soul of Man, common to that with the Brutes, should be also affirmed to be immaterial; for by what knitting together, can two independent Souls subsist in the same Body; being from thence separated and Combined, by no common Bone, into what place can they depart severally? Certainly as to reason, it is more probable, and to the Humane government more agreeable, to affirm that one most subtilly Corporal Soul, is joyned immediately to the Body, and is intimately united, and that by the intervention of this Soul, another immaterial, residing in its Bosom, inhabits the Body, and is the supream and principal form of the whole Man: But that after Death, the Corporeal Soul being extinct, this survives and is Immortal.

That

The Preface.

That the Corporeal, Flameous, and lucid Nature of this Soul, and its Parts and Affections, may be the better known, I have thought it necessary to describe the Vital Organs, both of all Kinds of living Creatures, by the Action of which the Lamp of Light is maintain'd; and also to shew plainly laid open, even to their intimate recesses, and least and secret Passages, the Brains, both of the more perfect Brutes, and also of Man. The Anatomy of which being manifold; not being able to perform it only with my own hand, and Skill, being also almost continually interrupted by my Practice, the Famous and Skilful Anatomist and Physician Dr. Edmond King was much helpful to me, by his assiduous and notable assistance and labour. Also that learned Man, and my most intimate Friend, Dr. John Masters, Skilful in Physick and Anatomy, imployed much of his Labour and Diligence in the same Business. Out of this various Zootomie or Anatomy of the more perfect Beasts and many-flower'd dissection, the wonderful things of God are very much made known, for as much as in every the smallest and vilest little Animals, not only the Face and Members, but also the inward Parts, as it were the Hearths and Altars for the continuing the Vital Fire, shew them to be of a most Elegant and Artificial and plainly Divine Structure.

As to our Pathology or Method of Cure, I must confess, that in delivering the Theory of Diseases, leaving the old way, I have almost every where brought forth new Hypotheses: but what being founded upon Anatomical Observations, and firmly stablished, better solve all the Phænomena of the Sick, (viz.) They declare more aptly the Causes of the Symptoms, and shew the Reasons of Curing, more accommodate to every Disease. But as to the Remedies and Therapeutic Method, altho we follow not exactly, after the manner of others, the Ancients, we have nevertheless rejected nothing ratified by grave Authority, or approved by daily Experience; and besides, we have added many things found out Emperically and Analogically by the Moderns; Altho it is neither our Hope or Ambition that these should be pleasing to all; yet (what is my last wish) I doubt not, but that this may be an help to many for the illustrating the Medical Science, and for the more happy Curing of Cephalick Diseases. Farewel.

OF

Che Soul of the Brutes,

The First Part

PHYSIOLOGICAL,

SHEWING,

Its NATURE, PARTS, POWERS, and AFFECTIONS.

CHAP. I.

The Opinions of Authors both Ancient and Modern are recounted.

With what Pleasures, and with what Delight, beyond other things, the Contemplation of the Soul hath drawn to it self the Wits of Men, and most profoundly Exercised them, appears even from hence, that almost none of the Philosophers, of whatsoever Sect they were, and of every Age, who have not laboured in the search of it: But indeed, how hard and abstruse it is, and with what dark Blackness, not less than the shades of Hell it self, this Knowledge of the Soul is over-shadowed, may be gathered from this; because they are opposite and uncertain, concerning it; yea, almost as many Men as there are, so many several Opinions have they Published; that truly 'tis no unjust Complaint of the Soul, that she understands all things but her Self. Nevertheless, in this Age, most fruitful of Inventions, when that so many Admirable things not before thought on, as it were another Ancient World unknown, are discovered, about the building of the Animal Body, when new Creeks are daily found out, new humours spring up, and altogether another Doctrine than what hath been delivered by the Ancients, concerning the use of many of the Parts, hath been instituted; why may we not also hope, that there may be yet shewn a new disquisition concerning the Soul, and with better luck than hitherto? Therefore, however the thing may be performed, I shall attempt to Philosophise concerning that Soul at least, which is Common to Brute Animals with Man, and which seems to depend altogether on the Body, to be born and dye with it, to actuate all its Parts, to be extended thorow them, and to be plainly Corporeal; and that chiefly, because, by the Nature, Subsistence, Parts, and Affections of this Corporeal Soul rightly unfolded, the Ingenuity, Temperament, and Manners of every Man may be thence the better known; as also the Causes, and formal Reasons of many Diseases, as of the Phrensie, Lethargy, Vertigo, Madness, Melancholy, and others, belonging rather to the Soul than to the Body, as yet hidden, may in some part be discovered: Then Secondly, because the ends and bounds of the aforesaid Corporeal Soul being defined, the Rational Soul, Superior and Immaterial, may be sufficiently differenced from it; nor is that Argument admitted so easily, confounding them together, whereby some deserving very ill of themselves, have affirmed the Souls of Man and the Beasts only to differ in degrees of Perfection; and so that either alike must be either Mortal or Immortal, and alike propagated *ex traduce* or from the Parent. Wherefore that the Dignity, Order, and Immortality of the Rational Soul, discriminated from the Corporeal, may be vindicated, and likewise that we may make a way to the remaining Pathology, or Method of Curing of the Brain and Nervous Stock, in which not only Parts of the Body, but often the animal Spirits, yea, sometimes the whole sensitive Soul, seems to be affected, (altho we have formerly unfolded according to our slender Ability, not after this manner, the Descriptions and Uses of the Brain and Nerves,) Therefore at present, we

The Contemplation of the Soul pleasant but difficult.

It Conduces to the knowing of the Manners of Men, and the Diseases of the Soul.

It distinguishes the Rational Soul of Man, from that other of the Brutes

B shall

shall endeavour to deliver a certain Doctrine of the Soul, previous to the shewing the Doctrine of the Diseases of those Parts. But here it will be first expedient to rehearse the Opinions of others, or at least the chiefest and most noted among them: From which, being put together, if not what the Soul truly is, may be made known; yet what many considering it have thought of it; and from thence a little more certain search of it, we may enterprize.

And indeed if we would grow wise concerning the Soul only out of the Pleas of Authors, and the Writings of Philosophers of every Age, we should be intangled in a Labyrinth of Opinions, following for truth mere Phantasms, and for the genuine Idea of the Soul, as it were the Apparitions of divers Specters. But that we may reduce the various Opinions, whatever have been declared, both of the Ancients and Moderns, to some certain Heads; it will be fit that we observe, some did affirm it to be Corporeal, others Incorporeal. In either Kind we meet with great diversity of Opinions. For first of all, *Some have affirmed the Soul of the Beast to be an Incorporeal Substance; to wit, the Platonists, and the Pythagoreans.* among those who thought it Incorporeal, some affirmed it to be a Substance existing of it self and immortal, others without Substance having only an accidental form. Those who believed the Soul an Incorporeal and Immortal Substance, differed also among themselves. The *Platonists* and *Pythagoreans* said, the Souls of all living Creatures, to be a certain Part of the Universal Soul of the World, and that they were depressed or immerged in this lower Body, as in a Sepulcher; and therefore, the Soul, when the Animal received Life, was not born but dyed; for as much as by this inferior Birth, it was divided from the simple and undivided fountain of Nature. Further they thought, that the same Soul so demersed, did wander from one Body being dead, to another, and so by a various *Metampseuchosis*, did inhabit or was a guest sometimes in the Bodies of Men, and sometimes of Beasts. The *Manichees* asserted, That all Souls being taken out of the Substance it self of God, did actuate Terrestrial Bodies, and going from hence again, returned into God himself. The *Origenists* different from either, taught that Souls were Created from the beginning of the World, and at first to subsist of themselves, then as occasion serv'd, that Bodies being formed, they enter'd into them being begun, and actuated them during Life, and that at length they returned to their private or singular Substances. The state of which Souls, tho some attributed it only to Humane Souls; yet there were others, who granted the like Immortality to the Souls of the Brutes, yea and of Plants.

Cap. 2. de Nat. Hom.

Others an Incorporeal form as the Peripateticks.

On the contrary, *Nemesius* (but untruly) saith, That *Aristotle* affirmed the Soul to be Incorporeal, but without Perfection and Mortal, when he had designed the *Entelechia* or Perfection of every living thing; as to wit, She as it were arising up of her own accord, from Power only of matter rightly disposed, understands nothing else, but its own Crasis or Temperament, resulting from the mixture; which as it adds nothing substantial to the præxisting Matter, the Soul it self seems to be from thence a mere *Ens* of Reason, and only an extrinsical denomination. Further, when the *Peripateticks*, from the Soul raised up out of the Grave of Matter (which they affirmed to be a simple form, without Extension and divisibility) do contend that the Members of the same Body, do perceive many things at once and together, they have introduced into the Schools that Plea or rather Riddle, to wit, *That it is whole in the whole, and whole in every part.* To this Opinion thus unfolded, that of *Dicæarchus* was a-Kin, who said the Soul was *Harmony*, and also that of *Galen*, who call'd it a *Temperament*.

Others affirm the Soul to be Corporeal, and either something out of the Elements or the Blood, &c.

Nor do we meet with a less diversity of Opinions, among the Philosophers of every Age, delivering that all Souls, or all others, the rational excepted, are Corporeal. To pass by those who have affirmed the Soul to be either Fire, or Air, or Water, or something made out of many of these Elements; some, as *Critias* and *Empedocles* have said, that it was *Blood*. Which Opinion the Sacred Scriptures in some places plainly favour, where the eating of Blood is forbidden, because it is the *Life* or the *Soul*: Moreover, there are not Reasons and Arguments wanting, which conclude this to be very near, or very like to Truth; as shall be shewn anon.

The Opinion of Epicurus, that the Soul is made out of Atoms.

To these may be added, the Opinion of *Epicurus* delivered of old, and of late revived in our Age, which introduces the Soul plainly Corporeal, and made out of a knitting together of subtil Atoms, and asserts, citing *Laertius*, ὅ τί ἡ ψυχὴ, &c. which according to the mind of *Gassendus*, is as much as to say, *That the Animal is as it were the Loom, in which the Yarn is the Body, and the Woof the Soul.* From thence *Laertius* describing more fully its Corporeity, saith, ἐξ ἀτόμων, &c. which is, that the Soul is Composed of most light Atoms, and round, not much different from those out of which fire is. Other *Epicureans* describing the Nature of the Soul, otherways, depaint it as from something hot, flatuous, and airy, we need not to unfold any further this Opinion, nor shew out of *Laertius* and *Lucretius*, by what Rite the Assertors of the *Epicurean* Philosophy, do accommodate such an Atomical Composition of the Soul, to all the Actions and Affections of the Function, or Animal Government, which are to be performed.

Upon

Upon this Hypothesis of the *Epicureans*, as it were its basis, the Philosophers of this latter Age have built all their doctrines of the Soul, tho very divers, and I may almost say opposite. For as the soul of the Brutes, is affirmed by most of them, to be Corporeal and divisible, yet she is by some of them deprived of all Knowledg, Sense, and Appetite; in the mean time, not only Sense, Memory, and Phantasie is granted to her by others, but the use of a certain inferior Reason. And what is more to be wonder'd at, the same end of their Assertion is proposed by either Sect; to wit, That the Soul of the Brutes, both as it may be deprived of its gifts, and also as it is most notably adorned by them, may be very much distinguish'd, *or* (that I may use the Idiom of the Schools) diversified from the humane Soul. *The late followers of the Philosopher Epicurus have affirmed the Soul to be made of Atoms.*

The first Assertor of the former Opinion was *Gometius Pereira*, who affirmed that Beasts wanted all Knowledg or Perception; whom in our latter Age, the Famous Men *Cartesius* and *Digby*, with others Exactly followed; who endeavouring as much as they could, to discriminate the Souls of Beasts from the humane, affirmed them, to be not only Corporeal and Divisible, but also meerly passive; that is, that they were not all moved, unless that they were moved by other Bodies, striking some part of the Soul; from whence it followed, that every action of the Brute Consisted in it, as it were an artificial Motion of a Mechanical Engine, to wit, that first some sensible thing affecting the animal spirits, and Converting them inwards, stirs up sense; from which by and by, the same spirits being moved, as it were by a reflected undulation or wavering, return back again, and being determinated for the fitted order of the organs and parts of the Fabrick it self, in certain Nerves and Muscles, they perform the respective motions of the Members: For otherwise, if Cognition be granted to the Brutes, you must yield to them also Conscience, yea and deliberation and Election, and a Knowledge of universal things, and lastly an incorporeal and rational soul. *Others of them deny it to have Sense and Perception, as Gometius Pereira.*

Whilst these famous Philosophers suppose Brute Animals to be only certain Machines wonderful made by a Divine Workmanship; to wit, which without any Knowledg, Sense, or Appetite, perform only Corporeal Motions, and the Acts of their Faculties, according to the fitted structure of parts, and the precise direction of the spirits, within Certain measures or bounds of the Animals; yet some of them differ in their Opinions, about the structure and model of the Machine or moving Engine; to wit, for as much as the figure and properties of the Atoms, out of which the same is supposed to be made, are assigned one way by these, and after a divers way by those. The most illustrious *Cartesius*, unfolding all things by matter and motion, asserting the Souls of Brutes to consist altogether of round and highly moveable Atoms, which he Calls the Elements of the first Kind; affirms, That nothing else is requisite for all its acts to be performed, than that the fibres and nervous parts being struck by a stroke of a sensible thing, they receive a motion after this or that kind of manner, and transfer it by a Continued affection of the sensitive parts, as it were by a Certain undulation or wavering, into the respective parts: But our *Digby* supposing mobility of the particulars of this kind, out of which the Soul is made, adds further, That certain most thin Effluvia's, falling away from the sensible Body, do not only affect the Exterior sensories, but entring into the more interior recesses, mix themselves with the spirits, and moving them into Various fluctuations, do produce sense, and divers sorts of local motions: Moreover, that out of these Extrinsical Atoms, so entring into the nervous parts, and the Brain it self, do proceed not only Extempory Actions; but out of those left in the feeling body, and retaining the former Configurations, are Constituted the remaining Idea's, in the memory of things formerly done. It would be too prolix a business to recount particularly what appertains to the aforesaid Hypothesis, concerning the souls of Brutes, or animal Actions; or to Examine the Reasons of each; also to shew by what manner of Solutions of that Kind, those operations of the Brutes, which seem to be made by a Certain Judgment and Ratiocination, are wont to be unfoulded. *Cartesius. Digby and Others.*

But indeed these Solutions of difficult *Phænomena's*, and the Reasons for the mechanical provision of living Creatures, and their Souls, tho artificially formed by these Authors, seem not to satisfie a Mind desirous of Truth: And whilst every one expounds so the Works of the Creation, according to the model of his Wit, they seem to say, That God is not able to make any thing beyond what Man is able to Conceive or Imagine. Wherefore others, also renowned Philosophers, both Ancient and Modern, professing themselves no less adverse to Atheism than the former, Challenge in the behalf of the Beasts, not only the operations of an external and internal Sense, with Perception, Appetite, and spontaneous motions; but besides, grant to them a certain use of Judgment, Deliberation, and Ratiocination. *Others attribute to the Corporeal Souls sense and Perception; and further, the use of an inferior Reason; as*

Nemesius an ancient Philosopher, discoursing of the Cognation or Propinquity of all Created things, after he had shewed from Minerals, that some things came near towards the *Nemesius.*

De Nat. Hom. Cap. 1. the natures of Vegetables, and some of Plants, and Animals, ὁ δημιυργὸς (saith he) μεταβαίνων, &c. which is, The Common Architect passing from irrational Creatures to that rational Animal Man, hath not effected this suddenly, but first has referred certain natural Knowledges, and Artifices, and Subtilties to other Animals, so that they appear near to rational Creatures.

Phys. Sect. 3. Membr. post Lib. 8. Cap. 4. Peter Gassendus, a most Skilful and Cause-Expressing Man, in his late Experimental Philosophy, when he had enumerated very many Instances, by which the Cunning and Wonderful Sagacity of brute Animals were declared; and also the Epithets, whereby these kind of Animals are noted by Philosophers, to wit, that some are called *Excelling in Knowledg*; others *Artificial*, these Dexterous and Compleat, or Crafty and Wise, at length the Author adds, that, *These things could not deservedly be attributed to them, unless they granted them a certain kind of Reason. However it be, we may seem at least to be able to distinguish, by a ready way, that as Commonly a two-fold Memory, To wit, a Sensitive and Intellective, is distinguished, so nothing forbids to Call Reason Sensitive and Intellectual. And truly, as we understand by the Name of* Reason, *the faculty or beginning of Ratiocination, and that to Reason is nothing else, than to understand one thing by the Knowledg of another thing, there is nothing more Easily to be observed, than that Brutes do Collect one thing out of another, or what is the same thing, do reckon or recount, and therefore are indued with Reason.* From these we may easily understand, what dignity, and beyond the powers of any Machine, causing its Efficacy, he affirms to be in the Souls of Beasts. But in the mean time, if it be marqu'd, what Hypostasis, or formal Idea, he hath assigned them; it doth not so Easily appear, how that such Choyce Priviledges, do agree with those Souls, so slenderly gifted, *Who asserts the Soul, to be a little flame, or a Certain fire.* as to their Substances. For when from the Opinion of *Epicurus* he had shewn these to be Corporeal, and their Bodies to be made up of most light and round Atoms, out of which sort fire and heat is Created; at length he Concludes; *The Soul therefore to be a Certain Flame, or a Species of most thin fire, which as long as it lives, or remains inkindled, so long the Animal lives; when it no longer lives or is Extinguished, the Animal dyes.* But indeed, concerning his Hypothesis, he ought to have unfolded, by what means this Fire *Intelligent* and *Artificial* (to speak like the *Stoicks*) could be; or how a flame within certain bounds and Organs of the Body, however framed with the most excellent artificie, being inkindled and dilated, can be able to produce the Acts of the animal Faculty; This I say, most difficult Problem, this most Learned Man came to, and pass'd over its Knot as it were purposely in that place.

CHAP. II.

The Opinion of the Author Concerning the Soul in General,

That the Soul of the Brute is Corporeal and Fiery.

After having thus recited the chief Opinions of others, It now remains that we propose our own Opinion, or rather Conjecture, in so hard a matter. Where in *Why the Soul of the Beast seems not to be an Incorporeal, and immortal substance.* the first place, I am not easily led to believe, That the Soul of the Beast is an Incorporeal Substance, or Form: For as to what relates to that *Platonick* Fiction, concerning the Soul of the World, that, and also the Heresie of the *Manichees*, hath already been refuted and clearly exploded, both by the Ancient and Modern both Philosophers and Theologists, that there remains no further dispute about it. Further, neither can I Consent to those *Origenists*, who have affirmed the Souls of all Living Creatures to be immaterial, and also to subsist before and after their Bodies. For, tho I should be little solicitous, for the almost infinite multitude of the more perfect Beasts, which have liv'd, and do live, yet where do so many Myriads of Souls, even innumerable, of Insects and Fishes, which are dayly produced, subsist, and what do they? The Bodies of very many of these serve only for Food to other Creatures. And for that the Souls to these Bodies, serve chiefly to preserve them only for a little time, and as it were pickle them to keep them from putrefaction, there is no need that these should be therefore immaterial and immortal. Besides, when of old, *Egypt* was infested by Divine Punishment, with Swarms of Fleas, Flyes, and other Various Kinds of innumerable Insects, and that the same also abounded every where, it is not easily to be Conceived, from whence so many Souls were so suddenly Called, and into what places, the same being by and by seperated, could be placed. Moreover, as Heaven, the Kingly Palace of the Great God, challenges for it self Angels, *Gen.* 2. and pure Souls, free from all spot, to be its Inhabitants:

but

but the Earth, as it were a Certain sink, draws forth and extracts the feces of things, and from its bulk, ruinous Bodies; it seems more agreeable to the fitted Oeconomie of the World, that all immaterial things (with the humane Soul, which we have noted to be placed in the Confines of Nature, that it might be the fastning and knitting of either System) should be ascribed to the Air; but the other Animals, Condemned to the belly, and prone to the Earth, to this Glebe; so that the Souls of those, may be said to be born and dye with their Bodies, and to be altogether Corporeal. Yea if that Reasons and Arguments of greater weight, fight for this Opinion, than those we have seen on the opposite side; wherefore should we not rather follow this, and pass farther on into its parts?

And indeed, that the Soul of the Brute, even as the inferior of Man, Is material and divisible, yea Co-extended with the whole Body, seems to appear from many things; both first, because we perceive many and divers animal Acts, to arise at once, from divers members and parts of the Body: For Examples sake; in the same instant, that the Eye sees, the Ear hears, the Nose smells, the Tongue tasts, and all the Exterior members Exercise the sense of feeling and motion, and in the mean time, all the Inwards and the *Præcordia* perform their offices. Wherefore, since there is no medium between the Body and the Soul, but that the members and parts of the Body, are the Organs of the Soul; what can we think else, or affirm, but that many and distinct portions of the same Extended Soul, actuate the several members, and parts of this Body? Besides, it is seen in several living Creatures, whose Liquors, both the Vital and Animal (in which the Soul as to all its parts immediately subsists) are viscous, and less dissipable, that the Soul is also divided with the Body, and exercises its Faculties, to wit, of Motion and Sense, in every one of the divided members, layd apart by themselves. So Worms, Eeles, and Vipers, being cut into pieces, move themselves for a time, and being pricked will wrinkle up themselves together. *It is shown that it is Material and Co-extended with the Body.*

But that we have affirmed the Soul of the Brute to be not only Corporeal, and Extended, but that it is of a certain fiery nature, and its Act or Substance is either a Flame or a Breath, neer to, or a-Kin to Flame, besides the large Testimonies of Authors, both Ancient and Modern, Reasons and Arguments almost demonstrative, have also induced me to it. Some of the Chief of these, we have of late Exposed in the Treatise concerning the Inkindling of the Blood; there remains many others of no light moment to be added hereafter. As to what appertains to the suffrages of others, that I may not seem to stand upon the Authority of one *Gassendus*, who has maintained this Hypothesis; I shall here Cite many both Ancient Physicians and Philosophers. For not to mention *Democritus, Epicurus, Laertius, Lucretius*, and their followers; *Hippocrates, Plato, Pythagoras, Aristotle, Galen*, with many others, tho disagreeing about other things, in this Opinion, to wit, That the Soul was either a Fire, or something analogical to it, they all shook hands; to whom also have joyned themselves of the Moderns, *Fernelius, Heurnius, Cartesius, Hogelandus*, and others: and lately *Honoratus Faber*, hath delivered in Express words, *That the Soul of the Brute is Corporeal, and its Substance Fire it self*: But indeed he far otherwayes Explicates his saying, than is propounded in our Hypothesis. For having shewn this Soul to be material, and supposed all sublunary matter to be nothing else but the four Elements, he therefore Concludes the Soul of the Brute, because it is not seen to be any thing Compounded out of the rest of the simple Elements, or of many of them, *That it is mere Fire, Tract. 2. l. 2. pr. 33. ad 38*. I shall take notice of one or two of our Countrymen. The most noble *Verulam*, chiefly distinguishes animals from inanimals, in this respect, for that the spirits of those are otherways inflamed and inkindled, than the spirits of these. *Natur. Histor. Cent. 7*. The most Learned and Famous Physician *George Ent*, in his Apology against *Parisanus*, That Blood even as Fire, desires two things, to wit, Food and Ventilation, hath most clearly demonstrated. Wherefore, after so many Learned Men, it will be no Paradox to affirm, *That the Soul lying hid in the Blood, or Vital Liquor, is a certain fire or flame*; which Opinion agrees well enough with right Reason, as appears by what follows. *The Suffrages and Reasons of very many Authors, perswade that the Soul of the Brute, is not only Corporeal, but Fiery. The more Ancient Philosophers and Physicians have so affirmed. Also many Moderns of great Note. Hon. Faber. Tract. de Plantis et gener. anim. &c. Arguments and Reasons perswade the same thing.*

Indeed if Fire and Flame are to be defined or unfoulded, not by those External accidents of burning, glowing, and of heat, (which are not its proper Passions) but by intrinsic Causes; we conceive very easily, the substances of them to be even as the Souls of the Brutes, or altogether of the same sort. For truly, Fire, if we would describe it according to its Essence, it signifies an heap of most subtil Contiguous particles, and existing in a swift motion, and with a continued generation of some, renewed by the falling off of others; which indeed Conserves both its motion and substance; for that its Food, on which it continually feeds, is perpetually supply'd from the subject matter, which is Sulphur or some other nitrous thing in the Air, that Compasses it about; for from thence, out of the Food of either, the Particles being most minutely resolved, and agitated *The diffinition of Fire and Flame by its Causes and Essences, agrees also with the Soul of the Brute.*

tated with a moſt rapid motion, the forms of Fire and Flame (which differ only in more or leſs) reſult. Since we have in another place diſcourſed largely enough of theſe things, it will not be needful to add any more here.

The Souls of all Brutes after the manner of Fire, want a two-fold Food, to wit, a Sulphureous and Nitrous.

What if we ſhould in like manner ſay, That the Souls of Brutes, are an heap of theſe ſorts of moſt ſubtle Atoms, heaped up together, and extreamly moveable ? To wit, which being ſtirred up with Life into motion, as it were an infiring, Continue the ſame, and likewiſe its ſubſiſtance, ſo long as Nutriment, out of the appoſite matter, which is by degrees Conſumed, within Sulphureous, and without Nitrous, from the ambient medium, is granted to it. For that we ſay, That the Souls of all Brutes, ſo long as they live, and flouriſh after the manner of fire, do want Conſtantly either kind of aliment; to wit, Sulphureous and Nitrous: That this is true, is ſhewed hereafter, as well concerning Inſects and other bloodleſs Creatures; alſo concerning Fiſhes, and the more frigid bloody Creatures, as well as in the more hot and perfect Creatures, that have blood: Which Conditions however, are required to the Act and Subſiſtance of no ſubject beſides. But no motion, either of Fermentation, Ebullition, Vegitation, or of any other thing, (beſides Life and Fire) is immediately ſuppreſt, by reaſon of the taking away of the Air.

There are three things to be Conſider'd of - Concerning the Soul of the Brute. Its Subſiſtance or Hypoſtaſis.

Concerning the Corporeal Soul in general, theſe Three things firſt fall under our Conſideration: *viz.* Firſt, What kind of Subſiſtence or Hypoſtaſis it is of. Secondly, In what its Life or Act conſiſts: And Thirdly, What are its primary Offices or Operations.

As to the firſt, we may believe, That the Brutal Soul doth conſiſt of Particles of the ſame matter, out of which the organical Body is formed, but that they are choyce, moſt ſubtle, and highly active, which, as a flower ariſing out of the groſſer maſs, do mutually come together, and do conſtitute fit paſſages, which they produce thorow the whole frame of the Body, having got one continued Hypoſtaſis, to wit, very thin, and as it were Spirituous, and equal, and extended to the whole. For indeed, ſo ſoon as any matter is diſpoſed towards Animation, by the Law of Creation (and not by a Fortuitons Concourſe of Atoms) at once, the Soul, which is the form of the thing, and the Body, which is called Matter, begin to be formed under a certain Species or Kind, according to the Model or Form impreſſed upon them. Wherefore, the more nimble and Spirituous Particles, rowling away from the reſt, heap themſelves together, and by leaſure grow Turgid. Theſe being thus moved, ſtir up others more thick, and diſpoſe them into deſtinated places, where they ought to ſtay and to increaſe, and ſo they frame the Body, according to its deſtinated Species. In the mean time, this heap of ſubtle Particles, or the Soul, which explicating it ſelf more largely, and inſinuating its Particles into other more thick, and weaving them together, frames the Body, and is exactly formed according to the dimenſion and figure of that Body, is Co-extended with it, and fitted exactly, as to a little Box or Sheath, actuates, inlivens, and inſpires the whole, and all its parts: Further, on the other ſide, the ſame Soul, being apt preſently to be diſſolved from it ſelf, and to vaniſh away into Air, is Conſerved by the Containing Body in its Subſiſtance and Act.

So indeed, the Soul, altho moſt thin, yet Corporeal, ſeems to be as it were the Specter, or the ſhadowy hag of the Body : Further, this ariſing together with the Body, out of matter rightly diſpoſed, receives its Hypoſtaſis or Subſiſtence, no leſs than the Body, according to the Idea or Pattern fore-ordained to it, by the Law of Nature; But altho intimately united to the Body, and is as its prop or ſtay, Yet being made of a moſt ſubtil texture, and as it were of a moſt ſlender thrid, it cannot be perceived by our Senſes, but is only known by its Effects, and Operations. Moreover, when as by reaſon of hurt hapning to it, or to the Body, that the Life of the Soul periſhes or is deſtroy'd, preſently its Particles being ſnatched away from the Concretion, or its mutual adheſion, they are altogether diſſipated, without any footſteps or marks left : In the mean time, the Body being made exanimat or Soul-leſs, by and by tends to Corruption, but indeed, if it be more groſs and more Compact, its Principles waiſting or unrolling themſelves leiſurely and by degrees, it is not Corrupted but of a long time.

In its Life or Act.

2. The Exiſtency of the Corporeal Soul, depends altogether on its Act or Life; and in this reſpect it ſeems moſt like to Common Flame, and only like it; to wit, for as much as the ſubſtance of either, as ſoon as it Ceaſeth from all motion, it is no more, and can by no means be made whole again in the ſame number. Wherefore, the Eſſence of this begins altogether from Life, as it were the infiring of a Certain ſubtil matter; to wit, when many active, and chiefly ſpirituous, and ſulphureous Particles, with ſome other ſaline, being prædiſpoſed to Animality or Life, come together, in a fit Furnace or fire-place, take Life, ſometimes being as it were inkindled by another Soul, ſometimes of their own accord, which, from thence being ſupplyed, conſtantly (as we have ſaid) by a ſulphu-

sulphureous food within, and a nitrous without, Endures for some time; until at length, by the defect of Either of these, or by reason of some Violence or Injury hapning outwardly, the same as it were being Extinct, perisheth quite. The Act of the Corporeal Soul, or the inkindling of the Vital matter, in the more perfect Brutes, being indued with an hot Blood, appears so clearly and openly by noted heat, by the Exhalation of its fumes or sut, with other Accidents and Effects proper to the Kitching flame, that any one Considering or weighing them, may well believe that the blood doth truly flame forth, and that Life is not so like to flame, but even a flame it self, as we have formerly shew'd at large: But indeed in others less perfect or frigid Animals, altho we do not say the Soul is properly flame; yet (which is next to it) we say it is a most thin heap of subtil Particles, and as it were fiery, to wit, a certain spirituous breath; this being shut up in the Body, agitates its thick bulk, actuates all its members, and arteries, and in some with wonderful agility, goes thorow and inspires the same, more than in the more perfect animates, as appears in some Reptils and Insects. Further, that there is a firey Vigor in these Kind of Souls, may be even Collected from hence, because, whilst they live and do not lye asleep, they have no less need of Food and access of Air, than the more hot living Creatures; as shall be declared anon.

3. As to the Operations in General of the Corporeal Soul, we say, That as soon as it Exists in Act, that it performs chiefly these two offices; *viz.* First, to frame the Body as it were its domicil or little house, and then that Body being wholly made, to render it apt and fitted to all the Uses necessary both to the Kind, and to the Individuum: for which Uses it is furnished with a manifold Guard or Company of Faculties or Powers; also according to the Various instincts and suggestions of Nature, it exerts or puts forth as it were predestinatedly the Acts of a Various Kind, altho almost after the same manner. It will not be an easy matter here to rehearse, all the natural Powers and Habits with which all Corporeal Souls are wont to be gifted, to wit, because they are not in all after the same manner; But as living Creatures are more or less perfect, some than others, also according as they being destinated for the Various Scene of this worldly Theatre are diversly figured, and ought to live, their Souls also are furnished by a divers manner of provision of Faculties: The speculation of these things, tho very pleasant and profitable, is too copious and large for us to divert our selves within this place; But for the illustrating of our Psychologic or Doctrine of the Soul, it may not be amiss to recite the chief Kinds of Living Creatures, and to reduce them as it were into certain Classes or Forms, and then to describe their Chief Species, together with the Various degrees of the Souls, that inhabit them.

In its Offices and Operations.

CHAP. III.

The Various Kinds of Brutes, together with their respective Souls, and the chief Species of each of them, are rehearsed and described.

FOr as much as the Brutal Soul ought to be proportionate to the Organical Body, it easily follows, that as there are Various kinds of Bodies, in the divers Habitacles of this world, and offices of those Bodies destinated to life, so also Various Souls, by which they are actuated, do exist, and are indued with a Divers Gift of Faculties. If we would consider the perfect Sence of these, it were first needful to write the History of all Animals, and to deliver the Anatomy of each of them. But as that will be a business of an immense and tedious labour, it seems much more to the purpose, to reduce here, all the Bruits to certain Kinds, according to some certain affections in many of them, and thence to describe some chief Species of those Kinds, and their Various Compositions and Structures, in respect of the Vital parts.

Living Creatures may be distinguished or reduced into certain Classes, either First, according to their Various Organs of Respiration, which in some are numerous Branchiæ or Gills, and these dispersed thorow the whole Body, as in many Insects, or they are appropriated Branchiæ or Gills, in Fishes; or lastly, Lungs, common besides to divers animals, with Man. Or secondly, the rehearsal of the Brutes may be made according to the Various Constitution of the vital Humour, in which respect, they are either First, without Blood, or Secondly, of a less perfect or frigid Blood, or Thirdly, of a more perfect or hot Blood: And to this partition, as the more Known, insisting here, we shall run thorow the several members of it in Order, and briefly Notifie in them the Fabricks of the Blood.

Animals are reduced into Classes either according to the Organs of Respiration, Or according to the Vital Humour; and they are either without Blood, or of frigid Blood, or hot Blood.

the chief Vital parts of the Body, and the Constitutions of the Souls, Inhabiting them.

Bloodless Creatures are either of the Earth or Water.

First, Bloodless Creatures, are either belonging to the Earth, in which number are very many Insects; or belonging to the water, of which Kind, besides some certain Kinds of Insects, are also found various Fishes, which are wont to be divided into Soft, of which sort are the Cuttle Fish, the Sea Woolf, &c. Shelly, as Oysters and Cockles, &c. And Pargated or other thinner shell'd Creatures, as the Lobster and Crab: We will examine in either sort, some chief Species of these Bloodless Creatures, as to the States of their vital Parts, and their Souls.

It appears that Insects have fiery Souls, because they want Sulphurous and Nitrous food.

First, Therefore in earthly Insects, altho indued with a small bulk that they have great Souls, their Actions testifie, which indeed are performed by some of them, as the Silk-worm, the Bee, the Ant, or Emmet, the Spider, to admiration: Further, That the Souls of these are of a certain fiery nature, no less than those of the more hot and perfect Brutes; we from hence deservedly suspect; because they stand in need of a Copious Food, after the manner of an inkindled Flame, and of the access of much Air. The first appears by common Observation, for as much as Insects often devour all the Corn, and Leaves of Plants, and so take away the grateful greenness of the Summer. Besides, it appears from hence, that their Lives require a constant afflux of Air, because as it hath been experienced by our noble Mr. *Boyle*, Insects being put into a glassy Globe, quickly

Malpigius de Bombyce, p. 28.

dye, after the Air is suckt out. This Learned *Malpigius* hath more fully declared in his most ingenious Tract of the Silk-Worm: where he Observes, *That Insects have not only Lungs, but so abound in them, that every little ring or section of them is indued with two, yea and that every part also of the Viscera or Inwards, delight in the derived Lungs.* For as in the sides of Insects, the whole length of the Body on both sides, black spots or pricks appear, he hath found, that these were indeed tunnels or breathing holes, leading from so many Wind-pipes or asper Arteries, which by and by, being branched forth into the Heart, Ventricle, Spinal Marrow, and all the other Inwards, and Internal parts, carry

These have Lungs, or numerous wind-pipes, the Orifices of which, if stopped up by Oyl, presently death follows.

in and out air to and from them all. Moreover, if these orifices be all smeared over with Oyl, or Hony, the Worm presently dyes; but if only a part of those breathing holes be so stopped, the neighbouring parts being by and by Convulsed, and then resolv'd or loosned, sink down or flag, the rest keeping their motion: But if the orifices of the *Trachea* or Wind-pipe be untouched, and that the Head, Mouth, Belly, or any other parts be sprinkled with Oyl, neither death nor any trouble of the Sense will be induced; and what is yet more wonderful, the Insects that have oyl or the like poured into their Wind-pipes, so suddenly dye, that tho the Heart keep a motion for some space, yet they can never be revived. These *Phenomena* happen alike not only in the Silk-Worm, but in Wasps, Bees, Grass-hoppers, Locusts, Caterpillers, and other the like Insects, which certainly, I believe, gives very much Light concerning the use of Lungs, in every Animal: But first let us inspect some other Parts of Insects, described by a most accurate Anatomy.

The Heart of the Silk-Worm is long, unequal and stretch'd forth thorow the whole Body.

Therefore he says in the Silk-Worm, and the like in others, That the heart is placed all along the Back, between the Muscles and the Lungs, here and there appending, and that it is stretched forth from the top of the Head to the extreme part of the Body; This consisting of their Membranes, as appears as it were one Tube or Pipe, but unequal, to wit, sometimes broader sometimes narrower, continuing from the Tail to the Head, so that for their inequalities, they seem as so many Eggs, or little Hearts, one laid by another, and continued by one passage. These little Hearts, or the aforesaid parts of the Heart, do gently drive forward, not at once but successively and slowly (after the manner of their membranes) being bound and dilated from heart to heart sometimes upward, sometimes downward, the contained vital humour, which is limpid or clear, and so (as we may believe) a certain portion of the vital humour, being squeezed forth into the Arteries (which are so small and few, that they cannot be seen) is agitated by the Circulation of the rest, contained almost only within the oblong Cavity of the Heart.

The Brain is wanting the Spinal Marrow being sufficiently large.

As to the head, this most diligent searcher observed, that Insects had no Brain within the Skull, its Cavity being filled with the Muscles of the Eyes, and some others, but its Spinal Marrow sufficiently large, and divaricated in many places, for the going out of the Nerves, and as it were protuberated with knots, is extended from the Head to the Tail; and what is worthy to be noted, in the whole passage, branches of the Trachæa or Lungs were superinduced to this Spinal Rope, and inserted to it in very many places. I omit what he most learnedly discourses of the members, ventricle, and other Inwards of Insects, lest it should seem impertinent, or too much Plagiarism: But that the discourses may be the better understood, concerning the vital parts of Insects, it will be convenient here to borrow the draughts of the heart of the Silk-Worm; and of the Trachæa or Wind-Pipes, both of that and of the *Grass-hopper*, and Locust (in which the Tra-

chæa

chæa or Wind-pipes are like to other Insects) most diligently delineated by *Malpigius*; which shall be added at the end of this Chapter, with other Figures of other Animals; but these the first Table shews. Further, as to what belongs to the Doctrine of the Soul, we may with the Authors lieve Philosophize, or at least conjecture, concerning the Phænomena of the Heart and Lungs by him described.

Therefore, for that Insects first having such copious Lungs dispersed thorow all the Viscera or Inwards, Heart, and spinal Marrow, to which that each might come distinctly, they have many distinct Trachæas or Wind-pipes, with so many gaping orifices, on the superficies of the Body, it appears from hence, that the use of the Lungs in these little Animals, is not for the refrigeration of the Blood, or its exact mistion, nor for the suscitating the motion of the Heart; because, neither the Vessels carrying the Blood or Vital Humour, accompany the Trachæa or Wind-Pipes, nor is such a humour to be rapidly Circulated, but seems to be only carryed and placed gently into all the parts. *The Use of the Parts is exposed.*

But that the orifices of the Wind-pipes being stopped, presently Life is extinguished in these (as also in a glassy Globe empty of Air) what can one imagine else, but that this access of Air, is required for the sustaining of the Vital Flame, as it is wont to be for that of the Chimney? Wherefore, because the vital humour (which is not at all or only slowly Circulated) cannot be carried all quickly to one Fire-place of accension, as in more perfect Creatures, therefore very many Lungs gaping every where outwardly, and dispersed every where inwardly, are framed for the bringing of Air to the several portions of the vital humour, planted on all sides; for that not only the Heart, but also the Ventricle, Genitals, spinal marrow, and all the other parts of the Soul dispersed, growing with a kind of silent Fire, are inspired with the admitted Air, to every one a part. *Why such numerous Wind-pipes.*

Besides, when as the vital humour cannot be Circulated into all the other parts, and from these into that, with a rapid motion therefore, instead of a Conick Muscle, which receiving the watering juyce, may be able to explode it presently, and to cast it forth a great way on every side, a Tube or as it were a membranaceous Sack or Bag is made, to wit, which by a long tract stretching it self nigh to all the parts, and to which it might by degrees bestow what might suffice, and in the mean time gently moving the provision chiefly contained in it self, preserves from stagnation or putrefaction. Further, the little Branches of the Trachæa, deeply inserted into the Membranes or Coats of this, inspire or rather inkindle the humour contained with vitality. *Wherefore the Heart is so long.*

As to the aquatick bloodless Creatures of the other kind, *viz.* some soft Fishes, also many, perhaps all shelly and crusty Fishes; I have not yet happened to see the former, but *Severinus* being my Author, the *Sepia* or *Cuttle* Fish is made with an heart and gills, and the *Polypus* or *many feet* with it and Lungs: what is to be met with that is more curious in the framing of them shall be omitted. Concerning the other two Fishes, to wit, the shelly and crusty, we shall add some Anatomical Observations, such as we have search'd out in their vital parts, and other beginnings, truly weighed, and what the souls are of these sort of bloodless Creatures. *Bloodless Creatures belonging to the Water.* *Soft Fishes.*

Of the testaceous or shelly, though it hath been dissected by many, we shall make choice of the Oyster. The body of this Fish, though it seems rude and wholy without shape, yet it hath all its Viscera and parts, and especially the Præcordia, for, as it were the hearth and Tunnel of the Vital Fire, most curiously framed. As we shall describe some of the chief of these, we will begin with the shells, which are born with them, from Eggs, and are first soft, and as they encrease in bulk they are by degrees hardned: A robust Muscle being implanted in the middle of the Oyster, grows by its tendons to either shell. The moving Fibres of these (which seem as it were a little bundle of Chords or Strings) ascending rightly, whil'st they are drawn together, strictly shut up the shells; but being relaxed, they suffer them to be opened and lifted up; to which Office of opening the shells, another Muscle adjoyned to this, is required. Besides these upright Muscles, and perpendicular to the planes of the shells, there are two Circular, stretched forth by the brims of either shell; which in the same place comprehending in themselves Gills, serve chiefly for their motion; as we shall shew by and by. *The Anatomy of the Oyster.* *The Muscles opening and shutting the shells.*

On the top of the Oyster, the Circular Muscles being united, make a thing as it were a Vail for the covering of the head; then being a little divided below, they include four superiour Gills: In the middle of which, a gaping chink leads by an oblique process to the mouth of the Oyster. From the Mouth there is a short and strait passage to the Ventricle. The Cavity of this large enough, is endued with little holes, leading into darkish bodies, fixed on either side of it. These bodies seem to be in the stead of the Mesentery and Liver, and to perform their offices; to wit, for that they receive the *Circular Muscles moving the Gills.* *The Mouth of the Oyster.* *The Ventricle of the Oyster.* *The Liver and Mesentery.*

C

the more pure part of the Chyle, by and by from the Ventricle, and deliver it, being made clear from dreggs, to the vital humour. The like is in crustaceous Fishes, and perhaps in some Brutes; to wit, in such as a simple and only Intestine, without folds and Meseraick or milky Vessels, is produced from the *Pylorus* to the great Gut or Ars-hole.

The Intestine. For so in the Oyster, the Intestine beginning from the bottom of the Ventricle, descends with a plain and equal Tube, towards the right Angle of the streight Muscle, where being rolled and retorted in it self, it ascends again towards the Ventricle and Liver; being from thence demersed, and bending back towards the left side, goes towards the border of the strait Muscle, till it ends in the great Gut or Arse-hole: After this manner in the Oyster, a simple and only Intestine is carryed about, with a most long compass, more than in many other Animals, by which indeed they may be able the longer to retain their Dung ; to wit, lest that when they are dry, that being more importunely put forth should polute (by mixing with it) the water, for the food of life, included in the shell.

An Intestine in an Intestine. Which perhaps is the Spinal Marrow. This Intestine being dissected and opened longways, in the bottom of it arises an hardish and almost round body, which ascending from the Arse to the Ventricle arises there, and stretches under the *Oesophagus* towards the Head : The like to this is found in a Worm, which hollowness in it we think to be in the place of the Mesentery and milky Vessels: but otherwise in the Oyster, this hard and compacted body being less apt for such an office, seems not unlike to the spinal Marrow: But we shall shew the Chyliferous passages do supply the darkish bodies, hanging to the Ventricle.

Its Pericardium with the Heart and Vessels. Below the Ventricle, the *Pericardium* is placed, including the Heart, being whitish with a large black ear, which being opened, that is beheld to beat, and at every *Diastole* to admit the vital humour, out of the hollow vein, into the little ear ; then at every *Systole*, to drive the same forward into the *Aorta*, placed on the contrary side; then by tripartite branches of this Vessel, a certain part of this humour tends upwards, towards the Head, Liver and Stomach ; also a certain portion is reflected into the strait Muscle; in the mean time a great part of it being delated from the great Trunk of the Artery, to the *Branchiæ* or Gills, it is there unfolded, *The Gills.* within most small and numerous passages, as it were little Rivers, that it might enjoy, according to all its parts, little nitrous bodies inspired from the water. And that this may be the more plentifully done, we observe that the water, as in bloody Fishes, did not only wash the outward superficies of the Gills ; but that it *The Description and use of them.* every where did enter all the more intimate recesses, and deeper passages ; yea these Gills expansed largely thorow the Hemisphere of the Oyster, exceed in bulk, all the other Viscera, also almost the parts. So that in Fishes, because they breath but little in the water, it is so provided that in many places together, the food of respiration should be afforded them.

There are Four hairy tufts of Gills, and as it were two Lobes of either of them ; to wit, the upper more broad and thicker, and the lower which is thinner and a little more contracted ; in all the passages of them, every one is two-fold, and contains two series of little Finns, seen to grow together ; to the several Gills belong two Vessels, the Artery and the vein ; which being deposited in the heaps of the hairy tufts, dispose the small moots of either kind thorow all the borders. But besides these Four orders of Vessels, there are found also so many series of little breathing holes, lying between these Vessels; which also by manifest passages open in the places between the Finns : and from thence they deduce the waters sup'd up by the inferiour mixture or joyning of the Circular Muscles : The like is in crustaceous Fishes, as we shall shew by and by.

The motion of the Gills depends upon the Circular Muscles. As to the motion of the Gills, it is clear by ocular Inspection, that the Circular Muscles, which are knit to either shell, for the shutting them, when relaxed, do reach to the extream brims of the shells; whereby at that instant, also the Gills being relaxed, do imbibe the Waters, and together from them draw the nitrous food ; and by and by being contracted, they are drawn inwardly, and together compel the Gills, to the pressing forth the Waters newly admitted.

Shelly and crusty Fishes, contain waters in their whole bodies, to wit, whereby they may be able to live out of the Waters. If the Reason is asked, why shelly Fishes (which also holds with the crustaceous, as we shall shew anon) have besides the Vessels carrying about the vital humour, also Passages or open Chanels, by which the Waters are carried to their most intimate recesses ; it seems to be because both these sorts of Animals, though they reside at the bottom of the Sea, yet oftentimes they happen to remain dry, therefore that they might then breath (the most wise Creator so providing) they contain plenty of water within their own frame, as it were reposed in Wombs ; by the during provision of which,

which, they live as well in the open Air, as in the Waters; But these Waters being taken away, shed, or evaporated by heat, both these sort of Fishes quickly dye: By reason of these Waters, these live longer then others out of the Waters. Further, as the Noble Mr. *Boyle* hath observ'd, the Oyster and the Sea-Crab, being put into a Glassy Globe, after the Air was suck't forth, did not presently expire like many other Animals; to wit, because part of the Intestine Water being rarified, quickly supplyed the defect of the exhausted Air; at least, that being detained within the proper frame of the Fish, affords an inkindling or matter for respiration. It is sufficiently known, that the Oyster, when it is taken out of the Waters, hath a great quantity of Waters shut up within its shells: as also the Lobster (which we intend to consider of among the crusty Fishes) doth the same thing, as shall be declared. In the mean time, for the illustration of this our Anatomy of the Oyster, *Tab. 2d*, shews the Figures of its parts aptly represented.

The *Lobster* and other Fishes a-Kin to it, *viz.* the *Crab*, *Sea Creevish*, *Shrimps*, &c. As they retrograde, or rather swiming backwards, so their parts and Viscera in respect of other Animals, seem to be inverse or opposite: For as to the members and moving parts, the bones are not covered with flesh, but the flesh with bones: wherefore, almost all the Muscles of the Feet, Arms, Head, Back, Tail, and other parts, either moveable or moving (excepting those that are temporal) are shut up every where with a crusty covering: Indeed it is so ordained by Divine Providence, that as these Animals inhabit among Rocks and sharp Stones, lest they should be in danger of being dashed too hard by the force of the Tides, they are fortified with Bones, planted outwardly, as it were with Armour: Moreover, lest that the crusty Covering should more sharply compress the Membranes, or the Flesh underneath, or should rub against them, the same is every where covered within with a thick Purple Muck or Stuff, as it were lined with a soft cloath: I do believe this purpuling in crusty Fishes, otherwise than in soft (who also are besmeared with muck) to happen through the greater plenty of Sulphur. *The parts and Viscera of Fishes swiming backwards are inversed.*

As their Bones and Flesh, so their *Præcordia* and *Viscera*, are observed to be *Hysteron Proteron*, topsie turvie; for the Liver, Stomach, and Womb is placed above, and the Heart below, yea contiguous to the Back: yea, and the spinal Marrow lyes not close to the Back, and above the Viscera, but under them, and to the prone part of the Body, in its whole passage; and is included in the bones or jointings of the Sternon, or meeting of the Breast.

But that the Parts and Viscera of the Lobster may the better be beheld, let the armed coat with the red Muck and Membrane lying under it, be taken away; then in the top of the head, appears the Brain but meanly large, of a greenish colour, and as it were two-fold; from which the mammillary Processes, and the Optick Nerves ascend, and two shanks of the oblong Marrow descend into the spinal Marrow, and in its whole process, they are sometimes divided, and sometimes placed together, now united, and then again seperated one from another. *The Brain of the Lobster. The Nerves and spinal Marrow.*

The *Oesophagus* tends from a two-fold mouth, by a strait and short passage, into the Ventricle, this large indued with a thick and strong Membrane, has three Teeth within its Cavity, by which its aliments are chawed or bruised: further, for the work of Chawing and brusing, two pair of muscles are framed, in the neighbouring parts, to wit, one temporal or belonging to the Temples, and another hanging to the sides of the Stomach; from the sides of the Stomach or Ventricle, grow too glandulous Bodies, stuffed with many Vessels and various passages, as it were certain little thin Intestines, and from thence being by degrees sharpened with two Lobes, they descend into the lowest Trunk of the Body; from the Stomach into these Bodies, on either side, passages lye open, so that wind being blown into it by a Pipe, presently it runs into these and makes them swell up: These parts in crusty Fishes (as also in the shelly) are commonly called the Liver, and indeed they seem to perform the Offices both of the Liver and Messentery; to wit, for as much as they receive the more pure portion of the Chyle fresh digested in the Ventricle, and commit that by and by, being made purer, to the vital humour. *Malpigius* observes in the Silk-Worm, and in other Insects, that certain diversified Vessels, analogical to these Bodies, are stretch'd out through the back of the Ventricle, and from thence to reach lower upon the Intestine; which (as he probably thinks) receive the more thin portion of the meat already macerated and loosned in the Ventricle; and deliver it, the juyces perhaps being not much changed, to the Heart, or at least to the Skin and other parts of the Body. Truly by observation, after what manner these parts which supply the place of the Liver and Messentery, in some Fishes and Insects are made; something may be thence gathered concerning the uses of the Liver, and of the Vessels both Miscraick and Milky, in bloody Brutes. *The Oesophagus. The Ventricle from which there is a passage into the Liver and Messentery. De Bombic. p. 40. Things answerable to the Liver and Messentery in Insects.*

In

Spermatick Bodies.	In the Male Lobster, above the beginnings of the aforesaid parts, on either side, from the sides of the *Oesophagus*, the spermatick Bodies begin, which being sent down towards the bottom of the Trunk, and there being more compacted and made smoother, after
Two Yards in the Male.	the likeness of the *Epididimis* or thin covering of the Testicles, are terminated in two Yards; the Tops of which have their going out thorow holes forged in the last little feet but one. In like manner in the Female Lobster, two nests of Eggs on either side of the sides of the *Oesophagus* and Ventricle are placed, and pass into two Wombs planted in the lowest Trunk of the Body, and into those, thorow the holes
Two Wombs in the Female.	forged in the last little Feet but one, there lyes a passage to the genital Members, also a passage from the Womb for the laying of Eggs: so that it appears how these living Creatures are most fruitful, with a multiplyed Issue, when as nature seems to be careful and industrious about their genital parts, being double and greater than in many other Brutes; to wit, that as they being both at once double, they might produce both by the works of Generation, Conception, and bringing forth not only always Twynns, but almost *Miriads* of *Twynns*.
The Pericardium and Heart.	Below the Ventricle, yea and lower also then the beginnings of the other Viscera, the *Pericardium*, in which the beating heart is included, is placed in the bottom of the Back; the *Systole* and *Diastole* of the heart are strong and swift, as in Creatures of Blood; this appearing of a whitish Colour, is indeed a *Conick* Muscle, whose Cavity being sufficiently large is framed with Fibres or Columns, also with many strong and
The Aorta.	various little Furrows: The *Aorta* going forth from its top, is cleft presently into two Branches, which go towards the Gills; The *vena cava*, one ascending, the other descending, meet together from the bottom of the Heart, and there enter into its little ear. The Heart whilst it is relaxed, receives the vital humour from the vein, and by and by when it is contracted, drives it forward into the *Aorta*.
The Gills.	The crusty Fishes, even as the shelly altho without Blood, are indued with numerous and large Gills, which are instead of Lungs; to which, that all the Vital humour may be frequently carried, therefore not as in earthy Insects, are they dispersed thorow the whole Body, but on either side, under the brim of the armed coat, and being gathered together in one place, are made into certain little bundles: The inferiour and utmost part of the Gills, which are broad and obtuse, is fixed to the *Sternon* or meeting of the Breast, with hanging little feet; the upper part ascending under the Coat is loose and free, and by degrees grows sharp; otherwise than in Fishes with Blood, whose Gills are tyed together, being solid at either end.
The Gills of the Lobster have three Bosoms.	In all the Gills of the Lobster, Three Bosoms are found, of which two seem to be made for the carrying in and out of the vital humour; because a black Liquor being injected into the heart, passes to the Gills, and there passing first thorow one Bosom, returns by and by thorow the other. We will speak by and by of the third: from these Bosoms appear productions of small Vessels, as if it were feathery, arising on every side, thick set and short, like jagged welts or fringes; which being spongy, sup up the
Two of these carry about the Vital Humour.	Waters continually flowing to them, at every turn of the *Diastole*, and press them forth by *Systole*: to wit, for the end, that whilst it is there unfolded within the small passages, the food for the vital humour may be inspired. The Third Bosom being carried from the top of every Gill, to its Basis ends in the common Channel, in all the Gills of the same side, which nigh to the insertion of the highest Gill (which beats perpetually) gapes with a large gap; Any one may easily perceive this, in a
The third receives, and casts out the Waters flowing to it.	live Lobster, whilst it breathes out of the water; for in every *Systole* or pulse of this supream Gill, one may see a bubble of water break forth out of that hole. Further, if into that hole a black Liquor be injected, by and by entring under that Common passage, it passes thorow from thence, both into all the Gills, and the small and feathery Bosoms of them, and also into the Arms, and all the little feet (the Cavities of which the Muscles do not fully stuff) yea, and into the Cavity of the Body. In like manner wind being blown into that hole, all the aforesaid parts will be inflated or blown up.
Shelly and Crusty Fishes receive the Waters, that when they remain dry, they may be able to live.	From hence we may guess, that hole, with the common channel, and the three bosomes of Gills, to be a certain *Trachea* or Wind-pipe, into which plenty of water entring at every *Diastole*, is returned back at the next *Systole*: In the mean time, these waters in this passage, do not only Communicate with the Vital Humour, abounding between the Gills, but besides, are laid up between the Cavities of the Members and the Trunk, that they may supply these Fishes, whilst they are kept dry with matter for respiration; and therefore, they not only longer subsist in the open air, but also live for some time in a place void of all air.

In Crusty Fishes, for that, for the agitating the Gills as it were with Lungs, the Ribs belonging to the Sides, the Muscles of the Breast, and other things are either wanting,

According to their Vital Parts.

or by reason of the stiffness of the neighbouring parts, are made unable; it is performed by an admirable artifice, as whilst the Gills, for the most part being loose, and are left easily moveable, the several little bundles of them, about the basis of the bony little Foot, being included with the Muscles, within their Cavities, as it were so many hanging Ribs, are fixed, being drawn forth far beyond the Trunk of the Body; which, as so many distinct Pendulums, by the help of the Muscles, which they include, being almost continually shaken, cause also continual *Systoles* and *Diastoles*, for the inspiring and exspiring of the Gills. *The Gills of Crusty Fishes, hanging from the Sides or Ribs, are moved as it were by shaking Pendulums.*

But it may well be doubted, whether we ought to assign Souls of the nature of fire, to these bloodless Creatures inhabiting the waters; because they rejoyce in an Element that is deadly to fire it self, and to the Lives of more perfect Brutes: But this Problem shall be satisfied by and by, when we have first discours'd of the Use of the Gills in Bloody Fishes, as also concerning the *Præcordia* of these, and others, of a more frigid blood: In the mean time, the Third Table shews the Figures, representing to the Life the parts of the Lobster. *Whether there be fiery souls in bloodless Creatures.*

Secondly, After the bloodless Brutes, their second Class, and of a little higher degree, is that of the more cold bloody Creatures; in which for that the vital Humour or Liquor, being dyed with a reddish tincture becomes bloody, it seems to proceed from a greater plenty of Sulphur, and chiefly destinated for living Creatures, for the increasing their bulk and strength; For where blood is, though in a mean Plenty, their Muscles, Inwards, Præcordia, Brain and more strong and compleat Organs of the senses exist. We have observed it otherwise among most Insects, whose little Bodies being ordained to subtle and small actions only, are made up of very little Sulphur, as their *Analysis* or the unfolding them shews, but of plenty of Spirit and of volatile Salt. *From whence the vital humour becomes bloody.*

But that among the Bloody Brutes, some are hot in Act, and others are frigid or cold, the reason may be, both from the quantity of Sulphur, to wit, with which they are only meanly or very much imbued; also from the Kind of life which they live, either in the Air, or in the Waters, or within the Earth: Wherefore, the Inhabitants of the latter Regions do not grow hot in the Act, yea 'tis scarce possible they should; for how, or which way should heat subsist, where it is in danger to be damped or overthrown by a more potent Cold? Wherefore, the blood of Animals destinated to these places, is tempered with little Sulphur, lest otherwise growing hot above measure, it should be forthwith suffocated; yea and we suspect the Souls of these, tho of a firy nature, to have not a flamy *Hypostasis*, but a breathy, to wit, which consisting in Vapour, hardly or not at all inkindled, like an *ignis fatuus* or false fire, is destitute of sensible heat. *Why the bloody Brutes, are some of them more hot Animals, others more cold.*

The more Cold bloody Creatures, altho all of them have a *Conic* Heart, very fibrous and thick, to wit, that being strongly Contracted, it might drive forward the Vital Liquor, by a certain Circulation, into all the parts, and from them into it self: yet this Heart in some is two bellied, and to it always the Lungs are hung; in others it hath but one belly; and in many, in the place of Lungs are Gills, but in some there are numerous Wind-pipes, and dispersed thorow the whole Body: We shall consider the different ways and buildings in each of these. *Why some are indued with an heart, with a twofold Belly, & Lungs; others with one Belly, and Gills, or Wind-pipes dispersed.*

Among the Brutes of Cold blood, The Earth-Worm, tho of the lowest order, may be rightly placed; for that its humour appears by occular inspection to be bloody: This little living Creature, tho it be esteemed Vile and Contemptible, hath allotted to it vital organs, as also other *Viscera* and Members, made most admirably by a Divine Workmanship; the frame of the whole Body (even as of many bloodless Insects) is a chain of ringie Muscles, the orbicular fibres of which being Contracted, render every Ring first large and dilated, and then more narrow and longer. For then, when the superior portion of the Body being made long and stretched forth, is extended to a further space, and is there affixed to the plane, the inferior portion of the Body, being relaxed and abbreviated, is easily drawn to it, as to its Centre. A four-fold series or rowes of little feet are placed thorow the whole length of the Worm; with these, as it were with so many hooks or claws, he fixes now this part, now that, to the plane or superficies, whilst he stretches forth the other, or draws it after him. Above the opening of the Mouth, he is indued with a snout, with which he diggs thorow and thrusts up the Earth. *Description of an Earth-Worm. Its local motion. The little Feet. Its Snout.*

The Earth-Worm, being laid on its back, and fixed with Bodkins to a Table, let it be cut up long ways, then the Sides being layd apart, its parts from the head to the tail easily shew themselves to your view. Above the opening of the Mouth, the Brain appears in a very little Bulk, and whitish like a bubble: Then a little lower, the *Oesophagus* being placed with the Muscles, descends thence with a streight passage to the Ventricle. *It's Brain. Oesophagus.*

Nigh

Pericardium and Heart.

Nigh to the top of the *Oesophagus*, the Heart beating is placed, having reciprocal turns of *Systole* and *Diastole* or pulses, as in more perfect Brutes: from either side of the heart, and from thence a little lower, are framed whitish Bodies, and something globous or round, and on either side distinguished as it were into Three Lobes. The Two superiour of these, shine more bright and are smaller; the lowest little Globe, greater in a double measure then either of the other, is long and like a Sawsage; between these whitish Bodies, and more backward, other lesser little Globes as they were small and little yellowish whelks, are placed in a two-fold series, to wit, on either side, now Four, now Five, or more. Noted Blood-carrying passages go thorow the midst of these Bodies, and in them a notable pulsation, as it were in the neighbourhood of the heart, is beheld.

White Globes which are Spermatick Bodies.

By what names I should call the aforesaid parts, and for what uses they served, I was a long time in doubt, because in the dissection, or by blowing them up with a Pipe, I could find no Cavity in them; but some of the little globes being opened and squeesed, there dropt out of them a milky humour, from whence I presently suspected, that they were spermatick Bodies; which seemed likely, because these parts were not formed after the same manner in all the Earth-Worms. Further, it was sufficiently obvious, that Earth-Worms Coupling together, do not strain themselves as most of the other Brutes, by a direct planting of either Sex about the Tails, but on the contrary, by mutual embraces about the Head. At length, after I had often and narrowly inquired into the matter, it appeared past doubt: For by chance dissecting a certain bigg-bellied Worm, I found the greater white shining Bodies, and the longish like a Pudding or Sausage, stuffed with very many Eggs: Moreover on the other side of these Bodies, in the Breast of the Earth-Worm, appeared two white shining little Paps, with holes, which seemed to be the privy members of the Earth-Worm. *Malpigius* hath observed, in *some Insects, and especially in the Beetle and Imperatus's Mole, certain little whitish Globes about the Ventricle* (like as it seems to these in the Earth-Worms) *to be found, and a portion of it, to be incompassed with plenty of them*: It is very likely that these Bodies are also spermatical in them.

The like to these in other Insects.

The Ventricle, of which there are three Bellies &c. The Intestine.

Below these whitish shining Bodies, the Ventricle, of a noted bulk, is placed, indued with a large Cavity, and divided into three Regions or Bellys. From the lowest of these, the *Intestinum* proceeding, is carried by a streight and long passage, even to the Tail, and in the whole space is so compressed, by the several interspaces of the anulary Muscles, that it appears like the *Colon* or Arse-Gut in perfect Animals, divided as it were into very many little Cells. This *Intestine* being dissected long ways, and the dung removed, in its bottom was placed a vessel, in its whole passage, of a yellowish Colour, from the Tail even to the Ventricle; but in the same place arising up, and creeping thorow the walls of the Stomach, Is stretched forth even to the Head: This Vessel is in truth a *Tube*, which being blown up by a Pipe, shew'd an ample Cavity; and that which *Malpigius* noted to be stretched forth upon the *Ventricle* and *Intestines* of Insects, seems answerable to these passages and vessels, and we may well suspect it to be in the place of the Liver and *Mesenterie*. In some Earth-Worms about the Tail, on either side of the *Intestine*, we found sometimes very many Eggs, ready to be lay'd, which indeed were seen to have descended thither, from the genital parts, and were cast out by the Passages lying open into the Arse.

An Intestine in an Intestine, which is in the place of the Liver and Mesentery.

The holes in the back of the Earth-Worm, which seem to be Wind-Pipes.

So much concerning the internal parts of the Earth-Worm, opened with its Belly upwards: If the same be held down with its Belly downwards, on the top of the Back, near the brim of every Ringlet, little holes are continued; almost in the whole Passage, from the Head to the Tail; into which, if you blow with a Pipe, presently the underlying parts swell up, the dung of the *Intestine* being driven up and down here and there, backward and forward: From these holes, if they are pressed, a white, viscous, and sometimes a milky Humour drops forth, which seems to be muck or stuff besmearing those Cavities, and fortifying them against the inclemency of the Air.

Without doubt these little holes are so many Wind-Pipes, which as in bloodless Insects, being numerous and dispersed thorow the whole Body, supply the place of Lungs, and draw in the nitrous Air for the inspiring the Vital Liquor, and by and by sends it forth being spent. But against this it may be objected, That little and sometimes almost no respiration serves the Earth-Worms. Because they sometimes lye hid in the depth of the Earth, for above three Months, and are able so to ly and to live; yea, if the holes of the Wind-Pipes be smeared over with Oyl, they do not presently dy like the bloodless Insects; but being immersed in Oyl they swim in it unhurt, and live a long while; but if you apply heat to them, tho moderate, they dy presently: The same thing we have observed almost of Fishes, and especially of the Shelly and Crusty, who bear the defect of Air or Water, better than the presence of Fire, or Heat.

The

The reason of this (that we may defend our *Hypothesis*) we shall indeavour to shew; we have shewn in a late Tract, That altho Fire and Flame necessarily require, besides Sulphureous food from the matter of the Subject, something nitrous from the Air, which being denyed or withdrawn, they are suddenly extinguished; yet, if that the matter be inkindled of Sulphur and Nitre (as is wont to be in Gun-Powder) together mixed with the Concrete, that Fire or Flame will burn in the midst of the Waters, or in a place Empty of Air; to wit, because either food being contained within, they do not presently desire supplyes from without. In like manner we suppose it may be concerning the *Hypostases* and accensions of Brutal Souls: For altho many of these being inkindled in their vital humour, draw in altogether from the ambient Air, a Nitrous, and from within a Sulphureous Food; Yet in the blood of some of them, which are destinated to the Waters or to the Earth, much of Sulphur thick and Earthy, with little of Nitre, and very little only of spirit and volatile Salt, may be so temper'd that it being inkindled into Life, may burn with a silent and almost suppressed fire; neither requires from without the access, either of much or continued nitrous Food, but, as it hath a certain intestine task, its burning is more securely performed in the Earth or Waters, than in the open Air: For that indeed from this, there is danger of too much inkindling the sulphureous Particles, and so quickly of overturning the *Crasis* or disposition of the Soul: Wherefore, these kind of Animals greatly abhor fire or external heat, which may make the internal Sulphur to work, and too much to burn. However, altho the Souls of these are not contented with fire, and it sometimes as it were hid in the Ashes, suffers them to be nummed or stiff; yet notwithstanding, Organs of Respiration are given to them all, for the continuing it aslong as it pleases, and as occasion serves for the increasing or repressing it. And indeed the Creatures of a more frigid blood, appear to be constituted or imbued with plenty of Sulphur, tho sparingly inkindled, because Earth-Worms and Fishes, quickly putrifying, yield a most stinking smell; and the putrified flesh of some of these, by reason of the very many Effluvia's of Sulphur, shine in the dark like a live Coal. Moreover, it hence appears, that the saline Particles, which make up the temperament of these, are for the most part nitrous, and bestowed for the food of Life; because from the bodies of these, dissolved by Chymical operation, you can neither draw a Volatile Salt, as out of all Other Animals, nor a Fixed. The Images of the Earth-Worms, shewing their Anatomy, are described in the Fourth Table. *Earth-Worms and Fishes, abound in nitrous Salt, being almost wholy destitute of a fixed and Volatile Salt.*

In the next degree of the more frigid bloody Creatures, above Earth-Worms, Fishes are placed, indued with one belly'd Heart and Gills. If indeed Lungs be wanting to these, the other bosom of the Heart were superfluous. But most Fishes want Lungs, both for as much as living in the Waters (whose medium is not fit for sounds) they have neither voyce, nor make a noyse, and chiefly, because the water ought not to be emitted thorow the Wind-pipe, into all the Cavities of the Lungs, if they had them; for that by watering them, or overflowing them, it would presently overthrow them, and fill them to a stiffness: But as in Brutes with Lungs, the Air being admitted within it, slides thorow all the blood-carrying Passages every where; that entring the little mouths of the Vessels, every where gaping, it inspires the Blood with nitrous food; so the Gills in Fishes, which are substituted as so many Lungs, or rather inverted, are so placed without the Cavity of the *Thorax*, that the Waters continually flowing to the Passages of the Vessels, and their little Mouths being outwardly planted, whilst the Gills are inlarged, they inspire something nitrous, or what is like it, to them; the remains of which, being by and by spent, the Gills being contracted, is sent away again; and so by Continued reciprocations of Inspiration and Expiration as in hot Animals, the Life or the Flame of the Blood is Conserved. *In the next degree of the more frigid bloody Creatures are Fishes. They are indued with an one Bellyed Heart and Gills.*

We have not much to say concerning the structure of the Gills, they being already sufficiently describ'd by several: As to their fabrick, they are bony semi-circles, planted on both sides of the bottom of the Mouth, nigh to the opening of the Gill holes, which are made hollow quite thorow, with little ditches, as it were quilly, that they may receive the Vessels sent to them and much branched forth, and defend them against injuries. *The Structure and use of the Gills.*

The Vessels belonging to the Gills, are Arteries, and Veins; which in the Sturgion, Salmon, and Cod, are found to be made after this manner: The *Aorta* going forth of the Heart, and ascending towards the Chin, or end of the lower Jaw, sends forth branches to the right and the left; some of these presently growing forked, accommodate an Artery to two Gills of the same side, which by and by being again divided, puts thorow two arterous shoots, thorow the Bow of every Gill, near to the bony Basis; then from them, others smaller thick set shoots, tend into the sides and midst of every Come-like Finn: After the Gills being passed thorow, all the arterous Branches meet together again, and Constitute the same Trunk, which being by and by reflected, has a

prospect

prospect to all the other parts. The Trunk of the *Vena Cava* or hollow Vein descending, applyes it self and enters near into the *Aorta* ascending into the Gills. Further, in the several Finns of the Gills, lesser shoots, as in the Bows, answer the greater passages of the Venous, with so many Arterous shoots. Besides, from the several parts on both sides the Gills, a veinous branch is inserted into the descending Trunk. This plainly appears, because if you open the branches both veinous and arterous, lying on the Bows of the Gills, there will appear a series or row of holes leading into the Finns; Moreover, a black Liquor being cast into those Arteries, will return by the Veins. Yet I have observed, part only of that injected Liquor to turn aside thorow the holes into the Finns, but another part to pass directly thorow into the Channels, and thence to flow into the descending Trunk of the *Aorta*, which the Gilly Branches being at length all united do frame: From hence I gather, That the Blood in Fishes, (not as in Brutes with Lungs) is carried at every Circuit, or passes thorow the Vessels, between the organs of respiration, not all, or whole, or is carried from the Arteries into the Veins, whereby the hole might be inspired anew of the Air; but for that they, as we have shewn, enjoy in themselves a nitrous food partly intestine, therefore it suffices them, that the blood only be by parts exposed to the External Nitre flowing to it.

Not all the Blood, but a part only, is carryed thorow between the Gills, at every Circulation.

Fishes breath by the Gills.

From these also it seems to appear, That Fishes do breath by the Gills, or draw what is nitrous from the Waters, and do enjoy it as it were the necessary food of Life; which also many other Reasons do manifestly declare: To wit, for that the Waters where Fishes dwell, standing still a long time, tend to putrefaction; or if by too much Heat or Cold, or other means, by which the nitrous Particles are wont to be driven away or perverted, they be affected, they Choak their Inhabitants. Further, if Fishes be shut up in little water, or with too strait limits, also if more than should be in the same Fish-Pond, tho large enough, tho they have plenty of food, they will dye for want of the nitrous food, which also argues the Cause of their death, for before they dye, they will shoot forth of the waters, putting forth their mouths and heads, to take in the naked Air: so that it may from hence be Concluded, That there are also in these Inhabitants of the waters firic Souls; to wit, the *Hypostases* of which are an heap of most subtil Atoms, which being stirred up into motion, by a certain inkindling, do require, for the Continuing of their substance, besides the Sulphureous Aliment within, which they feed on, another nitrous from the ambient Medium.

wherefore Fishes rejoyce rather in the Waters, than in the Air.

But that Fishes rejoyce in the region of the Water instead of the Air, where any one would think that their Flame should be rather extinguished, than inkindled, we gave the reason of it but now, to wit, as certain Animals are destinated to these places, their Souls were so temper'd, that as the matter made up of Sulphur and Nitre mixt together, they burn or grow hot under the waters, yea they there live more securely; to wit, for as much as there is in them plenty of Sulphur, it is suffer'd to be only sparingly inkindled, and to burn forth. Further, altho some nitrous Particles seem to enter into the intrinsick and ordinary food of the vital fire, and left the flame, by the defect of these, should expire, new suppliments are daily instilled through the Gills: yet indeed, by reason of the divers Constitutions of Souls, living Creatures do respire after a several manner, and some require this medium more thick, others moderate, and others more thin. And for this Cause, some living Creatures, whilst they remain in the same number, sometimes change their sphere or ambient medium, and sometimes go out of the Waters into the Air, and sometimes from this into them. A certain Insect called the watry *Phryganion*, in some places in *England* a *Caddis*, at the first of the Spring is cloathed with a Coat of a sprig or small rind of wood, and creeps into the depth of the Rivers, in the shape of a Mite or rather a Maggot; afterwards, when its Soul begins to be sublimed, he gets to the tops of the Bulrushes, and in the Month of *May*, rising up to the superficies of the water, puts off its Coat, and having wings, flyes into the Air, and there lives during Life. Who knows not that Frogs live at first in the Waters, in the shape of a Tadpole, altogether; then all the Summer do leap about in the Meadows, and that at last in the Autumn, returning to the Waters, do bury themselves in the Mud? After this manner, many more Insects, do not only change the Region, but also vary their Species or Kind, and of Reptils become flying Creatures.

Certain Animals change the Regions of the Air and Water.

Brutes of a more cold blood, which are framed with a Heart with a two fold Belly, and with Lungs.

Thirdly, A little more superior degree of Creatures of a more frigid or cold blood, is those who are gifted with a doubl'd belly'd Heart, and with Lungs; of which sort are Serpents, Lisards, and some Amphibious Creatures, that is such as live on Water and Land, as the Frogs, and some Fishes, to wit, the *Polypus*, the *Sea-Calf*, with many others. To these former, Lungs are necessary, because they oftentimes live in the open Air, which always ought to be deeply admitted into the *Præcordia* themselves; Moreover, because they put forth a certain sound, for which a Wind-pipe is required; but

for

for as much as Lungs are granted to them, so also a two-fold belly'd Heart, without which the blood passes not thorow the Lungs. As to what respects the *Amphibious* Creatures, which at their pleasure now live on the Land, and now in the Waters, tho it appears that these cannot stay always, or very long under the water, yet it is to be wonder'd at, how in the mean time they breath; for if they open the Wind-Pipe, the Waters rushing presently in, would drown the Lungs. *Bartholinus* easily untyes this doubt, by asserting, That in these Brutes, an Oval hole as in *Embrio*'s, is kept open all their life-time. *Cornelius Consentinus* affirms it after the same manner to be in Divers, or such as dive under the waters; and he shews the manner whereby some men may be made able to dive; to wit, if whilst they are Infants, they be provoked often to Cry, they are suffered a long time to restrain the spirit, from hence there will be a necessity of casting forth the Blood thorow the oval hole or navil, and for that reason will hinder its Coalition or Closing up.

But indeed in these Brutes, as to such a Conformation of the *Precordia*, the most skilful Anatomist Doctor *Walter Needham* did doubt, and desired to have found it in some of them by an ocular search, after many dissections.

However it is, we are to suppose these living Creatures do not breath, whilst they are under the Waters; and from thence the Course of their Blood is by and by made more slow, and smaller: In which Condition it matters little, whether it so growing torpid or sluggish, creeps from the hollow vein into the *Aorta*, by the navil hole; or whether lying quiet, it creeps forward by a gentle or slow pulse of the Heart; for either way, there will be a necessity, that the Vital fire, for defect of aerial food, would be presently diminished, and as it were depressed into a halituous or breathy substance: Notwithstanding in the mean time, that it may not wholly Expire or be Extinguished, these two things are done, *viz.* *On which the faculty of diving depends.*

First, Because in these Animals (and as in all Fishes) the Vital fire, together with a certain Sulphureous and also Nitrous food within (as we have shewed) is injoy'd; therefore it is able a long time to want its external supplement from the Air.

Then Secondly, in some of them the *Hypostasis* it self, or Constitution of the Soul, consisting of less subtle Particles, is not so suddenly dissolved; but that its parts stick together more strictly among themselves: nor are they wont to be dissipated presently, by any force, as in more hot Animals. Further, as their Souls, as to the greater part by much, subsist in the Brain and Nervous stock, more than in the Blood, it comes to pass, that however this fire being diminished and almost suppressed, the Animal faculties remain still lively enough: and indeed, far otherways than in hot Living Creatures, whose blood being obstructed about the *Precordia*, presently there follows an Ecclipse of the Animal faculties. Notwithstanding, Frogs, Eeles, and Serpents, after their Hearts are taken forth, will live for some time, and leap about; yea, by reason of the animal spirits being intangled with a viscous matter, and not easily dissipable, retain for a little while motion and sense, after their Bodies are cut in pieces, and the several portions divided, and lay'd apart; as we have shew'd before.

The Third and highest Form of Animals, Is that of Creatures of an hot Blood, all which are framed with a two-Belly'd Heart, and Lungs. The Anatomy of these being already so accurately performed by many, and commonly known, there needs not any description of the History and Uses of the Vital or Animal parts, in these kind of Creatures or Brutes. *In the highest form of Animals are those of an hot Blood.*

The chief Species of this Kind, are Fowls and Four-footed Beasts, and in the same Class or Rank, we place with the Souls of the later, also the Inferior or Corporeal Soul of Man; and that rightly, because there is the same Conformity in either of their *Pracordia*, of their Brain, and also of their nervous Appendixes; which notwithstanding differs from that of Fowls or Birds. What kind of difference this is, between those and these, as to their Animal parts, we have formerly declared at large; and now we shall notifie what difference happens between them, as to their Vital parts. *They are furnished with a two-fold belly'd Heart and Lungs.*

The Lungs of Men and Four-footed Beasts are every where shut in the outmost superficies, that the Air entring by the *Trachea* or Wind-Pipe, and by and by entring into its Chanels, quickly blows up all the Lobes of the Lungs, and distends them, but it goes no further: But in Fowls, the Lungs being full of holes, admit the inbreathed Air into the whole Cavity of the Belly, which by the Muscles of the *Abdomen* or lower part of the Belly, is exploded thence. The reason of this I suppose to be in some part, that there may be a greater plenty for singing, and (in some) for the longer tuning of the Voyce, or for the more strong or longer breathing forth of the Air. Besides, (for that all are not singing Birds) it is so provided for, in these Brutes, that by reason of the Trunk of the Body being filled, and as it were extended with Air, they may the more easily fly, and are more easily held up, by the outward Air, by reason of that within. *How the Lungs differ in Birds and four footed Beasts.* *For what end the Lungs are perforated in Birds.*

D Indeed

Indeed Fishes, that they may the more lightly swim in the Waters, have in their Bellyes Bladders blown up with Air. In like manner Fowls, by reason of the Trunk of their Body, being full and as it were blown up with Air, whilst they rely on the open Air, become less heavy, and so fly more lightly and faster. Hence it comes to pass, that men being in danger of drowning, whilst they swim, receive great help by restraining the spirit, and inflating the Breast as much as may be: yea Dead Carcasses being drowned, after the breath or fumes begotten by the inward putrefaction, and shut up within, blow up the fallen Cavities of the Viscera, and extend them more, rise up again, and swim on the surface of the Water.

That the Souls of the more hot Brutes is chiefly Fire.

If we inquire into the Souls of the more hot Brutes, without doubt, it was at first in respect of these, that the Ancients did declare the Soul to be Fire, and the more modern Fire or Flame, these placing it in the Heart, those making it to be inkindled in the Blood: And indeed, since we have granted Souls, as it were fiery, to Bloodless Creatures, and those of a more cold Blood (which also the Lord *Bacon* grants to Plants) it is not for us to deny the same dignity, in Creatures of a more hot Blood: For besides, that the Souls of those, like Flame, require absolutely either sort of Food; *viz.* the Sulphureous and the Nitrous, and cannot be a minute without them, the very hot Blood also, is seen, by mere accension (for as much as we cannot shew how it can become so hot after any other way) to boyl up, yea and the Lungs, hanging to the two-bellyed Heart, to be the fire-place, chimny, or breathing hole, of the Flame cherished within them. Therefore, as the Soul of the Brute of a more hot Blood, being the perfectest in its Kind, is as it were a Rule or Square, by which others more inferior ought to be measured, and as the same actuating and vivifying the humane body, is subordinate to the Animal, and is the immediate substance of it, (as shall be more fully shown) it remains now, that we inquire into its Nature and Essence, and first of all, that we search into, what parts, powers, and affections she has, which shall be the chief Members of our Psychology or Discourse of the Soul.

In Man the Corporeal or fiery Soul is subordinate to the Rational.

The parts of the Corporeal Soul.

The Explanation of the Figures.

The First Table,

Contains certain Figures taken out of *Malpigius*, in which the Vital Organs of the Silk-Worm and of other Insects are represented.

The First Figure

Shews the Navil-hole, of which two being planted in the sides of every Section or little Ring (except in the three uppermost) are the Doors or Openings of the Wind-Pipes.

A. A. *The Extremity of the hole, which being black, and a little reflected, is united to the Contained Head of the Wind-Pipe.*

B. B. *The Head of the Wind-pipe, filling the Hole, in whose middle is a Cleft.* C. *To which little fibres, like an hairy space, being brought, draw together the gap, or dilate it, that the Air may go out and in at its pleasure.*

The Second Figure

Shews some interior Branchings in the Silk-Worm.

A. A. *A gaping, where the head of the Wind-pipe opens into the oval hole or Navil.*

B. B. B. C. C. C. *The foldings or ramifications of the Wind-pipe, distributed into the Viscera and other neighbouring parts.*

D. D. *Greater Branches, reaching from the lower and upper head of the* Trachea *or Wind-pipe, towards the other infoldings.*

The Third Figure

Shews the Ramifications of the *Trachea* or Wind-Pipe in a Grashopper.

A. *The head of the Wind-Pipe opening outwardly into the Hole, by and by is branched forth inwardly into various shoots.*

B. *The*

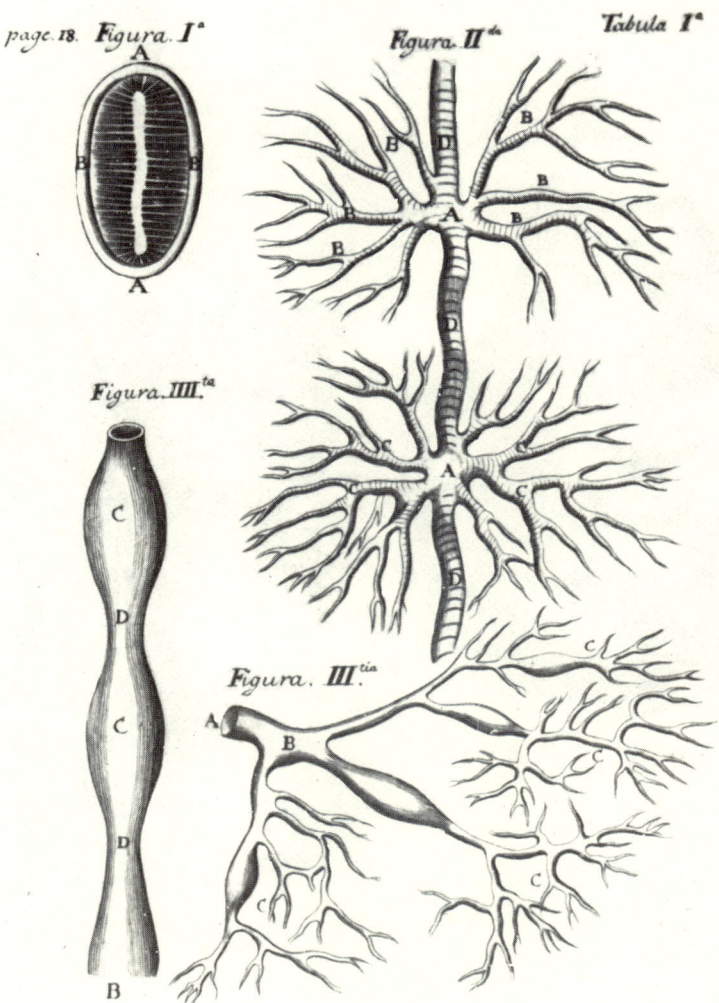

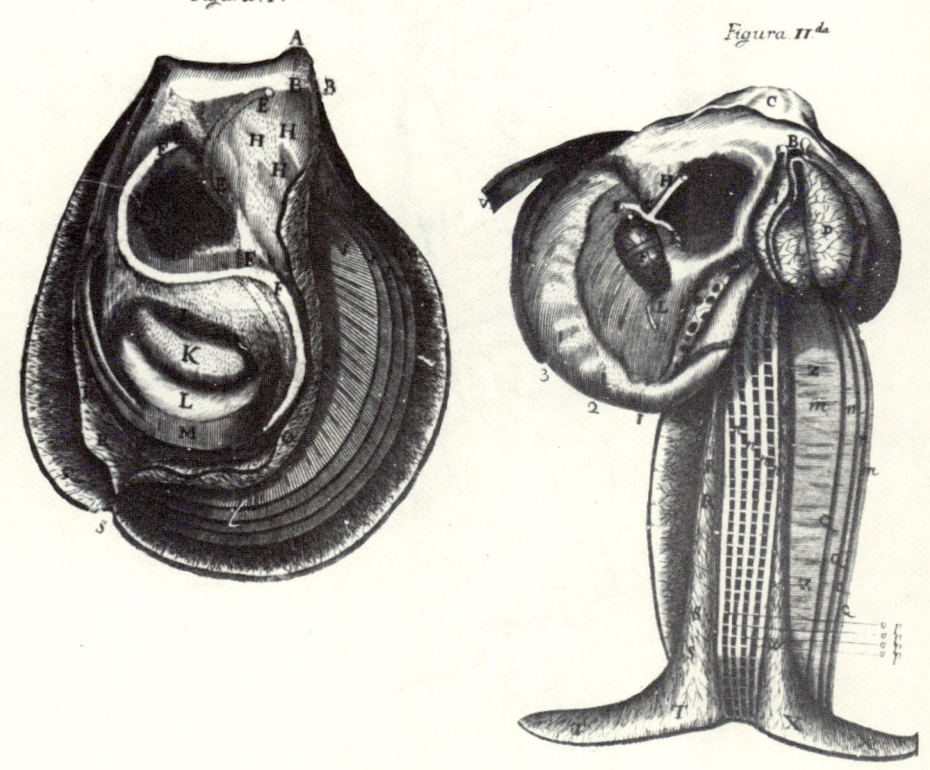

The Explanation of the Figures.

B. *The greater shoots of the Wind-pipe, being extended by degrees into the Ovals, as it were into bladders.*
C.C. *The lesser shoots going from those greater.*

The Fourth Figure,

Expresses the Heart of the Silk-Worm, which seems to be made oblong and unequal, as if into many little oval Hearts.

A. *The upper part of it nigh the Head.*
B. *The lower part nigh the Tail.*
C.C. *The broader part of the Heart.*
D.D. *Its narrow portions.*

The Second Table,

Of which

The First Figure

Shews the Oyster taken forth and whole from the shell, that his parts may be seen as they are in their natural situation.

A. *The Head of the Oyster, in the Corners of which,*
B.B. *The Circular Muscles, going about the whole Body are terminated.*
C. *The gaping or Chink leading between the Muscles and Gills to the Mouth.*
D. *The superior portion of the Liver, of a brownish colour, leaning to the Ventricle.*
E.E. *The Oesophagus leading from the Mouth to the Ventricle.*
F.F.F.F. *The Intestine, descending from the Ventricle towards the Corner of the strait muscle, which being from thence bent inward and rolled about, ascends above the Liver, being there hidden, arises again in G: and is terminated in the Arse.*
H.H.H. *The skin with the glandulous flesh and fat hiding and lying between the Viscera.*
I. *The Cavity in which are the Pericardium, Heart and Vessels.*
K. *The strait Muscle, with the perpendicular fibres, opening the shells.*
L. *The other strait Muscle, the Tendons of which growing to either shell shut them.*
M. *The thickness of the same Muscle, and the altitude of the fibres, are denoted.*
N.N. *The Circular Muscles including the Gills from the right side.*
O. *The superior Circular Muscle leaning to the Gills, being rolled out of its sight, that the Gills may be beheld.*
P. *The inferior Circular Muscle lying under the Gills.*
Q.Q. R.R. *The Parts of the same Muscles placed on the left side of the Oyster.*
S. *The Bosome, where both the Circulary Muscles, and their right and left parts coming together, Constitute the Passage, for the admitting the waters to the Gills, and for the shutting them forth from thence.*
T.T.T.T. *Four inferior Tufts of Gills which are thinner and broader.*
V.V.V.V. *Their superior Tufts thicker and more contracted.*

The Second Figure

Represents the Oyster open, and unrolled, that its Viscera and internal parts may be seen.

A.A. *Two Gills dissected from the uppermost, and removed out of their places, that the Mouth of the Oyster may be plainly seen.*
B. *The Mouth of the Oyster.*
C. *The Veil or Covering of the Mouth.*
D.D. *Two other superior Gills in their proper site with the Creeping Vessels.*
E. *The superior brownish portion of the Liver under which the Ventricle lies hid.*
F. *The Heart made bare from the Pericardium with the broad and blackish Ear of it.*
G. *The Aorta, by and by from the going forth of it from the Heart, divided into three branches.*
H. *The first Branch ascending towards the Head.*
I. *The second towards the strait Muscles.*

K. *The*

K. *The third Branch tending into the Gills.*
L. *The Trunk of the hollow Vein, entring into the little ear of the Heart.*
M. M. M. M. *The Inferior Gills, with the Circular Muscles, cut off from the Body of the Oyster, where they stuck to it, and spread forth, that their Passages and Cavities might be beheld.*
N. N. N. N. *The yoakings, or beginnings of the Gills on which lye the several Vessels, viz. Veins and Arteries, O. O. O. O. and the holes lying between, P. P. P. P.*
Q. Q. Q. Q. *The Extremities or fringes of the same Gills.*
R. R. *The Inferior Circular Muscle of the right side, out of its site and inverted, that it may be seen.*
S. S. *A portion of the same by which it sticks to the bottom of the Oyster.*
T. T. *A portion of the same which Compassing the left side of the Oyster sticks to the portion* V.
W. W. *The upper Circular Muscle of the right side, folded and contracted, that it may not hide the Gills.*
X. X *A Portion of the same which Compassing about the left side of the Oyster, sticks to the Portion* Y.
Z. Z. *The superficies of the Gills, in which the Finns or streaked Passages, for the ingress and egress of the Vital humour and the waters, appear.*
1. *The lower border of the Oyster, from which the Yoakings and the Circular Muscles are cut off.*
2. *A Portion of the Intestine ending in the Arse.*
3. *The Arse.*

The Third Table.

The First Figure

Shews the Lobster open in the back, that the Brain, Viscera, Vital, Genital, and other interior Parts may be seen.

A. A. *The Brain double, the Hemispheres of which being distinct, are separated one from the other, also a little from the oblong Marrow.*
B. *The Head of the oblong marrow, out of which the optick Nerves* b. b. *and the Mammillarie Processes under them, proceeds.*
C. *The Cerebell.*
D. D. *Two shanks of the Oblong Marrow, which pass into the Spinal, and as it were two greater Nerves, meet now and then in their descent, and now and then separate, and then again come together.*
E. *The Carotis Arterie.*
F. F. *A portion of the Oesophagus.*
G. *The Opening of the Ventricle.*
H. *The upper Orifice.*
I. *The Bottom and Lower Orifice near which are three Teeth.*
K. *The Temporal Muscles out of their place.*
L. L. *Muscles appendixes of the former.*
M. M. *Bodies stuffed with pipes and Glandula's or little Kernels, into which passages lye open, from the Ventricle, to whose Sides they grow; these seem to be in the place of the Liver and Mesenterie.*
m. m. m. m. *The same Bodies brought lower from either side, and ending in the processes,* μ. μ.
n. n. *Spermatick Bodies arising on both sides of the Ventricle, which descending under the Pericardium, are terminated in the processes,* n. n.
o. o. *Processes out of the Spermatick Bodies, like to the* Epididymis, *from which are two Yards.*
p p. *Two Yards, in the tops of which, thorow the holes made in the last little feet but one, a passage lyes open.*
q. *The hole in the little Foot for the going forth of the Yards.*
R. *The Pericardium, with the Heart included.*
S. *The little Ear of the Heart into which the Vena Cava enters.*
T. T. *The ascending Trunk of the* Vena Cava.
V. *The Aorta going out of the Heart, cleft into three branches.*
W. *The first Branch to its Head.*
X. X. *Two other Branches in either Side sent thence to the Gills.*

Y. Y. *The*

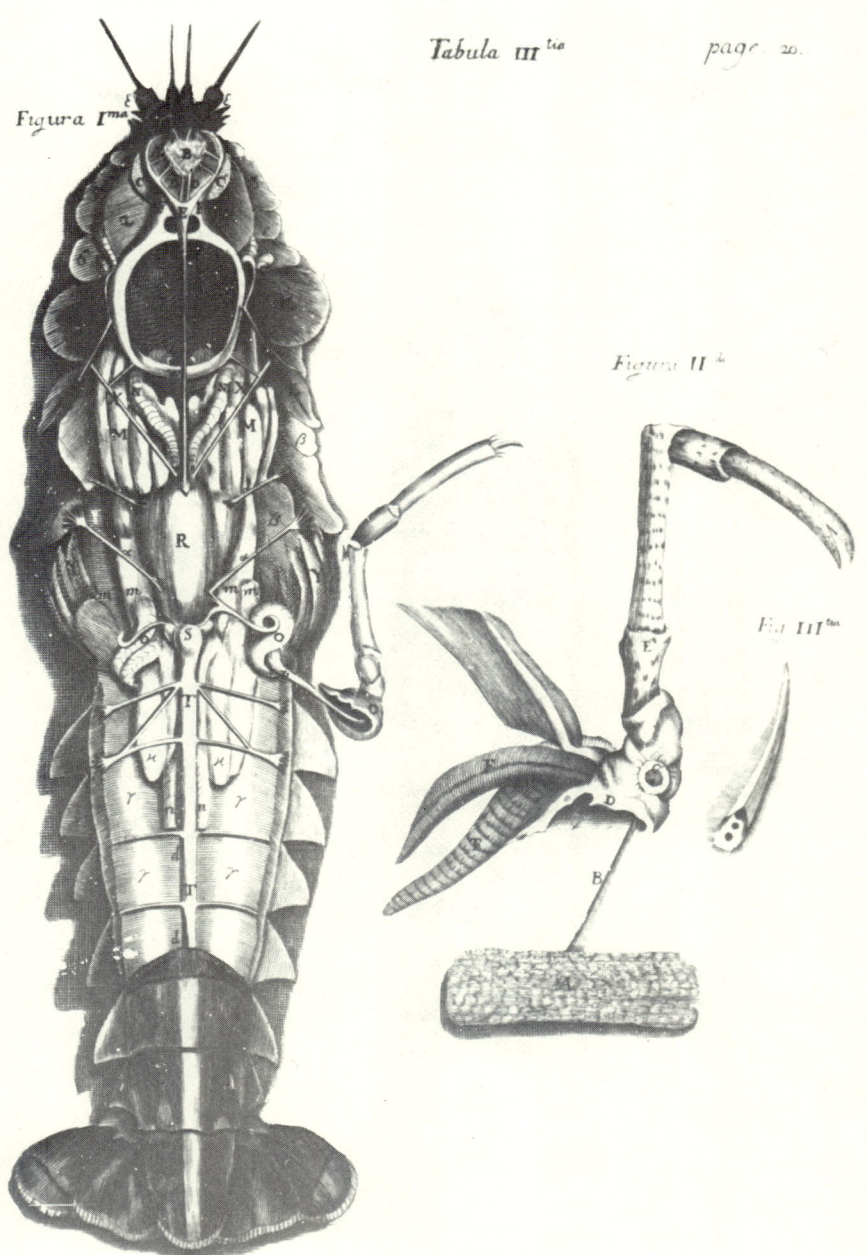

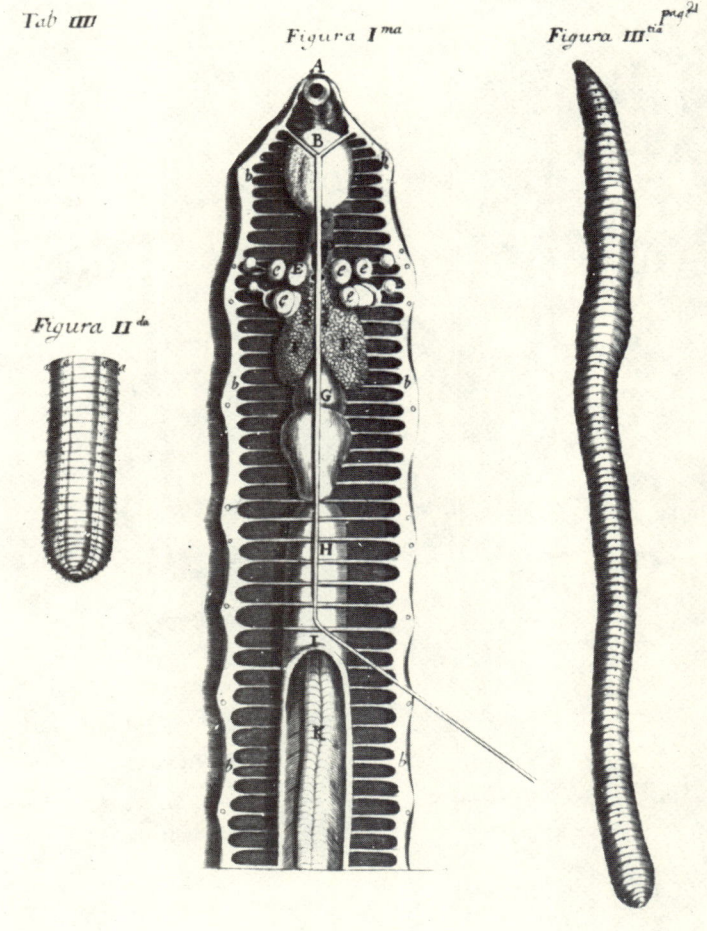

An Explanation of the Figures.

Y. Y. *The Tops of some of the Gills in view.*
1.2.3.4.5.6. *Some portions of the Muscles.*
α. α. α. α. *Ligaments from the Pericardium to the Muscles of the Breast.*
β. β. β. β. *The Muscles of the Belly, and Breast.*
γ. γ. γ. γ. *Muscles belonging to the Tail.*
δ. δ. *The Intestine from the Ventricle to the Arse.*
ε. ε. *Tubes or Pipes, within which, the Optick Nerves are brought to the Eyes.*

The Second Figure

Shews the Womb of the Lobster, and its Neck, and Privy Member, or aperture made thorow the hole in the last little Foot but one, together with the little Foot it self, and the affixed Gills.

A. *A portion of the Womb or place of Eggs, full of Eggs.*
B. *The neck of the Womb.*
C. *Its Orifice in the hole of the little Foot.*
D. *The Basis of the little Foot.*
E. *The little Foot, the shaking of which moves the Gills fixed to it.*
F. F. *Two Gills fixed to the basis of the little Foot, with Finns or spongy borders.*
G. *The appendix of the Gills, which like a bladder or membranous bagg, may be blown up and distended.*

The Third Figure

Expresses a portion of the Gill cut off, that its three Passages or Cavities may appear.

The Fourth Table.

The First Figure

Shews an Earth-Worm laid with its belly upwards, the greatest part of it dissected and lay'd open, that the Brain, *Præcordia, Viscera*, and other Parts may be seen.

A. *The Mouth and Chin of the Worm.*
B. *The Brain, in the superficies of which, an Artery Expansed or stretched out, descends to the Heart, and from thence to the Tail.*
b.b.b.b. *Annulary or ringie Muscles opened and unfolded with their Tendons.*
C. *A portion of the Oesophagus.*
D. *The Heart.*
E. e.e.e.e. *The upper little white shining Globes, both the greater and the lesser.*
F. F. *Two lower Globes, bigg and full with Eggs.*
G. *The Stomach, of which there are three Bellies, 1. 2. 3.*
H. *The Intestine, descending from the Ventricle, which being bound by the Tendons of the ringie Muscles, appears like the Gut Colon in perfect Animals.*
I. *A portion of the same Intestine opened, that the Body included in it, or the Intestine in the Intestine may be seen.*
K. *That interior Body, which seems to be in the place of the Liver, and Mesenterie.*

The Second Figure

Expresses a portion of the same Earth-Worm, with the Tail cut off, that the rowes of little Feet, which are 4, to wit, *a. a. a. a.* may be seen.

The Third Figure

Shews the whole Earth-Worm prone, or with its back uppermost, that the ringie Muscles, and the Wind-Pipes in them, may be seen.

CHAP. IV.

Of the Parts or Members of the Soul of the Brutes.

A double Subject of the brutal Soul.

THE Corporeal Soul in more perfect Brutes, and common to Man, is extended to the whole organical Body, and vivifies, actuates and irradiates both its several parts and humours, so it seems to subsist in both of them eminently, and to have as it were its imperial seats; But the immediate subject of the Soul, are the Vital Liquor or the Blood, Circulated by a perpetual Circulation in the Heart, Arteries, and Veins; and the Animal Liquor or Nervous Juyce, flowing gently within the Brain and its Appendixes: The Soul inhabits and graces with its presence both these Provinces; but as it cannot be wholly together at once in both, it actuates them both, as it were divided, and by its parts: For as one part living within its Blood, is of a certain fiery nature (as we have shown) being inkindled like flame, and the other being diffused thorow the animal Liquor, seems as it were Light, or the rayes of Light, flowing from that Flame; which from thence being Excerpted, and manifold ways reflected and refracted, by the Brain, and Nerves, as it were by Dioptrick Glasses, are diversly figured, for the Exercises of the Animal Faculties.

The blood or vital Liquor.
The Nervous juyce or animal Liquor.
From hence two parts of the Soul.
Flamy and light.

There are therefore Corporeal Souls, according to its two chief functions in the Organical Body, *viz.* the Vital and Animal; two distinct parts, to wit, flamie and lucid, for what belongs to the said natural function, that indeed is involuntary of the Animal, and is performed by the help of the Animal spirits.

To which may be added another the Epiphysis or dependence of the whole Soul, viz. the Genital part.

But besides these two members of the Soul, fitted to the individual Body, a Certain other portion of it, taken from both, and as it were the Epitomy of the whole Soul, is placed apart, for the Conservation of its Species: This as it were an Appendix of the vital flame, growing up in the Blood, is for the most part Lucid or Light, and Consists of Animal Spirits: to wit, which being Collected into a certain band, and having got an appropriate humour, *viz.* the genital, are hidden within the spermatick Bodies; to the end indeed, that, when opportunity shall serve, that Band of spirits, as it were a little Brand not yet inkindled, may be able from thence to be drawn into fit fire, and to be inkindled into another Vital Flame, the formatrix of a new animated Body.

The parts or Members of the Soul.

Concerning these three Members of the Corporeal Soul, two, to wit, the Vital and Animal, fiery by Act, and the other, *viz.* the Genital, lay'd up for a future firing, it should have been particularly and fully here treated on: But since we have already sufficiently discoursed of the two former, I shall only add briefly, by way of Suppliment, the Summ of what I have said before, and then we shall also briefly discourse of the begetting part of this Soul.

The Flamy part of the Soul in the Blood.

First, It appears, that the part of the Corporeal Soul rooted in the Blood, is truly flamy, as to which we need only to refer you, to what we have wrote lately in a particular Tract of the Accension of the Blood: For there having shown, the heat of the Blood to be necessarily required, to wit, whereby a greater plenty of spirits may be instilled into the Brain, from its frame being very much loosned; by and by we prove, from those three ways, by which all Liquors whatsoever are only made hot, none can agree with the blood, besides accension or inkindling: For neither by heat put to it, nor by reason of Salts and Sulphurs, which are Corrosives of a divers Kind being put together, can the blood be made to boyl; wherefore it follows, that it is inkindled like the spirit of Wine, and so as it were flames forth and boyls up. Further we shewed, that it is truly inkindled in hot living Creatures, because the proper Passions of Fire and Flame, are found only besides in the Life of the Blood; for in like manner both to this, and to them, there is need constantly of an Internal Sulphureous Food, together with the External nitrous; yea, and either Flame, alike, to wit, the Kitchin and Vital, whil'st they burn desire Eventilation. To these may be added, that the Life and Flame of the Blood, as to their Various ways of production and extinction, there particularly described and rehearsed, are wholly after the same manner. Lastly, the analogie or agreement of either Flame, being sufficiently unfolded, we have declared, by what beginnings, the Vital Flame arises, by what degrees it increases, and, after its hight, is diminished; Further, we have shew'n reasons, wherefore this is not visible and destructive as the common Flame, but as it is Subordinate to the Corporeal Soul, as to a Superiour Form, it admitting a proper Species, and serving to the uses of Nature, destinated by the Creator, silently burns with a gentle and friendly heat, like a Fire shut up in *Balneo Mariæ*, apart by it self; and as it so destroys not the Blood, but inkindling the Liquor

Which we have shewed to be truly inkindled.

even

even so its Superficies, wholly dissolves the frame of the whole mixture; it follows thence, that some particles being burnt, others of a various Kind being manumitted or let go, they are Variously imployed in the offices of the others; but of these, those which are chiefly Subtil, as it were Beams of Light sent from a Flame, are, as it were distilled into the Brain and Cerebel. These most subtil particles are called the Animal Spirits, and first of all entring the Cortical Substances of those parts, and from thence flowing into the *Meditullia* or middle parts of either of them, and into the Oblong and Spinal Marrow, and further into all the Nerves and Nervous Fibres, dispersed thorow the whole Body, Constitute the other and more noble part of the Corporeal Soul, commonly called the Sensitive, by us the Lucid or Etherial; into whose Nature, as also into the ways of its Subsisting, Acting, and Suffering, we shall now in the next place inquire.

Secondly, The sensitive part of the Soul, even as the Vital, is extensive and divisible; whose *Hypostasis* when as the Animal Spirits, as to the Integral parts, do Constitute, a great and difficult question arises, concerning them; of what sort of substance they are, and from whence they are indued with so notable an Energy or Power? I shall say nothing to those, who wholly deny these Spirits, for that the existencie of which, is almost palpable, and may be proved demonstratively by the effects; nor am I much solicitous of those, who arguing Contend, that the Senses and Faculties of living Creatures, however perceptive, cannot be but from an Immaterial and Immortal Substance, and therefore without any necessity, multiply almost to Infinity; and I know not for what end, not only Essences, but also immortal Souls of Brutes, yea, of Fleas, Flys, and of other, more vile Insects. Against these Opinions there needs no other Argument, than that any one may consider truly in every Brute or Man, the Organs of the Animal Faculties, than which certainly nothing in the whole nature of things, can be made more Mechanically, and with a more neat Artifice. The Brain and Cerebel, the two Roots of the Lucid part of the Soul, or rather the Fountains of the Primary Spirits, are placed in the top it self of the Body, into which, when the Animal Spirits are distilled, from the Blood, placed above and round about, as it were by a descent; they from thence flow forth through the Medullary and nervous Appendixes, as it were by Bills or Pelicans placed here and there, into all the inferiour parts. Either head consists of a double Substance, *viz.* a Cortical or Barkie, which for the most part serves for the reception of the Spirits; and a Medullary or Marrowy, which serves for their dispensation and exercise.

Further, as the Animal Spirits, for divers uses of the Animal Faculties, ought to obtain Tendencies or Stretchings-forth of a divers sort, within their distinct and peculiar passages, either Medullary and nervous Processes, is cut every where into Various tracts of Labyrinths, as it were so many Conclaves and Chambers; all which Medullary tracts, the Cortical part every where lies between and fortifies; From these, as it were Primary Palaces of the Soul, the Oblong and Spinal Marrow, like spacious Courts are stretched forth, which also are furnished, by reason of the Medullary substances variously lying between, with many Porticoes and Walks, planted here and there, for the necessary works of the Animal Function: From these Marrows, Nerves arising, are carried to the several parts of the whole Body, as it were so many distinct paths; then from these many other small Shoots or nervous Fibres, being on every side sent forth, as it were so many smaller or lesser Paths, are almost innumerable; at the ends of which, others secondary Fibres, Membranaceous and Musculous, are disposed, though thick Series, as it were so many martial Fields, in every one of which is placed a Maniple or Band of Spirits. In this most ample and highly intricate Labyrinth of Cloysters, and Animal passages, the Medullar or Nervous Processes, how small soever, being most thickly set, variously implicating one another, and ordinarily cutting cross one another, yet all of them distinct, and designed to certain offices, allways agree mutually between themselves, and intimately conspire together; So that every Impulse or Instinct, is carried from one end to another presently, yea, from every part to all the rest, sooner than in the twink of an eye. Further, from the effects it is demonstrated, that within these several tracts, some subtil particles do flow, and cause Animality or Life in all; which tho they be most thin, invisible, and nimble, we rightly call the Animal Spirits, and the Constitutive parts of the sensitive Soul.

Altho it appears plain, that such like Spirits are the Authors of the Animal Function, and do constitute the *Hypostasis* of the Soul it self; yet what they are according to their proper essence, seems hard to be unfolded; because we can hardly meet with any thing in Nature, to which they may be compared in all things.

The comparing of these, with the Spirits of Wine, Turpentine, and Harts-Horn, and such like, does not quadrate or agree. For besides, that those Chymical Liquors, neither represent the Images of their Objects, nor are indued with any Elastic Virtue, as the &c.

The Parts or Members of the Soul.

the Animal Spirits; those also are less Subtle than these, and less Volatil, for as much as they may be powred forth out of one Vessel into another, or may be distilled; but the Animal Spirits presently vanishing, after life is extinct, leave no Foot-steps of themselves. Wherefore, it is better, according to our *Hypothesis*, that we liken these Spirits sent from the Flame of the Blood, to the Rays of Light, at least to them interwoven with the Element and the Air. For as Light figures the Impressions of all visible things, and the Air of all audible things; So the Animal Spirits, receive the impressed Images of those, and also of Odors, and tangible qualities, and stay them at the first Sensory. But the Air, or Aerial particles, whilst free and unmixed, create nothing of force or tumult, yet they being more strictly pressed together, shut up in Clouds or Instruments, or imbued with Sulphureous, and other Elastick Bodies, being become presently raging, they often break forth into Meteors, *viz.* Winds, Hurricanes, and horrid Thunder. After the same manner, the Animal Spirits, whilst pure, are carried in the open spaces of the Head, and its Appendixes remain quiet enough; but they being shut up within the Muscles, and there being mixed with Sulphureous Particles from the Blood, and sometimes in other places, with an heterogeneous matter, become very impetuous, to wit, Elastick, or Spasmodick or Causing Cramps, as we have declared formerly at large.

Better to the Rays of Light interwoven with the Air, or the Element.

Therefore the Animal Spirits, according to this *Analogy*, (to wit, which thing of them happens chiefly and almost only with other things) we say are most subtil Bodies, and highly active, instilled from the inkindled Blood into the Brain, and its Appendix, which partly of their own nature, for as much as they are lucid and aerial, and partly from the agreeable furniture of the Organs, for that they are shut up within Passages, as it were Pipes and other Machines, abound with both an objective Virtue, by which many rays of Light promptly meet together in the Images of all sensible things, and effect the sension of every Kind, and also, an Active, by which the loco-motive powers, and also the acts of the Spasmodick Affections, are performed, beyond the forces or Instincts of wind, or any blast shut up in machines.

The Animal Spirits abound both in an Objective and an Active Virtue.

In Mechanical things, Fire, Air, and Light, are chiefly Energetical, which humane Industry is always wont to use, for the greatly stupendious, and no less necessary works. This the Furnaces of Smiths, Chymists, and Glass-men, and of other boylers of several Kinds, Dioptrick Glasses, Musical, Warlike, Mathematical Instruments, with many other Machines, never enough to be admired, do testifie. In like manner we may believe, that the Great Workman, to wit, the Chief Creator, from the Beginning, did make the greatly active, and also the most subtil Souls of Living Creatures, out of their Particles, as the most active; to which he gave also a greater, and as it were a supernatural Virtue and Efficacy; from the Excellent structure of the Organs, most Exquisitly laboured, beyond the Workmanship and artificialness of any other Machine.

As Fire and Light in Mechanical things so in Animals, they are chiefly Energetical.

We have described these Parts formerly in Plates, so that we need not here repeat their Anatomy, but only add a few things that were omitted. In the Animal Government, altho the Spirits are disposed, as it were an Army spread abroad thorow the whole Field, yet we say, that they obtain Orders and Offices, one thing in this part, and something different in that. In every one of these we have noted, as it were a double Aspect or Gesture, in the Provinces in the Medullary shanks of the Head, in the Nerves and also nervous Fibres, to wit, one of Begetting and Dispensing, and another of Exercise and Government.

A two-fold Action of the spirits in the Brain and its Appendix, 1. Of begetting and dispensation, 2. Of Exercise and Government.

As to the first, we have shown, that the animal spirits being procreated wholly in the Cortical or Barky substances of the Brain and Cerebel, do descend by and by into the middle or marrowy parts, and there are kept in great plenty, for the businesses of the Superiour Soul; in the mean time, a sufficient stock of these, gently flowing from this highest Province into the oblong and Spinal Marrow, and thence into the Nerves & Nervous Shoots, actuates all these passages, and blows them up into a certain Tensity. Lastly, a sufficient plenty of Spirits, distilling forth from the ends of the Nerves, enter into the nervous Fibres, planted in the Muscles, Membranes, and Viscera, and so constitute them, the proper and immediate Organs of the Sence and Motion. After this manner, the Region of the whole Sensitive Soul being viewed, if we would describe its *Idea* or Image, we must altogether represent the same Figure and Dimension, and the whole Head with its System and Appendix; so that as we may behold all these parts, shaddowed in the same Image, we ought to frame at once, the *Hypostasis* of this Soul, adequate and Co-extended to them.

The reason and manner of the former.

As to the several sorts of Offices and Exercises of the Spirits, so planted in distinct Provinces, First, we deservedly attribute to them a two-fold Aspect, to wit, inward for Sense, and outward for Motion: But more particularly, we may conceive the middle or Marrow part of the Brain, as it were the inferiour Chamber of the Soul, glased with

The distinct Offices of the spirits in various Provinces.

with dioptric Looking-Glasses; in the Penetralia or innmost parts of which, the Images *The perception of Sensions in the streaked Bodies.* or Pictures of all sensible things, being sent or intromitted by the Passages of the Nerves, as it were by Pipes or strait holes, pass first of all thorow the streaked Bodyes, as it were an objective Glass, and then they are represented upon the Callous Body, as it were upon a white Wall; and so induce a Perception, and a certain Imagination of the thing felt: Which Images or Pictures there expressed, as often as they import nothing besides the *The Imagination, P.... in the Callous body.* mere Knowledg of the Object, then by and by further progressing, as it were by another waving, from the Callous Body towards the Cortix or shell of the Brain, and entring into its folds, the phantasie vanishing, they Constitute the memory or remembrance of a Thing: But if the sensible species being impressed on the Imagination, promises somthing of Good or Evil, presently the spirits being Excited, respect or look back upon *The memory and remembrance of a thing or reminiscency within the folds of the Brain.* the Object, by whose appulse they were moved, and for the sake of embracing or removing it away, by other spirits flowing within the Passages of the Nerves, and successively by others implanted in the Members and moving Parts, they swiftly give their Commands of performing the respective motions. So the Sense brings in the Imagination; this the Memory or the Appetite, or both at once, and at length the appetite stirs up *The series and order of their powers.* local motions, performing the prosecution or driving away of the appearing Good or Evil. For the several Kinds of these sort of Animal Functions, yea for the Various Acts of either Kind to be performed, the Animal Spirits, who are the immediate Instruments of them all, obtain peculiar and distinct tracts or paths; within which, if there be any let or bar to hinder, presently some function is hindred, or some member of the sensitive Soul, being as it were cut off, becomes impotent.

Who can sufficiently admire the innumerable series of nervous Fibres, distributed in *The tracts or paths of the Spirits, are distinct within the head it self, even as within its nervous Appendixes* a most wonderful order thorow the several parts of the whole Body; in which the animal spirits, like Soldiers sent abroad, perpetually running up and down, on this side and on that, perform the offices of Sense and Motion. Further, those who dwell within the Head it self, the superior Legion of the sensitive Soul, altho more freely ranging, yet lye not disorderly or loosely, but its numerous Company, being limited with certain Bounds and Cloysters, as it were within the narrow space of One Chamber, perform infinite Variety of Actions and Passions.

Concerning these, discoursing formerly more fully in our description of the Brain and Nerves, we did distinguish the Seats of all the Faculties, yea we did shew the Commands of the Animal Function voluntary and involuntary, to be divers in themselves, also to belong to divers Governments of the Brain and Cerebel, with their respective appendixes of the Nerves. Further, we shewed that those Spirits, the Authors of either function, not only within the narrow Channels of the Nerves, but also in the large meet- *Every where the various Medullary tracts, are distinct from the Cortical.* ing places or *Emporiums* of the Head, have peculiar paths, to wit, the medullary tracts, as it were intrinsick Nerves, most curiously stretch'd forth here and there. But indeed, because it is objected, that I have not described all, and perhaps not exactly enough; therefore, that those medullary Passages may be the better beheld, we have lately instituted another more accurate anatomy of the Brain; to wit, by gently scraping with the *A more exact Anatomy of the Brain, through its Cortication or Shelly part.* point of a Pen-knife its parts, we removed every where the softer and brownish substance, a-Kin to the *Cortex* of the Brain, the whiter and more hard being left; by which means, in several places of the Brain and the Oblong Marrow, many Medullary Chords or Strings, as it were distinct Nerves, wonderfully Communicating among themselves, and with other white or medullary Bodies, were brought into sight. For as much as this Anatomical Administration, render'd the more secret passages of the Spirits, and the motions *The Common passages, and the private pathes of the Spirits.* belonging to the Arcana's of the animal Government, very Conspicuous; we shall here shew a new Figure or two of the Brain rolled forth, and the flesh when taken off in the chief places; in which are plainly beheld, both the Common Passages, and the Private paths of the Spirits, and which carry them backward and forward, immediately thorow the beaten way of the medullary tail, and which lead thorow the by-paths of the Prominences, into the streaked Bodies.

Therefore, in the Brain taken out, and rolled abroad according to our Method, let there be a dissection so made, between the Orbicular Prominences, to wit, between the *To wit, which thorow the orbicular prominences, are the Testes and Nates.* *Testes* or Testicles, *Nates* or Buttocks, that when they being whole, and divided in the middle of the Pinal *Glandula*, the parts are layed by themselves, the streaked Cavity of either may be lay'd open. (As in the 6th Table, Fig. 1. A. b, E. A. b. c. c. D.) Then it will easily appear, that the said Prominencies, called the *Testes*, are marrowy *Epiphyses* (or additions) of the oblong marrow, which sticking to the tails of the Cerebel, from thence look towards the Brain, and a Commerce is seen to be maintained between this and that.

This last *Ephiphysis*, passes from the parts of the Brain, into the next *natiform* (or of the form of a Buttock) *B*. which is an adjunct, or some Augmentation of that: To this

E   Medullar

Medullar *a.a.* in a Sheep, Ox, and many four-footed Beasts, grows a Cortical substance *B.B*. But otherways in a Man, Dog, Fox, and other more sagacious Creatures, it is marrowy thorow the whole; the reason of the difference, I have shewed in another place.

The description and use of them. This medullary *Epiphysis* reaching above the *Testes* and *Nates*, and going under the Pineal Kernel, tends towards the Chambers of the Optick Nerves; approaching which (*F.*) by and by it is cleft into two Branches, as it were Nervous, one of which *G*, is carryed to the Cone of the streaked Body, and the other *H.* towards its Basis, and in its oblique passage, sends a shoot into the midst of the Border of the streaked Body: this Branch going to the basis of the streaked Body, behind the root of the *Fornix*, is inserted into an Angle of the streaked Body.

From these Medullary tracts into the streaked Bodies. As to the Use of these Parts, we have proposed our Conjectures in our Tract of the Brain; and truly nothing seems more probable, than that by this side-path of the Prominences, and by the Passage of the Medullary Passages, there are Commerces held between the Brain and the Cerebel; for as often as it happens, that Impressions or Instincts meerly natural, follow spontaneous Affections and Motions, or are joyned to them, all that, within those private Tracts, is occupied. See our *Anat. of the Brain*, p. 176.

And wherefore. Further, whereby every such Impression from the Viscera or Precordia, by the mediation of the Cerebel, are carried from them in the same way forward and backward, into the streaked Bodies, and on the contrary every force and perturbation; The Medullary passage, which is for their commerce, enters in three places, *viz.* In the middle, and at either end, into the streaked Bodyes.

To the orbicular Prominences, succeed the Chambers of the Optick Nerves. To the Prominences which are called *Nates* and *Testes* succeed the Chambers of the Optick Nerves *E. E.* as also above the Medullary Trunk, certain *Epiphyses* or Additions, serve for a private office *viz.* only for the visive Function. For as the sight is a most noble faculty, and as the Organ of the eye is highly curious, so it obtains a very spacious Furniture or Porch, and also a very strait, to the common Sensory, *viz.* the streaked Bodies: Because the Optive Nerves coming together, under the Trunk of the oblony Marrow, and being by and by disjoyned, they climb up his sides, where going under the appropriate Protuberances, they go into a numerous company of hairy threads, which *The description of them.* are every where interwoven with the cortical Substance. *Fig. 2. Tab. 6.* These Medullary or Nervous structures or bindings, which without doubt the visible Species pass thorow, are all parallels, which being stretched forth Strait, are brought to the streak-*The use.* ed Bodies, every where, through their whole Compass. *Fig. 2.* Hence it is probable, the causes of the Sandy drops or Spots, yea, and of the sight otherways depraved or lost, do lie hid, not only in the Eye and Optick Nerve, but sometimes in these parts; for as much as those Filaments or Nervous threads, being obstructed or bound together, the visible Species are not able to beam themselves to the streaked Bodies. I knew one, being affected, by his Imagination and Memory being grievously hurt, that those diseases vanishing, fell into blindness: The reason of which accident seems to be, that the morbifick matter occupying at first the superior frame of the Brain, being slid thence lower *The Mamillary Processes, are carried by a private passage, to the streaked Bodies.* by the Cortix, at length enter'd into the Optick Chambers.

There remains yet a private passage of another sence, to wit, of the smelling, to the common Sensory, *viz.* the streaked Bodies; The mamillary Processes being entered into the Prominences of the Inferiour Brain, go under its Basis till they come to the border of the streaked Body on both sides, then being a little bent inwards: they proceed by an oblique passage towards its Basis, where they are inserted. *Fig. 1 Tab. 6.*

The common passage of the Spirits, to the streaked Bodies, is made by the shanks of the oblong Marrow. As to the Impressions of the other Senses, and to the force and Instinct of every Spontaneous motion, carried up and down, there is a necessity, that all these Kinds of Commerces, between the streaked Bodies and the Nervous Appendix, should be made by the Shanks of the longish Marrow: The tops of these being large and broad, Stick to the hindermost borders of those, so that from these into those, and so on the Contrary, a going and returning is easily performed. Further, that the many and divers motive and sensible Forces and Impressions together, may be carried without confusion, by this beaten and common way, the whole frame of the Medullary Shanks, appears thorow the whole to be made with Nerves or Medullary strings compacted together; as if they were so many distinct paths, in this common passage of the Animal Spirits, for the inculcating the Various acts of the Senses and of Motions. The Sixth Table represents these parts to the Life.

An accurate description of the striated or streaked Bodies. The chamfer'd or streaked Bodyes, consist of a most exquisite and greatly to be admired Fabrick: The figure of either, coming something near the Cone, appears like a Cone reflected and bent inward; the outmost and superior Superficies is round and Barkie, thorow which creep Blood-carrying Vessels, and a portion of the *Choroedal* Infolding hides it; The middle and Inferior frame of them consists of a Medullary Substance, with a Cortical mixed between. *Tab. 8th l. m.* The sides or either border of these, both the

Superior

Superior and Inferior, are for the most part Marrowy, and look white like the greater Nerves; n. K. Between these streaks or Marrowy strings, thick set, and of a divers magnitude, being stretched forth like the greater Nerves, Knit together, both the Borders: The anterior Border n. n. is every where knit to the Callous Body; so that whatsoever is to be carried forward and backward by either, *viz.* from one to another, we suspect they have for it this passage between those Medullary passages. The hindermost Border of the streaked Body, in its upper part, receives the Medullary Processes sent thither from the round Prominences, and also the Optick Chambers, into its Bosome: In the middle and lowest part, either Border is fixed to the Shanks of the oblong Marrow; and nigh to the Basis of the Fornix, the inferior Border of one streaked Body, is continued into the other Border; to the end, that these Bodies also might have between themselves a mutual Commerce, which is also observed almost of all the rest of the Parts of the Head, that they are double, and do communicate among themselves, by certain passages; so that if one part should be faulty, its defect might be made up by the other being whole.

As to the Offices and Uses of the streaked Bodies, though we can discern nothing with our eyes, or handle with our hands, of these things that are done within the secret Conclave or Closset of the Brain; yet, by the effects, and by comparing rationally the Faculties, and Acts, with the Workmanship of the Machine, we may at least conjecture, what sort of works of the Animal Function, are performed in these or those, or within some other parts of the Head; especially because it plainly appears, that the Offices of the Interior Motions, and Senses, as well as the Exterior, are acted by the help of the Animal Spirits, ordained within certain and distinct Paths, or as it were small little Pipes. *The use or Offices of the streaked Bodies.*

As therefore it appears from what we have said, that the chamfered or streaked Bodies are so placed, between the Brain and Cerebel, and the whole nervous Appendix, that nothing can be carried from these into that, or on the contrary be brought back hither, but it must pass thorow these Bodies; and as peculiar passages lead into these most ample Diverfories, from the several Organs of Motions, Sense, and the other Functions; and further, as Passages lie open from these into the Callous Body, and into all the Marrowy Tracts of the Brain, nothing seems more probable, than that these parts are that common Sensory, that receives and distinguishes the Species, and all Impressions, transferrs them, being ordained into fit Series, to the Callous Body, and represents them to the Imagination there presiding; that also transmitts the Force and Instincts of all spontaneous motions, begun in the Brain, to the Nervous Appendix, to be performed by the motive Organs. By reason of these manifold and divers offices, so many Marrowy streakes or internal Nerves are produced within the streaked Bodies, for the Various Tendences and Beamings forth of the Animal Spirits, it may very well be concluded that the Sensitive Soul, as to all its Powers and Exercises of them, is truly within the Head, as well as in the nervous System, meerly Organical, and so extended, and after a manner Corporeal. *They receive the Impressions of sensible things: and convey the Instincts of Motions.*

The Explanation of the Figures.

The Fifth Table,

Shews the Figure of the Brain of a Sheep roled forth, and derased, and as it were made bare of the Flesh, in many places, that the Marrowy Tracts may be seen.

A. A. *The Medullary Protuberances called Testes, which being certain Epiphyses or excrescences of the oblong Marrow, and joyned to the Trunks of the Cerebel look thence towards the Brain.*

B. B. *The Natiform Protuberances, the Substance of which in a Sheep, a Goat, and many others, is partly Cortical,* a. a. *partly Marrowy,* b. b. *in a Man, Dog, Fox, and others it is wholly Marrowy.*

C. *The Cavity or Ventricle, lying under the Prominences, which is lay'd open, these being dissected and opened.*

D. D. *Two Marrowy Chords or Strings of the Medullary Trunk, going strait to the streaked Bodies.*

E. E. *The Chambers of the Optick Nerves.*

e. e. *The parts of the pineal Kirnel, cut thorow the midst, and laid apart.*

F. F.

F.F. *The Medullar or nervous passage proceeding from the Prominences, which presently becoming forked, sends forth one branch G. to the Cone of the streaked Body, and the other H. to its Basis.*

I. *A shoot from the medullary Branch, going towards the Basis of the streaked Body, reaching into the midst of its Border.*

K. *The latter border of the streaked Body, receiving the nervous passages, and under the root of the Fornix, united to its like Border of the other side.*

L. *The whole streaked Body with its Vessels creeping thorow its Cortex or shell.*

M. *The other streaked Body, with the shell scraped off, that the Nerves or marrowy Tracts may appear.*

N.N. *The foremost border of both the streaked Bodyes, Conjoyned to the Callous Body.*

O. *The Basis of the Fornix.*

P. *The Trunk of the Fornix Cut off, and with the Brain rolled out, removed at a distance.*

Q.Q. *The two roots of the Fornix.*

R.R. *The interior superficies of the Callous Body, noted with transverse medullary streaks.*

S. *A medullary hedg or mound, dividing the streaks of one side, from those of the other.*

T,T. *Portions of the Brain Cut off and rolled forth, which (as also its whole Frame) appears with a marrowy, and a Cortical substance intermixt.*

V,V. *Portions of the divided Cerebel lay'd apart.*

W. *The Portion of the Oblong Marrow situated beyond the Cerebel.*

The Sixth Table,

Shews the Basis of a Sheeps Head, in certain parts of which Derased, and in others Exposed naked, the Streaks or Medullary Tracts, as so many Nerves, appear.

A.A. *The Mamillary Processes carried to the Basis of either Streaked Body, and inserted into them.*

B.B. *Some remaining portions of the Brain cut off from it greater bulk.*

C.C. *The streaked Bodies derased, and as it were made bare of flesh, that the Medullary streakes may appear also in its lower parts.*

D.D. *The Chambers of the Optick Nerves, in which the strait and thick set Medullary streakes, are reached forth, towards the streaked Bodies.*

E. *A Tract leading to the Tunnel of the Brain.*

F. *A Kirnel placed behind the Tunnel, which is twofold in man.*

G.G. *The Trunks of the Optick Nerves divided, and removed, from their joyning together before the Tunnel.*

H,H.f.f. *The Shanks of the oblong Marrow lying under the Orbicular Prominences, in which strait and most thick streakes are also stretched forth towards the chamfer'd Bodies.*

I.I.I. *Transverse Medullary Tracts distinguishing the regions of the oblong Marrow.*

K.K. *Ringy Processes compassing about the oblong Marrow, nigh the Cerebel.*

L. *The extremity of the oblong Marrow going into the Spinal.*

M. *The Top of the Spinal Marrow.*

The Seventh Table,

Shews the orbicular Prominences, and the Optick Chambers Erased, and as it were made bare of Flesh that their inward Frames may be beheld.

A.A. *The Testes, which thorow the whole being Medullar, are marked with strait Fibres.*

B. *The Nates, one of them being Derased, in which the strait and thickest Medullary streakes, are stretched forth towards the Brain.*

C. *The Medullary Hedg or Mound, dividing the Natiform Prominences from the Optick Chambers, and from which, one Medullary Process is carried into the Basis of the streaked Body, and the other into its Cone.*

D. *One Optick Chamber scraped, that its straight and most thick-set streakes, stretched forth towards the streaked Body, may appear.*

page. 27. Tabu V.

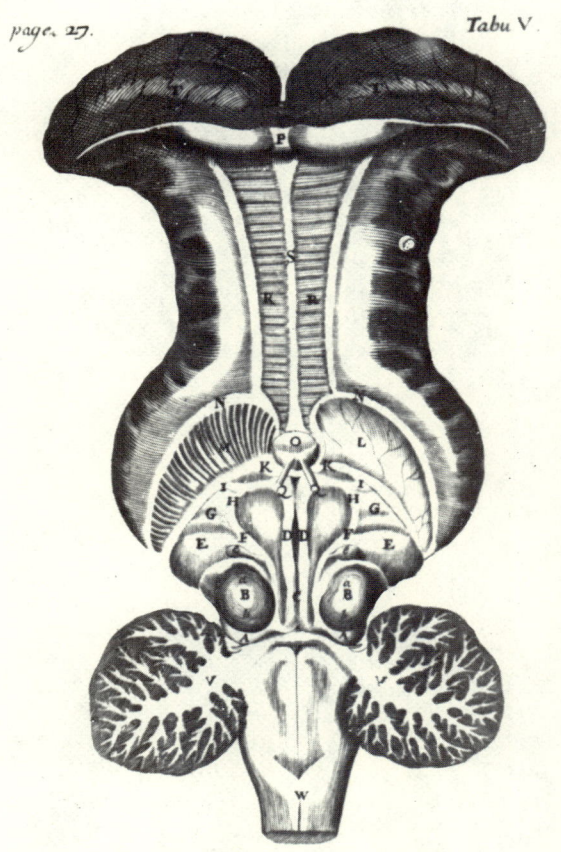

page 28   Tabu. VI.

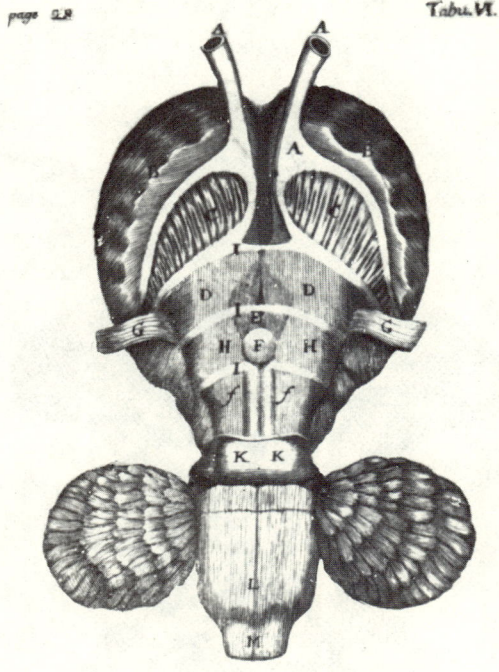

page 28   Tabu. VII

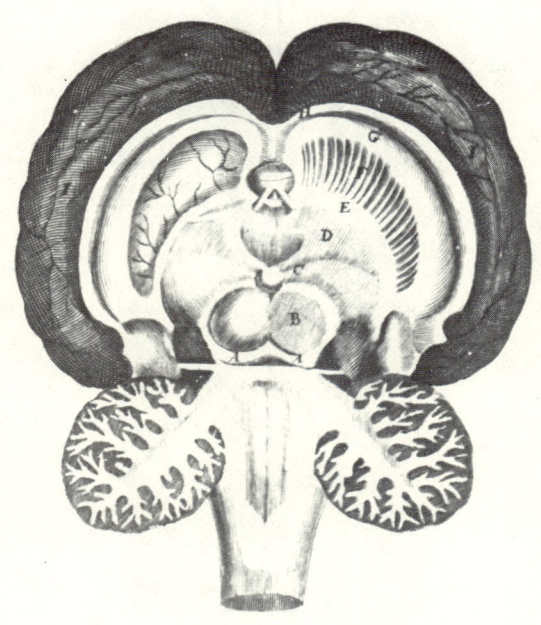

E. *The hinder Border of the streaked Body, receiving the Optick Medullar streakes and other Medullary Processes.*
F. *The Streaked Body decreased, whose little Medullary Nerves and Passages, are explained in the 5th. Table.*
G. *The foremost border of the streaked Body.*
H. *The Bosome, leading from the Mamillary Process into the Ventricle of the forepart of the Brain.*
I.I. *The Hemisphear of the Brain opened and seperated by it self.*

The rest here described are explained in the former Figures.

CHAP. V.

The Beginnings and Increase of the whole Corporeal Soul; also some Innate Habits and Inclinations of it are noted.

FRom what has been said, concerning the *Hypostasis* and Members of the Corporeal Soul, or of the more perfect Brutes (which is also the inferiour Soul of Man) it will be easier to trace out the Original, and the Increase of the whole. From hence also we may collect its figure and dimensions, as also the proportion, habits, and inclinations of its parts, in respect of it self, and the members of the Body, together with its Various ways of acting and suffering.

As to the first beginnings or original of the Corporeal Soul; this, (like as a Shell-fish forms and fits its shell to it self) exists something a little sooner, and so more nobler than the organical Body; Because a certain heap of animal Spirits, or most subtil Atoms, or a little Soul not yet inkindled, lies hid in the Seminal humour; which having gotten a fit cherishing or Fire-place, and at length being inkindled from the Soul of the Parent acting, or endeavouring, or leaning to it, as a flame from a flame, begins to shine forth, and to unfold it self, a little before the Foundations, or first ground-work of the body is lay'd: This orders the web of the conception, agitates and inkindles the applyed matter, disposes, and by degrees forms the Figure, designed by the Archetypal Law of Creation. In this stupendious Fabrick, together with its bodily bulk, being daily increased, and Imaged into the due Species of each animal. the Soul also takes its increase, and still renders it self like to the Body, which it forms. For when as the more thick particles, from matter continually put together, are bestowed in the Corporeal Organs; in the mean time, the more subtil and spirituous being loosned, and more rarefied, by the burning of the others, they dilate the *Hypostasis* of the Soul, and together with the Body unfold, and equally extend it. But that after this manner, the Seeds of the Soul being laid, from the beginning, together with those of the Body, do rise up to a due figure and bulk in either, it ought not to be attributed to the fortuitous concourse of Atoms, nor to the proper Energie of the Soul it self; but the beginning of all things, proceeds wholly from divine Providence, directing Generations, to the Ends and Ideas of Forms, according to the original Types primitively ordained by the same.

The beginning of the Brutal Soul.

Frames it self before the Body.

And increases likewise with it.

Secondly, As the Increase of the animated Body, and the first marrying together of the Elements proceed from this Soul, informing and disposing the matter; so the duration and subsistence of the same Soul, is the Bond of its Mixture or Concretion. For the flame of the Soul being extinct, or the inkindling and motion of the subtil particles ceasing, presently the frame of the Body it self begins to be dissolved and loosned, so that in a short time, the Elements being loosned and laxed one from another, fly away, and by degrees break their Concretion: wherefore this Soul, as it were salt or pickle preserves the fleshy bulk of the Body from putrefaction; yea, the same is almost in an animated Body, as the Flower or Spirit in Wine, which indeed being present, and unfolding its spirituous Particles thorow the whole, the Liquor continues still generous and flourishing; but as soon as this Spirit of the Wine flies away, forthwith the remaining water or liquor degenerates into an insipid and dead thing.

The duration also of the Body depends upon the Soul.

Thirdly, So long as this Soul subsists in the Body, according to an ancient saying of *Hypocrates, It is always Born, even till Death*; In which respect also, it seems to be most like flame, or rather the same thing, which is continually renewed almost every moment: Some parts of eithers subsistence, in like manner are consumed by burning, and fly away, and others in the mean time are laid up anew, from the Food continually laid in: For as the

The Soul always Born.

more

more Crass or thick Particles of the nourishing juice, wrought in the Viscera, fill up the losses of the Corporeal bulk, so the more subtil make up the layings forth or wastings of this Soul ; which, as they come to the blood, are as it were Oyl to a Lamp, and being perpetually inkindled within its bosom, restore to the Soul both Flame and Light, which would otherways perish. For whilst the purer part of the nourishing Liquor, cherishes the flame of the Blood, and sustains it, the most spirituous Particles falling off by its burning, are instilled into the concavity of the Head, which there propagate and nourish the other part of the Soul, to wit the Sensitive ; So the making of Blood, is owing very much to Chylification, or the making of the Chyle, and Animality or like to this ; notwithstanding which offices, the Animal Function payes back to the Vital, and both to the Organs of Chylification; for as much as the Animal Spirits, bestow a pulsifick force to the Heart and Arteries, whereby the Blood may be agitated and carryed about, to the places of accensions or inkindlings : yea, the Viscera of Concoction, receive heat which they want, from the flame of the Blood, and a motive and sensitive virtue, which they have need of, for their Offices, from a Constant afflux or flowing in of the Animal Spirits ; so the Brain is indebted to the Heart, and both of them to the Stomach, yea, and on the other side, this Region to that, and both to the third. To the end that the *Hypostasis* of the whole Soul might the longer continue, the Tributes of all the Parts are Compensed with mutual Offices one to another, and so at once the members both of the Body and of the Soul being conjoyned, by a Circular necessity, they desire and shew their mutual Labour.

The Offices of the Organs and Faculties, are reciprocal towards one another.

Fourthly, The Soul of the *Brute*, as it is Fire, according to Philosophy, has these two innate Dispositions by the Law of Creation, to wit, that it should defend it self, or delay its proper inkindling long, for whose sake it is still careful of taking of food; and also, that it might propagate its Species, or produce other Souls ; for which end, it Continually lays up from its provision, an incentive matter, and Continually desires to expose it to an inkindling.

It is natural to the Soul to defend it self, and to propagate its Species.

It is natural for every Animal, without guide or example, to take its proper food, and to Swallow it down, both that the web of the Body being daily increased, might grow to its due magnitude, and also that the Soul , as it were its woof , being daily supplyed with new plenty of Spirits , may be able to be Coextended or stretched forth equally with the Body , and able to perform lively the Acts of its Functions. Then assoon as the Lineaments, both of the Body and the Soul, being sufficiently drawn forth, and the Compass and Bulk of each Compleated, some Animal Spirits, superfluous from the individual work, begin to abound, and so seperate into the genital parts, with a Subtil humour, picked from the whole Body, as it were into a Store-house, destinated for the propagating the Species, and there being lay'd up, forme the Idea of the Animal, which afterwards is transferred into a fit Matrix, for to be perfectly formed.

Hence the young one as soon as it is born, seeks for food.

When the Individuum is made the genital humor, for the propagating the Species, is lay'd up.

The genital Humour, is not, as *Hippocrates* formerly taught, and as now commonly believed, carried from the Brain into the Spermatick Vessels ; for no peculiar passages lye between that, and these Bodies far remote ; but without doubt , the bloody mass it self, sends its most noble part into the Genitals, as well as into the Brain. Wherefore, when as there are no Nerves that reach to the Testicles, and that there are noted Arteries sent, and admirably made thorow wandering Passages and frequent engraftings of the Veins ; to wit for that End, that they may carry the most pure flower of the Blood, as it were thorow the winding Chanels of an Alembick, distilled by a long passage, and so wrought and made most highly subtil, into those parts : what is superfluous of this or less clarified, the Veins do not only receive and carry back, but also because from the much Spirit, a great quantity of Serous water (which serves always for its Vehicle) abounds , therefore the Water-Carryers are produced in these parts abundantly more than in any others.

The Genital Humor, not from the Brain, but from the Blood.

But that a great loss of the genital Humor doth hurt very much the Brain and the Nerves, and bring to them a notable debility ; the reason is, because the blood as it makes up the losses of the seed , destinated for the propagating its Species, carries thither and bestows whatsoever is most precious of its own ; in the mean time, as the Brain is defrauded of its due provision , by the great plenty of Spirits being carried into the Spermatick Bodies: yea as the blood is not able sufficiently to impart to the Genitals, out of its proper store, it remands or snatches its Tribute from the Brain and other parts, that it might be there bestowed ; so that not seldom the strength of the whole Soul and Body is consumed, on the mad insatiate fulfilling of Lust or Venus; and in these desires, every one, or the unskilful, complains of Flames, and feels the blood not only to flame forth, but a greater fire increasing, to make hot the marrow, yea oftentimes it is known to burn up the Flesh, Inwards, and Bones, and to reduce them to a rottenness.

why the loss of seed disturbs the Brain and Nerves.

As

The Dispositions and Habits of the Soul. 31

As to that most quick and Intimate Commerce of the brain, with the genital Members, for as much as the Venerian imagination Causes presently an insurrection in these parts, and on the other side a swelling up of the seminal humor, stirs up the Venerial Imagination, the Cause is, not an Instinct thorow the private passages of the Nerves, (which are wholly wanting) reciprocated from this to that; but, because for the Act of Generation, greatly necessary, and performed with a most vehement Affection, one part of the soul by it self, or one part after another is not moved, but the whole *Hypostasis*, together, and on a sudden, and is inclined or snatched towards the Genitals; hence every most light incentives of Lust, are most swiftly powred forth thorow the universal parts of the Soul, fiery of themselves, and Extreamly perclive or apt for such fires. *From whence is this Wonderful Commerce of the Brain, with the Genital Members.*

Whilst this Corporeal Soul, being inkindled like flame, in the animated Body, on every side diffuseth Heat and Light, we may take notice of its various tremblings, shakeings, inequalities, and irregular Commotions; these sorts of Irregularities, to be observed, concerning the *phasis* or appearance of this Soul, of which we treat, tho they are more perspicuous in Man than in Brute Animals, yet they altogether respect the inferiour Soul of Man, which is Common to him with the Brute Animals. But that we may briefly handle some of these Affections of the Corporeal Soul, first it is to be noted, that its flame does not always flame forth equally: For besides that its food is sometimes afforded more plentifully, and too sulphureous, sometimes more thinly and less inflameable, so that the Flame is inlarged or Contracted, its accension also, in the præcordia, tho of it self moderate and equal, is wont to be variously shaken, by the fanning of Passions, so that it is carried forth sometimes into an Excessive burning, as from Anger and Indignation; sometimes this vital flame is in danger to be always blown out, as by sudden Joy, and another time almost suffocated, as by sudden fear or sadness; In like manner the *Systasis* or Constitution of the Soul, from the rest of the Affections, being exposed as flame to the winds, is diversly changed in its appearance, as will more clearly appear, when we shall speak particularly of its Affections. *The Soul, like Flame, has in equalities Trendations &c.*

The Flame of the Soul is sometimes enlarged by passions.

Nor do these sorts of Inordinations only proceed from the sudden impulses of Passions, but sometimes, the Vital flame, habitually becomes decayed, weak, and as it is were half exstinct, as by intemperate Cold, and also as is observed in the phlegmatick disease, the dropsie, longing of maids, and other diseases; in whom the Blood being too watery, like moist and green wood, sends forth but a small and inconstant flame and almost overwhelm'd with fume and vapour: But sometimes the bloody Liquor being more sulphureous than it ought, is almost wholy inkindled, as happens in a Choleric Complexion, and in an intemperate Feavor: According to either of these hights, as the inkindling of the vital flame is altered, so the lucid particles, which flow from it, to wit the beamie texture of the Animal spirits, diversly shines, and breaths forths from the decayed or bound up inkindling of the Blood, the sphear of the sensitive soul is seen to be straitned, and to be drawn in, within the limit of the Body, and to be immerged or sunk down so that it doth not sufficiently actuate or illustrate the whole frame of the Brain, and its Appendix: On the Contrary, when the Vital Fire is very strong (so it doth not burn forth too much and feavourishly) the Constitution of the Animal Spirits being made greater in it self, is much inlarged forth far beyond the Compass of the Body, so that any one exulting for Joy, or blown up with pride, is seen to grow very great, and not be able to be contained within its proper Dimension. *Sometimes Contracted.*

The same habitually is now decayed.

Now intense or strong.

Also the lucid part of the Soul shines diversly.

And is altered on the part of the Fame.

Besides these Kind of Alterations, which the Soul properly sensitive, or the lucid part, receives, from the Vital and flamie, variously changed; many other things happen, which disturb its *Systasis* or Constitution, and its wonted manner of Order, immediately both from a certain affection of the Brain, and Nervous stock, and also from external Objects because in the night, the Brain it self, from a too great infusion of the nutricious Juce, or from the black darkness, or vapours, is filled, so that the lucid part of the Soul in sleep, is wholly obscured, as it were with darkness; not seldom from a morbific matter somewhere gathered together, and as it were obstructing the Spirits, or the ways of their Beams, there arises an Eclipse of some or more of their faculties; sometimes the Animal Spirits themselves are not light or airey enough, but are infected with heterogeneous effluvia's, to wit, either Saline, Vitriolic, Nitrous, or otherwise Cloudy, which deform the sensible species, change them into some affrightful thing, and excite inordinate Motions: Hence it comes sometimes that the whole Soul suffers various Metamorphoses or Changes, and puts on strange species's, as often happens in Melancholy diseases, or to mad men. *Also from the various affection of the Brain and Nervous stock.*

As to the various gestures of the Soul, by which for the variety of sensible objects it expresses now Joy and Pleasure, by and by loathing and trouble, it is observed, that sometimes it is allured more outwardly by the Organ of this or that sense, and as occasion serves almost wholly to wander into the Eye or Ear, Palate or any Sensory meeting with *Also from the various incursions of sensible things.*

some-

something pleasant ; sometimes on the Contrary, for the fake shunning or flying away from some approaching evil, that she retires inwardly, and leaving her watch, hides her head ; so that we think or Imagine nothing without being touch'd , but that the whole Soul almost is moved , and trembles at every apprehension of the sensible object, and its *Systasis* is variously agitated, as it were the leaves of a Tree, exposed to the blasts of Winds.

Alterations of the Flamy part of the Soul impressed by the Lucid.

Nor do these sensible Impressions induce Metamorphoses only to the sensitive soul, or the beamy Texture of the Animal spirits ; but undulations or waverings being brought to it, presently they go forward; and impress alterations on the vital Soul, lying in the blood, and move about its flame, as it were with blasts, driving it hither and thither, and unequally inkindling it. For as we mentioned before, the same moment, in which an object carried from the sense or memory, stops at the Imagination, as that Comes under the shew of good or evil, it affects the Animal Spirits destinated to the Motion of the Precordia, and causes the Precordia, by the influx of them, to be variously Contracted or dilated, and for that Cause it is , that the inordinate motions, and inkindling of the Blood , are so performed. But of these there will be a more opportune place of treating, when we shall speak especially of the Affections of the Soul.

CHAP. VI.

Of the Science or Knowledge of Brutes.

WE have hitherto spoken of the Original Nature and manner of the Soul of the Brutes, subsisting in the Body, as also of its various degrees or species, and as it hath in the more perfect Living Creatures Parts or Constitutive Members. Further, the *Hypostasis* figure, and dimensions of the same Soul , being rightly delineated, we have Considered, how that she is capable of Impressions from outward Objects, also to what passions and alterations besides she is obnoxious : yet from all this furniture of the Corporeal Soul, and of its powers being put together, it doth not plainly appear, what the same is able to do beyond the Virtue or force of any other machine, and to perform by its own proper Virtue or strength. For altho an Impression of an Object driving the Animal spirits inwards, and harmonizing them by a certain peculiar manner, causes sensation ; and the same spirits, for as much as they leap back from within outwardly , as it were by a reflected undulation or waving, stir up local motions ; yet it is not declared how this Soul, or any part of it, perceives it self to feel, and is driven according to that perception into divers Passions and Actions , directed to the Appetite or desire of this or that Action ; and sometimes, as we have generally observed in some Beasts, for the prosecution of the desired thing doth pick out and choose Acts, which seem to flow from Council, or a certain Deliberation. In Man indeed it is obvious to be understood, that the Rational Soul, as it were presiding, beholds the Images and Impressions represented by the sensitive Soul, as in a looking Glass, and according to the Conceptions and notions drawn from thence, exercises the Acts of Reason, Judgment, and Will. Yet after what manner in Brutes, Perception, a discerning or discrimination of Objects, Appetite, Memory, and other species or Kinds of Inferiour Reasons as one may say, are performed, seems very hard to be unfolded ; therefore, when some could not solve this Knot or difficulty, they attributed to Brutes Immaterial Souls, and subsisting after their Bodies. Which if that were true I Know not, why Four footed Beasts should not be indued with reasoning and understanding as well as man, yea and might learn Sciences and Arts ; for as much as in either, besides their immaterial souls alike, there is altogether the same Conformation of the Animal Organs ; upon which indeed it appears, that the Rational Soul whilst in the Body, hangs or depends as to its acts and habits, because the Organs being hurt, or hindred, a privation or an Eclipse of these succeeds : wherefore that the Soul of the Brute using the same Organs as man , can Know nothing clearly, nor rise above the Acts and material Objects , it planly follows , that she is different from the Rational Soul and also that she is much inferiour and Material.

But that it is objected, that all matter whatsoever is not only insensible and sluggish, but also meerly passive, therefore incapable of sense and animal activity, omitting here many instances of æquivocal productions, the *Epicureans* affirm to be equally

The Soul of the Brute is strong in sense and motion as a Machine.

But wonderful how by perception.

If the Soul of the Brutes be immaterial, it is also rational.

equally stupendious and inexplicable, of which we shall discourse anon; we shall propose as to the former, this one thing, as very Consentaneous to our *Hypothesis*; to wit, that there is not much more difference between an insensible and a sensible Body, than between a thing uninkindled, and a thing kindled; and yet we ordinarily see, this to be made from that; why therefore in like manner, may we not judge a sensible thing, or Body to be made out of an insensible? Every matter, as it is not Burnt, so not animated; but being disposed, by either of the active Elements, it behoveth it to be indued with Spirit chiefly, with Sulphur and Salt: Combustible things, as Oyl, Rosin, Wood, and the like, of themselves torpid and sluggish, lye unmoved without fire, heat, or some agitation of the parts or particles: But as soon as they have taken flame, from some incentive being put to it, by and by their Particles being rapidly moved, and as it were animated, produce a shining with Heat and Light; and not only make light all about them, but Create innumerable Images, of all things that are seated near them, and thickly object them on every side: In like manner, the Vital humour in an Egg, remains torpid and sluggish in the beginning, and like to unkindled matter; but as soon as it is actuated, from the Soul being raised up, presently like an inkindled fire, it excites Life with Motion and Sense, and in the more perfect Creatures with heat. Further, the Animal Spirits as Rays of Light, proceeding from this Fire, are Configured according to the Impressions of every of their Objects, and what is more, as it were meeting together with reflected irradiations, cause divers manner of motions. *A sensible thing or Body, is produced from an insensible, as an inkindled Body from one not kindled.*

Then what is vulgarly delivered, that Matter, out of which Natural things are made, is meerly passive, and cannot be moved, unless it be moved by another thing, is not true; but rather on the contrary, Atoms, which are the matter of sublunary things, are so very active and self-moving, that they never stay long, but ordinarily stray out of one subject into another; or being shut up in the same, they cut forth for themselves Pores and Passages, into which they are Expatiated. *That matter is not meerly passive.*

Yet it may be argued, That if the Soul of the Brute be Composed out of these, whilst the same is Extended and is Corporeal, it cannot perceive. For it admits the Species of the Object into its whole self, or into some part of it self, not the first, because then neither the Senses would be distinguished one from another, nor any of them by a perception or common sensation of these: But if (as indeed it is) it shall be said, that all the sensible Species being received by appropriated Sensories, to a certain part of the Soul, to wit, the first or common Sensory, where they are perceived: Then it may be again objected, That so manifold and divers Species or Images of sensible things, which at once are Conceived, from Objects, cannot be painted forth in a certain small part of the Brain, but that some should obliterate or blot out, or at least Confound others: I say none ought to wonder, who hath beheld the Objects of the whole Hemisphere, admitted thorow an hole into a dark Chamber, and there on a sudden upon Paper exactly drawn forth, as if done by the Pencil of an Artist: Why then, may not also the Spirits, even as the Rays of light, frame by a swift Configuration, the Images or Forms of things, and exhibit them without any Confusion or Obscuring of the Species? *But sometimes too active. The common Sensorie is not the whole Soul, but a certain part of it. This receives all species without Confusion.*

But yet, tho it be granted, That the Images of sensible things are represented in a certain part of the Soul, to wit, actuating the Brain it self; to which there happens a most speedy Communication, with the whole, and also with the several Parts: however, we are yet to inquire of what Kind of power that is, which sees and knows such like Images there delineated, and also according to those Impressions there received, chooseth Appetites, and the respective Acts of the other Faculties. *How this perceives that het self feels or knows.*

That we may go on to Philosophize concerning this matter, I profess indeed, whilst I consider the Soul and the Body, to wit, either of them by it self and distinct, I cannot readily detect, in this, or in that, or in any material subject, any thing, to which may be attributed such a Power, with a self-moving energy: But indeed, when I consider the animated Body, made by an Excellent and truly Divine Workmanship, for certain Ends and Uses, nothing hinders me from saying, That it is so framed by the Law of Creation, or by the Institution of the most Great God, that from the Soul and Body mixed together, the same Kind of Confluence of the Faculties doth result, by which it is needful for every Animal, to the Ends and Uses destinated to it.

In most Mechanical things, or those made by humane Art, the Workmanship Excels the matter: who would think there could be an Instrument made out of Iron or Brass, being most fixed and sluggish Mettals, whose Orbs like to those of the Celestial, without any external Mover, should observe almost continual motions, the Periods of which being renewed at a constant turn or change, should certainly shew the spaces of Time? No Body admires that a rude and simple sound is given by wind, blown into a Pipe; but indeed, by Wind sent into musical Organs, and that being carryed variously thorow manifold openings of Doors, into these or those pipes, that it should create a most grateful *As in mechanical things, so much more in an animated body the work is more excellent then the matter.*

F

ful Harmony, and Compoſed Meaſures of every Kind; this I ſay deſervedly amazes us, and we acknowledg this Effect, far to Excel both the matter of the Inſtrument, and of the hand of the Muſitian ſtriking it. Further, altho the Muſical Organ very much requires the labour of him playing on it, by whoſe direction, the ſpirit or wind being admitted, now into theſe, anon into thoſe, and into other Pipes, cauſes the manifold harmony, and almoſt infinite Varieties of Tunes; yet ſometimes I have ſeen ſuch an Inſtrument ſo prepared, that without any Muſitian directing, the little doors being ſhut up, by a certain law and order, by the mere Courſe of a Water, almoſt the ſame harmony is made, and the ſame tunes, equal with thoſe Compoſed by Art. And indeed Man, ſeems like to the former, in which the rational Soul, ſuſtains the part of the Muſitian playing on it, which governing and directing the animal ſpirits, diſpoſes and orders at its pleaſure, the Faculties of the Inferior Soul: But the Soul of the Brute, being ſcarce moderatrix of its ſelf, or of its Faculties, Inſtitutes, for Ends neceſſary for it ſelf, many ſeries of Actions, but thoſe (as it were tunes of harmony produced by a water Organ, of another Kind) regularly preſcribed by a certain Rule or Law, and almoſt always determinated to the ſame thing.

A ſelf moving muſical Organ.

To which the ſoul of the Brute is like.

This indeed holds good, concerning the more imperfect Brutes, in whoſe Souls or Natures are inſcribed the types or ways of the Actions to be performed by them, which they rarely or never tranſgreſs or go beyond; and that according to the vulgar ſaying in the Schools, *They do not ſo much act, as are acted*: yet in ſome more perfect Brutes, whoſe Actions are ordained to many and more noble Uſes, there are far more Original Types, and to their Souls there ought to be attributed a certain faculty of Varying their Types, and of Compoſing them in themſelves; for the Brutal Soul it ſelf, being ſo gifted naturally, as ſhe is Knowing and Active, concerning ſome things neceſſary for it; ſhe is taught through Various Accidents, by which ſhe is wont to be daily affected, to know afterwards other things, and to perform many other, and more intricate Actions: But how all this may be done, (without calling an immaterial Soul into play) to wit, by what helps, whether innate or adventitious, or acquired, the Science of the Brutes is gotten or polliſh'd, will be worth our Labour to ſhew a little more fully: that it may appear at length, what is the utmoſt thing that living Brutes can know or do, and how far that is below the power of the Rational Soul.

The more perfect Brutes are indued with knowledge.

Therefore, that we may ſeek out as it were the ſeveral footſteps, by which all brute Animals are imbued with the Knowledg of things; we ought firſt to diſtinguiſh here, that ſome of their Knowledg is born with them, as we but now hinted, to wit, for ſome Uſes needful for the lengthning of Life, being infuſed by the moſt high Creator, and impreſſed like a Character, from their firſt formation, on the beginning, or on their very Natures themſelves, which is wont commonly to be called *Natural Inſtinct*: But others acquired, to wit, which by degrees is learned, by the incurſion of ſenſible things, Imitation, humane Inſtitution, and other ways, and is carryed to a greater degree of Perfection in ſome than in others; yet in ſome, this acquired Knowledg, as alſo Cuning, depend wholly on the natural Inſtinct, and being poliſhed by frequent uſe and habit, and Carried a little further, ſeem to be certain additions only.

That is either inbred.

Or acquired.

Firſt, As to what regards natural Inſtincts, it is a great and moſt ancient Notion, That there is in all Living Creatures, an innate Conſervation of themſelves, to wit, that every Individual might preſerve it ſelf as long as it can: This is a Law of Divine Providence, inbred in all Creatures, which gathers together the Principles of Life like a Bond, otherways apt to be diſſipated and to depart one from another, and on which, as the Baſis, the Duration or Continuance of the whole World ſtands.

What natural inſtinct is.

This being ſuppoſed, it neceſſarily follows, that all Animals ordained for this end, are furniſhed alſo with certain fit means, for following the ſame, wherefore they ought to know by Natural Inſtinct, whatſoever things are Congruous and benign, and what are incongruous or hurtful to them, and that they ſhould follow theſe with hatred and averſion; and thoſe with Love and delight. Hence it is, that every one of them are able to chooſe Food proper for themſelves, and to ſeek it being abſent, and remote from their Eyes; And from an implanted diſpoſition of their Nature, are skilful to know and oppoſe Enemies, to love their Friends, to get a female fit for themſelves, and to make ready whatever may conduce to the Procreating and Cheriſhing their Young; beſides many other Kinds of powers and habits, granted to us not without Learning and Study, are originally fixed on the *Præcordia* of the Beaſt.

What it brings to the Brutes.

And truly, if we look upon the Ingenuity and Proprieties of all Animals, we ſhall find theſe Kind of Effects after a manner in all: For many of them are no ſooner brought to light, but they ſeek and greedily embrace remedies againſt hunger and Cold, without any guide or ſhower; then being ſomewhat grown up, tho Carefully Kept from all their Companions, yet without any one to ſhew them, or any example, they

Some examples and inſtances of it.

they of their own accord perform the peculiar Actions of their Kind. A Lamb just brought forth, and scarcely out of the after-birth, presently snatches at and sucks the Duggs of its Dam. A Chicken, as soon as out of the shell, will pick up grains of Corn, hides it self under the wings of the Hen, and flyes from the approach of the Kite. Cattel feeding in the Pastures, are more Skilful than Men, about the Virtues of Herbs; for they easily discern at the first tast, what are for food, what for Medicine, yea, what is to be shun'd, being imbued with poyson and death; when we in the mean time, unless taught by experience, are wholy ignorant of their Virtues or poysonous force: so that Pliny Complained, that it was a shame, that all Animals Knew what was healthful for themselves, besides Man. *Natural Instinct dictates to Brutes, what is wholesome and what unwholesome.*

Neither does what some object otherways determine this matter, that the means of these Kind of effects, depend only upon the similitude or the dissimilitude of Patricles, which are in the sensible and the Sensory, without any intention of the Beasts, or End of their Acting; because we have observed, that Brute living Creatures, by the Virtue of natural Instinct, perform not only simple actions, stirred up by one Impression of the External agent, as when the heat of the Sun invites to take the Cool of that shade, but they perform and do manifold works, and Continued by a long Series. Birds by reason of the Influence of the Spring, being instigated to the begetting others apply themselves to that business, without any other provoker or director, as it were Consultingly and premeditated; for they enter into wedlock, as it were by a solemn manner of Espousals, they choose a fit place for the building their nest or habitation, where they make it most artificially beyond the skill of humane Architecture; then they lay Eggs, and by sitting on them bring forth young ones, and then carefully nourish them with food which they get for them. We might here also take notice of the most admirable Republiques of Bees and Ants, in which, without any written Laws or promulged Right, the most perfect ways of Government are exercised. But as in all these without any Variety, one thing is always and wholy after the same manner administred, it is a sign, that these Kind of principles or beginnings of the Brutes, are not stirred up either by external objects, whose Impulse is still various and divers, nor from an internal proposition of the Mind, which is more mutable than the wind; But excited from a more fixed and Certain principle, determinate always to one thing, which can be only Natural Instincts: The World is full of Examples of this sort, which testifie the native indowments and implanted Ingeny of Brutes: For in all Animals, there are by Nature a Certain Ingeny and habit born with them, by which they are instigated through a secret impulse and blind power to the performing of Actions, which respect both the Conservation of themselves, and the propagation of their Kind; and these Gifts being originally granted, constitute as it were the first lineaments or groundwork of practical Knowledge, with which the Soul of Brutes are wont to be imbued: then an acquired Cognition being superadded to those rudiments, fills up the vacuities of those things drawn forth, and adds a perfection to the former foundation. *Leads not only to simple Actions but also to very Complicate Actions.*

But yet those always, and in all, of one Kind only.

For Secondly, besides the natural Instincts, living Brutes are wont to be taught by sensible species, to wit, to profit in the Knowledge of several things, and to acquire certain habits of practice: But this happens not equally to all nor at all times. For in many Animals newly brought forth, natural Instinct is of some force, but then the Impressions of sensible things little or nothing affect the sensitive soul: Because, altho the flamy part of the Soul is enough inkindled in the Brain, yet because the Brain and its Appendix, abounds with much humidity, therefore the Spirituous Effluvias, or the lucid part of the Soul which ought to irradiate these Bodies, is very much obscured, as the beam of the Sun passing thorow a thick Cloud: Wherefore at this time, the strokes of sensible things, being not deeply fixed, are presently obliterated, and in them local motions hardly follow: yea in some Beasts, in whom the Blood being continually and habitually thick, and who have a less Clear Brain, tho through their whole Life some acts of the Exterior Senses and Motions are performed, yet few Characters are left, of any interiour Knowledg. Wherefore, we shall here inquire only concerning Brutes, that are more docil, to wit, in whom are besides local motions, and the five Exterior Senses, Memory, and Imagination; and in these we may conceive this kind of Introduction, or Method of Institution, concerning the Exquisite Knowledge, by the sense with which they are wont to be imbued. *2. Brutes, in some things, are taught by the Impressions of sensible things.*

Therefore, as soon as the Brain in the more pefect Brutes grows Clear, and the Constitution of the Animal Spirits becomes sufficiently lucid and defecated, the exterior Objects being brought to the Organs of the Senses, make Impressions, which being from thence transmitted, for the continuing the Series or Order of the Animal Spirits inwards, towards the streaked Bodies, affect the Common Sensory; and when as a sensible Impulse of the same, like a waving of Waters, is carried further into the Callous Body, *The direct sensible Species creates in them the Phantasie and the Memory.*

and thence into the *Cortex* or shelly substance of the Brain, a Perception is brought in, concerning the Species of the thing admitted, by the Sense, to which presently succeeds the Imagination, and marks or prints of its Type being left, constitutes the Memory; But in the mean time, whilst the sensible Impression being brought to the common Sensory, effects there the Perception of the thing felt; as some direct Species of it, tending further creates the Imagination and Memory; so other reflected Species of the same Object, as they appear either Congruous or Incongruous, produce the Appetite, and local motions its Executors; that is, the Animal Spirits looking inwards, for the Act of Sension, being struck back, leap towards the streaked Bodies; and when as these Spirits presently possessing the Beginnings of the Nerves, irritate others, they make a desire of flying from the thing felt, and a motion of this or that member or part, to be stirred up: Then, because this Kind, or that Kind of Motion succeeds once or twice, to this or to that Sension, afterwards, for the most part, this Motion follows that Sension as the Effect follows the Cause: and according to this manner, by the admitting the Idea's of sensible things, both the Knowledg of several things, and the habits of things to be done, or of local Motions, are by little and little produced: For indeed, from the beginning, almost every Motion of the animated Body is stirred up by the Contact of the outward Object; to wit, the Animal Spirits residing within the Organ, are driven inward, being strucken by the Object, and so (as we have said) constitute Sension or Feeling; then, like as a Flood sliding along the Banks of the shore, is at last beaten back, so, because this waving or inward turning down of the Animal Spirits, being partly reflected from the Common Sensory, is at last directed outwards, and is partly stretched forth even into the inmost part of the Brain, presently local Motion succeeds the Sension; and at the same time, a Character being affixed on the Brain, by the sense of the thing perceived, it impresses there, Marks or *Vestigia* of the same, for the Phantasie and the Memory then affected, and afterwards to be affected; but afterwards, when as the Prints or Marks of very many Acts of this Kind of Sensation and Imagination, as so many Tracts or Ways, are ingraven in the Brain, the Animal Spirits, oftentimes of their own accord, without any other forewarning, and without the presence of an Exterior Object, being stirred up into Motion, for as much, as the Fall into the footsteps before made, represent the Image of the former thing; with which, when the Appetite is affected, it desiring the thing objected to the Imagination, causes spontaneous Actions, and as it were drawn forth from an inward Principle. As for Examples sake, The Stomach of an Horse, feeding in a barren Ground or fallow Land, being incited by hunger, stirs up and variously agitates the Animal Spirits flowing within the Brain; the Spirits being thus moved by accident, because they run into the footsteps formerly made, they call to mind the former more plentiful Pasture fed on by the Horse, and the Meadows at a great distance, then the Imagination of this desirable thing, (which then is cast before it, by no outward Sense, but only from the Memory,) stops at the Appetite: that is, the Spirits implanted in the streaked Bodies, are affected by that Motion of the spirits flowing within the middle part or Marrow of the Brain; who from thence presently after their former accustomed manner, enter the origines of the Nerves, and actuating the Nervous System after their wonted manner by the same Series, produce local Motions, by which the hungry Horse is carried from place to place, till he has found out the Imagined Pasture, and indeed enjoyes that good the Image of which was painted in his Brain.

After this manner, the sensible Species being intromitted, by the benefit of the Exterior Organs, in the more perfect Brutes, for that they affix their Characters on the Brain, and there leave them, they constitute the Faculties of Phantasie and Memory, as it were Store-houses full of Notions; further, stirring up the Appetite into local Motions, agreeable to the Sensions frequently, they produce an habit of Acting; so that some Beasts being Taught or Instructed for a long time, by the assiduous Incursion of the Objects, are able to know and remember many things, and further learn manifold works; to wit, to perform them by a Complicated and Continued series and succession of very many Actions. Moreover, this Kind of acquired Knowledg of the Brutes, and the Practical habits introduced through the Acts of the Senses, are wont to be promoted by some other means, to a greater degree of perfection.

For in the third place, it happens to these by often Experience that the Beasts are not only made more certain of simple things, but it teaches them to form certain Propositions, and from thence to draw certain Conclusions. Because, draught Beasts, having sometimes found water to be Cooling, they seek it far as a remedy of too much heat; wherefore, when their Precordia grow hot, running to the River they drink of it, and if they are hot in their whole Body they fearlesly lye down in the same. In truth, many Actions which appear admirable in Brutes

came

came to them at first by some accident, which being often repeated by Experience, pass into Habits, which seem to shew very much of Cunning and Sagacity; because, the sensitive soul is easily accustomed to every Institution or Performance, and its Actions begun by Chance, and often repeated, pass into a Manner and Custom. So it happens sometimes by Chance, among Hounds, that one had caught the prey, not exactly but by following a Shorter way; this Dog afterwards, as if he were much more Cunning than the rest, leaves the Hare making her turnings and windings, and runs directly to meet her another way.

Living Brutes are taught by Example, by the Imitation and Institution of others of the same or of a divers Kind, to perform certain more excellent Actions. Hence it is that the Ape so plainly imitates Man, that by some, it is thought a more imperfect Species of him. For this Animal being extreamly mimical, as it is indued with a most Capacious and hot Brain, it imitates to an hair, almost all the Gestures that it happens to see, presently with a ready and expeditious Composing of its Members, and is furnished with a notable Memory, and retains all its tricks which it has once acted very firmly afterwards, and is wont to repeat them at its pleasure. They are very admirable habits, which Horses, Doggs, and Birds get, being carefully instructed by the Discipline of Man; and not only from Men but being taught first by their Companions, they imbibe altogether new and more Excellent Customs: so one Dog ordinarily teaches another to hunt, and one Bird another to compose harmonious notes and various tunes. It were an Easy matter to bring very many Instances of this Kind. But we shall hasten to other things. *4. By Example, Imitation, and Institution also*

Having thus enumerated the Chief Helps from Nature and Art, by which living Brutes do profit in the Knowledg of things, and are instructed by the Habits of Acting, we shall now inquire, to what hight most of them or all of them put together, can arrive. *How far it is that Brutes are able to Know.*

First, from what we have said 'tis clear, that Living Brutes are directed to all things which belong to the Defence and Conservation of the Individuum, and that are to be done for the propagation of their Kind, by a natural Instinct, as it were a Law or Rule fixed in their Hearts: when as therefore we behold for these ends, ordained by Divine Providence, Brutes to order their matters wisely, and as it were by Council, no man Esteems this the work of Reason, or of any liberal faculty; yea they are led into these enterprises, by a certain Prædestination, rather than by any proper Virtue or Intention.

Secondly, The Natural Instinct of Brutes, happens, not rarely, with notions acquired by the sense, and being Complicated with them conduces to the Propositions or Assumptions to be done, Concerning many things, and the Deductions to be drawn from thence. A Dog being by a staff struck, or by the flinging of a stone, perceives the hurt received by the senses, and easily retains the Idea in his Memory, but the Instinct dictates to him that the like stroke may be shunned afterwards, wherefore, when he sees a staff held out before his eyes, or a stone taken up, fearing thence the like hurt, he hastily flies away. *How natural Instinct is wont to be Compacted with acquired Notions. With the Impressions of sensible things.*

Thirdly, sometimes Instincts, and also all other acquired Knowledges, are mixed together, either with the Example of Habits, or with the general Institution of things learnt: And when as notions so arising from one faculty or power, answer to Actions drawn from another, from thence is produced a certain Kind of Discourse or Ratiocination, and often times it is continued by a certain Series or Thrid of Argumentation. Many admirable Histories are reporte concerning the Subtilties and Craft of the Fox, which he is wont to perform for the getting of his living. This Creature, that he might allure the Hens within the Compass of his Chain, with which he was tyed, lying all along, his legs stretched forth, feigns as if he were dead, then they coming near him, he readily leaps upon them. Moreover, I have heard it told, that a wild Fox, that he might get into his clutches a Turkie Cock roosting in a Tree, running round the Body of the Tree, with a swift Motion, continually beheld the Bird with an intentive Eye, by which Means, as the Turkie still followed the Fox thus running Round with his eye, carrying his head about till being infected with a giddiness, he fell down from the top of the Tree, into the mouth of his Enemy: I say, it was natural to the Fox, that he should desire domestick Fowl, as his prey; but that he should frame these Kind of Snares for them, this he must have by former acquired Knowledges, from Sence, Experience, and Imitation, and complicated with natural Instinct. It is very likely that the Fox had learnt by former Experience, that the Hens did not fear him lying as dead, which might happen by Chance, when being wearied, or to sleep, he had lay'd himself on the ground: In like manner, perhaps, when he had run about the Tree, seeking some way to get up into it, the Prey might fall down into his mouth; Wherefore afterwards when he would take his prey, he repeated the Series of the same Actions; because, what he *With Habits learnt from Example or Institution. With notions learnt from Experience and Imitation.*

he had known to be done before, he presumed might be done again. In both Cases, and in others like them, the reason of the whole thing done, or the Endeavour, is resolved into these Propositions; The Fox thinking, now to take the Prey, that is before his eyes, after what manner he may, remembers how he had taken the same formerly, by these or those sort of Cunning ways or Crafts, found out by some chance; These are the Premises, the former of which is suggested from Nature, and the second from Sense and Experience, from whence a Conclusion follows, Therefore Foxes for the taking of their Prey, use again the same Wiles. According to this sort of *Analyzing*, the most Intricate Actions of Brutes, which seem to contain Ratiocination, may be explained, and reduced into Competent notions of the sensitive Soul.

The Syllogisms of Beasts.

CHAP. VII.

The Corporeal Soul, or that of the Brutes, is Compared with the Rational Soul.

FRom what we have said is to be understood, how much it is that Brute Animals are wont to do with the whole furniture of the Corporeal Soul, and to obtain towards the use of Reason: But now we shall endeavour to shew, how far they are below it, and how much less they are able to do than Man, endued with a Rational Soul. The means of observing the difference between these Souls are commonly to be had, being noted by divers Authors both Ancient and Modern and both Philosophers and Theologists, till it is almost worn thread-bare, yet we will take leave to shew you only some few select things, which for Methods sake, we shall reduce to these three Heads: viz. 1st. It is shown, That man using expeditiously and freely the Powers of the Superiour Soul, of the Intellect, Judgment, Discourse, and other Acts of Reason, shews them far excelling any Faculty or Science of the Brute, and the whole power of the Corporeal Soul. 2. By what Knitting the Corporeal Soul, and the Rational are joyned together, in the Humane Body, by what means they agree in the same habitation; also what offices they perform each. 3. Shall be declared, for what means, and for what occasions these Souls differ among themselves, yea sometimes are wont to dissent and move more than Civil Wars.

Three heads of this Discourse viz 1. *It is shown that the Rational Soul far excels the Brutal.*

2. *How both Souls are joyned in Man, and*

3. *How they frequently disagree among themselves.*

The eminency of the Rational Soul above the Brutal or Corporeal, shines clearly by comparing either, both as to the Objects, and to the chief Acts or Modes of Knowing. As to the former, when as every Corporeal Faculty is limited to sensible things, and every one of these to certain Kinds of things, the object of the humane Mind is every Ens, whether it be above, or sublunary, or below the Moon, Material or Immaterial, true or fictitious, real or Intentional; wherefore *Aristotle*, who seemed to hesitate something about the Nature of the Rational Soul, hinting its acting Intellect as if it were Immaterial and Immortal, doth pronounce it not only separable and without Passion, but also unmixt because it understands all things. *Lib. de Animâ* 3. *Cap.* 4.

The Priority of the Rational Soul as to

1. *The Objects which are Every Ens.*

Secondly, The Acts or degrees of Knowledg, Common to either Soul, are Vulgarly accounted these three. To wit, simple Apprehension, Enunciation, and Discourse; how much the Power of the Rational, excells the other Corporeal in each, we shall consider:

2. *The Acts of Knowing.*
The first Act of either Soul is simple Apprehension.

First, The Knowing Faculty of the Corporeal Soul is Phantasie or Imagination, which being planted in the middle part of the Brain, receives the Sensible Species, first only impressed on the Organs of sense, and from thence by a most quick Irradiation of the spirits delivered inwards, and so apprehends all the several corporeal things, according to their Exterior Appearances; which notwithstanding, as they are perceived only by the sense (which is often deceived) they are admitted under an appearing, and not always under a true Image or Species. For so we Imagine the Sun no bigger than a Bushel, the Horizon of the Heaven and the Sea to meet, and then the Stars not to be far distant from us in the Horizon, and that in respect of us, there are no Antipodes; further we may think the Image in the Glass, or in a Fountain delineates it self, that the Eccho it self is a Voyce coming from some other place, that the shore moves being on the water, yea and many other things, being received by the Sensories, whilst Phantasie is the only guide seem far otherways than indeed they are: But indeed, the Intellect presiding or'e the Imagination, beholds all the Species deposited in it self, discerns and corrects

The power of this in Brutes is Phantasie or Imagination-
Which is often deceived.

In man it is the Intellect presiding or'e the Imagination.

corrects their obliquities or hypocrisies the Phantasie there drawn forth sublimes, and divesting it from matter formes universal things from singulars; moreover, it frames out of these some other more sublime Thoughts, not Competent for the Corporeal Soul: so it speculates or Considers both the nature of every substance, and abstracted from the Individuals of Accident, viz: Humanity, Ratiotinality, Temperance, Fortitude, Corporeity, Spirituallity, Whiteness, and the like; besides, being carried higher, it Contemplates God, Angels, It self, Infinity, Eternity, and many other notions, far remote from Sense and Imagination. And so as our Intellect, in these kind of Metaphysical Conceptions, makes things almost wholly naked of matter, or carrying it still beyond every sensible Species, consider or beholds them wholly immaterial, this argues certainly, that the Substance or Nature of the Rational Soul is Immaterial and Immortal: Because, if this Aptness or Disposition were Corporeal, as it can conceive nothing Incorporeal by Sence, it should suspect there were no such thing in the World. *Which discerns the errors of this.*

Sublimates its notions, & divests them from Matter.

Contemplates immaterial Substances.

Secondly, It appears clearly, from what was said before, that Phantasie, or the Knowing facultie of the Corporeal Soul, doth not only apprehend simple things, but also Compose or Divide many things at once, and from thence to make enuntiations: Because living Brutes, in various objects together, which are for food, discern things Convenient from others Inconvenient or unfit; moreover, they choose out of these, things grateful before others less grateful, and get them sometimes by Force, sometimes by Cunning, and as it were by stealth. A Dog knows a Man at a great distance; if he be a Friend, he runs to him and fawns on him; If an Enemy and fearful, he barks at him or flies at him, but if armed or threatning him, he flyes away from him. These kind of Propositions the Brutes easily conceive, for as much as some Species of the sensible thing being newly admitted, meets with Species of one thing or other before laid up in the memory, or being suggested by a Natural Instinct, associates with them or repulses them. But indeed, how little is this, in respect of the humane Intellect? which not only beholds all enunciations conceived by the phantasie, but judges them, whether they be true or false, Congruous or Incongruous; orders and disposes them into Series of Notions, accommodated to speculation or practise: Moreover, it restrains the phantasie it self, being too instable and apt to wander through various phantasies; it calls it away from these or those Conceptions, and directs it to others, yea it keeps it within certain limits at its pleasure, lest it Should expatiate or divert too much from the thing proposed: Which out of doubt is a sign that there is a Superior Soul in Man, that moderates and governs all the faculties and Acts of the Corporeal. But the Intellect, not only eminently Contains every Virtue of the phantasie; but from the Species perceived in it, deduces many other thoughts altogether unknown to the sense, and which the Phantasie in it self could no way Imagine. For Besides, that it conceives the formal notions of Corporeal things, abstracted from all matter, and attributes to them prædicates meerly Intentional yea and understands axioms or first principles alone, and as it were by a proper Instinct, without recourse to Corporeal Species; the humane mind also beholds it self, by a reflected Action, it supposes it self to think, and thence Knowing a proper existency, not to be perceived neither by Sense nor by Phantasie; when in the mean time, neither Sense nor Imagination (of which no Images are extant) do perceive it self to know or imagine: Besides these, the Rational Soul comprehends, as it were by its own proper light, God to be Infinite and Eternal, that he ought to be Worshipped, that Angels or Spirits do inhabit the World, Heaven, and places beneath the Earth, that there are places of Beatitude, and Punishment, and many other notions meerly Spiritual, by no means to be learnt from Sense or Phantasie.

The Second Act of either Soul is Enunciation.

What and how slender this is in Brutes.

The rational judges, discerns, and directs the propositions of the Phantasie.

It deduces from these others more sublime thoughts.

It beholds it self by a reflected Action.

And Contemplates other things remote from sense, as God &c.

3. The perogatives of the Rational Soul, and the differences from the other Sensitive or Corporeal, may be yet further noted, by Comparing the Acts of Judgment and Discourse, or Ratiocination, which it puts forth more perfectly, and often time demonstratively, when these Kind of Acts, from this power in the Brutes, are drawn forth imperfectly, and only analogically, we have already declared the utmost that Brutes can do, and how far they can go towards the exercise of Reasoning and Deliberation, through innate faculties, and acquired habits; which truly, if the whole be compared with the functions of the humane Intellect, and its Scientifick Habits, it will hardly seem greater than the drop of a Bucket, to the Sea. For to say nothing of that natural Logick, by which any one endoued with a free and perspicacious mind, probably and sometimes most certainly concludes, Concerning all doubtfull things, or things sought after, if that we mind how much the humane mind being adorned by Learning, and having learnt the Sciences and liberal Arts, is able to work, understand, and search out: it would be thought, tho in an Humane Body, to be rather living with Gods or Angels. For indeed here may be Considered, the whole *Encyclopædia* or Circle of Arts and Sciences, which

The Ratiocination of the Brute, what and how vile.

The humane Mind immensly more excellent.

Is imbued with a natural Logick.

(excepting

Of the Science of Brutes.

It hath Created all Arts & Sciences (except Theologie)

excepting Divinity) hath been the Product or Creature of the Humane Mind, and indeed argues the Workman if not divine, at least to be a particle of Divine Breath, to wit, a Spiritual Substance, wonderfully Intelligent, Immaterial, and which therefore for the future is Immortal. It would be tedious here to rehearse the Subtil Wiles of Logick,

Logick.
Physick.
Metaphysicks.

and the extremely curious web of Notions, or of the Reason of Essences, or Beings, where the things of Natural Philosophy being unfolded by their Causes, are dissected as it were to the Life; the most pleasant Speculations, the profound Theorems or rather Celestial, of the *Metaphysicks* or supernatural things; yea and the grand Mysteries of other learning first found out by humane Industry. But above the rest, is it not truly ama-

Mathematicks.

zing to see the most certain Demonstrations of the Mathematicks, and therefore a-Kin and greatly alluding to the Humane Mind, its Problems and Riddles how difficult soever to be extricated, with no labour, yea and many things of it attained, and most glorious

Algebra.

Inventions. What is it below a Prodigy, that *Algebra* from one Number or Dimension, which at first was uncertain and unknown, being placed, should find out the quantity of another altogether unknown? What shall I say concerning the Proportions of a Circle, a Triangle, a Quadrangle, and other Figures, and of their Sides or Angles variously measurable among themselves, being most exactly computed? what besides, that the Humane Intellect having learnt the Precepts of *Geometrie* and *Astronomie*, takes the

Admirable things of Geometry and Astronomy.

spaces of inaccessible places, and their heights, the floor or breadth of any superficies, and the contents of solids, yea the dimensions of the whole Earthly Globe: measures exactly the spaces of hours and days, the times of the year, the Tropicks, by the progress only of a shadow? yea it measures the Orbs, Magnitudes, and Distances of the Sun and Starrs, for a long time to come, Calculates, and exactly Foretells, their risings and settings, motions, declinations, and Aspects one to another; we should want time, should we go about to enumerate the several portentous things, either of the practice or specula-

The humane Mind does wonders in mechanical Things.

tion in the Mathematicks. Then, if passing over to Mechanical things, We shall consider the several Works and Inventions of Workmen, and the artificial Smiths-Works wonderfully made, there will be no place for doubting, but that the humane Soul, which can so famously understand, invent, and find out, and effect, I had almost said, Create things so stupendious, must needs be far above the Brutal, Immaterial and Immortal; especially because Living Brutes obtain only a few and more simple Notions and Intentions of Acting, yea and those always of the same Kind, and not determinated but to one Thing, altogether ignorant of the Causes of things, and know not Rights or Laws of political Society: further, they make no Fires or Houses, nor find out any mechanical Arts, they put not on cloaths, nor dress their food, yea unless taught by Imita-

In respect of Man, how little is it that the Soul of a Brute Can do?

tion, they know not how to number Three. When therefore we have plainly detected in Man, besides the Corporeal Soul, such as is Common with Brutes, the prints of another superiour, meerly spiritual, we shall next seek out by what bond, and by what necessitude, these twins are conjoyned, and intimately come together, in the same Body.

Some of those, who have shew'd the difference, between the Souls of the Brute and of Man, affirming the Irrational or Corporeal peculiar to them, would have the Rational Soul of Man, to perform not only the Offices of the Intellect and Discourse, but also the other Offices of Sense and Life, yea to do and administer the whole Oeconomy of Nature:

That there are two distinct Souls in Man besides many other of latter Time there are for Authors

To which opinion (however it may have prevailed in our Schools) the opinions of most learned men of every Age has been clearly opposite. That I may not be tedious, in rehearsing of many, I shall cite only two Authors (but either of which is worth a Multitude) in the Confutation of this Assertion. One is, that famous Philosopher, *Peter Gassendus*, who *Physic. Sect. 3. lib. 9. Cap. 11.* differencing the Mind of Man, as much as he could,

Gassendus

from that other Sensitive Power of his, by many and very remarkable notes of discrimination, yea (as 'tis said in the Schools) by Specifick Differences, he has (as they say) divided the whole Heaven between: Because when he had shewed this to be Corporeal, Extensive, and also Nascible or that may be born, and Corruptible, he saith that the other was an Incorporeal Substance, and therefore Immortal, which is Created mediately by God, and infused into the Body; which opinion he shews *Pythagoras*, *Plato*, *Aristotle*, and many ancient Philosophers, besides *Epicurus*, very much to have favoured; excepting however, that they, for as much as they not knowing the beginning of the Soul they judged Immortal, affirmed it, taken from the Soul of the world, to slide into the humane Body, and it to be refunded again either immediately into that Soul of the World, or mediately at length, after a Transmigration thorow other Bodies. The other suffrage concerning this matter is, of the most Learned Divine, our *Dr Hammond*, who unfolding that Text of St

And Hammond.

Paul to the *Thessalonians*, 1 chap. 5. v. 23. *The whole Body Soul and Spirit*: says, that man is divided into three parts, to wit, First into the body, which is the Flesh and Members:

Secondly

Secondly, Into an Animal Life, which also being Animal and Sensitive, is common to Man with the Brutes; And Thirdly, into Spirit, by which is signified the rational Soul, at first Created by God, which being also Immortal, returns to God, *Lib. Annot.* on the New Testament, *p.* 711. He Confirms this his Exposition, by Testimonies taken from Ethnick Authors, also from the Fathers. And truly it is most evidently plain, from what hath been said, That Man is made, as it were an Amphibious Animal, or of a middle Nature and Order, between Angels and Brutes, and doth Communicate with both, with these by the Corporeal Soul, from the Vital Blood, and heap of Animal Spirits, and with those by an intelligent, immaterial, and immortal Soul. And indeed, Reason persuades us plainly that 'tis so, to wit, for as much as we find in our selves, as by and by shall be more fully shown, the Strifes and Dissentions of one Soul with another, sometimes this, and sometimes that getting the Rule, or being in Subjection. But as it is said, That the Rational Soul doth exercise of it self all the Animal Faculties, is most improbable; because the Acts and Passions of all the Senses, and Animal Motions are Corporeal, being divided and extended to various Parts; to the performing which immediately, the incorporeal and indivisible Soul seems unable, so that it would be finite. Then as to what respects that Vulgar Opinion, that *the Sensitive Soul is subordinate to the Rational, and is as it were swallow'd up of it*, as that which in Brutes is the Soul, is mere Power in Man; these are trifles of the Schools. For how should the Sensitive Soul of Man, which subsisting at first in Act, was material and extended, foregoing its Essence at the coming of the Rational Soul, degenerate into a mere Quality? if that it should be asserted, That the Rational Soul by its coming, doth introduce also Life and Sensation, then Man doth not generate an animated Man, but only an inform Body, or a rude lump of Flesh.

This also Reason dictates.

The Rational Soul does not exercise the Animal Faculties.

Obliterates not the Sensitive Soul by its Coming. Nor transmutes it into a mere Power.

Therefore, supposing that the Rational Soul, doth come to the Body first animated by another Corporeal Soul, we shall inquire, by what Bond or Knitting, since it is pure Spirit, it can be united to it, for as much as it hath not Parts, by which it might be gathered to, or cohere with this whole, or any of its Parts. Concerning this, I think we may say, with the most Learned *Gassendus*, That the *Corporeal Soul is the immediate Subject of the Rational Soul, of which, as she is the Act, Perfection, Complement, and Form by her self, the Rational Soul also effects the Form, and Acts of the humane Body.* But for as much, as it seems not equal nor necessary, that the whole Corporeal Soul, should be employed by the whole Rational; therefore we may affirm, this purely Spiritual, to sit as in its Throne, in the principal Part or Faculty of it, to wit, in the Imagination, made out of an handful of Animal Spirits, most highly subtil, and seated in the Middle or Marrowie part of the Brain: Because, when as the Species, or every sensible Impression, of which we are any ways Knowing, being inflicted any where on the Humane Body, is carried to the Imagination or Phantasie, and there all the Appetites or Spontaneous Conceptions, or Intentions of things to be done, are excited, the Intellect or Humane Mind, presiding in this Imperial seat, easily performs the Government of the whole Man. For (as *Gassendus* properly has it) *As there is no necessity for a King, to be in his whole Kingdom, but only in his Palace, to which place, are carried whatever happens in the Kingdom; so the Phantasie is the Kingly Palace of the Intellect, to which may be brought whatsoever are acted Spontaneously and to our Knowledge, in the whole Body.* But as to what has relation to the Functions merely Natural, which being done by a constant manner of Oeconomy, as it were by a Law from the Creator, are performed unknown to the Animal, it were not fit, that the Imagination, much less the Intellect, should attend on these lower Offices: altho also, the faults of these, as often as they are amiss, lying hid to the Imagination, the Intellect most often finds them out, and procures them to be amended. As to the Mode of the Intellect, by which the Phantasms of all sensible Things being drawn in the Imagination, is beheld, it may be said, That this is done not by percussion from the Corporeal Species, (for this is repugnant to the Corporeal Faculty) but by an Intuition into it self, expressed in the Phantasie. But as the Rational Soul, will stay and preside in the Court of the Phantasie, there is no need that she should be shut out from thence, or bound by any Bond; because destinated to this by the most high Creator, to wit, that it should be *the informing Form of Man*; and also her self is very much inclined, to the Inhabiting this House; because, whil'st in the Body, it depends very much, as to its Operation, on the Phantasie, without the help of which, it can know or understand nothing. For it draws its first Species and fundamental Idæa's, by which it rears all its manner of Knowledge, from the Imagination; wherefore, that the Mind of one Man understands more, and reasoneth better, than that of another, it does not thence follow, that Rational Souls are inequal, but every disparity, concerning the Intellect, proceeds immediately from the Phantasie, but mediately and principally from the Brain, being variously disposed. For as this being affected, by an Intemperate

By what Bond the Rational Soul is united to the Body.

That the Corporeal Soul is the Subject of the Rational. Gass. Physic. Sect. 3. Memb. Post l. 9. c. 11.

Gassend. Ibid.

The Seat or Palace of the Humane Mind, is in the Phantasie.

The manner by which the Phantasms are beheld by the Intellect, viz. Intuition, not Percussion.

The Rational Soul is inclined to the Body.

The Intellect depends upon the Phantasie.

G

By reason of the various Constitution of this, and the Brain, Souls seem unequal.

Intemperate or Evil Conformation, the Spirits being made more dull, or hindred, cannot irradiate and actuate in their due manner; therefore the Phantasms are difficient or distorted, and the Faults or Vices of these infects the Intellect. Hence it very often happens, by reason of some hurt coming to the Brain, that the Faculties or Habits, or Ratiocination or Reasoning, howsoever strong, are diminished or taken away: Because, as the most Skilful *Gassendus* tell us, That *the acquisition and loss of an habit, stands in the Power of the Brain and Phantasie, a subject purely Corporeal; but that the Intellect, as it wants Parts, cannot be wrought upon by Parts, but that it is from the beginning, and of its own Nature, a full and perfect power of understanding; which understands, not more by the coming of any Habit, but is rather it self an Habit, always ready to understand:* where-

How the Habits of Reasoning are acquired and performed.

fore he says, that Aristotle has hit the mark, when he says, *that his Agent having its Intellect, as it were a Light, had it therefore as it were a certain Habit: to wit, when this Intellect, as it were a Light, is ever ready to illustrate; therefore it would have it self like to an Habit, in a Workman or Artist, to whom, when you give an Organ or Instrument, as an Harp to an Harper, he is presently ready to Play;* by which it comes to pass, as he says, the Intellect also to come under such a Reason, like *as Art comes under Reason, as to Matter:* So we may say, *As an Harper has in himself the Skill of Playing on the Harp, and if he shews not his Art, there is a defect, not of himself, but by reason of the absence or*

Gassendus, Ib.

the depraved disposition of the Harp; after the same manner, the Intellect is aboundantly instructed, in its own Nature, that it understands, and uses Phantasies, and if it may not do it, the cause is not in it self, but is either in the absence of the Phantasms, or their Imperfection. For indeed, as the same Author afterwards adds, *The chief Function of the Humane Intellect seems to be like that of the Angels, that it is of its own Nature, merely Intelligent, that is, Knowing things by a simple Sight, not by Ratiocination; But that darkness is poured on it dwelling in the Body, that it doth not perceive all that it understands, simply, nakedly, and as it were through the means of Intuition; but attains it very much by reasoning, that is, successively, and proceeding as it were by degrees.*

From these we may probably Conclude, or at least Conjecture, after what manner the Rational Soul remains in the other Corporeal, and using as it were its Eyes, and other Powers, understands; yea, and this mediating or coming between, she is said to be united to the Body, and to be its informing Form. As to the first yoaking of the one Soul with the other, thô the Rational Soul it self, and this, is altogether ignorant of its Birth, we

That the Rational Soul is Created and poured into the formed Body.

may affirm notwithstanding, what is Consonant to Holy Faith, right Reason, and to the Authority of Divines, who were of the chiefest note; That this immaterial Soul, for as much as it cannot be born, as soon as all things are rightly disposed for its Reception, in the Humane formation of the Child in the Womb, it is Created immediately of God, and poured into it.

Not propagated Ex traduce.

But least some have said, That the Rational Soul is propagated *Ex traduce* or of its Kind, for as much as oftentimes the Son, in respect of Wit, Temperament, Ingenuity, the Affections, and other Animal Faculties, is exactly like the Father, it follows not; because these Gifts and Offices proceed immediately from the Corporeal Soul, which we grant to be begotten by the Father, together with the Body, but not the Rational Soul. In what State this at last exists, being freed from the Body, and what Kind of Understanding and Knowledge it enjoys, is not easie to be determined; but

Separate States.

since we shall be like the Angels, we may think, that the separated Soul doth see all Objects with a Simple sight, and by no Corporeal Species, and wants no Ratiocination, for the discovering any thing lying hid in them. But this Speculation being let alone, as too airy, we shall further Consider, other Gestures and Manners of the Rational Soul, whilst it lives in the Body; and as hitherto we have seen the Marrying together of it, with the Corporeal Soul, and the mutual Commerces and Friendships as to the Knowing Faculties of either, we will now consider the Disputes and Wranglings of

A Plurality of Souls in Man, is manifest by their differences.

these, which in respect of their Powers, often happen: because the Intellect and Imagination, do not agree in so many things; but that it, and the Sensitive appetite, are wont to disagree in more: from which Strifes may further be argued, the distinct means of the aforesaid Souls, both as to their subsisting and working.

3. As there is said to be in Man a twofold Knowing Power, *viz.* The Intellect and the

In Man a twofold Knowing Power, and a twofold appetite.

Imagination, so it is commonly affirmed, that there is a twofold Appetite, *viz.* The Will, which proceeding from the Intellect, is the Handmaid of the Rational Soul; and the Sensitive Appetite, which cleaving to the Imagination, is the Hand or Procuress of the Corporeal Soul. Which Opinion, thô it be founded on the Sayings of the Ancient Philosophers; for that by *Plato* and *Aristotle*, The *Will is attributed to the Rational Part, and to the Irrational Lust and Wrath;* yet it ought not to be so taken, as if the Rational Soul, for that it is immaterial, and therefore esteemed without Affection, should be obnoxious to the Affections of desires or aversations, from every shaking approach of Good or

Evil,

Evil, of that being turbulent; for this indeed is repugnant to its incorporeal Nature, and to its Dignity and Prerogative above other Powers. Without doubt, in the Contemplation of Truth and Goodness, and especially of that which is the sum of either, in the doing of good Works, in the Knowledge of things by their Causes, and in the Exercises of Habits, both Scientifick and Practical, great Complacency happens to this; and on the contrary a certain displeasure for the want of these. Moreover, the Love of God, of Virtue, and of all that is good, and the detestation of Vices, and of wicked Men; yea, and other pure Affections, and such as are Simple, coming without perturbation or trouble, belong to the Rational Soul: In the mean time, *That she* (according to *Plato*) *like the top of* Olympus, *might enjoy a perpetual Serenity, hath the whole heap of Perturbations below it self, and in the irrational part, placed like Clouds, Winds, and Thunder, in an inferior Region, and under its feet.* And truly, all the vehement Affections or Perturbations of the Mind, by which it is wont to be moved, and inclined hither and thither, for the Prosecuting the Good, or shunning Evil, belong wholly to the Corporeal Soul, and are seen to obtain the same seat with the Phantasie, within the middle or marrowy part of the Brain: (by what means the Passions also affect the *Præcordia* by consent, shall be declared afterwards) in the mean time, the Intellect, even as it beholds all the Phantasms, and Orders and Rules them at its pleasure; so it not only perceives, but whil'st it is its self, governs and moderates, all Concupiscences, and Floods of Passions, that are wont to be moved also within the Phantasie; and so, as it approves these Affections, and rejects those, now excites others, now quiets them, or directs them to their right ends, the Rational Soul it self is said to exercise certain Acts of the Will or Power, by these kind of Dictates of hers, and that she her self wills or wills not, the same thing, which by her Permission or Command, the Sensitive Appetite desires or hates.

The Rational Soul of it self without Affections; how it governs and orders the Phantasie and Affections.

But the Corporeal Soul does not so easily obey the Rational in all things, not so in things to be desired, as in things to be known: for indeed, she being nearer to the Body, and so bearing a more intimate Kindness or Affinity towards the Flesh, is tied wholly to look to its Profit and Conservation: to the Sedulous Care of which Office, it is very much allured, by various Complacences, exhibited through the Objects of every Sense: Hence she being busied about the Care of the Body, and apt by that pretext, its natural Inclination, and indulging Pleasures, most often grows deaf to Reason, perswading the contrary. Further, the lower Soul, growing weary of the yoak of the Other, if occasion serves, frees it self from its Bonds, affecting a License or Dominion; and then there may plainly be seen the Twinns striving in the same Womb, or rather a Man clearly distracted or drawn several ways, by a double Army planted within himself; to wit,

In things to be Known, the Corporeal Soul obeys the Rational, but not in things to be done.

The Corporeal Soul inclining her self to the Flesh,

——*Where Ensigns Ensigns meet,*
And where with Arms, they one another threat;

Fights against the Rational.

This Kind of Intestine Strife, does not truly cease, till this or that Champion becoming Superior, leads the other away clearly Captive. Altho in the mean time, to the Establishing the Empire of the Rational Soul, also for the Vindicating of its Right and Principality, from the Usurpation of the Sensitive Soul, the Precepts of Philosophers, and Moral Institutes are framed; and when these can do little, Sacred Religion gives far more potent helps, whose Laws and Precepts being rightly observed, are able to carry Man, not only beyond the Brutes, but himself, to wit, above his Natural State; for as much as they subject the Sensitive Soul to the Rational, and both to the most high God. But yet, such a Divine Politie is not erected in Man, without great Contention: Because, whil'st Reason using its proper force, and also Institutes and Sacred Ethicks, endeavours to draw the Faculties of the Corporeal Soul to its Party, she rising against it, adheres pertinaciously to the Flesh, and is hardly pull'd away from its Blandishments; yea, what is to be lamented, it seduces in us the Mind or Chief Soul, and snatches it away with it self, to role in the Mud of Sensual Pleasures: So that Man becomes like the Beast, or rather worse; to wit, for as much as Reason becoming Brutal, leads to all manner of Excess. But indeed, 'tis not always so with the Empire of the Mind, but that she returning at length, sometimes on her own accord, or awakened by some occasion, and knowing of its fall, arises up against the Sensitive Soul, as against an Enemy or Traiter, casting her out of her Throne, commands her to Servitude; yea, sometimes by reason of some wickedness committed, it compels it to torment it self, and its Lover the Flesh, and so to expiate as much as it may, its faults, by inflicting on it proper Punishments. Indeed, these kind of Acts and Affections of Conscience, near to Man, plainly shews, that there is in him either two Souls subordinately, or at least the Parts of the same are far different; to wit, when one of which opposes the other, and either strives for the obtaining of Proselytes, it happens that Man is hurried into contrary Endeavours, and is acted little less than like a Demoniack possess'd with a Legion. But

How it is reduced to Obedience.

It often seduces the Mind.

Wars are moved between them.

Affections of Conscience nigh to Man.

having

having proposed these things, concerning the Rational Soul, (which we have touch'd only by the by, as besides our purpose) we will return to the Corporeal, and as we have illustrated its Essence, Hypostasis, and Integral Parts, we shall now descend to the Explaining of its Affections, or Passions.

But in the mean time, as we have shewn, by comparing the Corporeal Soul of the Brute, with the Rational of Man, what vast difference there is between them, perhaps it might be to the purpose, to compare the Brains of either, and to observe their differences. But this Anatomy being elsewhere made, we have noted little or no difference, in the Head of either, as to the Figures and Exterior Conformations of the Parts, the Bulk only excepted; that from hence we concluded, the Soul Common to Man with the Brutes, to be only Corporeal, and immediately to use these Organs. But as we have shewn the description of a Sheeps Brain, dissected within the *Cortex*, and as it were made bare of Flesh, whereby all the Interior Parts might appear, we shall here also, to Crown the work, give you the Figure of an Humane Brain; so as all the inward Parts may be laid open.

The Eighth Table,

Contains a new Anatomy of the Humane Brain, where, by a Dissection with an Instrument made thorow the Bill, the Callous Body, and the Fornix or Arch, and their Parts being taken away and separated; the streaked Bodies, also the Optic and Orbicular Prominences, one side erased, and the other whole and plain, are Exhibited.

A. A. A. A. *The Hemisphear of the Brain divided and separated by themselves.*
B. B. B. B. *Portions of the Callous Body with the Fornix cut off, and removed apart.*
C. *The Basis of the Fornix, with its Roots, which cohered with its Trunk* Y Y; *divided Portions of which, with Cuttings off of the Callous Body, are laid apart on the right and left hand.*
D. *One streaked Body scraped or Erased, that the Medullary streakes or nervous Tracts may appear.*
E. *The formost border of this Body, sticking to the right Hemisphear of the Callous Body.*
F. G. *The Basis and the Cone, of the same Body.*
H. *The hinder Border of the same, in which the Optick streaks, yea and other Medullary Processes, are sent from the Orbicular Prominences.*
I. *The streaked Body of the left-side plain, with the Vessels creeping thorow them; whose Borders and Ends are made after the same as in the right.*
K. *The right Optick Chamber erased, whose Medullary streaks, being strait and thick set,* K.K. *are stretch'd forth, into the Border of the streaked Body.*
L. *The right Nati-form Prominence in like manner erased, with streaks stretched forth into the Medullary Process* M.
M. *The Medullary Process, which proceeding from the Testes, and compassing about the Nates, sends from thence other Medullary passages into the streaked Body, as more plainly appears in the left side being whole.*
N. *The Pineal Kirnel in its proper place.*
O. O. *The Orbicular Prominences called Testes, Marrowy thorow the whole.*
P. *The left Nati-form Prominence plain and whole, which is smaller in Man, and for the most part Marrowy.*
Q. *A Medullary Process, Compassing the Nates, from which is sent one Medullary Pipe or passage* R. *towards the Cone of the streaked Body, and another* S. *towards its Basis; of which by and by a forked branch goes forth, one* r. *to the middle of the streaked Body, the other* s. *to the corner of its Basis.*
T. *A Transvers shoot knitting together the aforesaid Branches.*
V. *The hinder Borders of the streaked Bodies, joyned together among themselves.*
W. *The Gap or Chink leading to the Tunell.*
X. *The Gap or Chink, leading into the Cavity, lying under the Orbicular Prominences.*
Y. *A Medullary Process, leading from the Oblong Marrow, into the Cerebel, which seems to be the root of this.*
Z. Z. *Separated Portions of the Cerebel cut off, that its Tracts both Marrowy, and Cortical or Barkie, may be seen.*
X. *The Cavity or hollowness lying under the Cerebel.*

CHAP.

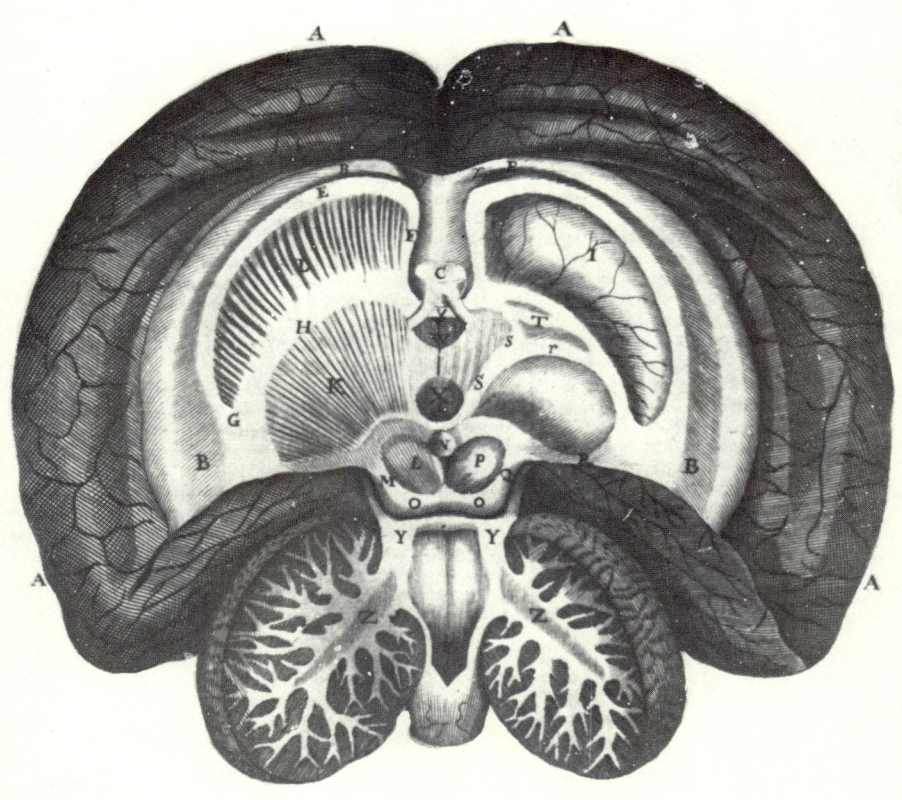

CHAP. VIII.

Of the Passions or Affections of the Corporeal Soul in General.

THe whole Corporeal Soul, so long as she is quiet and undisturbed, she is fittted to her *A Twofold state* proper Body equally, as to a certain Chest or Cabbinet, and waters all its Parts *of the Corporeal* gently, both with little Rivulets of Blood Circulating, and actuates and inspires them *Soul:* every where with a gentle falling down of the Animal Spirits; But it sometimes happens, *Tranquil or* that the whole Constitution of this same Soul, is so shaken and moved, that both the *Quiet,* Blood being interrupted in its equal Circule, is compelled into irregular Excursions, and *And Disturbed.* Recursions, and various Fluctuations; and also, that the Animal Spirits being snatched hither and thither, inordinately perform the Acts of their Functions: yea, the Animal *In which either* Spirits themselves, whil'st being moved irregularly, do shake the *Præcordia*, and flow *part of the Soul* into them in an undue manner, cause the Course of the Blood more to be perverted. Fur- *is moved.* ther, from the Corporeal Soul being disturbed, not only the Animal Spirits, and Rivers of the Blood, are driven into disorders, but they induce alterations both to the other Humors, and to very many Parts and Members of the Body, and to the Rational Soul it self, in Man. As there are manifold Examples of these kind of Perturbations, by which, the Corporeal Soul being too much swell'd up, or Contracted, or otherways distoited, it becomes as it were unequal, and not Conformable to the Body, the Chief of them may be referred to these two Heads. To wit, First, Sometimes this Soul, as it were *And is either too* leaping forth, erects and stretches out it self beyond measure, and so dilating its *Hypo-* *much inlarged,* *stasis*, desires to reach it self beyond the bound of the Body: Hence the Animal Spirits, being respectively moved, in the Brain, enlarge the Sphear of their Irradiation, and as they so shake the *Præcordia*, by a more full inflowing, they Compel the Blood therefore to be snatched together, and to be poured forth more freely into all the Parts. Se- *Or Contracted.* condly, Sometimes on the contrary, this Soul being struck, is more narrowly Compressed within it self; so that being drawn inwardly, and sinking down within its wonted Compass of Emanation, becomes less than the Body; wherefore, the Animal Faculties wonderfully flagg, and their Acts are either sluggishly or perversly performed: Moreover, the *Præcordia* also being destitute of their due influx of Spirits, almost sink down, and suffer the Blood to stay too long there, and to stagnate oftentimes. There are besides some other Gestures of the aforesaid Soul, by which the same departing from its equal Expansion, becomes not Congruous to the Body; and in these kind of Cases, chiefly the Sensitive Power, according to the received Impressions, affects a new Species, and brings the Brain and Imagination into its Party: Then by and by, by the passage of the Nerves, *The Trouble of* it affects the *Præcordia*, as it were with a certain stroke, and determinates them after her *the Soul, im-* measure; so that according to the Idea received from the Imagination, the Motion of *pressed on the* the Blood is Composed, as it were after the measures of a Dance: we shall add *Sensitive Part,* anon Instances and Examples of these, when we shall treat of the Passions parti- *by and by is* cularly. *Communicated* *to the Blood.*

In the mean time, that we may inquire into the Causes of the Passions in general, it plainly appears from what hath been said, that the Corporeal Soul is found under a twofold state, to wit, either of Quiet or Commotion: That she is like a Calm Sea, with a smooth Superficies, and squared altogether gentle and serene; or she becomes troubled, like water shaken into various Circles, and wavings by the blasts of the Winds, or by some solid things cast into it. The former state of the Soul is perceived, not only in Sleep, when the Spirits are bound up, or lye quiet of themselves; but often in Waking, *The quiet of the* to wit, as often as objects or sensible things, being brought from without, or imaginary *Soul happens not* things conceived within, do import nothing of Good or Evil to us, and that we only *only in sleep, but* know and apprehend them: for so, without any Trouble or Molestation, they pleasantly *often waking,* slide into the common Sensory and Imagination, and thence quickly pass away; but if *when pleasing or* the object is offer'd under the Species of Good or Evil, presently the Sensitive Soul pre- *unhurtful things* pares for the embracing or the avoiding it; and not only procures to its Endeavors the *are met with.* Animal Spirits, but also the Blood and Humors; yea, draws the solid Parts to help *On the Contrary* her. For as soon as the Imagination conceives any thing that is to be embraced or shunned, *when from the* presently the Appetite is formed by the Spirits inhabiting the Brain, ordered into a Se- *Objects, Good or* ries; then by an impression sent to the *Præcordia*, as they are either dilated or contracted, *Evil is promi-* the Blood is carried into various Motions of Fluctuations, and then by an instinct of the *sed;* Appetite transmitted to the proper Nerves, the respective Motions are drawn forth: *Then first the* And upon these kind of Furnitures and Affection of the Spirits and Humors, and of the *Imagination af-* *terwards the* *Appetite is mo-* *ved,*

solid

Of the Affections of the Corporeal Soul in General.

solid Parts, the Affections or Passions of the Mind wholly depend, we have elsewhere shewed, after what manner, and by what Trajection or Irradiation of the Spirits, within the Nervous Processes, such quick Commerces are made, between the Brain and the *Præcordia*, and between both these and other Motive Parts.

The Reason of Good and of Evil, either concerns,
The Corporeal Soul by it self. Or her united to the Body, Or her subjected to the Rational Soul.
Hence Passions are called either Physical, Metaphysical, or Corporeal.

But that we may yet more fully describe the Affections or Passions of the Corporeal Soul, as they are chiefly to be found in Man, it is here to be noted, That not every Species or Appearance of Good or Evil, does excite these Commotions of the Soul : because we behold undisturbed the prosperous or adverse things of others, not related to us : But further, 'tis requisite that the Goodness or the Malice of the Object belongs properly to a Man, altho what happens to our Friends or Relations, is as if it happened to our selves. Also besides, Good and Evil happen to the same Man after various ways, and under a diverse reason, both in respect of the Object, and also in respect of the Subject. Concerning the former we shall speak anon : As to the other, Good or Evil being brought to Man, either respect the Corporeal Soul by it self, and as it were abstracted from any other Relation ; or they respect her as conjoyned to the Body, and intimately dear to her : Or lastly, they respect her, as subdued by the Rational Soul ; so indeed, altho the Affection is continually poured into the Corporeal Soul, yet it respects Good or Evil, either of this, or that, or of another Subject, and is excited for the sake of that : And according to this threefold Relation of the Sensitive Soul, the Passions by which she is affected, are called either Physical, or Metaphysical, or Corporeal or Moral ; we shall discourse singly, and a little more plainly of these.

Passions merely Physical, are Sympathies and Antipathies.

First, Therefore, as to the Passions merely Physical, we say, That the *Sympathies* and *Antipathies* of a diverse Kind, which are as it were proper and intimate Affections, seem to belong to the Corporeal Soul by it self, and abstracted from all Relation : Besides, the highly attractive Species of Beauty and Fairness, by the sight of which this Soul is wont to be insnared, most certainly ; so that neglecting the Care of the Body, and laying aside the dictates of Reason, cleaves most closely to her Lover : Also sometimes less fair things which every whole Man would forsake, snatches this Soul, drawn as it were by Witchcraft, and leads it Captive ; as indeed, lost Lovers, though they see better things and approve them, yet follow the worse ; the reason of which is, that the Sensitive Soul enters into Friendships, of which the Affections are not knowing, with certain things in Secret, and inseparably and firmly loves them. Concerning *Antipathies* we meet with many things to be admired, as some sensible Objects, innocent of themselves, yea and grateful enough to many Men, and sought with delight, become most horrid to some o-

Some Instances of Passions merely Physical.

thers, and more Killing than the Head of *Medusa* at the sight only : So some abhor the presence of a Cat, others an Eel, or Toad, and others this or that Dish of meat made ready. Nor do they only fly things by the sight, but also received by the smell, yea, when they lye hid, and are not at all suspected, they suffer Swoonings and Fainting of their Spirits, by their secret Influence : These Kind of Affections without doubt, proceed from occult Enmities of the Sensitive Soul ; for when it happens this *Systasis* or Disposition of the Animal Spirits, by the meeting of some Object, to be driven into Confusion, it ever after that abhors the coming of the same, or its Contact by its Effluvia's.

Passions Metaphysical.

Secondly, Sometimes the Sensitive Soul receives the Superior Rational Passions, which we call *Metaphysical* ; and solicitously busying it self concerning their Good and Evil, it either draws forth or shortens the Compass of its Expansion. For indeed, the Rational Soul relying on the help and familiarity of the Spirits dwelling in the Brain, aspires to Metaphysical Notions, which having more fully learnt, it not only falls upon higher Speculations, but also exerts a certain Superior Appetite, to wit, the Will, and implicates it with certain Affections, as it were inspired of God ; the exercise of which sort of Sacred Affections are not performed by the mere Conceptions of the Mind : But their Acts being delivered from the Rational Soul into the Sensitive, do first employ the Brain with the Phantasie, then being transmitted from the Brain into the Breast, there, for that they produce in the Heart and Blood variety of Motions, receive their Complement or Perfection : Wherefore, in the Worship of God, Piety and Devotion are attributed very much to the Heart : Hence Repentance, the Love of God, and Hate of Sin, Hope of Salvation, Fear of Divine Vengeance, and many other acts of Religion, are wont to be ascribed to the work and endeavour of the Heart. The reason of which seems to be, for as much as the whole Corporeal Soul is Commanded by the Rational Power, that in Adoring God, she should very much bow her self before the Deity, and as it were lye prostrate on the Ground ; therefore, presently both Parts of it, *viz.* both the Sensitive and Flamy, do repress themselves, and restrain their wonted Emanations ; hence plenty of Animal Spirits being drawn from the Phantasie, for the more full actuating the Organs of the Senses, they bestow the Operations of the Nerves on the *Præcordia*,

By these first the Rational Soul.

Then the Sensitive and Sanguineous part of the other are affected.

which

Of the Affections of the Corporeal Soul in General. 47

which whil'st they are more straitly drawn together, and as it were constrain'd, cause the Blood to stay longer within the bosomes of the Heart; and so inhibit it, lest it should be too much inkindled within the Lungs, and left being inkindled by the Heart, in the whole Body, and chiefly should be carried rapidly into the Brain. For indeed, the Blood containing Life as a most precious Jewel in it self, is not only heaped up more plentifully about the *Præcordia*, in all Fear and Danger, and is there lay'd up as it were for defence sake, that it might better preserve its Flame: But further, in devout Affections, whil'st the Rational Soul orders the Spirits inhabiting the Brain into sacred Conceptions and Notions; by the Influence of the same Spirits, the Bosomes of the Heart are also so affected, that they cause the Blood to Centre, and to be more fully drawn into them, and there longer retain it, as it were an *Holocaust* to be offered to God: so as often as we Pray most earnestly, we endeavour nothing less, than that our Life with the Blood, be laid upon the Altar of the Heart. For truely, almost every body experiences in himself that in strong Prayer, the Blood is more and more heaped up in the Bosomes of the swelling Heart: wherefore, that the Vacuities of the Lungs might be supplied, we breath deeply, and so the Air being more fully drawn in, the Muscles of the Breast, and the *Diaphragma*, are detained almost in a continual *Systole*, or more often iterated; to wit, for this end, that the Vital Blood, to be offered as it were a Sacrifice to God, should be there kept, nor suffer'd to go from thence, or to be inlarged, till as it were by a long immolation, together with Prayers, lieve may be had from the Godhead. Yea, 'tis to be observed, that those religiously affected, are apt at all times to call back the Blood towards the *Præcordia*, and to repress it from a more plentiful Excursion, which may give a loose to Delights or Mirth: Because 'tis just, that this Vital Humor should be Conserved, even Holy and Pure for God; and as it is so restrained in the *Præcordia*, lest it should grow too luxurious, nor be carried towards the Brain with too impetuous a Rapture, the Conceptions also of the Mind, without much heat and distraction of thoughts concerning Divine things: Hence it is, that Drinking of Wine, Banquetting, and every Kind of Dissolute Life, because they render the Blood lawless, and not able to be restrain'd or bridl'd, are said to make hard the Heart, and to obstruct the Duties of Religion. Further, not only the devout Acts of Religion, and Pious Affections, are attributed to the Breast and *Præcordia*; but also the sober Counsels of Wise men, yea, and the Exercises of Virtues and Moral Habits, are ordinarily ascribed by Philosophers to this Seat or Subject: Hence Wise men are said to be *Cordati*, Hearty, or sage of Heart; but when one that is unwise or plainly foolish, doth a thing, it is said, That there is nothing leaps in the left part of his Breast: The reason of which seems to be, that when as the Animal Spirits (which are the immediate Instruments of thoughts) are procreated altogether from the Blood, not only their more excellent disposition, but their right and timely Dispensation, depends chiefly on the *Præcordia*. For to these are owing, that the Blood be inkindled in its due manner, and also Eventilated, that it may give to the Brain firm and stable Animal Spirits, which however Subtil and Active, yet may not be volatile beyond measure; and hence the Solidity of the Mind, and the sharpness of Judgment are produced: When on the contrary, by reason of the Blood more slowly passing thorow the *Præcordia*, or more swiftly than it should do, the Animal Spirits become too fixed, or volatile above measure, and therefore either a stupidity or lightness of Mind arises. But in truth, Wisdom is much rather ascribed to the Heart, for as much as from thence reins are put upon the Blood, apt for fiercenesses and Impetuosities, lest that rushing into the Brain, with an inordinate rapture, should not only disturb its serious Cogitations, but stir up enormous Motions of the Appetite, and mad Lusts. For truely, whil'st the Spirits inhabiting the Brain, are disposed by the Intellect, from thence presiding within the Imagination, into Series and Orders of Notions, the Blood about to break forth from the Heart, ought very much to be restrained, lest that growing luxurious, it should confound all things by an importune evasion of the Brain, and should agitate the Spirits, called away from this work into Commotions, and various Fluctuations; wherefore, from the immoderate drinking of Wine, for as much as by it the Blood is made more head-strong, and will not be repressed or contained by the Heart, Men become not only unable for Exercising the Acts of Judgment and Reason, but are found very prone to all manner of Wickedness and most filthy Desires.

Wherefore, and how the Præcordia are esteemed the seat of Holy Affections.

What it is to have the Heart hardened.

Wherefore the Præcordia are called also the seat of Prudence and Wisdom.

As to the Moral Passions, or by us called Corporeal, we may observe, that the Sensitive Soul is more often and easilyer affected, by reason of Good or Evil, which is of its Subject, that is of its Body, which includes its good Habit. Altho also, she hath her proper and occult Loves and Aversations, and is bound to shew due obsequiousness to the Rational Soul; for as much as it is united to the Body, as it were by a Conjugal Compact; therefore, all other relations being lay'd aside, it minds only this; Concerning the Care of it 'tis mostly solicitous, and by reason of its prosperous or adverse Affairs,

Three Corporeal or Moral Passions.

Affairs, it is wont to be affected with Pleasure or Grief, and other Passions depending on either of these.

For indeed (as we mentioned before) there are two Chief and Primary Gestures of the Sensitive Soul, as often as it is moved from its wonted and Natural State or Condition; to wit, either she stretches forth her self into a greater Compass, by profuse Pleasure, as if it affected to be dilated beyond the bounds of the Body: or being overthrown by Sorrow or Grief, she is contracted more narrowly, and runs her self within the wonted Sphear of her Emanations: from this twofold Affection of the Sensitive Soul, all the other Passions take their Origine. For truly Pleasure, or an Elation of the Soul, is its most pleasing Constitution, which desiring to gain for it self by any means, it follows all Objects promising it, with Love, Desire, Hope, Faithfulness, Boldness, and other means of getting it; On the contrary, Sadness or a Contraction or Dejection of this Soul, is a Gesture most ungrateful to it; what things then soever threaten or induce it, we endeavour to remove away far, by Fear, Hatred, Anger, Desperation, Shame, Pusillanimity, and other motions of shuning it. In the first place therefore, we will speak briefly of Pleasure and Grief, which are according to *Aristotle*, as it were a forked measure of the Sensitive Appetite, for the double Ladder of Affections, flowing thence, by which she is carried to this or that.

The two Primary Gestures or Affections of the Soul, are Pleasure and Grief.

First, Pleasure and Grief, because they bend or incline the whole Corporeal Soul after a diverse manner; therefore its two roots, to wit, the Brain and *Præcordia*, are chiefly affected. When the Soul is stretched forth in Pleasure, and is drawn to its utmost Sphear of Irradiation, the Animal Spirits being carried within the Brain, stir up most pleasant and pleasing Imaginations; and further, they actuating lively the Nervous *System*, Cause the Eyes, Face, Hands, and all the Members to shine, and as it were leap forth; Further, then more fully shaking also the *Præcordia*, by the Influence of the Brain, delivered by means of the Nerves, they thrust forth the Blood more rapidly, and as a Flame more brightly inkindled, they pour it forth with strength thorow the whole Body. On the contrary in Grief, whil'st the Soul sinks down, contracted into a more narrow space, the Spirits inhabiting the Brain, as it were struck down by flight, and troubled, put on only sad and fearful Imaginations, from whence the Countenance is cast down, the Limbs grow feeble, and the *Præcordia* being contracted or bound together, by reason of the Nerves carrying the same affection from the Brain, restrain the Blood from its due Excursion, which being therefore heaped up in the same place, with a weight, brings in a troublesome oppression of the Heart, and in the mean time, the Exterior Parts being deprived of its wonted afflux, languish and Contract a paleness.

They affect the two Roots of the Soul, to wit, the Brain and the Præcordia.

The aforesaid Affections of Pleasure and Sadness, which is wont, the Imagination being employed, to be poured from thence on the *Præcordia*, and by and by from that double Root into the whole Corporeal Soul; as to their first Originals, wholly depend upon the Sense. For from the beginning, Sensible Objects affect the Sensory with a certain sweetness or asperity, and there bring to the Spirits a certain Ovation or Triumph, or Confusion: from whence presently the Impression, like a waving of Waters, being Communicated to the Brain, excites the Spirits inhabiting it, into a consent either of the delight or trouble; and this Affection, being delivered from the Sensory to the Imagination, if it be short, there ends, and is not carried to the *Præcordia*: but if the stroke, being carried from the Sensible Object, is, like a more strong waving of Waters, impressed more vehemently, it reaches from the Sensory to the Brain, and presently thence to the Breast, that the Motions of the Heart and Blood, are intangled together with the disorder of the Animal Spirits, so as to the first Conceptions of the Affections, as well as Notions, there is nothing in the Imagination, or I may rather say, there is nothing in the Brain or Heart, that was not first in the Sense: But afterwards, when many Idea's of Pleasures and Griefs, are impressed on the Phantasie and Memory; then very often without any previous Sense, or feeling of Pleasure or Sadness, the Imagination being repeated, is wont to excite a Passion of the pleasant or troublesome thing; for when at any time we conceive in our Mind Good or Evil things belonging to us, not only present, but also past, or to come, that Conception employs the Phantasie, and not rarely very much exercises it: Further, being thence transmitted to the Breast, it inordinately either Contracts or Dilates the Breast, and so pours forth the Affection, together with the disturbed Blood, on the whole Body. A Wise and Strong man easily moderates the passions of Pleasure or Grief, lest these being brought, either from the Sensories, or suggested from the Memory, should affect the Phantasie and the *Præcordia*, by too great a waving; For the Brain and Heart, which are the supports of the Soul, ought not to be moved much, by the more light Objects of the Senses; nor are these principal Powers, at leisure to be present at every small thing: Hence some have born the torture of the Body, or the cutting off a Member, beyond Stoical Patience, undisturbed; whil'st others (in whom the sensible

Grief and Pleasure first of all arise from the Sense.

Afterwards, both from this, and also from the Phantasie, and Memory.

Some are more Pathetical, or moved than others.

Of the Passions in Particular.

sensible Species, being above measure increased, vehemently shakes the *Præcordia*) the skin scarce wounded, swoon away, or fall into fainting Fits. In like manner it is observed, that some are carried away by a most light Pleasure of the Senses into softness and Luxury, in the mean time others are scarce moved with any Pomp of Delights, or Exquisite Blandishments of Pleasures. It is observ'd in the fruition of a pleasing Object (which also holds of the appulse of a pleasant, or a painful sensible thing) there happens a certain reciprocation, between the Spirits of the Brain, and the Inhabitants of the Sensory. We imagine the Drinking of excellent Wine, with a certain Pleasure, then we indulge it; the Imagination of its Pleasure is again sharpned by the taste, and then by a reflected Appetite drinking is repeated: So as it were in a Circle, the Throat or Appetite provokes the Sension, and the Sension causes the Appetite to be sharpned, and iterated; this Kind of mutual reciprocation of the Animal Spirits from the Brain to the Sensory, and on the contrary, persists for some time, till the same, like twaving of Water, either leisurely vanishes, or is obliterated, by the exciting of a new waving: So indeed, Passions and Desires wear out themselves, or are consumed by time, or they are blotted out by the coming of some other Passion. When the Animal Spirits, desiring too much a sensible Delight, do often, and for a long time iterate and intend the Appetite, and Act of the pleasurable Sension, there is need of Reason to come between, whereby they being changed into Sacred and Moral Meditations, may be called away from their Carnal Genius; which Avocation however, they obey not but difficultly and unwillingly; for as much as to be expanded, and to enjoy pleasing Objects, is the Recreation and Food of the Spirits; and to be restrained or kept in, and very much to be employed about the works of the Mind, is to them a Labour, and a difficult task.

How the Affections are wont to be iterated, also how allayed or obliterated.

CHAP. IX.

Of the Passions Particularly.

Concerning the Number of the Passions, as it hath been variously disputed among Philosophers, so in famous Schools, this Division into Eleven Passions, long since grew of use; to wit, the Sensitive Appetite is distinguished into Concupiscible and Irascible, to the first, are counted commonly six Passions, viz. Pleasure and Grief, Desire and Aversion, Love and Hatred; but to the latter five, *viz.* Anger, Boldness, Fear, Hope, and Desperation, are wont to be attributed: But this distribution of the Affections is not only incongruous, for that Hope is but ill referred to the Irascible Appetite, and Hatred and Aversion, seem rather to belong to this, than to the Concupiscible: But it is also very insufficient, because some more noted Affections, as Shame, Pity, Emulation, Envy, and many others, are wholly omitted: Wherefore, the Ancient Philosophers did determinate the Primary to a certain Number, then they placed under their several Kinds, very many indefinite Species. Truely the Sensitive Soul, like a *Proteus*, is wont to be so diversly disturbed and altered, into manifold Kinds, with the various Fluctuation, and divers sorts of Inclination of the Animal Spirits, Blood, and other Humors, that a cense or view of all the Passions, can scarce be had; But however, that these, if not all, at least the chief of them, may be in some measure discovered; we will here ordain Pleasure and Grief for the extreams, or the opposite bounds of the Inclinations of the Corporeal Soul, then we will consider, after what manner, the Objects belonging to either, by what means soever may be applied, and what sorts of Impressions they are wont to fix on the Spirits, Blood, and solid Parts. The Corporeal Soul therefore, affecting Pleasure as the greatest height of its felicity, in which it would acquiesce, is moved at the appearance of any Good: if it be to come, and contrary to opinion, by and by for the getting it, Desire or Love arises; if with Opinion, Hope and Boldness; if Opinion esteems Fruition hopeless, Desperation is raised up; if this Good be past, or should be lost by our default, Shamefacedness or Repentance is brought in; if it be possessed by others, Emulation, and Envy; Love is busied about it being taken absolute, without respect to time or possession. Besides also there are other respects and habitudes of appearing Good, able to excite many other Affections with ease. In like manner on the contrary side, Grief or Trouble, is a Sickness of the Sensitive Soul, and a Disposition very much ingrateful to it; wherefore, at all the Objects apparently threatning its Induction, the Soul variously

The Number of the Passions uncertain.

Pleasure and what Affections are subordinate to it. Love, Hope, Boldness, &c.

Grief with the Affections subordinate to it.

variously Contracts her self, and is inclined hither and thither, that she might shun the approaches of the threatning Evils: wherefore there are so many Affections respecting Grief, and Subordinate to it, as there are means by which the Sensitive Soul, or the Disposition of the Spirits, composes her self for the shaking off or the shunning of any *Hatred, Aver-* Evil. Hatred is busied about Evil taken absolutely; that being absent, we prosecute *sion, Fear, &c.* with Aversion, by and by about to come with Fear; and unworthily brought, with Anger; falling upon our selves, we sustain it with sadness; inflicted on our Friends, with Pity. There are besides, many other Appearances of approaching Evil; for the shuning of which, the Soul is compelled into many Metamorphoses, and at the same time draws into the like Gestures, as it were Mimical, the Humors and Members of the Body, and oftentimes the Rational Soul it self: As it would be a business very tedious, and of immense Labour, to rehearse all the Kinds of Passions, and to unfold them, we have designed therefore to speak only of the Chief Species of the Passions, with their manner of affecting, in respect both of the Body, and also of the Superior Soul.

Next to Plea- Love and Hate follow next, and as it were at the back of Pleasure and Grief; because *sure and Grief,* the Sensitive Soul, being greatly prone, as hath been said, to Pleasure, Prosecutes all *are Love and* things apparently Good, without respect to Circumstances, with an Universal and most *Hatred.* ample Affection of Love; in like manner, shunning Grief or Trouble; it hates and detests all things apparently Evil, which may seem to induce Evil by any manner of way.

The Objects of The Good exciting Love, is objected after a twofold manner; to wit, either to the *these, are Sen-* Sense, or the Opinion: As to the first, Objects which consist of Particles Congruous *sible or Imagi-* and Curiously fitted to the Sensory, so that they stroke gently the Spirits there flowing, *nary things.* and cause them to run and to rejoyce together, these bring forth a desirable Sension, whose Impression being transmitted, by the passage of the Nervous Processes to the Brain, by pleasing there in like manner the Spirits, stirs them up into a pleasant apprehension of the sensible thing, and a desire of it: Hence these Spirits inhabiting the Brain, for the fruition of this Object, try several or manifold Endeavours, *viz.* Some being reflected towards the Sensory, desire to cleave more closely, and to be united to this Good: in the mean time, others flowing towards the Breast, sometimes dilate and open the Bosoms of *By what means* the Heart, that they may more plentifully receive the Blood, imbued with a certain Virtue *desirable things* of the Object, and enjoy it; and sometimes the Spirits draw together these receptacles *affect the Spi-* of the Heart, and drive outwardly the Blood, as if about to seek something more large- *rits, and the* ly of Good, from the Object, with which being filled at last, it is received by the heart, *Blood.* by and by dilated. Further, in this Affection of Love, concerning the sensible Object, if that it be very strong, the whole Sensitive Soul, or the whole *Systasis* of the Spirits is inclined towards the beloved thing, lifts up to it the whole Nervous *System,* and together with the solid Parts, draws, and leads the Humours; so, when we are indulged *A Pleasant Sen-* with a fair Aspect or Melody, the whole Soul seems to go out at the Eye or the Ear, and *sation is descri-* neglecting the other Sensories, Conspire with their proper Offices into those Acts of *bed.* Sension.

Love is excited It is somewhat otherways in Love excited through Opinion, because in this, the Spe- *by Opinion.* cies of the Object being represented by the Imagination, is erected as an Idol in the Brain; about this many Spirits being employed, at first they weigh the noted Beauty, and its various Ornaments, then they worship it; for whatsoever we love, we imagine it fair, profitable, pleasant, and far above what in truth it is; then by reason of these kind of feigned Attributes, we more earnestly fall in love with the thing beloved; Further, the *The Object of* Spirits inhabiting the Brain, invite all the rest, flowing in the whole Nervous stock, to *this, is set up,* the worship of the Idol erected by themselves: wherefore the Inhabitants of every Sen- *like an Idol, in* sory, watching for the works of the Senses, look hither; here also they wait for the Mo- *the Phantasie,* tions, Executors of the Limbs and Members; but they chiefly inspire the *Præcordia* with *And Worshipped.* the Love of this Imaginary Good; wherefore, these being variously dilated, and thrust together, greedily receive, sometimes the Blood imbued as it were with the Character of the thing loved, and as it were imbibe its Influence, sometimes they cast forth that Humor from themselves, towards the Brain, as it were to pick out something from the Image of the Good: This Kind of Image exciting Love, is impressed on the Imagination, either from the Intellect, or from the Memory and Phantasie, to wit, one of them only, or both together; and from thence a Passion of Love is brought in, either Metaphysical, or merely Sensitive, or mixt.

Hatred excited, Much after the same manner as we have said of Love, the evil Appearances also, which *by the Sensible* excite Hatred or the Aversation of the Soul, are objected to the Sense or Imagination: *or Imaginary* As to the former, when any incongruous and improportionate Object, is brought to *Species.* any Sensory, that distracts and drives the Animal Spirits into a certain Confusion; therefore afterwards, when such an Object comes again to the same Sensory, the Spirits mindful

Of the Passions in Particular.

ful of their former hurt, abhor the Contact and approach of this Evil, Contract as much as they can the Organ, and shut up the Passages and Doors; if they are strong they endeavour to remove the Enemy from themselves, by sudden and iterated Excursions; but if they are not able for such Assaults, they convey and hide themselves within, and reject the embraces of the hateful thing, by every manner of way. A rejection of the sensible Object happens, when stinking Odors of very unsavoury Meat strike the Palate, or Nostrils; and the like when incongruous things are offer'd to the sight, or hearing: But especially, when the breaking of the Unity happens to be inflicted by Fire, or a Sword, on the Skin or Flesh. Concerning these repulses of the approaching Object, not only the Spirits flowing in the Sensory, but oftentimes also by the consent of these others inhabiting the Brain, are irritated into Fury; so that the Imagination conceives a detestation of the thing; and the *Præcordia* being therefore disturbed, sometimes draws back the Blood, sometimes drives it outward towards the driving away the Evil, and stirs it up to its Expulsion. *How the first of these Affects the Spirits and Blood.*

When an Object apparently Evil, appears therefore hateful to the Imagination, presently the Phantasie fixes on it a Monstrous and very deformed Image; then stirs up all the Spirits, implanted both in the Brain and the Nervous Appendix, into a Detestation of this Imaginary Spectre, from hence the Brows are contracted, the Teeth gnash together, and the Face is writhed; but especially the *Præcordia*, variously open and shut themselves, that they might Eventilate the Blood, by driving in up and down, and Conserve it free from every Influence or Tincture of this Object. *The Imaginary Evil affects both the Blood, and Spirits.*

After this manner, the Passions of Love and Hatred are employed about Good and Evil, taken absolutely, and almost Indifferently; or rather about their Idea's: to wit, the Sensitive Soul, beholding the Image of appearing Good, received from the Sense or the Imagination, and admitting it into it self, presently she embraces it with a certain strictness, as it were with open and infolded Arms, and endeavours to be intimately united to it: But it rests not long in this fruition; for if this Image of Good be only Imaginary, and being embraced, vanishes like a Cloud, taken for *Juno*, the Soul, sensible of her Error, quickly lets go her empty Embraces: yea, if that Good were solid, after some time, its fruition brings forth a loathing, and the Complacency of the Object at first amiable, grows cold, by the enjoyment; and it is esteemed troublesome. For indeed it is so order'd, that we esteem nothing long in this Life, but being always wanting, whatsoever is obtain'd, we esteem less, seeking after new things; wherefore, we are perpetually incited to the desiring of absent Good, and to the flying from Evils hanging over us. Love or lasting Charity, is a Divine Passion, almost proper only to Heaven, as Hatred, standing and endless, is an Affection merely Diabolical, and ought to be esteemed peculiar to Hell. But in most Mortals, these are presently changed into Desires or Aversions; because the desire of any absent Good, which we seem to want, or the declining of any approaching Evil, obliterate the Idea of any Good or Evil before affixed to the Sensitive Soul, and adhering to it; even as the following waves sup up the former. *Love and Hate, are transitory Passions.* *Quickly changed into Desire, and Aversion.*

In truth the Sensitive Soul is chiefly employed with Desires and Aversions; these are perpetually suggested by heaps from our wants, either true or imaginary, and a very infinite Company or Succession of them exist. Concerning our Indigencies, from which these Passions are drawn, it is to be observed, that they proceed either from the Sense, or from Opinion, and so peculiar Desires or Aversions are excited: As to the former, the Animal Spirits in every Sensory, watch as so many hungry Guests expecting the Approach of an Object congruous to them, as it were food; to the meeting and snatching of which, they are often wont to go as it were to meet it, and be carried quite beyond the Confines of their Subject. But that the Spirits residing in the Organ of every of the Senses, do greedily Covet after this manner the sensible Object, as their Prey, happens by the mere Instinct of Nature, or is procured by Custom: The former is discerned, when hunger or thirst require the Supplies of Meat and Drink, and when the Coldness of a naked Body requires Cloathing: These sort of Desires, which Necessity puts upon Nature, are easily satisfied, and what are sufficient for the maintaining of Life, and obtained after this manner; to wit, the Animal Spirits labouring under a defect, in this or that part, do variously Contract, and so affect with a sense of trouble the Nervous Bodies, in which they flow, which Impression being presently Communicated to the Brain, it stirs up the Spirits inhabiting it into an Appetite or Desire, and then an inflowing being made into the appropriate Nerves; into a Prosecution of the desired thing; all this is performed without the Image of the Object, increased by the Imagination, also without any Perturbation known in the *Præcordia*, or the Blood. *The Soul is chiefly employed by these.* *Both proceed, either from the Sense, or Opinion.* *The desire of a sensible thing, is excited, either from Natural Instinct, or from Custom.* *The former is moderate, and easily satisfied.*

Of the Affections in Particular.

Desire got through Custom, despising moderate things aspires to new things.

It is much otherwise concerning sensible Desires got by Custom; for when as a Fruition once happens to the Spirits inhabiting this or that Sensory, of a more pleasant Object, having moderate things in Contempt, afterwards desire the same, and being not long Content therewith, still aspire to others more pleasant; so the Palate being accustomed to more delicate Victuals, loaths every thing unless spiced Aliments, and prepared with most exquisite Sawce: In like manner may be observed, concerning the Smelling, Sight, Hearing, and other Sensitive Functions; to wit, that the Appetite, proper to any of them, (for as much as it once exceeded what sufficed Nature) is always carried to more excellent Objects, and they for the most part only fresh; the reason of this seems to be, that the chief Pleasure of the Sensitive Soul, consists in a more lively Motion, and larger Expansion of the Spirits implanted in every part; but such a Motion of them, depends very much upon the Excellency, also the Variety, and Change of the Objects.

The reason declared, Because the Agent and Patient, ought to be unlike.

For whatsoever moderate or too familiar thing happens to the Spirits, it little affects them; for every motion supposes a Superior, and a Virtue of the Object, somewhat unlike to the Agent; wherefore, when any Object by daily use obtains a Similitude, or Equality with the Spirits, that is less apt to move them: therefore that the Activity, or the lively unfolding of the Spirits (which is the Effectress of Pleasure) may be continued a long time, leaving the Fruition of every old and worn-out Good, it always tends to new and more high things: After this manner, tho every Organ of Sense puts forth Desires, peculiar and proper to themselves, it reiterates them with a perpetual change; but for as much as Objects applied through Corporeal Contact, rather than by Effluvia, affect more vehemently the Sensory; therefore the greatest Company of Desires, arising from the Sense, are wont to be referred to Luxury, or Lust.

The Desires of sensible things, tend chiefly to Luxury or Lust.

The Desires of the Spirits dwelling in the other Sensories, for as much as they take only the Species, or the little Bodies, falling off from sensible things, and less thick Embraces; therefore they are more temperate, and are often directed to better uses.

Phantastic Desires are immense.

But our wants are chiefly Imaginary, and proceed from Opinion, and from hence a most plentiful Crop of Desires grows up. For indeed, every Man breaths after Felicity, or after a certain Divine State; wherefore, it seeks very much things apparently Good, which are said to Conduce to this State, and endeavours to obtain them: But having followed certain Goods, it finds not the desired Satisfaction in them; therefore it seems to want others, and then again others. So, for as much as Men always tend to the highest Good, or last end, and that he attains it not in his life-time, there is a Necessity of infinite Wishes, and Desires concerning the intermediate Goods: Hence it is, that whatsoever another has, yea, whatsoever of Good the Phantasie can conceive or feign, presently we believe we have need of it, and therefore we desire it, and wish for it.

But are chiefly carried to Riches or Honors.

So, though there is an immense Company of Concupiscible things, yet as most Men place their felicity in Riches or Honours, hence the Chief Species of Desires arising from Opinion; and therefore not to be satisfied, are Covetousness and Ambition.

Aversion is excited either from the Sense, or from Opinion.

As to Aversion, this Passion seems only to be the former inversed, and in like manner, to take its Original, either from a certain Defect, perceived by the Sense, or taken from Opinion; for a Sense or Opinion of want, calls to either, a declination of the same manner of State: Wherefore, when the Animal Spirits in the Sensories, are deprived of the Enjoyment of a necessary Good, or of what they were before accustomed to, they either conceive, or set before them the approach of its Contrary, and these being very unquiet, let go the Embraces of every present Object, and set themselves to perform, or enter into a new Confederation; until either the Sense or the Opinion, shall detect some apparent Good, to the desire and following of which, the same Spirits are busied; And so Aversion, being for the most part a Passion of it self Vain, and quickly perishable, terminates in the desire of Good, that may supply the Defect so carefully shun'd.

This Passion being frail, is soon changed into Desire.

Having shown after this manner for what Causes, and upon what Preparations or fore Occasions, the Sensitive Soul enters into Passions of Desire and Aversion: Let us now see after what manner or ways of Gesticulations or Gestures, she is Composed in either Affection. As to Desires begun from the Organs of the Senses, it is observed, that whil'st the Spirits there implanted, are carried towards the absent Object, all fruition being left, they, as it were naked and destitute of all helps, like Beggars ask an Alms, which as they most greedily desire, as it were about to take by force that Good, they exceed the limits of their Subject; and oftentimes, when the Desire is vehement, almost the whole Soul is drawn into Parties, and by a certain going out from the Body, wanders towards the desired thing, or at least emits a Portion of it self. That it is so, it plainly appears, in that mad affection of Lust, in which the genital Humor, containing Fragments picked from the whole Soul is poured forth. In like manner, in a

Sensible Desire affects both the Spirits and the Blood.

pleasant

Of the Passions in Particular.

pleasant Sight, Sweet Odor, and most pleasing Harmony, the Animal Spirits, as it were lifted up, role together out of the Sensories towards their Objects: but on the contrary in Aversion, they betake themselves inward, and sometimes forsake the Sensories themselves.

As to desires excited by reason of the Opinion of want, the Sensitive Soul being impatient of a Lot so poor, becomes very instable and unquiet, all the acquired Goods of its Body, it neglects and disesteems, also refuses to hearken to the dictates of Reason; yea being altogether precipitate in desires, she always looks outward, and as it were with wings is ready to fly to this or that apparent Good; hence, by the disorder of the Spirits, flying hither and thither the Nervous Parts are variously distracted, and Men betray their desires by their Countenance, and going; also the Breast and the *Præcordia* being moved together, the Blood, like the Sea working with the winds, is compelled into various Fluctuations, that those affected sometimes grow Pale, and sometimes are overspread with redness; also, from the same Blood, entring inequally and impetuously the Confines of the Brain, succeed inconstancy of Judgment, and frequent Changes of a thing proposed; as sometimes they will do this, anon that, as *if ten Minds were together by the Ears in one Man.* *What Alterations Imaginary Desire brings upon them.* *The Fluctuation of the Mind.*

According to the aforesaid Characters or Scheams, the Sensitive Soul is composed, about absent Good and Evil, and not quickly about to come; but when these seem to be at the Doors, the Soul alters her Position, and is respectively urged with Hope or Fear: Concerning which, First it is observed, that these Passions do not as the forementioned proceed equally from the Sense and the Imagination, but are founded only on Opinion; from whence, after entring into the desire of any thing, the Spirits being Solicitous concerning the following of it, and as it were depressed, when they upon some other Occasion, as the Drinking of Wine, are a little elevated with the fruition of another pleasing Object, and they begin to strengthen Opinion, forthwith doubtful desire is changed into a certain Confidence, that we hope shortly to possess the desired Good: In like manner, whenas Aversion beholds the absent Evil a long way off, the depression of the Spirits places it near, and by and by Causes a fear of its being about to come upon them. Indeed, Hope and Fear, are very near of Kin to Desire and Aversion, and either of these Symbolical Affections, denote only the more near, or more remote approach of the same Object. *Plato. Hope and Fear. Succeed to Desire, and Aversion.*

As to what appertains to the Provision and Exercise of Hope, when we desire greatly any absent Good, and that an Opinion arises, that we shall shortly obtain it, presently the Animal Spirits, who first like Soldiers sent before, carefully seek after, and observe the willed thing, forthwith returning towards the Soul, bring News of the Coming of its Guest, and prepare a Reception for it; wherefore the whole Soul is presently brought into an Expectation of its coming; all the Doors of the Senses are opened, that this Good, with all its Train, might enter thorow open Gates: In the mean time, the Spirits inhabiting every Sensory, are prepared to go forth to salute this approaching, and the Imagination doth forestall its Entrance; to wit, this frames an Idea of the wish'd for and coming Good, which it places within its Borders, as in a Throne, and confers on it Adornments and Splendor, borrowed from the Phantasie. Moreover, the *Præcordia* are Careful for a part of its Reception; for they being actuated with a more full Influx of Spirits, send forth the Blood more lively into the Exterior Parts, as it were for the meeting of this new Guest; hence, any one being full of Hope, feels in his whole Body, a certain Inflation, with the Spirit and Heat plentifully poured forth: Then, if by any accident, an occasion of fear or doubting is brought in, presently a sudden girding together in the whole, with a certain putting down of the Spirits, and a sinking of the whole Soul, ensues. *The Provision of Hope. Its Object, both the Sense, and the Imagination. Affects both the Spirits and the Blood.*

For in the Passion of Fear, the Sensitive Soul being first stretched out, being struck by the nearness of the approaching Evil, and being as it were prickt on every side, for as much as she conceiving her self taken by the Enemy, cannot fly away into this or that Part, she enters into her self, and that the Animal Spirits may be pressed together, she is Contracted most strictly, if the Affection be vehement, whilst the Animal Spirits suddenly go back, from the Superficies of the Body, they greatly bind up at the same time the Pores and Passages, as it were fastning the Doors, to shut out the Enemy: from this Constriction, the Pores of the Skin being drawn inward, oftentimes succeeds an erection of the hairs, or the hair standing an end; then the same Spirits being acted into Confusion, they are inhibited from performing the wonted Offices of their Functions, and not ouly want the helps of Reason; but sometimes the Locomotive Faculties fail, yea by a resolution or loos'ning of the Nerves, made in the Bowels, oftentimes the Excrements involuntarily flow out. Further, when the Animal Faculty languishes so much, the Motion of the *Præcordia* is tyred; hence the Blood stagnating within the Bosoms of the Heart, *A Character of Fear. How it Affects the Spirits, and all the Faculties. How the Blood.*

Heart, oftentimes a swouning follows: and when therefore it is not carried lively enough into the outward Parts, a Coldness and Paleness succeeds in them. In a sudden fear, we feel a certain stiffness, whence 'tis commonly said, that the Blood is curdled in the Body; but this happens, because, whil'st the Nervous Parts compassing about the Blood-carrying Vessels, are suddenly bound together, they at the same time repress the Blood from its Excursion, and so stop or plainly invert its Circulation.

It often passes into Desperation.
In the mid'st of fear, lest the Spirits being driven too much into flight, the Sensitive Soul should be wholly loosned, Reason is wont to interpose something of Hope, and so by degrees to lift up the dejected Spirits, and to animate them to stay, so that this Passion being alleviated by such a remedy, may more easily pass over; but if by the strong Evil falling on one, all means of Hope be cut off, then a greater Affection, to wit, Desperation, comes in the place of Fear, in which for the most part, this Soul yielding her self overcome, wholly sinks down, and being half dead, is drowned in her proper Body, as in a Sepulcher, or if she retains any strength, presently being carried into Confusion, all things being turned upside down, she Contracts, Melancholy, or Madness.

In like manner Hope into Audaciousness.
As Desperation follows Fear, all helps being cut off; so Hope, when it is joyned to more, and more certain, of the same, passes in Audaciousness: And in this Affection, the Sensitive Soul swells up, and opposes her self dauntless to any ensuing Evil; wherefore, the Spirits Guardian, by a more strong Connexion of themselves, every where extend the Muscles, and strengthen them, by a more full Inspiration, to the bearing or resisting any thing; hence the Breast being inlarged, and then strongly bound together, a bigger Voice is sent forth; the Fists being Contracted, the Arms lifted up, the Head erected, the Face grim and threatning, the Neck swollen, and the rising up, or the stretchings forth of other Parts, shew the Animal Spirits in the whole Body, unfolded and prepared for Battel, as if about to enter into Conflict: In the mean time, the *Præcordia* being moved most strongly, by a more full influx of the same Spirits, notably rarifie the Blood, and like Lightning, send it forth impetuously, and drive it into the outward Parts.

To which Anger is of Kin.
Anger is of some Kin to Boldness, in which the Sensitive Soul, by reason of the Evil unworthily brought to it, at the same time is made sad, and grows hot; wherefore, as she Contracts her self by reason of Sadness, so presently girding her self for Revenge, she is dilated; therefore, as here divers Contractions come together, this Passion is performed with a mighty Perturbation of Spirits, and of the Blood: for those affected, at *The Character of Anger.* the beginning wax Pale, by and by they are overspread with Red; the Forehead is wrinkled, the Lips quiver, the Tongue murmurs, the Countenance is sometimes cast down, sometimes lifted up, and threatning, but the *Præcordia* are especially agitated, with a notable heat and boyling up of the Blood: which kind of Various, and sometimes Contrary Symptoms, may easily be resolved; to wit, that the Soul at once conceiving Sadness and Indignation, like the Sea working with opposite winds, has Floods excited from every Coast, and striking one against another among themselves.

There are more than Eleven Affections.
Besides the Eleven Affections even now recited and unfolded, according to the Vulgar Opinion, there remains some others, excited according to the other manifold Affections and Gestures of the Corporeal Soul; the chief of which are Pity and Envy, Glory or Boasting, and Shame; which however are very near related to the afore recited, or are Composed out of them. For Pity is made out of Love and Sadness, by reason of the Evils of a Friend: On the contrary, Envy out of Hatred and Sorrow, by reason of the Good things of an Enemy: Glory or Boasting, is a certain kind of Joy and Exultation, conceived by reason of an Opinion of our Good, had from others; and Shame is a certain Sadness and Consternation of the Soul, by reason of an Opinion of *A Character of Shame.* our ills conceived by others. Further, Concerning this Passion 'tis observable, that when the Corporeal Soul being abashed, is enforced to repress its Compass, she notwithstanding being desirous, as it were to hide this Affection, drives forth outwardly the Blood, and stirs up a redness in the Cheeks, to wit, the Sensitive part of the Soul, as it were hiding its head, puts before her self a Portion of the Vital or the Bloody Soul, under whose wings somewhat stretched forth, the Confusion might be hid.

Pity, Envy, Boasting,

Shame, &c.

Innate Affections.
Besides we take notice, that the Corporeal Soul is not only affected by Objects, and their Impressions, and compelled into various Gestures, and the aforesaid Passions; but besides, she hath certain innate Dispositions, by reason of which, by the mere instinct of Nature, without any Influence of the Object, she puts forth her self, and is excited into certain Emanations or Spontaneous forces: Of which sort are first an amplification or inlarging the Individual Person, and then a Propagation of its Kind. It is Natural for every Animal without example or teaching, to seek for, and swallow down its food, both

Of the Passions in Particular.

both that the Body may be daily increased to its due Magnitude, and also that the Soul, being daily supplied with a new Store of Spirits, may be co-extended to the Body, and be able lively to perform the Acts of her Functions. Then, as soon as the Lineaments both of the Body and Soul being sufficiently drawn forth, and the Bulk and Compass of either are Compleated ; some Animal Spirits flowing over from the work of the Individual, begin to abound, and then being separated into the Genital Parts, with a subtil Humor picked from the whole Body, destinated for the Propagating the Species, as it were in a Store-house, and there layed up, they form there the Idea of a new Animal ; which afterward is transferred into a convenient Womb, to be perfectly formed. When the Seeds of a new Animal are so lay'd, the whole Corporeal Soul is drawn with all its Powers into this work of Propagating the Species, more than of the Conserving of the Individual : wherefore the Blood supplies the Testicles, no less than the Brain, with a most subtil and noble Matter for the store of Animal Spirits : and when after too great Expence, the Spirits are deficient in them, that presently the loss may be made up, oftentimes the Brain and Nerves are defrauded of their due Pension, and are suffered to languish, that in the mean time the Blood may pour forth more plentifully spirituous Particles into the Spermatic Vessels. Yea it is thought, that it doth sometimes snatch the Animal Spirits from the Brain it self, which it bestows on the Genitals, in the Act of Venery : For it appears so, when by immoderate Venery, the Brain presently labours with a want of Spirits ; for as much as from thence there is no passage for them, to the Spermatick Vessels, but by the Blood ; if that the Animal Spirits superabound with a Prolifick Humour, Swelling up within the Genital Parts, presently the whole Corporeal Soul, as it were incited, to the begetting of a young one, is inclined to Concupiscence or Lust : The Incentives of Lust, even against the Mind, are sought for, and they are lay'd hold on, however brought by any Sense ; the Blood boils up, the Marrow in the Back grows hot, the Eyes are inflamed, the Genitals are inflated, so that there wants little (unless Reason coming between recalls her, and Prohibits her from the Beastliness of it) but that the whole Corporeal Soul, on every occasion, should be dissolved in Lust. In these kind of Affections of Concupiscence, may be most clearly discerned the distinct Strivings, and contrary Endeavours of two Souls : because, whil'st the Corporeal Soul being incited to Lust, inclines her self wholly towards the Genital Members, and Compels thither greater floods of the Blood, and greater store of the Animal Spirits, the Heart and Brain being left wanting of Provision ; on the contrary, the Superior Mind, rising up, and shewing the Commands of Reason and Religion, shews a receipt to the other, and Commands that the Animal Spirits return to their tasks, to be performed within the Brain, and also that the raging Blood should be recalled towards the *Præcordia*, and being there suppressed, might be restrained from disorderly Excursions ; Hence, the flame of Lust being re-extinct for a time, and the Powers of the Inferior Soul being reduced into Order, the Acts of Sobriety, Prudence, and of other Science, and Discipline may be exercised ; but if the reins of Reason be let loose, or new incentives of Lust are brought, the Corporeal Soul, shaking off the yoak, snatches her self again to the like Enormities.

There remain yet some other Affections of the Corporeal Soul, as Sleep and Watching, Grief and Pleasure, excited in private Members; which, for as much as they respect not the whole Soul at once, but this or that Portion of the Body, or Peculiar Powers of it, and chiefly the Sensitive or Locomotive ; therefore we shall handle these anon, and shall next proceed to the Sense and its Kinds.

Viz. in largement of the Individual.

A begetting of its Kind.

Venus an Enemy to the Brain and Nerves.

The madness or fury of Lust.

Reason suppresses its flowing.

CHAP. X.

Of the Sense in General.

THe Vital or Flamy part of the Corporeal Soul, being rooted in the Blood, seems not much to know or perceive what things are offer'd outwardly to, or acted inwardly in the Body : So, altho the Blood have life, yet 'tis scarce sensible or knowing, for this which ought to be always employed, with a perpetual Motion, and even inkindling, for the Offices for the sustaining of Life, cannot be at leisure to mind any smaller Matters, or outward Accidents. Indeed great Passions also in some measure disturb the Blood, and pervert and variously drive it from its wonted Course, and like violent Blasts, shake not

The Blood is animated, but hardly sensible.

only

only the Leaves or Body of the Tree, but also sometimes pull up the Roots out of the Earth: So whatsoever mutations or alterations happen to the Blood, proceed either from the Complexion of its Liquor being changed, or from the impulse or incitation of the containing Bodies. But the other Sensitive part of this Soul, which being diffused within the Brain and stock of Nerves, is Co-extended or equally stretched forth with the Organical Body, and almost with all its Parts, is affected with every Contact, or with the meeting of other Bodies, she perceives all Impressions either outwardly objected, or raised up within; and as she is moved by these, every where diversly inflicted, she induces according to the various impulse of the Objects, various Gestures and Species in her self, and also draws the Members and Parts of the Body it self, with her wholly into the same Figures and Motions. For indeed it is the Energie or the Act of the Soul it self, from which every Function of the animated Body primarily and chiefly arises. If at any time any Stroke or Impression be inflicted any where to the animated Body, presently a certain Fluctuation or waving is stirred up in the *Hypostasis* of the whole Soul, or of the struck Member; by which, some Animal Spirits or subtil Particles, shut up in the Organical Parts, as a blast of Wind in a Machine, being struck, run hither and thither, and so produce the Exercises of Sense and Motion in the whole Body, or respective Parts.

The lucid part of the Soul, feels or perceives the impulse of all Objects, and is moved by them.

Truly, among the various Gestures of the Corporeal Soul, by which, she altering her Species or *Hypostasis*, brings a change to the containing Body, the Sensitive and Locomotive Powers obtain the chief place; for as much as they are Common almost to all living Creatures, at least to the more perfect, to which also all the rest of the Faculties may easily be reduced. These are the chief Advancers of the animated Body, upon which all the other Wheels of this Self-moving Divine Machine depend.

Sense and Motion, are the chief Advancers of the animated Body.

But the Internal and next efficient Cause, both of Sense and Motion, are the *Hypostasis* of the Sensitive Soul, or the Animal Spirits, instilled from the inkindled Blood into the Brain, and from thence diffused into the Nervous Stock which being distributed from the Brain, as the Fountain thorow the Nerves to the whole Body, imbue, irradiate, and blow up all the Parts, and bring a certain Tensity or stretching forth to each; so that the passages of the Nervous Bodies, like Cords stretched forth straitly on every side, from the Brain and its dependencies, reach forth into all the Exterior Parts, by which, so stretch'd forth, and actuated by a certain Continuity of the Soul, if one end be struck, presently the stroke is perceived through the whole, so that every Intention conceived within the Brain, presently performs the designed work, in every Member or Part; and on the other side, every impulse or stroke, which is inflicted from without to any Member, or to the Sensitive Body, is communicated instantly to all the Parts within the Head. If that an Impression or force tends from the Brain outwards, thorow the Nerves into the moving Parts, Motion is produced; but if they being made outwardly, are directed inwards towards the Brain, Sense arises. But whilst either of these are performed, it is not so to be understood, (as is commonly asserted) as if the same Spirits make haste, and leap back presently, as it were from one end of the Course or Circuit to the other; but as the Soul is stretched forth, thorow the whole, with a certain Continuity, its Particles, *viz.* the Spirits contiguous one with another are set like an Army in Array; for they after a Military fashion, whilst they move not from their station, and keep Order, perform their Offices; and whether they be set in Battel Array, or on the Watch, they perform the Commands carried outward from the Brain, themselves being almost immoveable, and effect Motion, and deliver presently to the Brain the news of any sensible thing impressed, whereby Sensation is made. So indeed, the same Animal Spirits, tho with an opposite and inverse tendency, and aspect of them, cause Motion and Sense: But both Faculties, as to the Exercises of their Acts, require something divers Organs; yea, the Animal Spirits planted within the same; for the performing the divers Offices of their Faculties, are ordered with a various Affection, and with a different manner of Orders. That each of these may be the more clearly illustrated, we shall first of all speak of the Sense, and of whatsoever belongs to it both in General and in Special, and then afterwards concerning Motion.

The efficient Cause of either, are the Animal Spirits.

A most swift Communication of them, implanted within all the Parts.

An opposite tendency of them, effect both Sense and Motion.

The Sense, as it is taken in a more strict acceptation (*viz.* for the proper Function in animated Bodies, and by which they are distinguished from inanimates) is wont to be described after this manner; *That it is the faculty of perceiving Sensible objects.* Because, the Sensitive soul, as hath been said, being apt to be affected or moved by every Contact, or Impulse of an exterior Body, forces its constitution to vary in the whole, or in part, according as it is struck: But exterior Bodies, because they consist of Particles, of a various Kind, and diversly figured, therefore, when some are applied to others, their approaches one among another, are not always made after one and the same manner, but after a manifold manner, and with notable variety; to wit, either by Corporeal Contacts,

What the Sense is.

The approach of the sensible Object, is made either by Contact, or by Effluvia's sent forth, or by reflected and repercussed Particles of the Air, Breath, or Light.

Of the Sense in General. 57

tacts, or by Effluvia's falling from them, or by Particles of Air, Breath, or Light, reflected from them, issuing from them on every side like Darts. Further, and to every one of these Kinds, many Species are attributed: Because, not only Concretes, but also various little Bodies of the same Subject, shew and impress manifold Types of their Contacts; several of which, as they are received and so known distinctly, by living Creatures, the Sensitive Soul using Corporeal Organs, hath many Sensories, fitted for such variety of Objects, and divers representations of things; in which several, both the Conformation of the Pores, as also the disposition of the Animal Spirits, are proportionated to the little Bodies, sent in from the Object, which are only of one Kind, fitly to be received. By this means sensible Impressions, at least that may be of use to any Animal, are perceived, and from this manifold way of Sension, proceeds the Knowledge of all things, according to that of the Philosopher, *All Knowledge is made by the Sense*; when on the contrary, if Bodies and their Particles, should strike the *Systasis* of the naked Soul, or part of it, always after one and the same manner, nothing at all would be known, because one thing or parts, from another, or these from those Members, would not be distinguished. Wherefore, that all the chief Objects and their Accidents, might be distinctly noted, it is so provided, that some Particles strike this Organ and not that; so that they affect their several respective Sensories only, the rest being untouched.

As these several are made manifold, they require divers Sensories.

All Knowledge from Sense.

From hence it is clear, that 'tis necessary that there should be many Sensories in perfect Animals; which may perform divers Actions, both for the preserving of Life, and propagating the Kind, and also for the knowing many things, and chiefly for the embracing of what things are Congruous to themselves, and for the shunning all incongruous things; for these things 'tis needful, that the Sensitive Soul should be affected by the Objects, after a various manner, and so perceive their manifold Influencies. How vile their Condition is, and how hard their Lot, that are gifted with the only sense of the Touch, appears from the Life and Operation of the more imperfect Animals, as Oysters and Lympins; then besides, how false is the Opinion of some, who say, That every Sense in all Animals is the feeling only; for although every Affection is made by Contact, from the Object to the Soul; yet neither is the same thing still employed, nor received after the same manner; but how many types soever of sensible things are to be found, so many Counterfeits remain in the Sensories.

In Perfect Animals, there ought to be many Senses.

That one of the Touch or Feeling, suffices not.

Nevertheless it may here be rightly Quæried, How it may be? for as much as the whole *Hypostasis* or Contexture of the Soul, is made up of most subtil and also most highly moveable Particles, that every one of them wheresoever implanted, are not indifferently moved, by every sensible stroke; when especially the Interior frame of the Soul, which is Common to all the Sensories, receives the Affections of every one, and so is mediately affected by every sensible thing: I say, why the Spirits implanted in the Eye, do not equally perceive Sounds and Smells, as they do Colours? for as much as they inhabiting the streaked Bodies, discern both these, and all other sensible things.

How the same Spirits receive sensible Species so very divers.

For the resolving of this Problem, these two things are to be suppos'd, to wit, first, That the Structure of every Sensory is so made, according to its Pores and Passages, that Particles only proportionate to them may be admitted in: wherefore as Light, and the Images of things, pass thorow Glass, and clear Bodies; not dark Bodies; so the same are received only by the Eyes, and not by the other Sensories: The same Reason holds of all the rest. For we may observe, when in the Circumambient Air, or in the Atmosphere, there are Bodies of a various Nature, and of a divers Configuration, that some things affect this, others that Sensory, and so the things which are of a several Kind affect the particular Organ of the Sense. As for Example, the Particles of most thin Air or Light, which seem to be of a Sulphureous Nature, being reflected from Bodies, Convey (as was said) their Images into the Organs of the Sight or Seeing; the little Bodies of Air which seem to be saline, being repercussed from Solids, shake the Drum of the Ear, by their leaping back; yea, and the same being made clammy by a sweet dew, or moistned, affect the taste; the Particles of the same Air, filled with sweet Exhalations, strike the Nostrils: And lastly, The same stuffed with warm or cold Effluvia's, move the Sense of Feeling: But in the mean time, the Particles of the same Air or Element, which are proportionate to one Sensory, are incommunicable to the rest.

That this may be done are required.

First a Structure of the Otmosphere can after a diverse manner.

But Secondly, the Animal Spirits themselves, which reside in the Organs of the Senses, and that are like Watchmen, are furnished for the respective meetings of the Objects, with a certain peculiar Provision, and an appropriate manner of Disposition: for when some Spirituous Particles, more pure than others, and more subtle exist, some more dull or blunt, others notably moveable, these Naked, those smered with Humor, and marked with many other Affections; it is so provided, that as the Naked Spirits, or those less gifted

Secondly, a Various Constitution of the Animal Spirits.

I

Of the Sense in General.

gifted suffice for the Sense of Feeling, these without any farther indowment are disposed every where in the Membranes, and fibrous Flesh; but the most pure Spirits, and as it were Chrystalline for the Sight, flow into the Eyes; those that are highly moveable are fitted for the Hearing, and the more Viscous, which are fused with a requisite Humour, for the Taste, and Smell.

After what manner Sension is made. These things being thus premised, concerning the Multiplicity and Difference of the Senses, and the Organs, we will now inquire into Sension it self; by what means, and after what manner it is performed. Concerning these we thus say in general, that the Object being applied to the Sensory, (whether it be done immediately, or the Particles of the Air or Element coming between) doth impress its Idea or Character on the Spirits implanted in that place; and in the same instant, by a continued Series of the Animal Spirits, as it were an Irradiation, the Type of its Impression doth pass from the Sensory to the Head; and whil'st the Spirits actuating the streaked Bodies, are in like manner affected by it, a perception of Sense, begun from the Organ, is formed.

All sensible Impressions do beam forth from all the Organs, into the streaked Bodies. That Sight is so performed, Dioptrick Experiments do plainly shew, by which, the same Species of any Body, by a Glass artificially placed, may be Carried or Reflected hither or thither, and may be figured and beheld at once in several places: why in like manner, may we not Conceive the Image of the Object represented in the Eye, as in a Glass, to propagate its likeness from thence further to the streaked Bodies? But as to the other Sensories the Business seems more hard to be unfolded, because the sensible Species, for as much as they are more Corporeal or thicker, cannot be conveyed to the Head with so quick a passage, and almost unperceiveable like Lightning; but as to these, it is to be understood, that altho' the Smell, Touch, and Taste, require more near and more Corporeal approaches of the Object, than either the Sight or Hearing; yet the Animal Spirits, which as it were *internuncii*, are placed within every Organ, and the chief Sensory, equally and as easily transmit the stroke or impulse of every Kind; Because as the Spirits are diffused thorow the whole Nervous System, and thorow the Head it self, as it were with a continued beaming, every Impression by the stroke of the Eye gets sooner from one bound to the other; yet the Character of the Object, is conveyed by the like Motion of their Neighbors, and as it were by a certain waving, even to the streaked Bodies.

In every Sension is required, First, That the sensible Species be impressed on the Sensory. Secondly, That it be carried thence, by the passage of the Spirits to the Common Sensory. Hence it follows, that for the Act of Sension, these two things are required. First, That the sensible Species be expressed, so as it may be impressed on the Sensory: And Secondly, That the Idea of the same Impression, be carried thence, by a like Affection and Motion, by the Spirits flowing in the intermediate passages, to the Common Sensory; for otherwise Sension is not performed, as it appears, when being intent on other things, we take not any notice of any Objects, tho they approach near to the Eyes, or the other Organs.

How the divers sensible Species are distinctly represented, in the Common Sensory. But here we may have a Cause of Doubting, how the manifold Species of sensible things, for the receiving of which, many Organs, and those diversly framed, are required; do all come together within, and are discerned in the same Common Sensory; For it is a wonderful thing, that the same streaked Body, consisting of a make not much unlike, should admit, and know distinctly in it self, the universal Idea's of Objects. As to this we may say, that the Images of things to be perceived by the Sense, are not distinctly painted in the Common Sensory, as on a Table; but every Impression there shown, depends on the Motion, as it were by a certain waving, of some Spirits separate from others, and within these or those peculiar Tracts of them: Nor is it irrational to affirm, that some Spiritual Particles are moved within the *Hypostasis* of the Sensitive Soul, and her the same Portion of it, whil'st others lye quiet, lying between them; for it plainly appears, and which afterwards is more largely shown, that within the Body of the Air, the lucid Particles are agitated, whil'st the rest lye at ease; yea also, that Sonorifick, yea and odorous little Bodies, and perhaps many others of another Kind, are moved by a distinct and peculiar Agitation apart by themselves, from the other texture of the Air; for both Images pass thorow, Sounds are poured out, Odors flow, warm or cold Effluvia's, and other little Bodies are variously carried; yet notwithstanding, others in the mean time are neither driven by force by some others, nor is the Consistency of the whole Air disturbed by some Singulars. Yea, various Impressions, not only pass thorow the Air unchanged, but also the Superficies of the Water; for we have observed in a River, or a Fish-pond, when many wavings have been stirr'd up, by various and divers strokes together, that all of them, however they meet one another, pass thorow, or cut one another, continue still distinct, and inconfused; why then may we not suppose, that in the Airy *Systasis* of the Soul, (which also is founded in a Watry Humor) there are Particles of a various and unlike make, and that manifold Species, by their

It is shown by an example of the Air, whose divers Particles have divers carryings forth.

Also by the example of Water, in which, many wavings being at once made, are all distinct.

Of Sense in General.

their passing thorow, may be at once brought to the Common Sensory, without Confusion? As for Example, Suppose that for seeing most Subtil and as it were Ætherial Particles, others almost Saline and notably moveable for the Hearing, and so for the other Senses, Spirits endowed after this or that manner, to be interwoven together, and every peculiar Sension to be produced, by a particular affection of them; to which it happens, that for the various passing thorow of the Spirits of so diverse a Nature, divers Tracts or Paths are produced, both in the Organ it self, and in the Common Sensory: and so, when the Animal Spirits are affected, which are of this or that Nature apart from others, which are of another Nature, and as there are beamings forth of several kinds, as it were within various Inlets or Passages; 'tis no wonder, if in divers Organs, distinct Acts of Sensions are performed; and that all of them, however different in Kind, and coming together from many ways, are shewn within the same Common Sensory, to wit, the streaked Bodies; because in this Marrowy Part, Spirits of every kind abound, and also passages of every sort of Conformation are found; therefore, every Impression impressed on any Organ from without, may be distinctly represented in this same Body. That it is so, it more clearly appears from hence, because both the streaked Bodies, and the way leading to these, consist of many white Ligatures, which seem as so many soft Nerves, or marrowy Tracts, for the divers ways of receiving the Impressions of sensible Species. *The like is in the Airy Hypostasis of the Corporeal Soul. For the divers Perceptions of which, together, in the Common Sensory, there are many and distinct Tracts produced.*

When a sensible Impression is brought through the Animal Spirits, being affected by a continued Series, from the Organ to the Common Sensory, if it be light it is there terminated, and the perception of the External Sense quickly vanishes, without any other Affection; but if (which more often happens) the impulse of the Object be stronger, the Sense excited from thence, like the vehement waving of waters in a Whirl-pool, both partly passes thorow the streaked Bodies, and going forward to the Callous Body, it oftentimes raises up two other Internal Senses, to wit, the Imagination and Memory, either one or both of them; and also is partly reflected from them, and from thence, by a declining of the Spirits, leaping into the Nerves, local Motions are made. *Sensible Impressions, as they are strong or weak, stir up other Powers, either more or fewer.*

For indeed Impressions of sensible things, from the beginning, furnish both the Imagination, with the Memory and Appetite, and induce the first attempts of local Motions. It is first effected, for as much as the sensible Impulse, is often propagated beyond the streaked Body, into the marrowy part of the Brain, or the *Cortex*, or the extream Confines of it. But local Motions ordinarily succeed to Sension, for as much as the Animal Spirits being struck back from the bolt or stay of the streaked Bodies, spring up outwardly, and as they enter these or those Nerves, by a certain Consequence, or by chance, they excite fortuitous local Motions, or depending on the previous Sense; for in the reciprocal exercise of these Faculties, to wit, of Sense and local Motion, (before Animals are imbued with Phantasie and Memory) almost the whole Animal Function consists; because Brutes or Men, whil'st they as yet know not things, want Spontaneous Appetite. So long therefore, they being destitute of the Internal Principle of Motion, move themselves or Members, only as they are excited from the impulse of the External Object, and so Sension preceding Motion, is in some manner the Cause of it. *All the other Powers of the Soul proceed at first from Sension.*

Therefore in every Sension, the Animal Spirits are moved; and their Motion being excited, in the utmost Sensory, from the approach of the Object, and harmonised according to its Impression, turns inwards, and (as hath been said) is conveyed to the first or Common Sensory: wherefore it is not to be thought, that the little Body's sent from the Object, do penetrate deeply, and enter the inward parts of the Brain it self (as some have asserted); but it suffices, that they being cast forth like Darts from the sensible thing, do affect the Spirits placed in the fore-front; and then, they from thence most swiftly pass thorow, by their Irradiation, the impressed Motion. As to the Parts, within which the Animal Spirits dwelling, do carry thorow, as it were by Pipes and Dioptrick Glasses, the impressed Species of sensible things; they are the Fibres, Nerves, and the Oblong Marrow, and chiefly the tops of it, to wit, the streaked Bodies. The Fibres being stretched forth in every Sensory, as it were Nets spread abroad, take the Particles of the Object, diffused and entring here and there, from which, whil'st the Spirits implanted in those Fibres, are affected, and are marked with the type or shaddow of the Objected thing, forthwith the same Character being expressed, by a continued Series of Spirits, passes forward, thorow the little Pipes of the Nerves, and the Medullary Trunk, into the streaked Bodies, and is there represented as upon a white wall; But the Rational Soul, easily beholds the Image of the thing there painted; or perhaps carried forward beyond into the Callous Body, the Imagination and Phantasie being excited, But after what manner Brutes perceive themselves to feel, and by reason of that Sension, they either imprint it in their Memory, or draw forth the Acts of the Appetite, we have shewn elsewhere. *The Animal Spirits pass thorow the sensible Species; and not the Effluvia of the Object, penetrate even to the head. The bounds and passages, by which, and into which the Species pass thorow.*

I 2 Con-

The Number of the Senses is well affirmed to be Five.

So many, and not more, are requisite.

Concerning the number of the outward Senses, we shall not recede from the vulgar Opinion, affirming them to be Five; for altho in some imperfect Animals, perhaps one Sense or two are only found; and thô it may seem, that the more perfect living Creatures may exercise many more than Five; because it is possible, that the Kinds of sensible things, far exceed that Number; yet it is seen, that those Five Organs of the Senses do abundantly enough supply the wants of all living Creatures: at least it seems good to the great Creator, not to grant to Man more than these, nor perhaps better than brute Beasts have obtained: Hence we may argue, that whereas the first Notions of all Simple things, are acquired only by the shewing of the Sense, and that Man, notwithstanding, is wont from thence to form Complicated Orations and Discourses, beyond what Brutes are able to do, that this is done by the Virtue and Operation of the Rational Soul in him, of which indeed Beasts are wholly destitute.

As to the Order or Method, by which we should treat of the Senses, particularly to be consider'd, if their worth or dignity be respected, it is confessed by all, that Seeing, and then Hearing should by right have the Prerogative; but indeed, because Knowledge more easily, and always more happily, proceeds from more Known things, to things less Known; therefore, I think to begin with the Touch or Feeling, as the most Common Sense; also for that the formal Reason of which seems to be most easily unfolded.

CHAP. XI.

Of the Senses in Particular, and first of the touch or Feeling.

The Sense of Feeling is more thick, but the most ample or large.

THe Touch or Feeling, tho it seems a Faculty of a lower Order, and as it were of a more gross Nature, because it apprehends not the object, unless it be brought near, and as it were pressed with its Arms; yet in some respect, it is more excellent by far than the rest; because this Sense beyond all others, receives and knows the Impressions of many sensible things, and those inflicted with greater variety; and so obtains a most large, and as it were a general Province. For since that the Sensible Qualities so called, are manifold and divers, to wit, Heat and Cold, Moisture and Dryness, Hardness, and Softness, and other Modifications of Bodies, their Make, Motions, Influences and Types, or Figures of Appearance, which in Concretes result from the mixtures and divorces, or the various Transpositions of the Elements, the greatest part of them by much, are the proper Objects of Feeling, and are discerned only by its Judgment, and as it were by its Will.

Exhibits Signs of Judgment to the rest of the Senses.

Further 'tis observ'd, That the Touch or Feeling, gives notes of Judgment to all the other Senses concerning uncertain Objects: for when the Sight cannot distinguish a Ghost or Spectre, from a solid Body, by the tryal of Feeling, presently the thing is put out of doubt; so likewise of the Smelling and Taste, which oftentimes put away sensible things brought to them, and fear their near Embrace, unless first tryed by handling.

It hath a mighty diffusive Sensory or Organ.

But this Power, as it enjoys great variety, as to its Objects, so it hath a most ample Sensory, and equally extended almost with the whole Body; That indeed few Parts, either within or without, but partake of this Sense. Further, this Faculty, for that 'tis of a general and common use, insinuates it self into the Organs of the other Senses, destinated to the private Office of every one: For both the Tongue and Nostrils, also the Eyes and Ears, perceive heat and cold, hardness and Softness, and other tangible qualities, no less than their proper Objects. If that we should further inquire, what the immediate Organ of Feeling is, in the several Members, or Parts? it may be said, that it is the Nervous Fibres, every where stuffed, and as it were distended with a Company of Animal Spirits;

Which are the Nervous Fibres.

which as the Strings of a Lute, as often as they are struck by the strokes of Tangible things, propagate the Impulse every where received, by the passages of the Nerves, forthwith to the Common Sensory. For as such Fibres being thickly set, are interwoven in the Skin, the fleshly Pannicle, the Membranes, and Musculous Flesh, yea, and with some of the Inwards, so that the Approaches of outward Tangible things, are not only felt in the Palm of the Hand, or the Superficies of the Body, but as often as

In all the Parts, both External and Internal.

sharp Humors are brought within into the Bowels, or that Preternatural Contents cause a pulling or hawling; a troublesome Sense of it is felt; wherefore the proper Organ of Feeling, is neither the Skin, nor the Flesh, nor the Membranes, as hath been asserted after this manner by some, and after that manner by others; but the

Fibres

Of the Sense of Feeling. 61

Fibres are that Organ, implanted in the whole frame or make of these or those Parts.

Altho many sensible Fibres are placed every where thorow the whole Body, also, thô there are divers and manifold Tangible qualities; yet it is not to be thought that these *Which Fibres,* Fibres, that they may be the better fitted for those qualities, are of a different Kind or *tho every where* Conformation; for neither are there some Fibres, by which heat, or others by which *of the same Con-* cold, or others different from either, by which other Tangible things are perceived; *formation;* but the same Fibres, are every where alike, and receive and distinctly carry the approaches of every Object, for neither do the sensible Fibres, planted in divers places or parts, acquire a diversity of Office, so that one Member should be the Index of heat, another of cold, or another of a several Tangible thing, but every one indifferently feel almost all Tangible things, from every Fibrous Part. The reason of the difference *Yet Exhibit va-* is, because the Fibres, thô of the same nature and frame, enter into divers ways of Con- *rious Species,* tractions or wrinklings, from the various strokes of sensible things; even as the strings *according to the* of an Harp, from the various strokes of the Musitian, give forth different Sounds; so *ches of tangible* also, the Fibres, which are the Instruments of Touching, are affected after a different *things.* manner, by the various impulse of Tangible things. For it seems, that these are irritated or provoked one way, with heat, and another way with cold, and so from the rest of the Qualities, after a manifold manner; therefore, the Animal Spirits implanted in them, enter into a peculiar way of Gyration or turning round, or of undulation or waving, according to which, the Spirits being harmonized, which flow within the passage of the Nerve belonging to those Fibres, do propagate the same Figure or Type of their carrying forth, to the Medullary Stock, and by its means, to the Common Sensory.

The Tangible Species being impressed after this manner, on the Nervous Fibres, or *Tangible Species* the outward Organ of the Touch, are not always carried from thence, or at least not *immediately* immediately to the same Common Sensory; for we have shewed elsewhere, that some *the Cerebel, or* Nerves spring from the Parts of the Brain, and others from those of the Cerebel; where- *to the streaked* fore, when they direct the Impulse, hap'ning outwardly immediately to the striated or *Bodies.* streaked Bodies, these latter convey the Sension from the Fibres, which are planted somewhere more inwards about the *Viscera* to the Cerebel; from which (without Knowledge of the Animal) oftentimes involuntary Motions are reported: as when Vomiting follows upon an Emetick Medicine, unknown, and against our Minds. If that this private Sension belonging to the Cerebel be a little stronger, and vehement passing thorow the same Cerebel, goes further even to the streaked Bodies; as when Medicines provoking the Stomach, more sharply, induce a Sension or trouble about the Heart, or otherways molestious, which they plainly give notice of.

Further, when the Tangible Impression arrives first and immediately at the streaked *And from thence* Bodies, if the same be light, it is there terminated, and the sensible Species presently *goes forward,* vanishes; but if the Impulse of the Object be somewhat stronger, it passes further to the *sometimes to the* Callous Body, and oftentimes to the Shell of the Brain; and therefore their Affections, *Viz. the Imagi-* Imagination, and sometimes Memory, gather'd from the touch of the thing, succeed: *nation, Memory,* and when, the sensible Species being also dilated to the Common Sensory, a divergency *and Appetite.* or bending down of the Spirits, from thence is reflected into the same Nerve, or others related to it, so it stirs up local Motions. These sort of Effects are sufficiently known by the Common Proverb, *Where the Pain is, there the Finger will be*: for it is implanted by Nature in every Animal, to rub or press the place with its finger or foot, where any sense of Trouble or Pain is.

As to the Kinds and Differences of Feeling, both are taken, either from the Objects, *The Kinds and* or from the various affection of the Sensory: the ways or means of the former, are so *Differences of* manifold, that they cannot easily be recounted; for hither ought to be referred (as we *Feeling, are ei-* said but now) the universal Tangible Qualities; By Tangible Qualities we understand *In respect of the* here, the various habitudes of Natural Bodies, which arise from the Crasis and Dispo- *Object,* sition of the Elements, of which they are made; as also from their Intestine Motion, or Effluvia's variously appearing in themselves; which kind of Modifications of Bodies, the Sense of Feeling chiefly finds out, and makes their knowledge or marks so certain, that when we do not believe the Scrutiny of the other Senses, we are wont to rest satisfied with the Examination of this.

Concerning the Species of Feeling, Constituted in respect of the Sensory, we shewed *In respect of the* even now, that the sensible Impression was immediately derived from the External Or- *Sensory.* gan, either to the streaked Bodies, or to the Cerebel: Therefore, for that Reason, Sen- *And so it is ei-* sion is either manifest, and knows plainly every thing; or private of which the Animal *ther manifest or* is scarce knowing: but the Consequence declares this Kind of Sension to have been stir- *private.* red up: for a Motion being made in any inward unseen, argues a previous sense of it to
have

62 *Of Tasting.*

Pleasant or Sad.

have been; as from the change of the Pulse, or a failure of Spirits, shews a certain Malignity to have affected the *Præcordia*, or the Cerebel.

In either of the aforesaid Kinds of Sension, to wit, whether the same be manifest or private, the Tangible Impression, either coming pleasantly to the Fibres, gathers together the Spirits implanted in them, and more nearly delights them, and strokes them with a soft and gentle rubbing, whence pleasure arises; or the Impulse of the same, pulling and wrinkling the Fibres, distracts and dissipates the Spirits one from another, and so Grief, Pain, or Trouble Succeeds: But concerning these Affections, *viz.* Grief and Pleasure, we shall have hereafter a more fit place to speak of them; so that it next remains, for us to proceed, from the Sense of Feeling, to its nearest Neighbor and Relation the Taste.

CHAP. XII.

Of the Taste.

The Taste a Kin to Feeling.

THe Taste is so like to the Sense of Feeling, that it seems to be a certain Species of it; and certainly the Object, in either Organ, ought to be brought near, and laid upon it; yea in tasting, to be admitted more deeply within the Pores and its passages.

The Sensory of the Taste discerns its Objects, and is delighted with those things that are Convenient.

Upon this Sense, depends chiefly both the Life and Vegetation of Animals; for this chooses and takes in Juice for nourishment convenient, and that by this Office it might be constantly and rightly performed, it is furnished with a faculty, or a certain implanted Judgment, whereby some wholesome and agreeable Aliments, fit for every Individual, are discerned from those that are disagreeable and hurtful; also further, as it were in reward of its work, it is delighted after a notable manner, with the Exercise of its Function; For unless convenient agreeable things, fit to be Eaten, move Spittle, and as it were prickle them with a most grateful pleasantness of Taste, the appetite of desiring or taking of Food is quickly extinguished, with oblivion or tediousness; so for the preserving the Individual, no less than the Species, Desire and Pleasure ought to be had.

Venus or Pleasure is necessary for the preserving of the Individual.

The Sensory of the Taste is not so diffusive, and almost Co-extended with the whole Body, as that of Feeling, but is limitted to one part only: yea, and its Sensible is of one Kind only, to wit, a Savoury thing, nor does it include, as the Tangible Quality, the Subjects of many Catagorical things. Indeed the chief and almost only Organ of the Taste is the Tongue; to which, after a manner, but obscurely, do consent the Palate and the Upper part of the Throat; But in all of them, the Nervous Fibres are the immediate Instruments of Sension; wherefore 'tis observed, that the Tongue is notedly more Fibrous than any other part, also consists of a very porous Contexture; for this end, that the savory Particles of the thing, might be more plentifully, and more deeply admitted, into the passages of the Sensory, and so meeting at once with many Fibres, might excite a more acute Sension: yea, it may be suspected, that whil'st the subtil Particles of the savory Humor are imbibed so deeply by the Tongue, the Animal Spirits do in some measure snatch the same, for their nourishment, and convey them inwardly, by the passages of the Nerves, towards the Brain; for it plainly appears, that in great Fastings or want of Food, and swouning or failure of Spirits, that a refreshment of them immediately follows, upon the first tasting of any noble Liquor.

The Organ of the Taste, is the Tongue, with the Palate, and Throat.

Eating is a certain Solution;

Wherefore one savour, oftentimes excludes another.

Eating is a certain Kind of Solution, whereby the savory Particles may be the better taken in, from the Food by the Sensory: Because, whil'st solid eatable things are reduced into bits, by Chawing, the Tongue, and other parts of the Mouth, and Throat, pour forth as it were a certain Menstruum, which washing and as it were Elixivating the savory little Bodies, carries them into the Sensory, and insinuates them into the Pores of the Tongue: Further, The savory Particles, because so impacted in the Sensory, do employ its passages, hence it comes to pass, that one savour not rarely excludes another; so sweet things being tasted, because they are clammy, and very obstructing, hinder or pervert the more exact taste of Wine; wherefore, that the hindred Faculty might be again restored, salt or sharp things are eaten, which may open the Pores of the Tongue, and clear away the sticking Viscousness.

As

Of Tasting.

As to the Nerves, which serve to the Fibres of the Tongue, thickly interwoven with it, and which carry the Impressions of Savours, to the chief Sensory, it seems, that they are of a double Kind: for as Nerves are inserted in the Tongue from both the Fifth, and the Ninth pair, and are every where distributed thorow its whole frame, with a most thick Series of shoots, it is very likely, that they are both Sensitive. Concerning the Nerves sent hither from the Fifth pair, the thing is out of doubt; and as from the same pair, other shoots are sent into the Nostrils, hence we may say, the reason is, of that Consent, which is between both these Sensories; but indeed, as to the Nerves bestowed also on the Tongue, from the Ninth pair, it may be something doubted, because it is commonly believed, that the Office of these serve to the Motion of the Tongue, and to Speech; wherefore, from the same pair are sent certain branches into the Muscles of the Tongue, and of the Bone called *Hyoides*, which without doubt are destinated for their Motion: Nevertheless, thô it be granted, that the Nerves of the Tongue and its Appendix, inserted from the Ninth pair, do bestow on them the moving Power (which indeed is necessary to this Part, as well for Tasting as for speaking; to wit, as the Tongue is very versatile, it takes in with delight the Savours from every corner or recess of the Mouth) yet what hinders, that however the same Nerves should not serve for both, to wit, Motion and Sense? For it appears, that many Nerves which serve for the Sense of Feeling, do in like manner serve for the performing of the Motions of those Parts to which they belong. Wherefore, as Tasting is a certain Species of Feeling, it is probable, that it enters in some measure through the moving Nerves of the Tongue it self; neither does it appear otherwayes, for what end Branches of the Nerves, derived from the Ninth pair into the Tongue, disperse such thick-set shoots into its whole frame, unless they should serve for the receiving of the Particles of Savours, coming from every Part. But for as much as after this manner, two Nerves of a distinct Original belong to the Tongue, and one of them arises from the Parts of the Brain, and the other from the Cerebel: Hence a Sension being carried inwards by the same, it is stay'd from either at the Common Sensory, and so according to the diverse Nature of the Object, a pleasant and delectable fruition, or an ingrateful and sad Aversion, at once in either Government the Imagination and the *Præcordia* are affected.

There is a sufficient indulgement to the Taste, for a reward of its necessary work, to wit, Eating; therefore its Objects are sought far and near, through the Regions of the whole World, yea and all the Elements are imployed. Further, as to its Ministry, all the rest of the Senses serve to this, for nothing pleases the Palate unless the Sight, and Hearing, Smell, and Touch approve it. 'Tis fit it should be so, for this Sensory, by which Food is conveyed for Humane Life, and that it might enjoy great variety, for the shunning of nauseous things; and use a guard upon the rest, for Discrimination; lest instead of Food, it might unawares take Poison.

The Speculation of Savours, (which are the next Object of Taste) contains in it self very many Pleasant, and no less Profitable things; wherefore I think it will not be from the Matter, to turn aside here a little into this Theory; and as we shall divide all Savours into Simple and Compound: First, we shall rehearse what Nature suggests of that Kind particularly, according to their several differences, both of themselves, and of the Subjects in which they are; Then Secondly, we shall add the Parallels, by what means, and by what service of Art, the same Savours in Subjects are produced anew, in which they are not by Nature; Thirdly, After what manner Savours both Natural and Artificial, are any way altered and changed in their Subjects, or wholly perish. It will be worth our while to discourse briefly concerning these, and lastly, somewhat of Compounded Savours.

Savours called Simple, are commonly counted to be Nine, *viz.* Sharp, Bitter, Salt, Acid or Tart, Astringent or Biting, Sowre, Sweet, Oyly, insipid or without Taste.

The first is sharp or biting Savour, such as is felt in Pepper or Pellitory, being chewed; which probably arises, as often as the Particles of any Body are smooth, and sharpned, and after that manner figured, like the stings of Nettles, that they may prick and very much dig into the Sensory. In Subjects indued with a sharp biting Savour, a volatile Salt, or an Alchalisat, or suffering a Flux from Fire, very much exceeds other Elements.

First, Concretes, which have by Nature Particles so figured, are accounted among Vegetables Hearts-ease, or Trinity-Herb, Pepper, Aron, Country-Mustard, Sea-Lettice, or Milk-thistle, Mustardseed, Pellitory, Ranunculus, *&c.* Of Minerals Arsneck, Sandarach, *&c.* Among Animals it is scarcely met with, nor among their Parts, a savour of this Kind, unless perhaps some Insects, as Cantharides, *&c.*

Secondly, Sharp biting Bodies produced by the help of Art, are Mercury Sublimate, Butter of Antimony, Strong-Waters, and Causticks, the fixed Salts of Herbs, made by burning to Ashes, Calcined Vitriol, the Rust of Brass, *&c.* The oftner things suffer

The Nerves sent to the Organs of the Taste, proceed partly from the Fifth pair.

Partly from the Ninth also, which serve for the Motions of the Tongue.

It is in like manner observed of the Touch, that the same Nerves serve both for Sense, and Motion.

Wherefore from the Taste of a pleasant thing, the Imagination and the Præcordia, are wont to be affected.

The rest of the Senses wait upon the Taste.

Savours the Object of Tasting. Simple or Compound: A Threefold Consideration of them, to wit,
1. *Whose Original are natural.*
2. *Artificial.*
3. *The Alteration or Abolition of either.*

Nine Simple Savours.

Sharp Savour.

1. *Which are sharp or biting of their own Nature.*

2. *Which are so produced by Art.*

Calci-

Calcination, and Fusion in the Fire, the more biting sharp they are made; because, by this means, the Pricks and Spears of the Particles are sharpned. An Example is in the fixed Salts of Herbs, calcined Vitriol, the Infernal Stone, &c. Bodies which are biting sharp, and Corrosives mixt together, and committed to the Fire, acquire a most sharp force of burning. An example is in Mercury Sublimate, and Stygian Waters, the reason of which is, because Salts of a like Kind, being mixed together, joyn their forces or edges, and are at the same time very much sharp'ned by the fire. It happens otherwise to Salts of a divers Kind, as are Spirits of Vitriol, and Salt of Tartar, mixed together; Sugar and Honey subjected to distillation, exhale a Caustick Water; also the Spirit of Wine highly rectified becomes biting sharp, and burning; because the Saline or Spirituous Particles, in both Substances being deprived of the sweetness of the others, put forth their Spears and Pricks.

3 By what means the biting sharpness is wont to be taken away, or altered.
Thirdly, Which was the Third Proposition, the biting sharpness in Bodies, both Natural and Artificial is put away or altered after various wayes. *Mercury* Sublimate highly Corrosive, if another quantity of live *Mercury* be added and sublimed, it takes away all acritude or biting sharpness, and it becomes insipid or without taste. The reason of which is, that when the Particles of the added *Mercury*, do grow to the little Spears of the Salts, they do thereby become more thick and obtuse. The Spirit of *Vitriol* and Salt of *Tartar*, being melted (which two are biting sharp and corrosive of themselves apart) if they be put together, lose all acritude; to wit, these Salts being of a divers Kind, viz. Fluid and Alchalisat; being put together, work mutually one upon another, by which means, the little Spears and Pricks of both are broken; even as if the edge of one Knife, should be rubbed against the edge of another. Plants and Herbs, which are naturally biting sharp, if they be macerated in White-wine, (or perhaps in any other Liquor) put away all their sharpness; and yet the Liquor becomes not at all sharp. In these sort of Concretes, all the acritude depends upon the volatile Salt, which being loosned, by the mixture, presently flyes away. For the same Reason, these sort of Herbs, being subjected to distillation, exhale almost an insipid water, and the dreggs of the Herbs remaining after distillation, is also insipid: Hence also some Herbs, which being green, abound with a sharp biting juice, being dryed, lose very much of their acritude; as Scurvy-grass, Water-cresses, and Brooklime, &c.

2. Bitter Savour.
Secondly, The bitter Savour or Taste, such as is principally in Gall and Wormwood, seems to be made, for as much as the Particles of its Body are planted with forked Pricks, which digging into the Sensory, not deeply, but only on the Superficies, cause a sad or sorrowful Sense; just as if the sharp-pointed fruit of the Teasle, should be sharply handled with ones hands. In Subjects indued with a bitter Savour, Salt, associated with Sulphur, and suffering an Adustion with it, Predominates.

1. Which are bitter of their own Nature.
First, Subjects which exhibit this kind of Savour naturally, among Vegetables, are Wormwood, Southernwood, Centaury, Colocynthida, Agaric, Fumitary, and almost all Herbs which grow in dry and mountany places; then Gumms, and Concrete juices, as Myrrh, Aloes, Opium, Ammoniac, &c. Among Minerals they are not easily met with. The Excrements of living Creatures, as the Gall, and Dung, the Liquor contained in the Bladder of the Gall; and so the Skins of some Birds are bitter.

2. After what manner, the bitterness may be produced anew.
Secondly, As to the second, Things which draw bitterness anew, they are Compounded Liquors; if in Cooking they are burnt, or are made too thick by Evaporation; hence Soot is bitter, and whatever things suffer adustion or burning. Sugared Aliments and sweet things are most easily Corrupted in the Stomach, and degenerate into a most highly bitter Humor.

3 By what means it is wont to be taken away, or altered.
Thirdly, As to the Third, a bitter Savour is most difficultly taken away, without the Destruction of the Subject, in which it is; as appears in Aloes, and Colocynthida, and Medicines prepared out of them. Yet New Beer, being something bitterish, by the boyling of Hops in it, grows sweet by clearing and a long fermentation: the reason of this we have shewed elsewhere. Further, Liquors, which grow bitter by reason of their Contracting an *Empyreuma* or burning to, if they be exposed for a long while in a moist Air, or distilled over again, mixed with Calcined Salt, they will partly lose their *Empyreuma*, or smatch of Fire, and bitterness.

3. Salt Savour.
3. Because Experience shews, that Salts for the most part do grow together, into many pointed, and diversly corner'd Figures, it is most likely, that the Salt savour is produced, when Particles of any Body, pointed with many Angles and Edges on all sides, do as it were cut into the Sensory, like as if little bits of broken Glass be strictly pressed in ones hand. In these Kind of Subjects, the Saline Principle excells the other Elements.

Salt things naturally.
First, Bodies naturally Salt, are scarce met with in the family of Vegetables, altho Plants and Herbs, almost all, owe their rise and growth to Salt. It is seen however that

Of Tasting. 65

that Sea Scurvigrass, and Capers have something of a salt Savour. Salt obtains the chief place among Minerals, and salsitude or saltness is chiefly eminent in Sea-Salt, in Salt that is dug up, Nitre, and Sal Gemmæ. The Excrements of Animals, to wit, the Dung, the Swet, the Serum, are Salt; Blood also participates something of the Nature of Saltishness.

Secondly, Those Salts which are made by an artificial means, are the fixed Salts of Herbs, made by incineration or burning to Ashes: Compounded Salts, to wit, Borax, Sal Ammoniac. A volatile Salt is drawn forth of Amber, Bones, Horns, and also out of the Blood of Animals, by Sublimation. *2. Things which are so made by Art.*

Thirdly, As to the Third, all natural Salts, if they be distilled often over again, pass into acetous or tart Liquors: The reason of which is, because these kind of Concretes suffer a divorce of the other Principles, by the fire, and so come more near to the Simple and Elementary Nature of Salt. Volatile Salts, at first white, if exposed to the Moisture of the Air, do melt into a reddish Liquor, not very Salt, and besides smelling like the stink of smoak or soot; because the mixture being loosned by the moist Air, the Saline Particles, for that they are volatile, many of them fly away, but in the mean time, the Sulphureous Particles, before subjugated, get the Dominion. *3. By what means saltness is wont to be taken away or altered.*

Fourthly, The Acid, or sour, or tart Savour or Taste, seems to be made, when the Particles of any Body are four pointed or corner'd (to wit, which appear with a smooth and acute point, and with a sharp Body, like a wedge made into a bigger bulk) so that which way soever applyed to the Sensory, they prick it, and by pressing it, something bind it up; and therefore they leave in it larger Incisions than any other Savour. This Kind of Savour, for the most part depends upon a fixed Salt, carried forth into a Flux. *4. The Acid or tart savour.*

First, Bodies naturally acid or sower, are among Vegetables, Pomecitrons, Oringes, Lemons, Berberries, Sorrel, Tamarinds, *&c.* Among Minerals scarce any to be met with, as I remember, nor is it easily to be found among Animals, unless perhaps the Melancholly Juice, the ferments of the Stomach, and Spleen, the Pancratic Juice, and also the fasting spittle of a Man, may be said to be something Acid. *1. Natural Acids.*

Secondly, Made Acids, are Vinegar, and the Spirit of it, or the Liquor distilled: The Melanchollic Humor preternaturally begotten in the Body, which often like the Spirit of Vitriol, becomes Acid, and almost Corrosive. Vitriol, Salt, and Sulphur, being whole, and tasted in their solid substance, shew no kind of acidity, if they be made subject to Chymical Operation, send forth a Liquor highly acid; the reason of which was shewed but now. *2. Made Acids.*

Thirdly, As to the Third, Chymists say, that acetous Spirits, to wit, of Sulphur, Salt, Vitriol, *&c.* by a long Digestion and Circulation, do grow sweet. All acetous Mineral Spirits, also distilled Vinegar, and the juice of Vegetables; if they dissolve any Body, by knawing or corroding it, as Corals, Pearls, or any Precious Stones, put away their acidness; because the Particles of the fluid Salt, in the acid Stagma or Menstruum, are fixed to the *Alchali* Salt in the mixture. Moreover, these Kinds of Spirits, and acetous Liquors, if they are mixed, either with Oil of Tartar, or with the fixed Salts of Herbs, loosed by Deliquium, loose their acidity. The Spirit of Vinegar being poured upon Salt of Tartar, and drawn off by distillation, becomes insipid. Spirit of Vitriol poured upon Quick-silver, and drawn off by distillation, putting away its acidity, acquires a taste like Allum; and if we may believe *Helmont*, passes by Coagulation into true Alum. Distilled Vinegar impregnated with the solution of *Minium*, or red Lead, grows wonderfully sweet. *3. By what means an Acid savour is wont to be taken away, or altered.*

5. The Sower, austere, or binding or astringent Savour, arises in Bodies, whose Particles are stuffed with very many little Spears and Hooks, which in chewing, being rolled upon the Sensory, are fixed to it, and greatly draw together, and pull its Fibres; not much unlike, as if a Comb, which Cards Wool, should be drawn up and down upon the hands. In substances indued with an austere savour, a fixed Salt, enwrapped with the Particles of the earthy Element, predominates. *5. Austere or sower Taste.*

First, Bodies naturally austere, among Vegetables, are the Fruit of the Medlar-Tree, of the Dog-Bryer, of the Cypress-Tree, Flowers of Pomegranat, Galls, Slows, Sumach, *&c.* Among Minerals Alum, Iron, Vitriol. Among living Creatures, or among their Parts, there is not as I remember, any austere savour to be met with. *1. Naturally austere things.*

Secondly, Bodies Artificially produced, which have an austere, sower or rough savour, are all made Vitriols, to wit, the Vitriol of Silver, of Steel, of Tin, of Copper, *&c.* The reason of which is, because in these Minerals, the Saline Particles, are very much intangled with Terrene, and they continue in the same state, when they are *2. Made austere savours.*

K drawn

66 *Of Tasting.*

drawn forth from their Substances, by the soluted Mixtion. Spirit of Vitriol being drawn from Mercury, by frequent Cohobations, acquires a Pontick or Aluminous Savour.

3. By what means an austere or rough Taste, is wont to be taken away, or altered.

Thirdly, As to the Instances, by which an austere, sower, or rough taste, may be taken away out of all Substances, it is to be observed, that Vitriol of every Kind, by long distillation and circulation with the Spirit made of Wine, grows sweet, and loses its astringent force. If waters impregnated with Vitriol, be poured into Oil of Tartar, there will be precipitated a certain thickish Matter wonderfully sweet. Steel, Tin, or Lead, being dissolved in Vinegar, and Coagulated by Evaporation, go into sweet Salts. Further, it is a common Experiment: If having before tasted Vitriol, you take the fume of Tobacco at your Mouth, the austere taste at first impressed on the Sense, is changed into a plainly honied sweetness; the reason of which is, because the Sea-salt Particles, such as are in Vitriol, being mingled with the Sulphureous, out of the burnt Tobacco, create a sweet Savour: from whence also we may Collect, that Sugar and Honey, are of a Sulphureous-saline Nature; which also clearly appears, by their distillation, for as much as they, like Salt Minerals, yield an Acid and very Corrosive Stagma.

VI. A sower Taste.

6. Of Kin to the austere, is the acerb or sower taste, the Particles of whose subject, are indued with little Tenters or Hooks, or Claws, but which are more dull and blunt, and with which they strike the Sensory, and stop up its little Pores, and being once fixed, they are not easily removed; whence a stupor or numness in the Teeth and Palat is caused; not unlike Burdocks, which being fixed to the Skin, become troublesome, and are not easily shaken off. In acerb or sower biting Bodies, a fluid Salt, implicated with an earthy Matter, excells.

1. Bodies naturally acerb or sower.

First, Bodies naturally sower among Vegetables, are unripe Fruits; as Grapes, Pears, and Apples, and most of all Wildings, Crabs, or wild Apples, tho kept till they are mellow: also sower Herbs: Among Minerals, or Animals, there is nothing easily to be met with, that has a sower Taste.

2. Made sower things.

Secondly, Bodies that are made sower anew, are chiefly Wine and Beer, degenerating into a deadness, through Age or Thunder; also Leaven, or Bread too much leavened. Broths and Milk-meats, if they Contract a settlement and hoariness, become sower: because in all those Concretes disposed to Corruption, the Saline Particles being exalted, and tending towards a Flux, carry forth also earthy Particles involved with themselves.

3. By what means the sower Taste, is wont to be taken away, or altered.

Thirdly, As to the taking away of this Taste, we have observed, That sower Fruits do grow sweet, either by the goodness of the Air, and Sun; in sower Fruits brought to maturity: or by the goodness of the Ground or Soil, as when wild Apples transfated to a good Soil grow sweet; the reason of either is, because the Spirituous and Sulphureous Particles before subjugated, at length Predominate over the Saline. If Wine degenerated into deadness, is impregnated with new Lees of *Tartar*, it shall recover its Vigor: The like happens, if a Can of good Wine be poured into a Vessel of sower Beer or Ale. Wine growing dead, if it be distilled, often yields a sweet Spirit, and in no less quantity, than if the Wine had been in its full strength: because the Spirits before subjugated in that Mixture, recover their Dominion by distillation.

VII. The sweet savour.

Seventhly, The sweet savour seems to be made, for as much as the Particles of any Body are so figured, into soft prickles, that they tickle the Sensory, with a soft rubbing, and from thence stir up a delightful Sense of Pleasure; like as if feathers were applyed to the Sides, or the Soles of the Feet. In these the Saline Principle seems to be associated, with Sulphureous and Spirituous, and when they are, in like manner are carried forth.

1. What are naturally sweet.

First, Those which are naturally sweet, are among Vegetables, first Sugar, and Manna; then Cassia, ripe Fruits, Grapes, Raisons, some Roots, as Parsnips, &c. Among Animals, some ascribe Honey, but others more rightly, say that is swet out of Plants, and gathered by Bees. Among Minerals nothing (that I know) hath naturally a sweet Savour.

2. Sweets prepared by Art.

Secondly, The things which have a sweet Taste, and are made by Art, are the Sugar of Lead, Salt of Steel, Lythargires, yea, and out of many other Bodies, Vinegar extracts a sweet Salt. Tasting Vitriol before-hand (as was said) and then taking a Pipe of Tobacco, the smoke grows sweet like Honey. In this, and in the former instances, whilst the Saline little darts grow to the Sulphureous Particles, or Saline of another Kind, both of them become more blunt. An *Alchalisat* Spirit, and the fixed Salt of any Body, being mixed, and circulated by a long digestion, acquire a sweetness. Barley soaked in Water, when it begins to sprout, and dried with a gentle fire, grows exceeding sweet: And Wheat in like manner also, if being wet, it sprouts yields a wonderfully sweet

Of Tasting.

sweet Meal; the reason of which is, because by that Artifice, the Sulphureous and Spirituous Particles, overthrown by the Earthy, get their Liberty.

Thirdly, There are many Instances, by which sweetness is abolished; for all sweet things too much boiled, grow bitter. Sugar or Honey, by distillation, yield at first an insipid Phlegm, then sharp and burning Spirits; In the dead Head remaining after distillation, is a burning Salt, and an insipid Earth, and whatever is sweet perishes. Further, Sugar or Honey being mixed with a great quantity of Common Water, and distilled through a Bladder, yield a burning Water, like the Lees of Wine distilled after the same fashion. In both these, and in the following Instance, the additional sweetnesses are bruised, by the saline little darts, Sugar of Lead being fused by the fire, melts into meer Lead; if it be distilled in a Retort, if we may believe *Beguinus*, it will produce a burning and sweet smelling Spirit. *3. By what means sweetness is taken away, or altered.*

8. The unctuous or oyly Savour, seems to be produced, when the Particles of any Body are very Spherical and round, which neither hawl, prick, nor tickle the Sensory, but only stroke it with a gentle and soft coming to it. In these, the Sulphureous Principle predominates. *VIII. An Oyly Taste.*

First, Bodies naturally Unctuous or oyly, among Vegetables, are ripe Olives, the Turpentine-Tree. The Larix, and some sweet smelling Gums naturally sweating forth. Among Minerals, Asphaltum, Bitumen, Amber, Sperma Ceti, and some fat Earths, and Ochers: Of Animals, and their Parts, the Sewet, Marrow, and Fat. *1. In which it is by Nature.*

Secondly, Unctuous things prepared by Art, are Butter, Cream, Oyls, press'd out of Fruits and Seeds, as Oyl of Nuts, of sweet Almonds, also Oyls drawn out of Seeds, Woods, Gums, and Resines by distillation. *2. In what things it is wont to be produced by Art.*

Thirdly, Altho unctuosity is most difficultly taken away from the Subjects, yet it is wont to be lessen'd: for so Unctuous Bodies, if they grow stale, or are too much boiled, or otherways grow hot by shaking, losing their smoothness, become rank, and prick and dig the Sensory. Further, Sewet and Fat, if they be long exposed to a moist Air, contract a settlement, and become hoary, and then are resolved into Water, or a corrupt Earth. In this, and in the former instance, whil'st the mixture of the Body is resolved, some Sulphureous Particles fly away, in the mean time the remaining lose their Dominion. *3. How it is taken away or alter'd.*

9. An insipid Savour or Taste, seems to be made, when the Particles of any Body, are indued with superficial little Darts, not at all sharp, but smooth and discharged; which enter not into the Pores of the Sensory, and no ways dig or hawl it. In these, the Principle either of Water, or Earth, predominate over the rest. *IX. An insipid Savour.*

First, Bodies naturally insipid or tastless, are Common Water, especially Rain Water, some cold Herbs, the raw white of an Egg, &c. Altho in the whole world, there is nothing insipid simply, yet Speech is wont to apply it to them things, in which some one of those Savours, are not eminently, which we have before recounted. *1. In what things it is by Nature.*

Secondly, That Savory things may become Unsavory, the more acute Particles ought wholly to fly away, or be very much broken. Herbs long kept, also many more things, if they be distilled by a moderate heat, yield almost an insipid Liquor. *2. How it is wont to be produced.*

Thirdly, Insipidness it self, sometimes is taken away; for insipid Water, if it stand long, that it putrifie, acquires a stink and mouldy Savour: The white of an Egg boiled hard, has something a sharp taste. In these kind of Instances, some active Elements, being before subjugated, get strength. *3. By what means it is taken away.*

Besides these Kinds of simple Savours, which are as it were the Elements of the rest, there remain yet many Complications of these simple ones, as the Savours rehearsed are conjoyned one among another: And for as much as by the Wisdom of Nature, to satisfie all Palates, and by the Luxury of Art, that she might please the Throats of some, manifold mixtures of Savours have been produced, that almost nothing to be eaten, is found simple and without Sawce or Condiment. The several Compositions of these, is a thing almost impossible to enumerate; it shall suffice for the present, that we note some of the more noted Conjugations, and their Affections, as they are grateful or ingrateful to the Palate. *Compounded Savours.*

The first Conjugation, and that most grateful to the Palate, is of acid and sweet, of which sort are generous Wine, Confections prepared out of Citron, Wood-Sorrel, Berberries, &c. Sugar'd things, and sharp things pickl'd, with Sugar. Secondly, Sweet and Astringent, as also sweet and sower, are well Consociated: as in Marmalade of Quinces, Candied Bulloes, Cyder drunk with Sugar, &c. Thirdly, Sweet and oyly yield a grateful Savour to the Palate, but that brings a nauseousness to the Stomach, as in Milk-meats, Sugar'd-meats, and Pasty-crust, &c. Fourthly, Sweet agrees not with biting, bitter, or salt Savour. Fifthly, nor doth a bitter Savour of it self, agree with any other: it is grateful to the Palate, well-tempered with the sweet. Sixthly, Salt-savour *Compositions of Savours, which are more or less grateful.*

savour best agrees with the biting sharp, as in flesh seasoned with Salt and Pepper, it is an ingrateful Sawce with the oyly. Seventhly, The Acid, Astringent and Sower, are well associated with the sweet, not with the rest.

There are more Kinds of some other Compounded Savours, which we have no time now to recount. But there are in respect of the Taste, as the Compounded Tunes of Harmony in respect of Hearing, in both sensible not simple Species of one Kind, but are carried manifold, and variously Complicated to the Sensory. It now remains for us to pass from the Taste, the Object of which we have largely handled, to the other Species of the Senses.

CHAP. XIII.

Of the Sense of Smelling.

IT seems that the Smell is a more Excellent, and a little more Sublime Faculty, than either Tasting, or Touching; to wit, because its Object is more subtle, and comes to the Sensory, with a thinner Consistency: for there is no need to put upon the Organ, the more thick substance of the mixture; but it suffices, that the Effluvia's or Breath, sent from odorous Bodies, thô at something a remote distance, be inspired into the Nostrils, together with the Air.

The use of the Smell, to discern Aliments as a distance.

Living Creatures are furnished with the Sense of Smelling for this end, to wit, that agreeable and wholesom Aliments may be known, and discerned from disagreeable and hurtful; for because it were an incongruous and dangerous thing, to take in presently into the Mouth, all things offered to be eaten, and to be examined by the Taste, lest perchance Venomous and Stinking things, carelesly taken in by the Palate, should bring loathing or hurt to it, the Smell examines first the thing at a distance, and refuses those rotten things, or guilty of any other very infestous quality, without receiving any hurt by the Contagion.

This is more excellent in Brutes than in Man.

This Kind of Primary use is seen more excellently in brute Animals, than in Man; for they by this Index only, most certainly know the Virtues of Herbs, and of other Bodies, before unknown, yea hunt out, and easily find their absent Food, thô hidden from them, by the Smell. But that the Noses of Men are less quick or sagacious, it ought not (as some would have it) to be ascribed to the abuse of the Faculty, but the Cause lyes in the defect of the Organ it self; for this is not so accurately required for the distinction of Humane Food, where Reason and the Intellect are present: For that Reason the inferior Powers in Man, exist less perfect by Nature, that there might be a place left, for the exercise and dressing of the more superior.

The Organ of the Smell described.

As to what belongs to the Organ of Smelling, we have largely enough unfolded it in our Discourse of the Nerves; to wit, we have shewed, that within the Caverns of the Nostrils, are placed tubulated Membranes or like Pipes, which contain sensible Fibres, most thickly interwoven. Into these Membranes, very many small Nerves are sent from either Mamillary Process, passing thorow the holes of the Seive-like Bones; but those Mamillary Processes, as they are plainly soft Nerves, arise in the Medullary Trunk, nigh the streaked Bodies; wherefore, when the odorous steams, strike upon the Fibrous, and very sensible Membranes, forthwith an impression of the sensible thing, is carried by the passage of the Nerves into the Mamillary Processes, and from thence into the streaked Bodies.

Further, We have formerly declared, why the Smelling Nerves, divided without the Skull are harder, but united within it are not only softer, but also tubulated or like Pipes, and for the most part in Brutes, filled with clear Water: There is no need to repeat it here again, nor what we have declared there, concerning other Nerves, coming from the Fifth pair, and inserted also into the Organ of Smelling: Of which certainly the Office is, to cause a certain Sympathy and consent of action, between the Smell and Taste, and something also between the Sight and it.

Nerves of a several Kind, serve for Smelling.

I know some attribute the office of Smelling altogether to these Nerves, arising from the Fifth pair, denying it to the Mamillary Processes, and from hence they render a reason, not only of that consent, between the Nose and the Palate, from whence it comes to pass, that the same Objects are embraced or refused, but also, wherefore it happens, that one Sense being lost, that oftentimes the other perishes; to wit the Cause of this

they

they say is nothing else, than that both Sensories do borrow the branches of their Nerves, from the same Trunk of the Fifth pair. But this Objection is easily overthrown, because the Nerves of a twofold Original, are bestowed not only on the Sensory of the Smell, but also of the Taste. For the Tongue receives more and greater Branches from the Ninth pair, than from the Maxillary Trunk of the Fifth pair: to wit, that if the Nerves of one Kind be obstructed, the Animal Function may be performed, by those of the other Kind. Concerning this then we may say, that the Principle Nerves serving to the Organ of Smelling, are derived from either Mamillary Process, also, that the Nerves on which the Sense of Tasting chiefly depends, are sent from the Ninth pair: Nevertheless, some secondary Nerves, or that are as it were taken in, are distributed to either Sensory, (as also to the Eye) far fetch'd from the Fifth pair: for this end, that there might be an affinity or mutual respect, between the Taste and the Smell, and between both and the Sight: hence therefore the Taste almost admits of no Object, unless that the Smell first approves of it: but both Faculties do require, that sensible things do first stand to the examination of the Eyes.

But that the loss of one of them, oftentimes brings in the defect of the other, as it is sometimes observed in a Pose, or Stopping of the Head, that losing the Smell, the Taste is lost also: the reason of it is, because either Sensory, being planted near, are both at once overthrown by the same serous Matter, poured forth from the Blood, and apt to be too much stopped: for both the tubulated Membranes of the Nose, and the frame or substance of the Tongue it self, are made of a very rare, and as it were spongy Texture: wherefore, the Pores and Passages of either Organ, are wont to be overflown by the serous flood, and the sensible Fibres in both, in like manner to be obstructed, which happens, because when as the Nostrils and Tongue ought to be moistned, with a continual Humor, either of them are punished more grievously than other Parts, by the shower of the Serum issuing forth, so both on every light Cause, become obnoxious to the same Evil. *Hence the reason it is had, of that Consent between the Smell and the Taste.*

Why one being wanting, the other for the most part is Defective.

CHAP. XIV.

Of the Sense of Hearing.

After the Smell and Taste, of which we have already treated, we shall next speak of Hearing; which as to the use, is far more Excellent than the other Senses; for as much as by its help chiefly, Sciences and Learning are acquired, also by whose instinct, the Passions are excited; yea, and are wont to be governed and allayed; further as to Activity, this Sense is much more Efficacious, because having got a larger Sphear, perceives its Objects at a great distance, and admits not the sensible Species, unless brought in a more thin consistency: For that it is the Interest of living Creatures, to know some remote things by Contact, and often placed out of Sight, because they may be timely prevented, if they should be inimical and disagreeable, but if thought amicable, that they may be come to, and apprehended; the Hearing serves for either Intention, and by its sign, the Marks and Symbols of approaching Bodies are received afar off. *The Excellency of Hearing, as to Use and Activity.*

Because the Hearing is always performed at a distance, and a sound comes often farther than the Effluvia's of a sounding Body, can be admitted; therefore, this Sense is supposed to be made even as Sight, by reason of a certain activity of the Medium it self, or by a Motion, and as it were a certain waving of little Bodies, which flow in it; so as the sounding Body, moves by its Vibration or shaking the Particles diffused in the intermediate space, and they being moved, at length affect the Sensory; but they conceive a certain Figure of their carrying forth, according to the Particles first agitated, and they propagate the same in others, and then in others, or move forward, as it were by undulation, and so the sound, still retaining the Character or Type of the first Impression, is continued even to the Ear. *Is performed at a distance, by reason of the Activity of the Medium.*

Altho by the consent of all, the Air is said to be the Medium, that carries the sounds, yet this ought not to be understood of the whole Atmosphear of the Air, and Breaths; for neither is the audible Species poured forth, by the Motion of this most fluid Body, as it were by a waving of Waters; because this much sooner runs thorow, than the Body or Consistency of the whole Air is wont to be moved, and propagate its Fluctuation, *The Medium carrying sounds is the Air, but not the whole frame of it.*

Of Hearing.

as may be difcerned plainly by the fucceffive blowing of the Winds, and bending of Trees, and the tops of Corn, which happens, becaufe any found, whether great or fmall, whether it comes with or againft the wind, is carried to a certain place, always with an equal time; which would be otherwife if it obey'd the waving of the whole Air, or fhould depend upon that: Further, That the whole frame of the Air doth not wave, by reafon of the tranfmiffion of the found, appears by this; becaufe, if a Lamp be held in a little Bell, whil'ft many other Bells being ftruck together, yield a mighty found, its flame will hardly fhake, much lefs will it be moved up and down hither and thither, by the moved Air.

The Sonorifick Particles feem to be Saline little Bodies, interwoven with the Air. Hence it follows, that fome Sonorifick Particles, or Caufing founds, are diffufed thorow the Air, and as they are more fubtil than the little Bodies of the Air, and are indued with a more rapid Motion, the Tranfmiffion or Propagation of the found, depends upon the peculiar motion and waving of thefe, made apart from the inclination of the whole Air. We have elfewhere fhewn, in the texture of the Atoms of the Air, that there are contained Luminous or Nitrous Particles, by the inkindling, and by the moft fwift trajection, and reflection of thefe, Light, the appearances of Colours, and the Images of all things are produced. And befides thefe moft thin and moveable Bodies, which feem to be of a certain fiery Nature, and interwoven with the Air, and by the private waving of which, the vifible Objects are carried to the Organ, it is likely, that certain other Particles of another Kind, and thofe perhaps Saline, are diffufed thorow the rare and moft fluid Conftitution of the Air, by which, whil'ft they are ftrucken and fwiftly moved, and apt to be figured, according to the Idea's of Sounds, the Organ of the Hearing is alfo affected, and by this means receives the Impreffions of fenfible things. For it feems, that the Sound-caufing little Bodies fwimming in the Air, and interwoven with a certain Continuity in its Pores, and thickly fet in its paffages, are placed after that manner, that when a Motion is impreffed, in any Portion of them, by the ftriking againft a folid Body, they being agitated according to the Character of the Impreffed Motion, move or fhake others planted round about, and they again others, which are next to them, and fo, when the fame Motion is propagated round on every fide, by a fucceffive affection of the fame Particles, (as when a Stone being caft into a fmooth water, many little Circles beginning after one another, and unfolding themfelves, create an Impreffion of the firft ftroke in every part) leffer types of the found, and almoft innumerable, take the place one of another, or fill up the room of the firft Prototype found, excited according to the folid Body, and from thence on every fide waved, according to the Symbolical Particles fucceffively moved; even after the fame manner, as when the rayes of

The Prototype of a found, by and by ftirs up innumerable Ectypes. Light are reflected from an Opacous or fhaddowy Body; for as much as they being fent at hand from every part of the Object, do meet together in a moft thick Series of Cones, in every place, and fo create infinite Images of the fame thing, vifible in all places: In like manner alfo, whil'ft the Sonorific Particles leap back from a folid Body, they caufe the audible Species to be every where reprefented, according to the ftroke there made upon them, in the whole Sphear of Vibration, whether by a like Contortion, or Gyration, or any other ways of Conformation in Motion, of the fymbolar Particles.

How the Sonorifick Particles, differ from the luminous. But altho there are found Sonorific little Bodies fomething like the luminous, they are differenced notwithftanding in many things; for firft of all, their Motion is much more flow than the luminous, which clearly appears from a Gun being difcharged at a diftance, for it is fometime after the flafh reaches the Sight, that the report comes to the Ears. But the luminous Particles, tho they eafily pafs thorow the more folid Diaphanous Bodies, yet not thorow thick fhaddowy or Opacous Bodies, tho they are made of a more thin or rare texture; or ftick in the chinks: On the contrary the waving of a

Thefe are carried only in ftrait-lines, thofe in all. found, does not fo eafily pafs thorow Glafs, but the fame is often heard within a Chamber, that is impervious of Light, or where Light cannot enter. Hence it may be conjectur'd, that the rayes or beams of Light, how fubtil and thin foever they be, are carried only in ftrait Lines; for whether they at firft ftream forth, or are broken in the altered Medium, or are reflected from an objected Body, they every where pafs forward, and obferve the Line of direction, and pafs thorow the oblique and winding paffages, not with a turning paffage or going thorow; but the founding Particles, being excited into Motion, infinuate themfelves within the bending pores and blind holes, like the flowing of Waters; but thefe Kind of little Bodies, which are the Vehicles of

Why they feem to be Saline. founds, I fufpect to be of a Saline Nature, for this reafon; becaufe the Particles of this Element, are moft of all Moveable and Active, next to the fiery and Nitrous Sulphureous; for it is feen, that Glafs, and Metallick Bodies, which abound with very much Salt, being ftruck, yield a found excelling all others: Alfo it makes for it, for as much as in a great Winter Froft, when the Atmofphear of the Air abounds with Saline Particles, a found becomes more clear, and is carried farther.

So

Of Hearing.

So much concerning the Sonorifick Particles, as much as we are able to get by Conjecture; concerning their Nature, Subsistence, and wayes of carrying forth, or of waving. As to these, what at first was propounded, concerning the Sense of Hearing it self, there remains yet to be unfolded, by what means, and for what occasions, these Particles interwoven with the aerial Body, are stirred up by a sounding Body into Act; then how the same being moved affect the Sensory.

As to the former, there are infinite ways, whereby the aforesaid Particles are stirred up into Act, or by which sounds are wont to be produced; whatsoever percussion of a solid Body, yea and almost every vehement Compulsion of the Air, when resisted, yields a sound. There are very many Varieties of these, but the Universal, or at least the chief Causes of sounds, may be not improperly reduced to two ways of being made; to wit, either that a solid Body being struck, and so affected with a Vibration or shaking, drives together the Air, and with it the Sonorific Particles, and the stroke being most swiftly repeated, causes them to shake or to wave; Or secondly, the Air, and with it the Sonorific Particles, being driven into a more narrow space, whil'st they go forth by Compression, are struck against the solid Body, and are driven by it into a vibration or shaking. By reason of the former way, all solid Bodies, struck by solids, yea and hollow Metallick Bodies, a Drum, the strings of an Harp, and other Musical Instruments, furnished with strings, when they are stroke, yield a sound; in all which, a vibration being excited from the stroke and shaking Body, and impressed on the Sonorific Particles, is the whole Cause of every produced sound, or of long Continuance, and also the but of a minutes durance or sounding. For both Metals, also Stones, and Wood, and other solids, being struck, make the Air to tremble and yield vibrations or shakings, in some measure like Bells, and the strings of an Harp: Wherefore, when by the Finger or any soft Body being lay'd upon them, that shaking is stopt, presently the sound is intercepted. In the latter Rank, to wit, where the Air is compelled or straitned, whil'st it strives for liberty, striking against the solid Body, produces a sound, ought to be placed sounds, which are excited by speaking, wind Instruments, letting off of Guns, and the passage of winds thorow strait places.

As it thus appears, by what means the Sonorific Particles are stirred up into act, there remains a no less difficulty, concerning the way, whereby they affect the Organ of Hearing, that by it a Feeling or Sension is produced. We shewed before, that by reason of the aforesaid Particles being interwoven with the Air, and successively moved with a continued Series, the Impression of a sound is diffused every where, into a Round or Orb; Further, we Note, that if their waving promotion meet with any stop, the same being thereby reflected, or forced by another thing, it in like manner affects other Particles, wherever met with, and so is still broken into more sounds, which are carried hither and thither into every part; which is the reason that sounds climb over Houses, being sent forth at hand, return back, enter into every hole and chink, and easily propagate themselves into secret places and recesses, where light cannot enter: In the mean time, all sounds, both direct and reflected, and which are diverted aside, and which become less and numerous, from greater refracted and divided sounds, and variously result, exactly bear the Character of the Prototype of the same sound: Hence it comes to pass, that the Hearing being planted in every place, it receives the same sound in specie, and oftentimes articulate.

But as to the second Proposition, for the manner of doing, whereby by the Sense of Hearing is performed, we think that first of all, the Structure of the Organ it self ought to be considered; in which, that which being utmost receives the first strokes of the sound is the Ear: This part being largely spread, by degrees grows narrow, till the hole made more narrow, leads inward to the den of the Ear. The use of the Ear is to gather together the Sonorific Particles, coming to it spread abroad and dispersed, and so many; that the Impression may be made more sensible, to direct it inwards towards the Sensory. In imitation of this natural Instrument, are wont to be made the Artificial whispering Instruments, which like a Pipe or Trumpet, by introducing many Sonorifick Particles, supplies the defect of Hearing. The Ears in most Beasts are moveable, that they might be turned every way, to any noise, and might receive a more certain notice of the sound, otherways uncertain; yea, it is probable, that mens Ears are moveable by Nature because they have hanging Muscles, but that by the continual use of the Head-bands, which they make use of in Infants, this faculty is taken from them.

After the Ears, follows the Cave or Den of the Ear, leading obliquely towards the inward Parts. Whil'st the Sonorifick Particles pass thorow the turning and winding passages of this, the same, by reason of the frequent strikings and refractions against the sides, encrease the sensible Species; after the same manner, as is seen in Cornets, and wreathed Instruments, by which the sound is very much strengthen'd. Also this

further

further appears, for that the Hollows or Cloysters in some Walls, are wont to be so artihcially made, that a low Voice whisper'd, being transmitted by the same, may be heard at a great distance. Moreover, the aforesaid Den of the Ear ought to be oblique and turning, that its more inward parts mought be defended from the easie meeting with of Injuries; and for this reason, there is there placed a bitter Wax, sweat forth from the little Arteries; so that if any little living Creatures, should by chance creep into the Ear, they might be there entangled, or at least driven away by the Bitterness, as Worms by Gall. This yellow stuff without doubt is of the same Nature with that which is destinated for the Bladder of the Gall.

The Drum. Nigh to the most intimate recess of this Den, a thin Membrane is placed, with a Circular Bone, fitted to the same, which wholly shuts up the Cavity of the Ear, and distinguishes the Interior Cloyster from the Exterior; so that the Impulse of the sound, shaking this Membrane like a Drum, delivers the Impression to the Sonorifick Particles planted beyond, and they being moved, affect the Fibres, with the Auditory or Hearing Nerve.

Three little Bones about the Drum, with the Muscle and Ligament.
The Hammer.
About this Membrane, three little Bones, with a Muscle and Ligament, and some other Parts, are placed; from which being throwly view'd, and truly consider'd, the Use and Offices of the Drum, and its whole Appendix, are clearly learnt. The first of these is a little smooth Bone, lying upon the more inward part of the Drum, and sticking to it, this is commonly called the Hammer, either from its figure, or rather because it is thought to strike and knock against the Drum; when indeed, this Bone affixed to the Boss or Shield of the Membrane, strikes not against it, but bends inward, and draws it with it. Also, besides this little Bone, is united with many other little Bodies, for the Tendon of the Muscle, which lifts it up, and bends it inward, is inserted into its sharp Process, and the other more blunt extremity of the Hammer, is ingrafted with the Anvil, so that the Hammer may be able to move round about upon the Anvil. This

The Anvil. Anvil is a Bone almost round, which leaning into the Cavity, hath two proper Shanks, one whereof being fixed to the Cartilage, is fastned by the same to the stony Bone; but the other shank of the Anvil is joyned by the Cartilage to a third Bone, called the Stir-
The Stirrop. rop; so that the Anvil being joyned by the Cartilage to the Stirrop, is also moveable; and the two shanks of the Stirrop are affixed to the Ligament, and by it stick to the stony
The Muscle. Bone. As to the Muscle, which lifts up the Hammer, (altho at first sight only its Tendon appears) if it be farther searched, it is seen to be big enough and round, planted in its proper Cavity, the Tendon of which is inserted into the sharp process of the Hammer, and lifting it up, and drawing it inwards, bends and distends the Drum within;
The Ligament. notwithstanding, lest this Muscle (if it should happen to be pulled) should be brought too near to the Drum, a smooth a transverse Ligament, is placed before the acute process of the Hammer, which strictly leans on the Hammer, and binds it; and lest it should be drawn beyond measure, by the Muscle, contains it in its due site.

The use of the Drum. From these it is easily to be understood, what use these Parts are for, which we described: For it is seen, that the Drum is the Preliminary, and as it were Preparatory Instrument of Hearing, which receiving the first Impression of the sound, or sensible Species, directs them in due proportion, and apt conformity towards the Sensory, which is placed more inward: It performs the like office in respect of the Hearing, as the Coats of the Eye, constituting the Pupel or Apple, in respect of the Sight; either Membrane break and as it were soften the sensible Species, and deliver them to the Sensory in proportion, to which if they should come naked, they might hurt or destroy easily its more thin Con-
The Drum hears not. stitution. Indeed the Drum does not hear, but contributes to the better and safer hearing. If this Part should be destroyed, the Sense may be still continued for a while, thô after a rude manner: because it appeared by an Experiment made in a Dog, that having boared both the Drums of his Ears, Hearing remained still for a time, which after three Months wholly ceased, to wit, after the Constitution or Crasis of the Sensory, suffering by outward Injuries, was overturned.

The use of the little Bones, as also of the Muscle, and Ligament.
But that the Drum might truly perform this sort of office of a Porter about the Hearing, its stretching forth ought to be bound or loosned, as occasion serves, to wit, as the Pupil of the Eye is wont, as the matter requires, to be either contracted or dilated. Wherefore, certain Machines or Braces, like to a Drum of War, are appointed for the Drum of the Ear, which render its Superficies sometimes more stiff, and sometimes more loose: For this, the three aforesaid little Bones, with the Muscle and Ligament, effect. The Muscle lifting up the Hammer, whilst it Contracts it self, the Drum is distended, when it remits its endeavour, that is suffer'd to be loosned; but the Ligament moderates the action of the Muscle, and hinders, lest the Hammer being too much drawn up, should distend the Drum till it break: But that the Rod or Beam (which is a part of the hammer) affixed to the Membrane, and drawing it to the Motion of the Muscle, is not

one

Of Hearing.

one Bone, but three little Bones joynted in one another; the reason is, both that the drawing of the Membrane be not too hard and stiff, but with a certain ceasing and flexibility of the Beam, without which the Drum, for that it is a most thin little skin, would be in danger to be broken; also, that by so many joyntings of the Beam, the motion of drawing might be determined, as occasion serves, into various parts, hither and thither: This part hath almost the same use as the *Hyodes* Bone, which is made of many little Bones joynted together.

As to the Action of the Muscle lifting up the Hammer, it seems that it is chiefly involuntary, and that 'tis acted by the instinct of Nature, according to the indigencies of the Bone; for when a sound too vehement strikes the Ears, this Muscle remits its indeavour, that the sensible thing might strike more strongly the soofned Drum; but if a smaller or duller sound enters, the Muscle being contracted, distends the Drum, that the Impression otherwayes obscure may become more sensible: If that many voices and confused sounds approach the Ears, it is probable, that the Drum disposes the Species brought to it, after a diverse manner of Action, and as it were admits them in, with a certain Choice. *The involuntary Action of this Muscle.*

Altho Hearing is not made by the Drum, as the proper Organ of Sense, yet this so much depends upon that, that oftentimes the Action of the Drum being hurt or hinder'd, a privation or a diminution of that Sense follows. For we meet with a certain kind of Deafness, in which those affected, seem wholly to want the Sense of Hearing, yet as soon as a great noise, as of great Guns, Bells, or Drums, is made near to the Ears, they distinctly understand the speeches of the by-standers, but this great noise ceasing, they presently grow deaf again. I heard from a Credible Person, that he once knew a Woman, tho she were Deaf, yet so long as a Drum was beaten within her Chamber, she heard every word perfectly; wherefore her Husband kept a Drummer on purpose for his Servant, that by that means he might have some converse with his Wife. Also I was told of another Deaf Person, who living near a Ring of Bells, as often as they all rung out, he could easily hear any word, and not else. Without doubt the reason of these is, that the Drum of it self being continually loose, by the impulse of a more vehement sound, is compelled to its due tensity or stretching forth, by which it might in some measure be able to perform its office. But we will proceed in Order, to the other Parts of the auditory Organ. *Deafness sometimes proceeds from the looseness of the Drum.*

Behind the Drum, the Den or Cavity subsists, in which the Ancients placed the inplanted Air, which received the impressed sound from the Drum: which thing indeed is not unlikely; for, because the waving of the sound ought to be conveyed still further towards the Sensory, it seems that the Sonorifick Particles, which are their Vehicle, are contained within this Den; and because it is needful, that the Sonorific Particles, included in this Den, should be in some measure consumed; therefore from this hidden place, there lyes an open passage into the Palate; but yet after that manner, that little doors being placed in its upper part, it admits the Air fetch'd from the Palate, as often as there is need; but the same being admitted into the Den of the Ear, its passage out by the same way is hindred. By reason of this Channel, it is, that the sound becomes rather sensible to the Palate of some deaf People, than to their Ears; to wit, when the office of the Drum is spoiled, the sensible Impression is carried, in some measure, to the Sensory, by this other way. *The Cavern containing the Air, placed behind the Drum. From this Den a Passage into the Palate.*

But from the aforesaid Den, placed behind the Drum, another passage leads towards that part, which is properly the Organ of Hearing; to wit, in the extream side of that Cavern, before-mentioned, there is a door, or certain round hole, covered with a thin Membrane, commonly called the Window, and beyond that hole, to wit, in the end or sharp process of the stony Bone, is the Shell contained: from whence we may think very well, that the impression of the sound brought through its next Chamber from the Drum, is from thence propagated, by an impulse made above the Window, into the Shell. *Another Passage from this Den (called the Navel hole, or the Window) leading into the Shell.*

But the Body of the Shell is an admirable Structure, which being framed in a peculiar recess of the stony Bone, is called by some the Labyrinth, by others the Shell; because its passage or hollowness, after the manner of a Snails shell, is carried about with a turning or spiral Convolution. There are two parts of this, or rather there are two Shells, the former being nigh the chief Oval hole, is less'ned by degrees, from the Spire or more broad Capacity, and ends in a very little one, then from the end of this, another Shell, beginning with a very small spire, is inlarged by degrees, in its progress, and its extremity opens with a greater aperture, into another Den or Chamber, placed beyond, with an open mouth; this is without any Membrane covering it. *The Description of the Shell.*

As to the Shell, the use of it seems to be, that the audible Species being brought thorow such turning and winding Labyrinths, and so receiving an augmentation by reflection, and manifold refraction, it may become more clear and sensible; then further, that every *The Use of it.*

L   Impression,

Impreſſion, carried about by this winding and very narrow way, may come more diſtinct to the Senſory : becauſe by this means, care is taken, that many confuſed Species together, may not be brought in. After the example and ſimilitude of this Shell, artificial Caverns, and arch'd Meanders, are wont to be framed by Architects, for the increaſing of ſounds, and for the diſtinct propagating of them to a wonderful diſtance. Further, there is another uſe of the Shell, no leſs noted, to wit, that the audible Species may be impreſſed on the Fibres and the ends of the ſenſible Nerves, inſerted in this place, not at once or at large, but by little and little, and as it were in a juſt proportion and dimenſion.

The auditor Nerves. We have elſewhere diſcourſed concerning the Hearing Nerves, which receive the ſenſible Species, and carry it towards the Common Senſory, and we ſhewed, that the ſofter proceſs of either of the ſeventh pair, is deſtinated to this office ; wherefore the end of this Nerve is terminated in the neareſt Chamber of the Shell, whence it is manifeſt, that the ſenſible Impreſſion, being diſpoſed from the Shell into this Chamber, is conveyed *Two Proceſſes of the ſofter auditory Nerve, one tends into the next Chamber of the Shell.* thence towards the Head, by the paſſage of this Nerve. But moreover (which we took not notice of before) it is obſerv'd, that this ſofter auditory proceſs, is cleft into two branches : one whereof is inſerted after the manner we have here deſcribed, into the aforeſaid Chamber ; but the other, no leſs noted branch, is implanted in the Shell it ſelf, about the mid'ſt of it, or nigh to the meeting of either Labyrinth ; ſo that this branch ſeems to receive the Depoſitum of the foremoſt Shell, and the other aforeſaid of the latter Shell.

The other into the Shell it ſelf. The extremity of either auditory Nerve, which are implanted about the end of either Shell, ending in ſlender thrids, ſeems to cover over the places of Inſertions, every where with Nervous Fibres ſpread abroad, as it were into a certain little Membrane ; whence it follows, that towards the end of either ſhell, the proper Senſory of Hearing ought to be placed ; for there is the Senſe, where the Nerve receiving the Idea of Senſion, is implanted ; but as the Shell is twofold, and that in like manner there is a double inſertion of the forked auditory Nerve, it follows, that in either Ear, there is a twofold Organ of Hearing : but for what uſe this is ſo made, does not plainly appear.

For what Uſes it is ſo made. That we may give our Conjecture concerning theſe, perhaps there is need for the audible Species, to be carried toward the common Senſory, that its paſſage may be the more certain, and that the perception of the ſenſible thing, may be put out of doubt ; but we rather think, that this Senſory is made double, that when oftentimes the Idea's of ſounds ought to be heard and perceived together, ſome might paſs this way, and others that way, without Confuſion. For it is obſerv'd, that the Hearing, not only as the other Senſes, receives many objects together ; and by and by whether united or confuſed, comprehends them, by the ſame act of the Senſe ; but moreover, this faculty in the time of Hearing, ſo diſtinguiſhes things often divers admitted together at the Ears, that it ſeems to hear one after another : It ordinarily happen'd, that in a confuſed multitude of voices and ſounds, that I have my ſelf taken notice to have heard the peculiar voice of a certain Man, and then a little after, I have known that I have heard, at the ſame time, ſome other words of another Man, that I did not perceive before ; the reaſon of which is, that this ſound, being received together with that, reached not at the ſame inſtant to the Common Senſory : wherefore, we may believe, that the ſenſible Species of the former ſound, paſſing thorow only one Shell, is by and by conveyed, by the firſt branch of the auditory Nerve, ſooner to the Senſory, but the other ſenſible Species, becauſe it could not be carried with it together by the ſame Nerve ; therefore it is carried by a winding about thorow the ſecond Shell, and at length to the ſecond branch of the auditory Nerve, and ſo coming later to the Common Senſory, is afterwards perceived.

A rehearſal of the Parts, which chiefly Organical ; Thus much concerning the Inſtrument of Hearing, and its parts, both Preparitory, and *ſerve for Hearing.* of the firſt ſort are the Ear, the outward Den, the Drum, and what belongs to it, the interior Den, and its two doors; to wit, one admitting inward thorow the door from the palate, the other emitting thorow the oval hole : Of the latter ſort are, The twofold Shell, with both the Branches of the auditory or hearing Nerves. Both the Parts, for the moſt part, are of like make in all Animals ; the greateſt mark of difference is, as to their Ears, which are variouſly figured, partly for ornament ſake, and partly for a diverſe uſe in reſpect of the inward Den, placed behind the Drum : for this is framed in a Calf, Sheep, and perhaps ſome other Animals, of ſpongy Bones, and long Caverns, having receſſes in themſelves ; In Man, and in Doggs, and perhaps in many others, *How they differ in Man, and in ſome four-footed Beaſts.* who are indued with a more acute Hearing, this Cavity is ſhut up with a round Bone, having a plain Superficies within, whence the ſound is reflected more ſtrongly into the Shell ; but in a Calf, and Sheep, the ſound ſeems to be much broken and debilitated, in theſe bony Caverns ; wherefore, theſe Animals are ſaid to have ſlow Ears ; for it is not expedient, for ſuch deſtinated for to be fatted for Food, to hear acutely, that they might be affrighted and provoked by every Noiſe.

CHAP.

CHAP. XV.
Of the Sight.

IF there be any strife for Dignity among the Senses, the Palm is given, almost by the consent of all, to Seeing, as the most noble Power; because this faculty apprehends things at a great distance, under a most subtil Figure, by a most clear perception, and with great delight; so this Sense acts, that is next in virtue to the Eternal and Immaterial Soul: To wit, it views and measures both Heaven and Earth in a Moment, and brings within its embraces whatever Bodies are situated in either, and that are far remote from our touch. *The Sight is the most noble Sense.*

'Tis needful that Seeing should be so performed at a distance, that visible things might diffuse, and every where propagate themselves by their Images far and wide; so that where-ever the Eye is stop'd, the Images of some Bodies objected are met with. But after what manner this is done, and by what means the sensible Species is received by the Organ, ought a little more deeply to be inquired into. *It acts at a distance by reason of the Species of visible things diffused afar off.*

As to the first, altho Light, Colours, and Images, are wont to be moved from place to place, and by the help of Glasses to be transferred hither and thither, and indeed affect the Eye with their Motion, yet it is manifest, that they are not meer Qualities, but certain Bodies, or consist of most thin little Bodies. These three are very much of Kin among themselves, and differ little or nothing one from another, as to their Essence; for indeed, the same Effluvia's or little Bodies, for as much as they proceed from a lucid Body, are called Light, for that they are reflected from an opacous or shaddowy Body, under a certain placing and meeting together, cause the Image of the Object; and for as much as it happens, the same rays of Light, in their reflection, are broken or turned in, from a dark or opacous Body, after this or that manner, they cause the Appearance of this or that Colour to be represented. *Light, Colours, and Images, are the same substance.*

As to the Rays themselves, or the passing thorow of little Bodies, the irradiation or beaming forth of which, shews the Representations either of Light, Colour, or Images, it is much disputed; whether they are only Effluvia's, darted from a lucid Body, and repercussed in their going forth, and reflected variously here and there, as is asserted by *Gassendus*, and some others; or whether Particles being sent forth from a lucid Body, move other the like Particles, implanted in the Air, and as it were by inkindling them render them luminous, and these at length others, and so a diffusion on every side of Light, or Images, is propagated as it were by a certain waving. *What the Rays are, which cause the visible Species. Whether they are Particles, streaming from a lucid Body,*

Against the former Opinion 'tis objected, that it seems impossible, that the Effluvia's of flame or fire, should be able to be unfolded so suddenly, and dilated or spread abroad to an immensity: for when a Candle being lighted, immediately the whole Chamber is illuminated, it can scarce be conceived, that the fiery little Bodies of that flame, should break forth so suddenly and so thick, that they should fill, in the twink of an Eye, so vast a space. For indeed, the new Motions and Increase of an inkindled flame, are more slow and perceivable to the Sight it self; how therefore can we imagine, the motion or dilatation of Light, for that this is but only a thinner flame, to be so incredibly swift? Besides, when in the same instant, in which a Light placed in an eminent place is inkindled, it is beheld at many Miles distance, none can think, that these Particles sent forth from it, can be able to be carried so long a space, at least in so short a time; but truly, how should it be supposed, that these Effluvia's streaming from a small Light, should presently possess the whole Hemisphear? Because the light enkindled in the whole Region round about, meets with the Eye where-ever placed. Besides, when from a Glowworm, a certain kind of Light or fire shines in the dark, and is perceived at a distance, if this apparition should be made by reason of the fiery little Bodies streaming from this little Creature, whence I pray is so much fiery Tinder supplied? From these and some other Reasons, we are led to believe, that when the Medium is so soon inlightned, besides the Effluvia darted from the lucid Body, others also interwoven with, and implanted in the Air, being moved by those Effluvia's, and as it were inkindled, contribute to illumination. *Or rather, whether inkindled Particles of Nitro-sulphureous Air.*

For the Explanation of this, hither ought to be referred what hath formerly been said concerning the Nature of fire and flame; to wit, we have shewed, that with the Sulphureous Particles, breaking forth from an inflameable Body, others Nitrous do come from the Air, and are inkindled with them, and so do not constitute fire or flame, unless both are *Which Opinion seems most likely.*

The differences of flame, and light.

are joyntly inkindled. The like reason may be given of Light, and consequently of Images, and Colours, most swiftly produced from Flame and Light: to wit, some Sulphureous Particles being carried beyond the compass of the Flame, joyn together with others Nitrous, and easily inkindled, and so produce a most thin Flame, *viz.* Light. For indeed, from an inkindled fire, many sulphureous Particles presently streaming forth thickly, lay hold on more, or at least the like Nitrous, and so constitute a more thick and almost dark Flame; this, for that it is fat and thick, passes not thorow the Pores of Glass, and thô it is apt of its own Nature, to be carried in direct lines, yet it is wont to be sent hither and thither, and to be made crooked by the blasts of Wind, yea to be carried within Tubes or hollow Pipes very crooked. But Light is made of fewer and more subtil sulphureous Particles, which passing beyond the first inkindling, fly away round about far and wide, and so meeting every where with many Nitrous, constitute a most thin white Flame, and without heat; this easily passes thorow Glass, and all clear Bodies: Its beams, for as much as they consist of more Nitrous than Sulphureous little Bodies, are carried only in strait lines, so that thô they are wont ordinarily to be broken or reflected, yet they cannot be made crooked.

Lucid Bodies, are either Cælestial,

Or Sublunary; In the light of which, we observe three measures.

Subjects emitting fiery and luciferous Particles, among the Cœlestials are the Sun, and Stars; but among the Sublunaries, whatsoever are filled with Sulphur, are apt to flame forth. Concerning the Sun we note, that wherever it may be seen in the Earth, it diffuses a clear Light, so do not the fixed Stars, because they are at too great a distance from the Globe of the Earth. As to the Sublunary Lights, we shall observe, as it were three Stadia or measures, in which they have their Beams after a diverse way; to wit, in the first place, the Flame consists within the compass of a lucid Body, which is both hot, and disperses heat every where round about, to what is near, not only by the open Air, but also by all Bodies, to wit, both diaphanous and dark, solid or rare. Secondly, In the extream Border of the Flame succeeds the Sphear of Light, which being more illustrious near the Flame, is by degrees attenuated, till it ends in plain darkness. Beyond the bound of the Light, the lucid Body propagates its Image or likeness a great way; for a Candle being inkindled, is beheld for many Miles in the dark: The trajection of which seems to be made, by reason of the Impression made on the Nitrous Particles, diffused thorow the Air; wherefore when the accension ends, about the border of Light, yet from thence it at a long distance transmits every way an Idea of the Flame or Light, by a most swift undulation or waving of them being moved.

Wherefore light, either reflected, or refracted, goes forward only in strait lines.

The trajection or the passing thorow of the Rays of Light, whether the same be direct, or reflected, or broken, goes forward (as we hinted but now) only in strait lines, and not in oblique, or turning about: the reason of which is, because the fiery or light-carrying Particles, how subtil or active soever they be, most easily pass thorow, and without any impediment, the Pores and Passages of the Air, and follow not its Course or Torrent. Further, as the fiery Particles (as it seems) are only of a Spherical Figure, and of a very small bulk, their irradiation or beaming forth, is made only in direct or strait lines: to wit, because, when the little Globes breaking forth from any fire, stream thickly forth on every side, and that the former are joyned to the latter, it is necessary, that they should be driven forward to the side, still without any declination: for as much as if Pricks be driven one from another, their progress create a strait line.

Light can pass thorow a Chamber in the mean time, not to be perceived.

But hence it happens, that Light does not as a Sound or Odors, pass thorow winding chinks, or passages of holes; yea, neither do we perceive the Sun or Stars, nor the Beams of a Sublunary Light, unless the same meet the Eye direct, or reflected, or refracted; for it may be made, that an handful of the Beams of Light, may pass thorow a Chamber whole, that in the mean time the Eye, placed in it, may perceive nothing of brightness. For Example, Let there be bored in one end of the Chamber a small hole, and in the other opposite a greater, in the space then without the less hole; if a Light or Lamp be placed, it shall illuminate that space placed without the greater hole, in the mean time, the Chamber between which the Beams of the same Light passes thorow, shall be seen dark: The reason of which is, because the Beams, passing thorow, for that they neither unfold themselves abroad, nor are reflected, meet not the Eye placed without the line, and therefore create no appearance of Light: also, for that reason it is, that when we look up from the bottom of a Pit, at Noon day, it is as if it were quite night, and we behold clearly the Stars themselves, without any appearance of Light.

Light Primary, or Secondary.

But althô Light is devolved into every Part round about, not by a waving fluctuation, but proceeds with only strait rays or strokes, yet these rays stream forth so thickly, and being reflected from Bodies after a manifold way, meet one another, mutually joyn, and are sent together, with so thick a Series, that not rarely almost the whole Pores or Passages of the Air, are possessed by them, either direct, or refracted, or reflected. Wherefore

fore Light is wont to be distinguished, either that which is Primary, which proceeds immediately from Light; Or Secondary, which is reflected from Objects, which sort of reflection of it, is wont to be many time reiterated.

Concerning the Primary Light we observe, that its Beams, from whatever Light they proceed, either Cœlestial or Sublunary, are almost the same; hence it is, when many of a diverse Original are mixed together, they are not easily known asunder, because the lesser Light is always obscured by the greater: But the Secondary Light, or Beams reflected from solid Bodies, that besides, by redoubling the illumination, they render the Medium more clear; also, according as they are variously modified from Objects, in their being reflected, they create the appearances of Images and Colours. *The differences of these.*

Concerning the Nature of Colours and Images, as the Philosophers of every Age, have disputed it, and that divers Opinions are delivered, by several Authors, none as I think has discours'd more ingeniously, or more like to Truth about this, than the famous *Gassendus*; wherefore, if it may be lawful to Plow with his Heifer, we will add the whole Matter in a short summary. *The reasons of Colours and Images unfolded.*

Every visible thing or Body is lucid, or illustrated from Light; That is beheld by its proper Light, and by direct Rays; This by another, and by reflected Beams; but the Medium is not seen purely perspicuous, because it emits not proper Beams, nor reflects others, by reason of its thinness. Concerning a lucid Body we observe, that this shining clearly and without any Impediment, appears under a bright form; wherefore Light in a fountain, is of a white shining Colour, but that it alters its Colour, it is nothing else than the intermixture made in its Beams, of shaddows or darknesses; but this is made either by reason of little Bodies, being between in the Medium, which avert some Beams: So the Sun seems red in the Horizon, by reason of Vapours which intercept many Beams, or the whiteness of a lucid Body degenerates, by reason of Particles, not lucid, intersperfed within its Body, and with the Beams themselves; so when Soot and Smoke stream forth with the inkindled Light, the Light becomes more red or darkish. *According to Gassendus, Every Body is either lucid, or illustrated. The Colour of a Light Body is white. Which is variously altered, by reason of interspersed Clouds.*

As a lucid, so also an illustrated Body, appears not pure, but altered, under the form of whiteness; for because the Rays are not all reflected, but by reason of the inequalities of the Superficies, some are wholly immerged, and others averted, therefore not a pure whiteness, but another Colour is seen in it. Indeed, as an illustrated Body is more smooth and polite, that it may reflect many Beams, the more bright and shining it appears, as is manifest by a Looking-Glass; but the more rough and rugged the Superficies is, that it hides many Beams, or averts them, the more the form of whiteness degenerates. *An illustrated Body, as it is either smooth or rough, reflects Beams variously, and therefore produces various Colours.*

Concerning the unequal Superficies of illustrated Bodies, two as it were extream dispositions are to be observed, by which the proper whiteness of reflected Light is very much altered; for either the Superficies of a Body is render'd unequal, by many Swellings up, as it were little hills or bubbles thick set, by which, tho many Rays are turned aside, yet by the divers faces of the little hills or risings, Beams are reflected in a more thick heap, than from a smoothed plane, therefore there is made a white Colour, coming near to the whiteness it self of Light. Or Secondly, The Superficies of an illustrated Body, gapes with very many Ditches or Pits, as it were Dens, in which the Rays entring, are wholly drowned, and are not reflected at all, from whence comes the black Colour, or a privation of white: after this manner, the two extream kinds of Colours, to wit, white and black, seem to be produced.

But as to the other intermediate Colours, besides the Light, being reflected with little shaddows, and variously intermixt with darkness, we ought to suppose, the divers manner of refraction of its Beams, to be partly also the Cause; of which there is a certain sign, for that in a Triangular Glass called the *Prism*, the Beams being refracted diversly, falling upon this or that Angle, are wont to shew Green, or Purple, or Yellow, or a Colour of some other Kind: In like manner we may believe, that also the Rays of Light being variously broken and turned inwards, in their reflection from an illustrated Body, and so cut and mixt together among themselves, do produce all manner of differences of Colours. This is not a place here to treat of the particular Splendor of every Colour, and the manner of their Production, but it may suffice, that we have mentioned in general the reason of their appearances. *The variety of Colours also depends, upon the refraction of Beams.*

But these things concerning the Nature of a visible Object, and the manner of its trajection, being thus premised, it behoves us next to shew, after what way Sight or Seeing is performed, by reason of the sensible Species being so sent from the Object, and received by the Organ. This commonly, and not improperly, is wont to be declared by the example of a Burning-Glass, which like a little Window is fixed before an hole made in the Wall of a shut up and dark Chamber; Because, from the Bodies every where *A Burning-glass placed before a dark Chamber, declares how Sight is made.*

where brought before that hole, the Rays of Light being reflected, meet together in the Glass, and in that passage cutting one another, spread themselves at last within the Chamber, and so upon a white Wall within, represent a Landschap of the whole visible Hemisphear. The Conformation of the Eye it self is much after the same manner, for in it may be discovered, both the shut up Chamber, and humors as it were Dioptric Glasses, which gather together the Beams, and break them after a manifold way, all artificially disposed; and lastly, as it were a whited wall, *viz.* the *Retine* Coat, or the Membrane of the Eye, on which the Images of visible things are Impressed.

The Organs of the Sight, are the Eyes, and the Optick Nerves.
Indeed the Eyes, and Optick Nerves belonging to them, perform the whole Act of Seeing; within the Cloysters of these, the Images of all visible things are formally painted, and by the passage of these, to wit, the Nerves, the perception of the Images there drawn is conveyed to the common Sensory: It now remains, that we consider both the Fabrick in either Organ, and the particular uses of the several Parts.

How the frame of the Eye, is fitted for Seeing.
As to the Frame and offices of the Eye, for the performing of which its Fabrick seems to be made, we shall take notice chiefly of three things to be done by it. To wit, In the first place, That the visible Species, or Rays of Light, sent from a lucid or from an illustrated Body, are intromitted by the Pupill, as it were thorow an hole. Secondly, The Rays so admitted being refracted, and artificially collected, through a fit Medium, are disposed according to the best Dioptrick Rules. Thirdly, That the Images of things, resulting from the due refraction and Coalition of the Beams, may be aptly represented, the interior Den of the Eye is formed, like a black Chamber with a white Wall, susceptible of the Images.

The Anatomy of the Eye, necessary for the Explication of Seeing.
If it should be further demanded, what kind of Fabrick it is of the Eye it self, and after what manner its parts are disposed, by which all its offices are performed, it will not be from the Matter, to shew here a perfect description of the Eye and its Appendix, together with the offices and uses of its parts, truly lay'd down. For truly, if any part of the whole Animal Body deserves a peculiar Anatomy, it is chiefly due to the Eye, which tho made of a very small bulk, contains in its Structure many admirable things, and is of most noble use.

But in delivering the Anatomy of this Member, many Authors, both Physicians and Mathematicians have already labour'd so exactly, that hardly any thing can be added in this business: but because, thorough the frequent Observations from others, made of the same thing, and then again from others, an easier apprehension, and more of certainty, yea, and a more accurate Knowledge is wont to be made; therefore it may be lawful for us, to subjoyn here our description of the Eye, not taken from the Writings of others, but by our own ocular Inspection, and observation of the Eye and its parts.

Why the Eyes are two.
We need not here mention that the Eyes are two, that there may be an help provided by one, against the loss of the other; also that the impression of the Object may be made more strong, and the more certain, which notwithstanding does not become double, being prevented by the Coalition of the Optick Nerves, before they are carried to the Common Sensory: nor is it behoveful to play the Rhetorician, by telling that the Eyes are placed like Watchmen, in an high place, and well fortified, from whence they may be able to move themselves hither and thither, with notable volubility, for the receiving from every part the met with Species, and to direct its Sight every where about:

The Parts of the Eye are either Exterior.
But that we may go about to describe the Fabrick of the Eye, without any Circumlocution; The Parts which belong to it are either Exterior, and as an Orchyard, which serve for Ornament, Defence, or Commodity of Action; of which sort, besides the round Bone, are the Eye-lids, with the hairs of the Eye-lids, and the Eye-brows, also the *Glandulæ* or Kirnels, with the Vessels, and Excretory passages; or its parts are Intrinsick, to wit, constituting the Globe it self of the Eye; which are again disposed, either about its Compass, as are the Muscles, and Vessels, with the fat lying between; or more intimate, which make up its Penetralia or inmost parts, to wit, the Coates, and Humours: In each of these, we shall note what is chiefly worth noting.

The Bone, Eye-lids, Hairs of the Eye-lids, Eye-brows, &c.

Or Interior, the Muscles, Vessels, Coates, Humors, &c.

For what use the Eye-lids serve.
Among the outward parts of the Eye, first is mentioned the Eye-lids, which are like a Membranous Vail or Covering, and cover or expose the Eye as there is occasion: as often as any injury is coming, these most swiftly hiding their Tenants, defend them; also when a relaxation is required from work, and that rest indulges the Animal Spirits, presently the Eye-lids shut their Windows, like an officious Servant; but when the Spirits are called back to watching, these Vails being again opened, the Impressions of visible things are admitted.

They are two in Number.
The Eye-lids are two, to wit, the Upper and the Lower; the motion of this is either none, or very obscure; yea, it is as it were fixed to the mound Bone, with which the other Upper Eye-lid meeting, causes the shutting of the Eye to be more firm. The
Upper

Upper Eye-lid, for the double Motion of opening and shutting, is furnished with two *There are two* Muscles, to wit, one strait, which arising near the Optick Nerve, with a broad and *Muscles of the* very thin Tendon, is inserted into the Margin of the Upper Eye-lid; this Muscle with *Upper.* its contracted Fibres, lifts up the Eye-lid: The other Muscle is Circular, which arising about the greater corner of the Eye, and from thence encompassing the lower Eye-lid, reaches to the Upper Eye-lid, nigh the other corner of the Eye, and coming under it, returns towards its beginning, this Muscle thus brought about, as it were into an Orb, draws down the Eye-lid, and so shuts up the Eye.

As to the Nerves which are inserted into the Muscles of the Eye-lids, we have shown *With what* elsewhere, that they are of a twofold Kind, to wit, some arising from the fifth Pair, *Nerves they are* others from the seventh; by virtue of these it comes to pass, that the motion of the Eye- *furnished.* lids accords with the Soul, and fitly answers to all the Passions; and that not only in opening and shutting the Eyes, for Sleeping and Waking, but in variously turning about, and composing the Eye-lids themselves, as is to be seen in Weeping, Anger, Joy, Sadness, Shame, and other Perturbations; which Kind of Pathetick motions of the Eye-lids, are for the most part involuntary, or are perform'd at least unthought of.

By reason of the Nerves of the seventh Pair inserted also into the Eye-lids, it may be known, wherefore we suddenly shut, or open, or any other way role about our Eye-lids, at any unaccustomed Sound, coming suddenly to the Ears. It is shewed elsewhere, why the Eye-lids being affected at the approach of Sleep, with a kind of heaviness or weight, desire to be closed whether we will or no, or thô we strive against it; where we treat particularly of Sleeping and Waking.

There is nothing to be observed but what is Common, concerning the Hairs of the *The hairs of the* Eye-lids, and Eye-brows; to wit, these hairy Walls or Mounds, like Ramparts, are *Eye-lids and the* constituted with a double Series or row of noted Pallizadoes, for the defence of *Eye-brows.* the Eyes, by which care is taken before-hand, lest any troublesom things should unawares fall into the Eyes, or lest that any thing should slide into them from the Head.

We will pass from the Eye-lids to the *Glandula's* or Kirnels of the Eye, which indeed *The Kirnels* stick to their Back, and put forth the Humour belonging to the Eye, thorow proper *are two.* Passages, which lye open within the interior Superficies of the Eye-lids; if that a superabounding serous Humor is poured forth, more than it ought into the Eye, that falling down into a Cavity like a Bason, nigh the greater corner, enters there two little holes, from which going out into a singular passage, is carried even to the end of the Nose, where it is sent forth of Doors at an open passage; besides, the serous Humour in a Man, being plentifully heaped up, nigh to the *Opthalmick* Kirnels, drops forth in Tears.

Indeed, the Eye leans on these two Kirnels, as it were soft stays laid under its round *Their Use.* Cushion; one of these sited nigh the greater corner of the Eye, is wont to be called commonly the *Lachrymal* Kirnel, thô the other better deserves the Name; To this be- *The Lachrymal* long Arteries, Veins, and Nerves, also excretory Vessels, which are of two sorts, to wit, *Kirnel is de-* out of this Kirnel, open two or three water-carriers; into the inward Superficies of the *scribed, with the* Eye-lid; out of which the watry Humor drops forth upon the Ball of the Eye; besides, *sages.* two passages also open into the Ditch of the inner Corner, which carry not thither the Water as some think, but sends forth what is there deposited, and superfluous, from the excretory Vessels, and received by them, and then it is carried forth of Doors by one Channel, which going thorow the Bone of the Nose, passes thorow its passage. This *Its use is hint-* Channel was first found out by *Nicholas Stenon*, who has ingeniously described its make *ed at.* and Use.

This little Channel, stretched forth from the Kirnels of the Eye, thorow the passage of the Nostril, even to its end, is like a Sink, which sends forth of doors the serous filth, apt to be too much poured forth on the Eye, by a secret passage: Hence is to be noted, that not only in Weeping, excited thorow Grief, but as often as Tears are pressed forth from the Eyes, by any thing bitingly pulling them, an humidity distils from the Nose. But as to the Vessels, which are properly Lachrymal, it is observ'd, *The Lachrymal* that three or four *Lymphæducts* or water-carriers, reaching from this Kirnel into the *Vessels.* Eye-lid, one of them opens into the Margent of the Upper Eye-lid, another into the Margent of the Lower Eye-lid, with a little Dam raised in either, and send forth the water in Tears or Weeping between the hairs of the Eye-lids themselves. I have sometimes seen in an Ulcerous disposition of this Kirnel, a filthy Matter to have dropt forth, by Compression, from those two Lachrymal Puncts.

The other Kirnel of the Eye, (commonly nameless, but deserves chiefly to be called *A nameless Kir-* Lachrymal) beginning at the lesser corner of the Eye, leaning on the back of the Eye, *nel rather to be* under the Upper Eye-lid, is carried forward, almost to the inner corner. As to its *called the La-* Figure, *chrymal.*

Figure, it is cleft into many Lobes, distinguished by various distances between; from every one of which, water-pipes ascend into the Eye-lids, and opening thorow the Lachrymal Puncts, within its inward Superficies, pour forth water requisite for the watering the Eye, both for its Motion, and for Weeping: The most Learned Doctor *Stenon*, has clearly and sufficiently described this Kirnel also, with the Lachrymal Vessels, and express'd them with apt Figures; whatsoever of superfluous Serum sweats forth through the Lachrymal Vessels of this Kernel, slides into the greater corner, for that it is seated in a steep place, and from thence is sent away, through the same excretory Vessels of the other Kirnel, as it were by a common Sink.

The Vessels of the Kirnels. Besides these Vessels, carrying the water from the Kirnels into the Eye, and the excretory of its superfluous Humor through the Nose; there belong to the Kirnels of the Eye some others designed for other uses, to wit, Arteries, Veins, and Nerves. From the *Carotid* Artery, gotten within the Skull, and about to ascend towards the Brain, a noted branch being sent into the Compass of the Eye, imparts shoots to either Kirnel, carrying Blood to them plentifully: To this Artery (which besides the Kirnels of the Eye, respects also the chief parts of the upper Jaw) is adjoyned a Vein, which reduces the Blood from them; yea, and to both these a Nerve is added for a Companion, to wit, the *Ophthalmick* Arm of the fifth Pair, which variously binds about and knits the sanguiferous Vessels, with many shoots, sent forth in its whole Progress, and also distributes many little shoots into the Kirnels themselves.

The Matter of Tears. From these we may easily gather, that from the Blood carried thorow the Arteries to either Glandula or Kirnel, a watry Humor, requisit both for the perpetual watering of the Eye, and also occasionally for the matter of Tears, is sifted forth, and there heaped up, for the aforesaid uses. As to the former, these Kirnels, even as others implanted elsewhere, imbibe the Serum carried to them for constant food; to wit, because the Arteries carry the Blood thither more copiously, than the Reins are presently able to sup back; wherefore what is watery is imbibed by the substance of the Kirnel, as it were a Spunge, the bloody Humor being sent away by the Veins. For this reason, because the Nerves bind these Vessels, therefore as often as the Serum abounds too much in the Blood, destinated for the Brain, these Arteries being provoked by the Nerves, and bound together, it is separated or bolted forth, and carried more plentifully than it was wont, towards these Kirnels.

The Causes of Weeping, and the manner of its being made described. But as to Tears, oftentimes poured forth in great plenty from these Kirnels of the Eye, that it may the better appear, by what means, and for what Causes this is done, it seems very opportune, to discourse concerning Weeping and Crying, and of the Causes and manner of its being made, which yet shall be done briefly and succinctly, because the more full Consideration of these, properly belong to the Doctrine of the Passions. In the first place therefore, concerning Weeping, we observe that it doth chiefly and almost only follow upon great Passions of the Mind, to wit, great Grief, Sadness, Pity, sudden Joy, and the like; to wit, whensoever the sensitive Soul, being struck by either a disagreeable or unaccustomed Object, is as it were compelled inwardly to shake, or to contract more near together its *Systasis*, or Constitution; so care is taken, that a greater company of Spirits, yea and a more plentiful flux of Blood, are compelled to the principal Parts, *viz.* The Heart and Brain, as it were the stays of Life: The Animal Spirits of their own accord leap forward to these places, as to the two fountains of Life, yea and the Blood is more fully heaped up in either; for as much as the blood-carrying Vessels, being bound together straitly by the Tract of the Nerves, drive forward swiftly to these places its Latex, and take it away, more sparingly from thence; therefore, whil'st an occasion is offer'd of Weeping, presently the Bosoms of the Heart, with the whole Neighborhood, swell up and are hugely inflated, by the Blood there heaped together, and (for as much as it is suffused with abundance of Serum) very much boiling; hence, both the Lungs are stuffed up that they can yield but a sobbing respiration; and the *Diaphragma*, that it might give place to their swelling, is depressed lower, with a stronger and more often repeated *Systole*, which is the Cause of Sobbing; in the mean time, for as much as the Air is hardly blown into the Windpipe, the Lungs and the *Diaphragma* being so distended, and at last hardly returned, that mournful sound in Crying or Lamenting is effected. The parts of the Face and Mouth, composed into a mournful Aspect, aptly answer to this Affection of the *Præcordia*; the reason of which we have shewed elsewhere; because the Nerves which Contract the *Præcordia*, are intimate Relations, and rejoyce in a mutual Sympathy, with those, which pathetically Compose the Face, in Laughing and Weeping. But whil'st these things are acted

Wherefore a bewailing, is often times joyned Weeping. in the *Præcordia* and Countenance, the business is carried no less tumultuously in the Brain; for here the Spirits being acted in Confusion, all things are upside down, and the Brain, by the too great influx of the Blood, is in danger to be either overturned,

turned, or drowned; which that it might not come to pass, and that madness follow not upon any Passion, the Nerves binding about the Truncks of the Arteries in many places, bind them strongly, and so repress the flowing of the Blood; and its Liquor being at first notably rarified, is thickned suddenly, and as it were melted, wherefore its Serosities running forth like a Flood, are disposed into the Kirnels of the Eye, destinated for this business by Nature: Then, because these Kirnels are pulled by the Pathetick Nerves, which are of the same stock, with those of the Face and *Præcordia*, and are strictly bound together, the serous Humors, by reason of these Passions of the Mind, being imbibed by the Kirnels of the Eye, are as it were stroked out from thence, and so distil in showers of Tears.

From hence a reason may be had, why Tears are wont to break forth in some, after a sudden Joy, because in great Joy, joyned with admiration, the sensitive Soul enlarges it self very much, and diffuses most amply its *Systasis* or Constitution; then as it were fearing a Dissolution, it again Contracts it self; wherefore, in such an Affection, the Blood flowing forth plentifully into the Brain, blows up all the Vessels, and by reason of its fulness distends them; then after its Channel being thus intumefied, the same Vessels being presently bound hard together, suffers a Flux, and as it were growing liquid, plentifully deposes its Serosities into the aforesaid Kirnels. *Wherefore Weeping comes upon sudden Joy.*

There remains another Consideration about Weeping, why Men or Man Kind only, or chiefly in bewailing, are wont to weep, or to shed tears? even for the same reason, which is given for Man's being a visible Creature, makes him fit for Weeping: To wit, Man is more fitly made for all Affections, and chiefly for the conceiving of Joy and Sadness, than Brute Animals; and as he is a sociable Creature, he ought to Communicate those sociable things, some signs naturally implanted in him, to wit, Laughing and Weeping: But as to the Organs, which perform these Kind of Affections, we have elsewhere observed, that there happens in Man, otherways than in Brutes, a wonderful consent between the *Præcordia*, and the parts of the Mouth and Face, by reason of the Conformation of the intercostal Nerve; so that as soon as sadness possesses the Breast, presently the Aspect of the Face, corresponds with the same Perturbation. *Why Mankind only or chiefly Weep.*

Thus much for the Kirnels of the Eye, and their Use and Action: Among the intrinsecal Parts of this Member, next follow the Muscles, concerning which, there is scarcely any thing rare to be met with, or that has not been already taken notice of by others. It is obvious for any to conceive, that so many Muscles ought to be constituted, as there are Kinds of spreading abroad, by which this Globe may be moved, as it hangs within the Compass of the Bone; for this is made after a fourfold way or manner; to wit, on that side and this side, upward and downward, and two ways obliquely, *viz*. By bringing it about both towards the outward, and inward corner. *The Muscles of the Eyes and their uses described.*

For these several Kinds of Motions are constituted so many distinct Muscles, which are found almost in all perfect Animals, and are easily seen in the dissection. Four strait Muscles are inserted into the Cardinal spaces of the Eye, to wit, the Muscle lifting it up, and pressing it down, its *Zenith* and *Nadir*, and drawing to, and putting from, as it were possessing the opposite points of the Horizon, to wit, East and West; the oblique Muscles compass it about like a Sphear, towards the Exterior and the Interior corner. I pass by here, that the Muscles of the Eye, do change their Names, according to the Passions of which they are Marks; wherefore, that lifting up, is called Superb or Proud, because that in Pride, it holds the Eye elate or lifted up, which however is more true of the Eyelid, and that Muscle deserves rather the Name of Holy and Devout, because it greatly lifts up the Eye in strong Prayer; wherefore it is the manner of Hypocrites, who affect the Habit of Sanctity, so to role the Eyes about, that they hide the Pupil of the Eye, and turn up the white to be seen: The depressing Muscle, by its action shews the mark of an humble, abject, and often of a Pious Mind also; that drawing inward, may not be improperly called Drunken, because Drunkards drawing their Eyes towards the inward corner, are wont to look asquint; and when one Eye is drawn in more than the other, for that by this means the Pole of the Sight is varied, they behold things as if they were double. I knew a young Man, obnoxious to the Palsie, when the drawing in Muscle was strongly drawn, the other Muscles of the left Eye being loose, by reason of the Eye being thus distorted, every object appeared double, nor could he distinguish the true one. The Muscle drawing from or outward, may be well enough called the Indignator, to wit, because in such an Affection, we bend our Eyes outwardly, with a certain aversion. The oblique Muscles may be called Amatory, because Lovers behold one another obliquely or side-ways, and as it were fearing the direct Sight of one another, they role about their Eyes like those of Cattel; hither and thither. *Four strait, two oblique.*

A Consent, and Sympathy, between them all.   That the Eye might rightly perform the Act of Seeing, there is required a Consent or Harmonious acting, between all its Muscles; to wit, that all acting together, may keep and continue its Globe, like the Tube of an Optic Glass, in a just Position for Seeing, for if any Muscle overcoming its Antagonist, acts more strongly than it ought, and draws the Eye too much to its part, presently the Sight becomes distorted; and by this means it is, to wit, by reason of overmuch strength of some one Muscle, whether it so happens by a Disease, by Nature, or by an evil Custom, that some are goggle-eyed, or
Whence squinting comes.   have them distorted or squinting; For squinting is wont to be caused by the fault of any one of the aforesaid Muscles; but especially the Muscle going about to the inward corner would Indanger the bringing in of this Vice, by its exorbitances, unless prevented by Nature; for as divers visible Species, being sent from Objects at a great distance, are received together by the Organ, every one is apt to turn about their Eyes, bending them forward : wherefore Infants, when many things at once are held before their Eyes, easily are brought to squinting : But lest this Muscle, inordinately rolled about, should cause in many this Evil, it is prevented with a wonderful Artifice, that its Motion may be still kept within just limits ; because, near the root of the Nose is hung a certain handle, like a Pully, which this Muscle passing thorow, there is a necessity for it to perform its trajection at a certain Angle, and as it were within a determinate compass.

Some Brutes are furnished with other two Muscles.   Besides these six Muscles which Man enjoys, and no more, and which are common to other perfect Animals, as well as him, some Brutes are furnished with two others for their peculiar uses. It is observed, that four-footed Beasts, who carry their Eyes prone or hanging down towards the Earth, have a peculiar Muscle, which holds up the Globe of the Eye, and which sustains it, lest by its weight it should be apt to slip beyond the compass of the Bone : with this Muscle are indued Kine, Horses, Sheep, Hares, Swine, and perhaps many other Animals, also a Dog is furnished with this, but has it made after another manner ; but to many who have the aforesaid hanging Muscle of the Eye, is granted another Membranous Muscle, which being placed nigh the inward corner of the Eye, when it is lifted up, hides almost the whole Globe of the Eye. The use of this seems to be, that when Beasts thrust their heads to feed among high Grass and Herbs, this Muscle hides the Pupil of the Eye, lest any thing should hurt it. The former Muscle is wont to be called the Seventh of Brutes, and this, that by which Brutes twinkle their Eyes.

The Globe of the Eye, with the Optic Nerve.   After that all the Muscles, with the Kirnels and the fat lying between, are separated from the Eye, its Globe remains naked, with the Optic Nerve inserted about its bottom : This Conformation, as we have formerly observed of the Brain, is after one manner in Man, and four-footed Beasts ; and after another in Birds and Fishes : for in these the whole compass of the Eye is not round, but depressed nigh to the more outward, and the posterior Superficies ; and almost like to a Platter or Shield rather ; but in the others, being perfectly round, it imitates the System it self of the World : The reason of the difference is easily known, by the divers framing of the Eye, which we shall show anon.

Its Figure in some is round, in others depressed.   We meet also with another notable difference in the Eyes of divers Animals, about the insertion of the Optic Nerve, for in Man, a Dog, and other more sagacious Creatures, the end of the Optic Nerve is placed directly before the Pupil, or is inserted to the Pole of the Eye it self : for the Beam, or the Optic Pole, passing thorow the Pupil or Apple of the Eye, and its middle Cavity, falls into the insertion of the Optic Nerve; but in a Sheep, a Calf, and many other four-footed Beasts, and besides in all Birds and Fishes, the insertion of the Optic Nerve being made in the Den of the most inward circular Cave, or side of the Hemisphear, is at a distance from its Pole, even as the Pole
The Insertion of the Optic Nerve, is after a divers manner, in divers Animals.   of the *Zodiac*, from the other of the *Equator*. This difference Dr. *Scheinerus* not perceiving, when he had found the Optic Nerve to be inserted into the side, in the Eyes of great Cattel, Oxen, and Swine, too soon concluded, that it was so also in Man, and in all Creatures besides; for he says in his Third Book, *Fundam. Optic.* p. 11. *That the Optic Pole does not fall into the Optic Nerve, with any Proportion,* the error of which Assertion, the Anatomy of a Man's, or a Dog's Eye, easily discovers.

It is placed either in the Pole, or at the Side of the Eye.   If the reason of this diverse Kind of Conformation be demanded, we say, that the Primary Organ of the Sight, to wit, in which the Image or visible Species stays, and from whence it is delivered to the first Sensory, is not the Optic Nerve, but the *Retina*, netty Coat, or fifth Membrane of the Eye, on every side spread out, by the Insertion
The reason of the divers Conformation inquired into.   of the Optic Nerve. Further, the Image projected within the bottom of the Eye, does not consist in the small Punct, neither is it determinated to the same individual space, but being variously drawn forth, is painted now bigger, now smaller, upon the *Retina*, or fifth Coat of the Eye ; yet so, as being placed nigh to the insertion of the Optic Nerve, it may presently be carried by it to the Common Sensory ; whenas therefore
the

Of Seeing.

the Optick Nerve is placed in the Pole of the Eye, the Images difposed round about upon the *Retina*, from every part of it, do fill the whole Circle of the painted Scene. But when the infertion of this Nerve, declines from the Pole, to the fide of the Eye, the apparition of the Objects ftands only below, and not at all above that Punct, and fo the whole apparition of vifible things, is concluded within a Semi-circle. This is clear to any thinking Perfon, that it is fit for fome Animals, that they receive many Objects at once, at one view, and that others but a few only; therefore the Optic Nerve, for the former, ought to be inferted about the middle of the Eye, and for thefe latter towards its fide. Man, a Dog, an Horfe, and perhaps fome other Animals, wont to be employed with various Matters, ought to behold all things in the whole Neighbour-hood placed together: but a Sheep, Ox, Hog, and many other fourfooted Beafts, and univerfally Fowls and Fifhes, to wit, fuch whofe chiefeft task is to get their Victuals, and to defend themfelves from Enemies, have no need to behold the whole Horizon, but only things placed near on the right and left hand; altho perhaps in fome of thefe, the paucity of the Objects, is compenfated with the fharpnefs of the Sight.

There is obferved another no lefs noted difference in feveral Animals, about the Pupil of the Eye; for this is round or fpherical in Man, a Dog, and in many other four-footed Beafts, in all Fowls and Fifhes; but in an Ox, great Cattel, a Goat, and fome others, it is oblong, like a great cleft; the reafon of this difference feems to be, becaufe that by a Man that is upright, and other Animals that are wont to lift up their heads, and to look round about on every fide, many Objects, coming from both above and beneath, and from either fide, out of the whole Hemifphear, are received by the Sight; wherefore the Pupil of the Eye ought to be round, that the vifible Species fent in from every fide, might be admitted in a round form: But Oxen, Cattel, and other Animals, almoft always carrying their Heads prone, and hanging down, need only to behold fuch things as are prefented before them, or a little of one fide: wherefore, the Pupil of the Eye is depreffed, and fomewhat long, for the receiving the vifible Species, that are only fhown at hand. Further, another difference is noted, about the colour of the Ball or Pupil it felf, which in Man, and in all Fowls and Fifhes is perpetually black, but in four-footed Beafts, it is either grey, or blewifh, like the Sky, or of a fhining red, or of fome other Kind, which colour notwithftanding being fixed, not in the Horney part, but in the Concave of the *Crocoideos*, fhines thorow all the Humors into the Pupil. Concerning the reafon of this, we may believe, that thofe indued with a black Pupil, fee more clearly by day-light, becaufe indeed the Image is rendred moft perfpicuous to the Eye, as it were in a Chamber wholly dark, but by Night they difcern little or nothing at all of any Objects; on the contrary, we have obferved, thofe furnifhed with a blewifh, or grey, reddifh, or fome other fhining Pupil, not to fee fo clearly in the day time, but much better in the night than the former; to wit, becaufe that fhining Colour of the Pupil, illuminates fomething the Cloyfter or Optic Chamber of the Eye, that fewer Beams being there gathered together from the darknefs they might conftitute the vifible Image.

The Pupil of the Eye in fome round, in other longifh.

The reafon of this inquired into.

The Colour of the Pupil in fome black, in others gray, reddifh, or otherways Coloured.

The reafon of this fhown.

Thefe things concerning the Fabrick of the Eye, and its divers manner of furniture, in various Animals, being thus premifed, it now remains, that we fhew its Anatomy, and that we unfold its feveral Parts, and the ufes of the Parts. We have already mentioned, what alfo is known to common Obfervation, that the Eye confifts of Coats, and Humors. The Coats or Membranes are as the containing Bodies, and conftitute the walls of the dark Chamber, with the little Window, and the Paper for the receiving the Images; but the Humors, are as *Dioptrick* Glaffes, fo placed within the hole of the dark Chamber, that they aptly break, and gather together, the Beams exhibiting the Images.

The Parts of the Eye, are the Coats and Humors.

The Coats of the Eye, like the Sphears of a Globe, are either Greater, which are ftretched forth thorow the whole Compafs, or its greateft part; or Leffer, which contain, or include the particular Humors.

The Coats greater or leffer.

The greater Coats of the Eye are three; which feem in fome meafure to arife from a threefold Subftance of the *Optick* Nerve; for in the Trunk of the Optic Nerve, may be found an Exterior Coat, arifing from the *Dura Mater*, with which it is included as with a fheath; Another more inward, cloathing the Membrane, lyeth under this, arifing from the *Pia Mater*; and within thefe Coats are found very many Fibrous Nerves, gathered together into one bundle. But this Nerve, being continued, to the Compafs of the Eye, its Exterior Coat being much inlarged, and ftretch'd out into a round inclofure, conftitutes the outmoft Wall of the Eye: This Coat, by reafon of its hardnefs, (becaufe it is ftrong, and is in the place of a defence againft Injuries) is called the *Sclerotick*: The hinder part in moft Animals is thick, and fpacious, except that in a Dog, and perhaps in fome

The greater are three.

The Sclerotick.

some others, it is thinner, and in some measure clear; but the Anterior part of this Membrane, that it may transmit the visible Species, is transparent and shining in all. But lest this should admit more forms than it ought, (by having a too broad, and too large a transparent opening) and so too confused together; another Coat, arising from the *Pericranium* grows to it, and covers it; excepting a hole left for the Pupil: This, from its Colour, is called the *Albugina* or the White, for besides that it determines the aperture of the *Cornea*, or horny or third Pannicle of the Eye, it firmly ties the Eye also to the sides of the bony Compass. The additional Coat, or the white Tunicle, besides the proper Membrane, is made up also of Tendons of Muscles, spread into a most thin Net; therefore, also it becomes white, because, when many diaphanous Membranes are thrust together, like thin cakes, they cause a shaddowing, and with it a whiteness, as may be perceived in the Bones and Horns of living Creatures, made up of a Pellucid Glew, also in the white of an Egg made hard by Boyling.

The Albugine grows to this.

The Figure of the *Sclerotic* Coat, is proportionate to the quality and disposition of the Humors, which are contained in the Eye; wherefore, in some (as we hinted before) it is round, in others press'd down, but in most its Anterior Part swells up, above the remaining Part of the Ocular Globe, by reason of the Watry Humor underneath, as it were a Portion of the outward Sphear, to wit, for this end, That the Compass of the whole visible *Hemisphear*, may be received together, by the Eye, as it were by a Convex Glass.

The Sclerotic Coat, is in some round, and in others depressed.

As to the Vessels which are inserted into this Coat, besides the shoots of the Nerves, sent from the fifth Pair, after they have bound about the Trunk of the *Optic* Nerve, they are bestowed on the bottom of the *Sclerotic*, whose Use or Office seems to be, variously to carry the Optic Nerve, with this outmost Chest or closure of the Eye, and to Compose it for the receiving the Species; there are also granted to this, noted Arteries, from the Trunks of the *Carotides*, before they reach to the Brain. It is observed, that the Artery destinated for this, falling in, nigh to the Trunk of the *Optic* Nerve, imparts to the same, in its whole progress, some small Shoots, which are certainly sufficient for Heat and Nourishment; then this Artery, spread forth at the bottom of the Eye, is divided into six Branches, like so many little Rivers, all which being brought upon the *Sclerotic*, towards the *Cornea*, divide the Exterior Globe of the Eye into so many equal and distinct Regions; from these, many little shoots, going thorow the *Sclerotic*, are inserted into the *Uvea*, and after a sort knit this to the other: The Arterous branches and shoots, are every where accompanied with Veins, by which the Blood is reduced towards the wonderful Net, and at length into the Trunk of the hollow Vein.

The Vessels of this Coat.

Within the *Sclerotic* Coat, or the outmost Coat of the Eye, follows the *Chorocoeides*, and is almost thorow the whole, Contiguous with it, and coheres to it, by some Fibres, and blood-carrying Vessels; this being perforated in the fore-part, leaves an opening for the Pupil of the Eye, which notwithstanding, as occasion requires, is wont to be either contracted or dilated. This Coat, being black in most Animals, is covered in the Superficies or Convex, or Concave, as it were with a black Paint, which is also fixed to the other contiguous Coat; the reason of this is, that it might render the inward Chamber of the Eye black or dark: But in some Animals, to wit, in most four-footed Beasts, a certain Interior Portion of the *Chorocoeides*, which is turned over the Pupil, shines with a diversified Colour, like the Rainbow, and according to this, the Pupil of the Eye seems to be coloured: but as this is wanting to Man, his Pupil is always black, according to the whole Picture of the *Chorocoeides*: But it appears otherways in a Dog, and otherways in a Cat, Ox, and the rest. In those also that have the Pupil round, this Signature is expanded round; those who have the Pupil stretched forth at length, like a chink, this Picture being as it were double, stands on either side of the Optic Nerve: The uses of this (as we said but now) is to illuminate the Pupil of the Eye, as it were with an inward Beam, that it may be able to behold things by Night, and placed in the dark; wherefore it is very shining in a Cat, but is wholly wanting to a Man, Birds, and Fishes.

The Coat Chorocoeides.

Is black in most Animals but not in all.

A Portion of this, in most Brutes, is of a diversified Colour, otherwise than in Man. The reason of this is shown.

Nigh to the opening of the Coat *Chorocoeides*, stands the Rainbow of the Eye, that is, nigh to the outmost border of this Coat, where the opening is for the Pupil, a certain Fringe, made up of Nervous Fibres, diversly coloured and disposed, covers it: These Fibres are called the *Ciliare* Processes, which like brows of hairs, being carried from the Pupil of the Eye, like rays from a luminous Body, are disposed into an Orb; These Fibres being placed in a thick row, are noted with a variegated or diversified Colour, outwardly, where they stick to the Corneous or horney Coat; in the mean time, where they are Contiguous to the brim of the Chrystalline Humour, and also to the border of the *Retine* Coat, they always appear black: These *Ciliare* Processes, do not only dilate and contract the Pupil of the Eye, but also they thrust forward, or draw backward the Chrystalline

The Rainbow of the Eye is described, and its use declared.

Of Seeing.   85

Chryſtalline humour, and bend it hither and thither into the view of the Objects. Fur- *The ſtrength and*
ther, there is in theſe Coloured hairs, or the Rainbow of the Eye, a certain vigor, and *irradiation of*
mighty conflux of Animal Spirits, by the Exertion of which, the Eye ſeems to beam *the Eye from*
forth, and to caſt forth outwardly certain darts like Lightning, according to the Inſtinct *the Rainbow.*
of the Paſſions : yea, hence we ſuppoſe Light to be diffuſed, and to illuminate the Medium; for which reaſon, Men diſcern in ſome meaſure Objects in the dark. I knew a
certain Man, indued with an hot Brain, who after a plentiful Drinking of Wine, was
able to read diſtinctly, in a very dark Night; the reaſon of which ſeems to be, be- *The Animal Spi-*
cauſe the Animal Spirits, being as it were inflamed, and ſo beaming forth from this *rits actuate it*
Rainbow, did illuminate the Medium, with an implanted Beam. Moreover, when by *very much.*
any ſtroke on the Eye, an apparition of flame, or ſhining appears; ſurely this proceeds
from a ſudden Concuſſion, and Exploſion of the Spirits, lying within the *Ciliar* or hairy Proceſſes. If it be demanded, by what paſſages the Animal Spirits run into theſe Fibres, we ſay; That from the Nerves of the ſixth Pair, which bind about the Optic
Trunk, certain ſhoots, entring the *Sclerotick*, and the *Corocoeidal* Coat, come alſo
to theſe Parts; beſides, the *Retine* Coat, which is wholly Nervous, ſticks to this
Rainbow.

Within the *Chorocoeides* or the *Uvea*, another Coat follows, whoſe Compaſs as it is *The Retine Coat.*
leſs, ſo it is ſhorter in breadth; for its Border, ſubſiſting about the lower brim of the
Chryſtalline Humor, is Contiguous to the lower Border of the Rainbow, and in ſome
part ſticks to it : This Coat, as it is white, ſo it is Medullary, and ſaid to proceed from
the Medullous and Fibrous Subſtance of the Optic Nerve, ſo that what is there of Nervous Fibres collected into a little bundle, is here like a Veil ſtretch'd forth of a Net-like
form. Indeed, if the whole Eye may be taken for the Flower which grows in the Brain,
thorow the Optic Nerve as its ſtalk; The *Retine* Coat is the Flower it ſelf, and the
two former, but the Stalk and Cup. The *Retine* Coat therefore being ſpread forth *Its deſcription*
within the Chamber of the Eye, or its inmoſt Conclave, is like a white Wall, which *and uſe.*
receives and repreſents the viſible Species, admitted thorow the hole of the dark Chamber; for doubtleſs this part, however Medullary and Fibrous, and ſo greatly akin to
the Brain, and to the Optick Nerve it ſelf, is the proper Organ of Seeing; to wit, on
which the ſenſible Species is impreſſed, and from which the ſame is communicated to the
chief Senſory; which ſhall more plainly be manifeſted anon, after we have unfolded
the Humors of the Eye.

Agreeable to the three Coats of the Eye, there are ſo many Humors of it, to wit, *The Humors of*
the Watery, Chryſtalline, and Glaſſy : The Chryſtalline Humor ſupplies the place of *the Eye Three.*
the Burning-Glaſs, placed within the whole of the dark Chamber, and the two other
Humors, conſtitute and fitly determine, the ſpaces only, or places between, which
ought to come between the firſt approaches of the beams into the Eye, and the place
or Organ of Sight, wherefore this is put behind, the other before the Chryſtalline
Humor.

But this Chryſtalline Humor it ſelf, within the aperture or opening of the *Uvea* Coat, *Chryſtalline.*
like a Glaſs placed before the hole, gathers together, and breaks the Beams coming thither on every ſide : The Subſtance of this is very ſhining, like glew, or the Gum of a
Tree, and is indued with a Conſiſtence like melted wax, yet if preſſed it will not willingly flow forth. Its Figure in Man, and moſt four-footed Beaſts, comes near to the
ſhape of a Lentil, whoſe utmoſt Superficies is more plain, and the innermoſt more
gibbous or bunching out; but in Fowls and Fiſhes, its Figure comes near to a Spherical ſhape; In theſe latter, where the Chryſtalline Humor is round, the whole Figure *Its deſcription*
of the Eye is depreſſed in either; But in the other, where the Chryſtalline Humor *and uſes.*
is of a depreſſed Figure, the Eye is found to be plainly Spherical. A reaſon of
the Conformation of either, ſhall be ſhown afterwards : The Chryſtalline Humor,
thô not apt to flow forth, yet is included with a proper little Membrane, for the Light-
neſs of it, called the Cobweb.

In Man, and in four-footed Beaſts, thô the Chryſtalline Humor be of the form of a *The watery Hu-*
Lentil, it doth not bear out enough, ſo as it might receive the Beams of the whole *mor and its uſes*
Hemiſphear, therefore the watery Humor is lay'd to it, as an addition, which thruſt- *deſcribed.*
ing forth the Cornea, or horny Coat, and rendring it more bunching out, encreaſes
outwardly the Convexity or bending forth of the Eye, which is indeed, that the viſible Species might be from this place, and from that, and on every ſide more plentifully admitted into it, as into a Window, made forth or butting out beyond the plane of
the Wall. Further, the watery Humor ſwelling forth with the horny Coat, breaks a
little the oblique Beams falling towards the Perpendicular; and ſo compelling them
nearer together, directs more together into the Convexity of the Cryſtalline ſwelling.
There is yet another uſe of this watery Humor, to wit, to temperate the Beams paſſing
                                                                            thorow

thorow it, being sometimes somewhat fiery, and so to render them more proportionate to the Sensory.

The glassy Humor.

On the other side of the Chrystalline Humor, to wit, on the back of it, the glassy Humor stands, like to fused Glass; this, much more plentiful than both the other, possesses the greatest part of the Optic Chamber; also, being less Compact in it self, is apt somewhat to flow out, and is included with a most thin little Membrane: this lyes upon the *Retine* Coat, and contains the Chrystalline within its Bosom. Its Primary

Its uses.

use is to separate the *Retine* Coat in a just space from the Chrystalline Humor, that after the Beams have past thorow this, as it were thorow the Burning-Glass, with a due Refraction, they may have in that, placed at a just distance, their habitation: Hence, in those who have the Chrystalline Humor in the form of a Lentil, and so the Beams passing thorow, can't come together but at a greater distance, have great plenty of this glassy Humor, and its plenitude causes the Spherical Figure of the Eye; But in those,

The Plenty of the glassy Humor varies, according to the Figure of the Chrystalline Humor.

who have the Chrystalline swelling round, that the Beams passing thorow, are more crooked, and have a dwelling or nest at a less distance, the quantity of the glassy Humor is found less; and its defect causes the depressed Figure of the Eye, or of the form of a Cheese. Further, the glassy Humor, according to *Scheinerus*, being somewhat a more thin Medium, than the Chrystalline Humor, breaks a little the Beams passing thorow, from the Perpendicular, and therefore somewhat enlarges or draws forth the Picture of the visible thing, otherwise more contracted, and shews the same more conspicuous in the *Retina*. Thus much concerning Seeing, and of all the Senses; in the next Chapter, we should speak of the other Power, to wit, the Locomotive: but being we have formerly largely discoursed concerning that; we shall handle in the following, certain Affections, belonging to the Corporeal Soul, as to the Exercise of the Motions and the Senses, to wit, Sleep and Waking.

CHAP. XVI.

Of Sleeping and Waking.

Sleep Necessary for all Animals.

SUch is the weak and instable Nature of all living Creatures, that they are not able, neither to Live perpetually, nor to Act and Labour continually; but that there is a Necessity for them (even as once, and at last to dye so) daily to repeat frequent turns of Sleep, as it were so many previous Monitors of Death. Though we have not experienced it, we easily know what it is to dye; to wit, when the vital Flame, like a Lamp, is either by degrees consumed, or violently extinguished, presently Heat and Light, and what flow from them, both all the Vital and Animal faculties, are abolished. But what is the formal Reason, Essence and Causes of Sleep, which we suffer, and daily experience, is almost wholly unknown. Concerning this, there are various Opinions, both of Ancients and Moderns, but they rather seem Dreams, than satisfactory Reasons: To wit,

What it is unknown, or greatly Controverted.

whil'st some affirm Sleep to be mere Privation, others a Bond of all the Functions; these place for its Cause a retraction, or introcession of Heat, those an assent of Vapours from the Stomach to the Head. Some assign for the subject the Brain, others the Heart, others the Stomach, and Spleen; and some again the Soul, others the Body by it self; and lastly, others both together, to wit, the whole Animal Body.

The Opinion of Schneiderus.

Among the latter Writers, *Conradus Schneiderus* hath of late been Eminent, who rejecting the Opinions almost of all others, and asserting Sleep not to be produced from Vapours, nor from any material Cause; nor to depend, either upon any affection of the

He affirms Sleep to be an inorganical faculty of the Soul.

Brain, or of any other part; affirms it to be, and Waking also, mere faculties of the Soul; to wit, innate, or born in it, and wholly inorganical. Also he saith, that the formal Reasons of either are, that the Soul, or its animadversive Faculty, sometimes withdraws, and as it were hides it self; and sometimes puts forth, and expunds it self. This Opinion, thô in some part it seems likely, does not easily deserve our assent, because, notwithstanding he asserts Sleep and Waking to be proper Faculties of the Soul, and these inorganical and independing of the Body, he further supposes, other chief Powers of the Soul, to wit, common Sense, Memory, and Appetite, not to be performed from the divers Organs within the Brain, nor to be distinguished by their Seats, but to be diffused thorow the whole Body.

Therefore,

Therefore, that we may the more rightly Philosophize concerning Sleep, we ought to consider, what are its Subject, formal Reason, Causes, Differences, and Effects.

First, As to the first it clearly appears, that Sleep is not extended neither to the whole Soul, nor to the whole Body: for the *Præcordia*, and Organs of respiration, are exercised with a perpetual *Systole* and *Diastole*, the Viscera, dedicated for Concoction, perform their Offices more, and better in Sleep than in Waking: Further, when as the aforesaid Parts are wont to alter their actions, according to the urgencies of evident Causes, (as may be argued by the Pulse and respiration variously changed, also from Vomiting, and sometimes a sudden loosning of the Belly) the exercises of the sensitive Power, as well as the Motive, ought to be granted to them in Sleep: But the Blood is circulated, and flames forth in quiet, the nourishing and Nervous Humors are dispensed, yea, and the superfluous, and what is excrementitious, are best separated or put forth: Hence, as it appears, perpetual watches are kept about the midst, or inmost part of the Animal Body. In the mean time it is observed, that Sleep urging, all the External Senses are shut up, also that all Spontaneous Motions whatsoever cease; so that the Bodies being wholly subjected to ease, lye as they were dead. Further, the Internal Powers, related to these, such as are the Common Sense, Phantasie, Memory, Appetite, conspire together with these External Powers, and either wholly omit their Acts, or exercise them but obscurely and confusedly. *The Subject of Sleep, not the whole Body.*

From these it may be plainly gathered, that the Animal Spirits, which are the next or efficient Instrument of Sense and Motion, are also the immediate Subject of Sleep; but, not all of them, but some Bands, as it were of a Superior Order, at those times keep Holy-day; but others, whose task is more assiduously required, for the Preservation of Life, are wholly inhibited. *The Animal Spirits are the immediate Subject of Sleep.*

Concerning these, that the reason of the difference may appear, and that the bounds of Sleep may be defined, we must note, that there is need for all the Animal Spirits (which constituting the *Hypostasis* of the Corporeal Soul, perform all its Functions) because they cannot incessantly exercise, or ever continue their Acts, to have frequent intermission; by which, being worn out and tyred, they might be refreshed: notwithstanding there is not granted a Vacation or rest to the Spirits of every Regiment, after the same manner, nor in the like dimension. *All the Spirits enjoy rest, but not in Sleep.*

For the Animal Spirits, which being born within the Brain, there constitute the chief Faculties of the Soul, and from thence flow into the Nervous stock, for the performing of the Spontaneous Acts of Sense and Motion, and effect the more hard and laborious tasks, are not tyed to the continual performance of them, but are permitted, after hard labours, to lay aside their work, and as it were to be idle; so that the Privilege of Sleep properly pertains only to these. But as to the Animal Spirits of the other Kind, which being procreated within the Cerebel, and there receive and emit the Instincts, and forces of Sense and Motion, merely Natural; and from thence flowing into the *Præcordia* and *Viscera*, perform the more assiduous Offices of the Vital and Nutritive Function; I say, that the Labours of these are more easie, and less laborious; but as they are absolutely necessary for the preserving of Life, that they ought not almost at any time to lye still, therefore the aforesaid Spirits, being busied about these Offices, are not suffered to keep Holy-day long, and to indulge themselves with Sleep, but it is sufficient for them, to intermit their tasks for a short space, and presently to resume them, and so to have, in stead of a longer Vacation, some broken times from their Labours: as chiefly appears from the pulse, and breathing, in which the times of motion and of rest, are reciprocal, and almost equal. Indeed the Spirits performing these tasks, seem as if condemned to the Stone of *Sisyphus*; to wit, that they still lift up the same burthen, then resting whil'st it slides down again, they presently, and so perpetually, repeat their Labour. Further, whil'st that the Animal Spirits influencing the *Viscera* of Concoction, propagate the Acts of Vermiculation, from Part to Part, receive and give place to motion, act mutually in themselves; which also is more amply performed when we Sleep soundly; in so much, that sometimes the work of more difficult Concoction, is not to be done but in Sleep. Therefore the Empire of Sleep chiefly and almost only belongs to the Animal Spirits, inhabiting the Brain, and the Executors of the Animal Function there, (of whose Acts we are knowing) and in the Appendix both Medullary and Nervous. If those Spirits arising from the Cerebel, as influencing some Pathetick Nerves, to wit, of the fifth and sixth Pair, seem to participate of Sleep, that happens by a consent, deliver'd from the Brain; to wit, by which the Commands, as of Motion, so of rest are conveyed to them. *The Spirits only arising from the Brain, and who are the Authors of voluntary Functions enjoy Sleep. Not those Procreated in the Cerebel.*

We affirm, That the immediate Subject of Sleep, is the greater Portion of the sensitive Soul, which being rooted in the Brain, and thence diffused into many Parts of the Body, is the Author of every Spontaneous Motion: But the Mediat, the Brain it self, and *The immediate Subject of Sleep, is the Knowing Part of the sensitive Soul*

The Mediate are the Bodies containing it.

and all the sensible and moving Parts, which Communicate with it. Also, on the contrary, the other lesser part of the sensitive Soul, which being rooted in the Cerebel, and thence stretched forth into the *Præcordia, Viscera*, and some other Bodies, is the Parent of the Vital and merely Natural Function, to wit, of whose Acts the Animal is not conscious, is freed from the Bonds of Sleep.

The formal reason of Sleep.

From these, that we may proceed to deliver the formal Reason of Sleep, let us conceive, that this greater portion of the sensitive Soul (the Animal Sleeping) doth lay aside its expansion like a Veil, sinks within it self, and hiding its head, as it were within its own Bosom, sees nor cares for nothing, that is without; so that both the Emanation of the Spirits into the globous Part of the Brain, and also their irradiation, into the Nervous stock, ceasing; the Act of spontaneous Sense and Motion, both outwardly and inwardly, is suppressed.

The beginning of Sleep, is in the Cortical part of the Brain, which is also the seat of the Memory.

If it be demanded, in what Part or Region these Spirits dwell, who first of all possess Sleep, and begin to be indulged with rest, before any others, it may be well supposed, that the Spirits first Sleeping, are those, which flowing within the globous part of the Brain, create the Acts of the Fantasie and Memory. To wit, these, either of their own accord, or by reason of the incourse of Strangers, falling down from the Pores of the Exterior Brain, in which they were wont to expatiate, convey themselves into its more deep Marrows, or middle Parts, where as it were lying down idely, intice the Spirits there implanted to the like slothfulness; and from thence flowing into the Nervous stock, recall others from their Efflux, and solicite them to idleness. Indeed, the Spirits irradiating the outer Brain, do first of all grow stupified, and begin Sleep in their recess, as appears from hence, because there is a Necessity, for these sometimes to be repressed from their expansion, and to be driven inwards, that there may be a place left, for the instilling the Nervous juice, or matter for new bands of Spirits, into the Brain; wherefore, those veterane, or old ones, being not only wearied, go from their Station, but being as it were drowned by the Humor, plentifully rushing in, are compelled from their watches.

The Causes of Sleep: First, what the final is.

From these things it will not be difficult to assign the Causes of Sleep; and first, that we may begin with the Final; (which is always the Key to the rest) If it should be demanded, for what end, the Animal Spirits going out of the globous part of the Brain, into its middle or marrowy Parts, are bound up with chains of Sleep, and so after a solemn manner, alter the vicissitudes, as of Exercise, so of Rest; this easily occurs; that the Animal Spirits (at least those who are wont to be more strongly exercised) lest they being wholly loosned should perish, and break the *Hypostasis* of the Soul, want for the sustaining of themselves a twofold prop, to wit, Rest and Food; by the former care is taken, lest the Spirits, for that they are highly volatile, should be very much drawn asunder, by too much Occupation, and acted into Confusion: wherefore, after that they have long and much laboured, they desire to rest, and be at quiet of their own accord; then by the other, to wit Food, the wastings both of themselves, and of the spirituous Liquor, with which they are washed, are repaired; therefore needful for them: But both these

To wit, a refection and quieting of the Spirits.

benefits, requisit for the Spirits, to wit, their sedation and refreshment, are granted (and almost only) to Animals in Sleep. For altho in Waking, pleasant sensible Objects do something please the Spirits, and that the nourishing Liquor, supplied from Aliments newly received in, may something cherish them, yet a fuller refreshment, and quieting, by which they are sufficiently fortified, for the lively performing the Animal Functions, are not obtained but in Sleep; for then the Spirits being at leisure for some time, from Motion, get to themselves new stores; and in the mean time the Brain, like a dry Sponge, imbibing most greedily the nutritious Liquor, takes it for Provision for it self; which after a little space, it dispenses to the several Parts, both of its proper Regiment, and also of its Appendix; yea, plenty of the Spirits, and their food, being somewhat exhausted, the Brain, as it were another Stomach, seems to be hungry after Sleep, greatly to desire it, and not to be satisfied, unless it daily enjoys it, and that in its wonted measure: for in the space of every Night, there is a certain Necessity of Sleeping for so many hours, as we have formerly accustomed our selves to; if at other times, as after Eating, an evil Custom indulges Sleep, we afterwards more hardly want it, than our Dinner; for the privation of due Sleep, or what often accustomed to, is as it were a fasting to the Brain, by which, if long affected, that, and its Nervous Appendix, languish as it were for hunger.

The formal Cause of Sleep, consists in the Rest of the Spirits, and in the watering of the containing Parts.

Therefore, for the taking of Sleep, by which the Brain may be filled, with the Nutricious Humor, and the Spirits, wearied or exhausted by Motion, may be refreshed, a certain Law of Nature, or Necessity is incumbent upon us, and calls it upon us oftentimes against our Minds: But this kind of Disposition being innate to most Animals, and chiefly to Man, whose Spirits are most of all employed, is the Final or *Procatartick*, or more remote Cause of Sleep; but its formal or Conjunct Cause, consists in these two things,

things, *viz.* in the Vacation or Rest of the Spirits, and in the Irrigation or watering the Parts containing them; by which (as common to either Affection) a relaxation follows, from a Tensity or Inflation of the Brain, and Nervous Parts.

As to the evident Causes or occasions, by which Sleep is wont to be introduced, first *The evident Causes.* we must distinguish concerning Sleep; That it is either Natural or Ordinary, which every one enjoys daily, for so many set hours, and its accession and duration depends upon either Conjunct Cause existing together in Act, *viz.* at the same time, the Spirits *Sleep either Natural, or not Natural, or Preternatural.* remitting their tasks, sink down, and the nourishing Humour flows into the Brain; then this being sufficiently watered, and they refreshed, Waking returns: Or Sleep is not Natural or Extraordinary, which for some occasions follows in an undue measure, and inconvenient time. Concerning preternatural Sleep, we shall speak more properly of it in another place; when we shall treat of Soporiferous or Sleepy Diseases. But as to the Non-natural, we have observed; that it is of a double Kind, according to the Complica- *Sleep not Natural, sometimes begins, from the Spirits being brought low.* tion of the Conjunct Cause; For either the Spirits first lye down, and so the Brain imbibes more copiously the apposite Liquor; or first the Brain is too much moistned with Humor, and so the Spirits being as it were drowned, are forced from their watches. For when the Blood every where washes the Cortex of the Brain, by almost innumerable Ramifications of Vessels, a certain spirituous Water from these bloody Rivulets, always stands at the Door, and is ready to be instilled into the Medullar Substance of the Brain; which, for as much as it is copiously received within, presently overwhelms the Spirits, and obstructs their passages, and so Sleep being call'd upon, every Animal Function ceases for a time; yet, lest this should be too frequently and untimely done, the Animal Spirits, *Sometimes from the Cortex of the Brain being too much watered.* so long as they are lively and active, inflate the Substance of the Brain, and keep it extended, so that the Spirituous Liquor, which is also Soporiferous, is not admitted, but only in a small quantity, such as may suffice for the exciting of Sleep. But if either the Spirits being weary lye down of their own accord, or are compelled by the boyling Blood coming impetuously to the borders of the Brain, to give place to it, the aforesaid Liquor, rushing in on heaps, produces almost invincible Sleep. Wherefore, according to which, either the Animal Spirits open the doors of the Brain of their own accord, or the Nervous Liquor besieging them, impetuously breaks thorow; The *Prophases,* or evident Causes of Sleep, are of this or that rank: there are many Kindes of both of these, and ways of being done, the chief of which we shall briefly touch upon.

First, In the first place therefore, there are many Causes, for which the Animal Spi- *For what Causes the Spirits lye down of their own accord. The force of Custom.* rits begin of their own accord to keep Holy-day, among which, the force or power of Custom obtains the chief place. For when we have accustomed our selves to Sleep at certain set hours, the Spirits about the same time, as it were dismissing the force of their Motion, leaving presently all work, and External Commerce, retire inward, and indulge themselves with Rest: The reason of which is, because the sensitive Soul, for as much as it is void of all Science, and proper direction, determinates this or that thing to be done, by outward Accidents and Circumstances; wherefore, the Animal Spirits, in what path they are once led, unless they be hinder'd, will repeat to an hair their former tracts, Hence it is, that we both Sleep, and also Awake, at set and wonted hours, also we expect and hardly can pass by, the same times of Dinner and Supper. So solemn the manner of Nature is to do the same thing which it did before, and till being taught new things, it is the manner of its Government, constantly and exactly to observe the old. An Example of this Kind of Natural assiduity is admirable, which was told me for certain, of a Fool living some years in our Neighborhood; who, thô he were silly and *A notable Example of Natural Custom or Assiduity.* foolish, yet did he know exactly, without any sign, the interspaces of the Hours, and as often as the space of an whole Hour was elapsed, as if he had been a living Clock, he would presently personate the like Number of the Hour, with so many hoarse sounds, and no business or employ about any other occupation, could make him omit this Task. He at the beginning was wont to imitate aloud, by making a noise, every stroke of the sounding Clock; and as often as he heard the sounding of the Bell of the Clock, presently he cry'd, *One*, *Two*, *Three*, &c. repeating successively the several Pulsations; hence it hapned afterwards, that the Animal Spirits, by daily imitation, being accustomed to be stirred up, to such a Motion, according to the set spaces of Time, at length they were able to distinguish the same Periods of their own accord, nothing directing, as if the sliding spaces of time, had been measured out by the wheels of a Clock.

Secondly, The Animal Spirits being wearied by the hard labour of the Body, or too *2. The Spirits being weary, lye down on their own accord.* serious intention of the Mind, indulge themselves with Sleep of their own accord: For when after immoderate exercise, by reason of Heat and Sweat flowing forth, the Spirits plentifully exhale, and those which are left being as it were poured forth and distracted one from another, as soon as those have left them, they presently lay aside all work, that they may Concentre themselves within, and recollect their forces; for the

like

like reason, after vehement study, or long Contention of the Mind, by reason that the Animal Spirits become very much tyred, we grow Sleepy; yea, sometimes serious Meditation, and when imployed with Hearing (chiefly of Sacred things,) and great Attention, procures an invincible Sleep; the reason of which is, not that the Spirits are so much consumed or wearied, but because they are gathered together in two great heaps in the Brain; and so with them too great plenty of the Nervous Humor is poured in, whereby the Brain is overflowed: Hence also it is, that if presently after Eating, Reading or Philosophical Lectures be attended to, they shall cause Sleep sooner than an Opiat; to wit, because these more grave Exercises of the Mind, both convey more plentifully to the Head, the Blood; and at the same time the Spirits Concentre together on every side towards the middle Part of the Brain; wherefore, from the Blood coming to its border, a mighty heap of Nervous juice is admitted in; by which the Spirits are presently overturned, and their spaces stuffed up; the contrary happens, as often as any one after a full Banquet shall go to the Theatres, to see Plays, for the Spirits being stretched forth by delectation, blow up and distend the Brain, so that the coming in of the Sleepy Humor, tho heaped up at the Door, is kept out.

The pleasing of the Senses, and the Phantasie, cause Sleep.

Thirdly, We may observe, that the Animal Spirits, when delighted with a soft Harmony, are invited inwards from the Organs of the Senses, and being there recreated, slide into Sleep. So a certain Musical and soft modulation of the Voice, the gentle murmur of Waters, the soft whispering of the Wind, also pleasant Fancies, as when we Imagine our selves to be in a green Meadow, or splendid Houses. because by this means, the Spirits gently Concentre together, Sleep is wont to creep upon one.

The Spirits are Compelled into Sleep, by Narcoticks.

Fourthly, There remains another manner of introducing Sleep, to wit, when the Animal Spirits are oppressed by *Narcoticks* or *Opiats* taken inwardly, or applied outwardly, and so are inhibited the exercise of their Function. For *Opiats*, because they Poison the Spirits, extinguish their forces, as Water poured upon Fire, or Sulphur laid on the Kitchin Fire, and cause a *Torpor* or Numness; wherefore, if they are more largely taken, that they cannot be overcome by the Spirits put to flight, who by little and little being recollected, renew the *Systasis* of the Soul, a deadly or perpetual Sleep follows.

Their Penury or want perswades to Sleep.

Fifthly, To this rank ought to be referred the Penury or evil Constitution of the Animal Spirits; for when they are either deficient in Plenty, or are dull and Torpid, that they can neither tolerate daily or hard Exercises, nor actuate the Brain, nor defend it against the Inundations of the serous Humors, from thence are wont to be induced a Torpor or Numness, and frequent Sleepiness of the Animal Faculty; as is to be observed in Dropsical and Scorbutical People: but the Consideration of this Kind of Torpor, we shall refer to another place, where we speak of Soporiferous Diseases.

By what, and how many ways Sleep begins from the Brain, first affected.

2. Another Kind of evident Causes, by which Sleep is introduced, consists in this, that the Brain is first affected; then by its Consent, the Animal Spirits being half overthrown, betake themselves to rest; these Kind of Effects are chiefly brought in when an heap of Serum is poured in upon the Brain from the Blood too much stuffed with a watery Humor, which watering it with too much moisture, rushes overs its Pores and Passages, and as it were drowns the Animal Spirits flowing in them.

When its Compass is overflow'd, by the Serum coming to it.

Such an Inundation of Spirits is produced, either from a too great taking in of Food, whence the Blood swelling up above measure, with the nourishing Humor, too much puts down upon the Brain the plentiful provision of Nervous Juyce; wherefore, presently after a more full feeding or drinking, men become Sleepy; or also, the Blood, as to its Temper, being made more watery, moistens the Brain, as it were with a perpetual shower, and so renders those affected continually Sleepy; as is wont to come to pass ordinarily in Dropical and Scorbutical People.

To which may be added, the imbecillity of the Brain, and loosness of the Pores.

To these may be added, and oftentimes is partly the Cause, the imbecillity or weakness of the Brain, and the loosness of its Pores, so that, they gaping too much, most easily admit the serous heap, whereby Sleepiness is brought in. For it is observed, That Drunkards, especially such as drink Wine, fall asleep with it, on the least occasion, and not only become Drunk, but also Drowsie or Sleepy. The reason of which is, that when the passages of the Brain, are more often and untimely unlocked, with the Particles of the Wine, at length become so feeble, that the Blood growing hot above measure, pours forth its Recrements upon the Brain, and so causes from thence a torpor or stupidness therein.

Sleep not from fumes or vapors.

These are the chief means, whereby Sleep is effected, when it is excited, by reason of the overflowing of the Nervous juyce, and as it were the over-turning of the Animal Spirits. But as to these, it hath been far otherways taught, by the Opinion of the Vulgar, to wit, that fumes and vapors are raised up from the Chyle, or Humors growing hot within the *Viscera* of Concoction, which cloud the Brain, and so cause a Numness. But this Opinion easily falls, since the Circulation of the Blood, and the more plentiful Suffusion of it on the Brain, have been known; and that the rather, because a passage

from

Of Sleep.

from the Stomach into the Head, thorow so many Inwards, and bony Cloysters, like stops, seem impervious, or not passable for the sending up of fumes. Without doubt, much the greatest part of the Humor, with which the Brain is watered, and the Spirits inhabiting it, over-turned, during Sleep, is carried by the Arteries, and distilled in immediately from the Mass of Blood. But altho we deny vapors elevated from the Stomach to the Head, to cause Sleep, yet by reason of some affections of the Ventricle, it manifestly appears, that Sleepiness is induced; for as much as Opiats being taken, they begin to operate oftentimes presently, and before the virtue or any of their Particles can come to the Brain, by the passage of the Blood. This also appears, because we become Sleepy from more gross Meats, and of ill Digestion, which stay long in the Stomach, and burthen it. The reason of which seems to be, because, when as the Corporeal Soul, or Sleepiness. a principle portion of it, is the immediate Subject of Sleep, and she entertains it, for as much as being restrained from Expansion, and as it were drawing a Curtain, she enters into her self, and sinks down on every side, towards the middle of the Brain; we say, that such a subsiding of the Soul, or its chiefest part, tho done in the Brain, is oftentimes excited, by reason of the Cause lying hid in the Stomach; because there is a mighty Sympathy, between this and that; or rather, the Animal Spirits, inhabiting the Ventricle, altho arising from the Cerebel, conspire so intimately with the desiring or knowing Soul (which is the Inhabitant of the Brain) that they are able to bend, exalt, depress it every way. The Appetite of necessary or delicate food, snatches it from any other proposition or desire. The frustrated longing of big-belly'd Women, causes an Abortion, or a Monstrous Birth. At the first taste of a draught of Wine, before the Liquor can be carried into the Blood, it lifts up and wonderfully chears the drooping Soul. In like manner on the contrary, Opiats or Sleeping Medicines, because they stupifie or mortifie the Animal Spirits, implanted in the Stomach, bring presently a Torpor to the Knowing part of the Soul, and sometimes an extinction to its whole *Hypostasis*, both flamy and lucid: For the same reason, undigested Aliments, because they fix and burthen the Spirits inhabiting the Ventricle, render the others Presiding in the Brain, for some time Dull and Torpid.

The Matter of Sleep, conveyed only by the Arteries.

Why raw and indigested meats induce Sleepiness.

That happens by reason of the Consent, which is between the Stomach and the Brain, and which it has with the whole Soul besides.

How Opiats cause Sleep, whilst they operate in the Ventricle.

But sleep seems to begin not only from the Ventricle, but for the most part from the Eyes; for when about to Sleep of our own accord, we our selves first of all shut our Eyes, & our Eyes being made heavy, and dull, Sleep creeping upon us whether we will or no, love to be closed; yea, if we would watch longer, we rub our forehead, and Eye-lids, and open them with a certain force, as if about to cast off Sleep chiefly there arising. Concerning these, we may say, that rest, being about to be indulged to Animals, may be the less disturbed, Divine Providence hath so provided, that the Windows being presently shut, the meeting with External Objects may be hindred. The Eyes ought to perform this Office especially, as the most noble Sensory; also that they may more certainly perform it; whilst the Knowing Soul withdraws it self, and Contract its Compass, the Spirits being recalled towards the middle of the Brain; the Sight, as the Organs of the other Senses, are destitute, and left flaccid and apt to fall down; and this happens chiefly and more certainly to the Eyes, because Sleep coming on, the Brain becoming full and swell'd with the flowing in of the Nervous juyce, at that time more uberous or plentifully abounding, very much presses upon the Optic Nerves, and those moving the Eyes, lying under its basis with a long passage, (different from any others) and so hinders the wonted inflowing of the Spirits into the Sensory of Sight.

How Sleep seems to begin in the Eyes.

Thus much for the Nature, Causes, and the various ways of inducing of Sleep; there yet remains for us to consider of the chief Effects and Alterations of it, which it is wont to bring to Soul and Body, and their Parts and Humors, and first, what it brings to the Vital or Flamey part of the Soul, radicated in the Blood.

Of the Effects of Sleep.
1. Towards the Vital or Flamey part of the Soul.

Concerning this, first of all we shall note, That the Blood is more inkindled, and much more plentifully burns forth in Sleep, than in Waking: the Truth of this is plain, from the standing Observations of such as have given it for Law, that Men Sleeping, exhale or breath forth a departure of a far greater weight, than Men Waking, tho they use Exercise and Sweat. Moreover, Reason and Experience dictate the same thing, for as a Combustible Matter, being placed near the Centre of inkindling, and heaped about it, burns more than if the same being divided into parts, smoaking and half inkindled, should be drawn out and planted here and there in various places; in like manner, it may be judged of the Blood, which being quiet in Sleep, being called aside or disturbed with no Passions, nor with the impulses of the Muscles out of the *Præcordia*, or detained out of doors, enters the Lungs with a more full Flood, and there more slowly passes thorow the Centre or place of accension; whence, there is a Necessity, that it should then be more plentifully inkindled, and burn with a greater flame, than if touch'd only with a more light burning, it should hastily pass thorow those places. But every one doth know

The Blood is more inkindled, and inflamed in Sleep, than in Waking.

Wherefore those that Sleep, are apt to be Cold outwardly.

by

by Experience in himself, that in Sleeping, the Præcordia grow very hot, and the External Parts are apt to be cold ; wherefore, there is need of covering them with Bed-Cloaths, whereby the Effluvia, deteined about the Compass of the Body, might warm it, whil'st in the mean time there is a Burning in the Breast, and from the Flame and Soot ascending from thence, the Tongue and Parts about the Mouth, as if roasted, are white : Hence in the Day-time those Sleeping in the open Air, or any where else, unless well defended with Cloaths, take Cold : for by reason of the Heat being drawn back, the Cold little Bodies of the Air compassing them, enter into the Pores, and stop them up; but on the other side, *Asthmatical* People, and such as have their Lungs stuffed or are otherways difficult to be moved, hardly Sleep within the Bed, because the ambient Heat so greatly increases the Flame, inkindled in the Præcordia, that for the eventilating it, and conveying it thorow the Arteries, the Lungs being weak, and growing tyred in the Motion, are scarce, nay, not at all sufficient.

2. Sleep allays the disorders of the Blood. 2. For as much as the Blood is more inkindled during Sleep, therefore then chiefly its disorders are allayed. But these are of a twofold Kind : to wit, either the Blood is variously agitated hither and thither by the impulses of the Conteining and Neighbouring Bodies, as in violent Passions, and Commotions both of the Body and of the Soul : Or it grows turgid, or swells up by its proper rage, after the manner of fermenting Wine, from the Heterogene, and heating Particles being mixed with it. As to the First, so long as we are Waking, the Course of the Blood being very much disturbed, is continually agitated as it were with certain winds : because the Fantasie, more strong Meditation, the Appetite, and the several Passions, drive the Blood sometimes more swiftly, sometimes repress it by their Influence, snatch it impetuously sometimes into these, sometimes into those Parts, and thence again repel it. Besides these Floods, *Whither they are induced by the conteining Bodies.* stirred up by the Mind, also the Motions of the Body and Members, render its Course yet more troubled and dangerous; because the Sanguiferous Vessels, being variously pressed, by the Motive Parts, and by and by released ; they variously transfer, and call back the Blood, and by and by snatch it elsewhere; hence, its Humour, so long as it rapidly runs from place to place, evaporates less, and so heaps together a greater stock of Excrementitious Matter, which being suppressed within, stirs up Preternatural Heat, and renders the Flame of the Blood unequal, more smoaky, and troubled, yea sharp and biting, and so troublesom to the Heart and Brain, and also to several Viscera, and sometimes to the whole Nervous Kind, all which notwithstanding Sleep allays ; yea whil'st the Animal Spirits lye quiet, like allayed winds, the Sea of the Blood presently becomes Calm.

The Internal boyling up of the Blood is also allayed by Sleep. Nor is the Blood, disturbed by reason of its proper Effervescency, less quieted by the Sleep: for when it grows hot from such a Cause, it flames not forth with a clear and bright Flame, but fumes up with Smoak and Soot, and therefore being less eventilated, diffuseth a very troublesom and sharp heat : which also is more infestous, because the Recrements of the Blood, to wit, the Serum, and adust, and otherways viscous Particles, being involved with its smoaking Latex, cannot be separated and carried away. But in Sleep, the Blood is soon quieted, and passes more slowly thorow the place of inkindling, to wit, the Lungs ; wherefore being there first more inkindled, it burns with a clearer Flame, and also more mildly, and so the smoak presently ceasing, and some Heterogenious Particles being burnt, all the rest extricating themselves from Confusion, what are profitable are imployed in their designed Offices, and what are unprofitable, are bolted or sifted forth, partly by Breathing, Transpiration, or Sweat, and partly thorow the other Emunctories.

The Blood performs its Offices, (which are the generation of the Animal Spirits, and the nourishing of the Parts) better in Sleep. 3. The Blood burning forth more clearly and plentifully in Sleep, at that time also performs better, yea chiefly, or almost only its Offices, the chief of which are, the Stilling forth of the Animal Spirits, and the Nutrition of the solid Parts. And first, it Prepares best of all Matter for both these, to wit, it well subdues, dresses, and ripens the Chyme, infused into its Mass : then it instills the more pure and more subtil Part into the Shell of the Brain, from which, the veterane Spirits, during Sleep depart, for the end that a way may be open, for the Nervous or Spirituous Liquor to restore their Stores ; and in the mean time, the other part of the Chyme, is conveyed every way by the Arteries, to the solid Parts, and whil'st they are quiet, it is best of all put upon them, and suffered to grow to them ; otherwise, by their too great Motion and Agitation (as in Waking) it is apt to be shaken and wiped off.

Sleep is not to be yielded to, presently after Eating. But that Nutrition, and the Production of Animal Spirits may be rightly performed, in Sleep, it is not to be presently indulged after Eating; for so the aforesaid Offices are wont, not only to be hindred, but perverted into Evil : because if any one Sleep with his Belly full, the Chyle as yet Crude, is snatched into the Blood : then before it can be there broken small, and mixed with the Blood exactly, it is exposed to a more full inkindling within the Lungs ; that from thence the Lungs themselves not rarely draw,

as

Of Sleep.

as from Juyces and Vapours there sent forth, from the Crude inkindled Matter (as it *Such Sleep* were from green Wood) an Evil: which thing indeed is observed of many, falling into *hurts the Lungs* the *Phthisis* or Consumption of the Lungs. Thirdly, At length from the *Chyme* so evilly *and Brain.* prepared, neither pure Spirits are dispensed to the Brain, nor laudible nourishment to *Makes the Spi-* the solid Parts; yea, that is obscured and made dull by Fumes and Vapours, and these *rits more dull* are disposed into a *Cachexie* or *Atrophie*. *nourishment.*

So much concerning the Effects and Alterations of Sleep, which indeed are wont to *What Sleep af-* be more immediately impressed on the Flamey part of the Soul, rooted in the Blood, *fords to the Lu-* but mediately on the Parts of the Body depending upon it: Now let us see next, what *cid part of the* this Passion brings to the other Part of the Soul, *viz.* the Lucid; and its Subjects, to *Soul.* wit, the Brain and Nervous Stock; Concerning these, we will shew what Sleep contributes to the dispensation of the Nervous Liquor, and to the generation of Spirits out of it, we shall also further Consider, what sort of influence it has on their Exercises and Government.

As to these, First, It is to be noted, which we before-mentioned, to wit, that the *It refreshes the* Spirits of the Regiment of the Brain, the Executors of every Spontaneous Function, are *wearied Spirits* employed only Waking; and that others arising from the Cerebel, both Waking *inhabiting the* and in Sleep: There is need for Sleep only for the former, whil'st they are well, that *Brain.* their Expences or consumed Stores might be by it repaired: yea, and that the languishing or weariness of those remaining might be refreshed. This every one experiences in himself, and feels that there is no farther need of explaining it: But if the *And allays* same Spirits, by some Morbifick Cause, being provoked, are moved into disorder, that *them, being out* they become irregular about the Acts of Motions, or of the Senses, whether Interior or *of order.* Exterior, and stir up a Delirium, Convulsions, or Pains, Sleep, like a Charm, fully quiets these Spirits, how mad and devilish soever they be: wherefore if it comes not of it self, in these Cases it ought to be fetch'd with Opiats.

But as to the Spirits, the inhabitants of the Cerebel, because, in Waking they are di- *The Spirits in-* sturbed by the business and tumult of the Spontaneous Functions, and being called away *habiting the Ce-* from their Labours are hindred; therefore, they perform their tasks better in the rest *rebel, are di-* and deep silence of the others: Hence the Concoction and the distribution of the Food, *sturbed, in Wa-* and the Separation of the Excrements, yea, and the *Oeconomy* of the whole Animal Fun- *king, with the* ction, is best performed by reason of Sleep: Hence, if at any time, too much Meat, or *Spirits of the* more gross than is wont, being eaten, molests the Stomach, and inducing fulness, nau- *other Regiment.* seousness, or bitter and acid belching to it, approaching Sleep, for the most Parts takes away these Evils, and facilitating the Concoction of the *Chyle*, clears it from its sharpness, foulness, and bitterness. The reason of which is, because the Animal Spirits, which *Why those being* actuating the Fibres of the Stomach, serve for Digestion, whil'st awake; being forced *disturbed, do* to bear its manner or guise towards the Brain, and its Parts, are distracted here and *perform their* there, and are called away from their proper work, so that the Meat being as it were *Offices better,* unfermented, and undigested, stays in the Ventricle. This every one plainly experien- *whil'st these lye* ces in himself, if presently he sits down after feeding to Study, or serious Reading, for *quiet in Sleep.* then the Brain being full and disturbed, the ponderous and heavy *Chyle* in the Stomach, is deprived of Digestion: But in Sleep, the Spirits inhabiting the Ventricle, being freed *Other benefits of* from the Businesses of the Brain, do best of all perform their task, and rightly digest and *Sleep are noted.* exalt by Fermentation, the *Chyle* in the Stomach, like an Elixir in a Furnace, with an equal and convenient heat. I might here enumerate other benefits of Sleep, for as much *Hence Chylifi-* as it refreshes the whole Faculties of the Soul, renews the vigour of the Intellect or *cation, and other* Wit, sharpens the Senses, stops the tumults of Passions, recollects the forces of the Co- *functions mere-* gitations, as often as they are either wholly enervated, or distracted by immoderate Stu- *ly Natural, are* dy, or long Waking, allays and quiets all things, and heals the weak Brain, and the *performed best* languishments of its Parts, yea, and of all other Parts and Powers, by giving to them *of all in Sleep.* new forces or strength, as it were Food to such as want.

The Nature, Causes, and Effects of Sleep, being unfolded after this manner, before we wholly leave its Consideration, it will not be from the Matter, to subjoyn something of Dreams, we shall here purposely pass over what manner of Signification they have, both Natural, as they indicate the intemperance of the Brain, and also fatidical, as if they were inspired by a *Dæmon*, and are affirmed to Prophesie things to come: we shall *Of Dreams.* only inquire by what Motion, and agitation of the Animal Spirits, Dreams are produced in the Brain. We say therefore, that the Animal Spirits, although they affect naturally alternate times of Motion and Rest, and whil'st they indulge Rest, instilling fresh Nervous Humor to the Brain, they suffer themselves to be bound together with Embraces, as it were with Chains, that they may not enter into Motion; yet it for the most part happens, that some Spirits easily cast off this Bond, and love to wander hither and thither, in the deep silence of the Rest. And indeed Dreams are only the Excursions of *What they are.*

some

some Spirits in the Brain, from their bond or tye, which, whil'st the rest are strictly bound together, wander about, without any Guide or Ruler; and repeat the types or shaddows of Motions, as it were Dances before learnt; and are wont to represent the Cogitations of things, though after a very confused manner. The Spirits which being got loose, variously run about, whil'st the rest are bound together, gain the Liberty of Motion, by a twofold means. To wit, some Spirits, fly from the Captivity of Sleep, for the most part, by reason of the Heat and Agitation of the Brain, as by Drinking of Wine, the fume of Tobacco, immoderate Exercise, as also by the Passions, and more hard study, is wont to arise: for by these means, the Spirits are stirred up, by a certain Stimulation or Provokement, and are driven as it were into rage, that, though Sleep creep upon them, all of them will not be bound or restrained, but that some of them will walk about the Sepulchers of the rest, like Spectres in a Church-yard, and cause stupendious Apparitions of things. Another Exsuscitation of some Spirits in the Brain, whereby Dreams are produced, is made by reason of some Spirits being disturbed in other Parts, as in the Præcordia, Stomach, Spleen, Genitals, &c. By which, whil'st the same Perturbation is Communicated by the Nerves to the Brain, perhaps one or two Handfuls or Bands of Spirits, there stirred up, causes various Phantasies to be represented. In the Disease called the *Incubus* or Night-Mare, when the Præcordia are stop'd in their Motion, or otherwise hindred, by reason of the Nerves being bound together, we Dream some Animal or heavy weight lying upon the Breast, stops our Breathing. The Genital Humor growing turgid or swelling up in the Vessels, and irritating them, produces immodest Dreams. Undigested and gross Meats, eaten at Supper, because they aggravate or lye heavy in the Ventricle, and trouble it, render Sleep also troubled, and infested with terrible and affrightful Phantasies; in like manner we might easily shew, that it is the same with many other Parts.

Whil'st as it were private Troops of Spirits, being excited in the Brain, carrying themselves hither and thither, exercise the Phantasie, their Divergency, or Excursions happen sometimes regularly, sometimes inordinately: and therefore Dreams, represent either the Series of things before acted, or only *Chimera*'s, or Notions altogether incongruous and disagreeing. Further, whil'st the Animal Spirits, being agitated by this means, within the Brain, produce Dreams or the Images of Cogitations, do often leap back, into the Nervous Stock, and there stirring up other Spirits, produce divers sorts of local Motions: wherefore some Men also, when they Sleep soundly, are wont to rise out of their Bed, to walk here and there, to remove the Houshold-stuff from place to place, oftentimes to put on their Cloaths, to open the Doors, go up Stairs, and to pass over Rocky places, which they could scarce go over when Awake; in the mean time if they meet with any Obstacle in their Progress, they either advisedly pass by it, or remove it out of the way. I knew a certain Man, who was wont after this manner to walk a-Nights like a Spectre, and to speak to others whom he met being Awake, would take them by the hand, and often-times strike them, then, unless he being roughly handled did Awake; returning to his Bed, and after Awaking of his own accord, knew nothing at all of what he had done. Yea, it is observed of most of these Night-walkers like Spirits, that being awakned, they scarce remember any thing of what they did, or acted in their Sleep; as if they suffer'd something that was different from other Dreamers; for these think that they perform local Motions, when indeed there is no such thing, but the others move from place to place, and yet know nothing of it. In Dreamers, the Spirits being stirred up, spread or are carried wholly inwards, towards the Callous Body, and affect only the Imagination and Memory: but in those walking in their Sleep, some handfuls or bands of them, being awakned, direct their tendency only outwards, towards the moving Parts, in the mean time, the Common Sense, Imagination, and Memory are not at all affected. It is wonderful, what ordinarily happens to Witches, or Wise-women; to wit, they, whil'st they lye Buried in a profound Sleep imagine that they are in very far and remote places, and that they have seen the Spectacles of Seas and Lands, and things wholly unknown to them, and shall exactly describe them; which without doubt is, because the Devil brings the Idea's of these things before the Phantasie, and so strongly impresses them, that they for a certain believe, that they had been in them: On the contrary, Walkers in their Sleep, wander about the whole House, and its Precincts, and truly perform divers Actions, of which, when they are Awake, they are wholly ignorant. If the reason of this Kind of Passion be inquired into, this first of all occurs; that those so affected, freely exercise, at that time, the Faculties, both Sensitive and Locomotive; because, they not only move their Feet and Arms, as it were in certain Measures and Numbers, as a Machine furnished with wheels and force is wont to do; but moreover, they hear with their Ears, see with their Eyes, and with a certain discretion vary their local Motions, according to the Impressions

made

made from sensible things. Wherefore, from hence we may lawfully conclude, that some Animal Spirits, being stirred up inordinately, within the hinder Part of the middle of the Brain, perhaps about the streaked Bodies, do strike upon the little heads of the Nerves, and so raise up other Spirits, implanted by a long Series, within the nervous Passages, and the moving Parts, and drive them into Motions before accustomed to; hence the divers movings of the Body and Members, are produced. But, because the tendency of the Spirits excited is made only outwards, and is not at all reflected inwards into the streaked and Callous Bodies; therefore, for that the Common Sensory nor the Imagination are affected, they neither perceive nor remember the Actions they had done. If it should be demanded, (for as much as the Common Sense at this time is stupified or asleep) by what instinct the Animal Spirits are determined, according to the Impressions of Sensible Things, for the performing of local Motions of this or that Kind; It may be said, That this reciprocation of Sense and Motion, depends chiefly upon Custom, *viz.* The Spirits being before accustomed to be ordered after this or that manner, and having gotten the Liberty of Action in Sleep, compose themselves of their own accord, for the performing of their wonted Measures; even as when an Harper, whil'st he is thinking of some other thing, his Fingers being before taught the Numbers of the Tune, exactly strike the Strings, with wonderful agility and discretion.

Therefore, the Cause of walking in Sleep, seems to consist in this, *viz.* That the Animal Spirits are too fierce and unquiet, and will not all lye down together, but that some of them, more fierce than the rest, leap forth of their own accord, and enter into Motion, like as perhaps one or two Dogs, starting out without government, leave the company of the rest and fall to Hunting: For that Cause also, the Spirits so apt to wander and roam about for Excursion, obtain their more free spaces in the Oblong Marrow, nigh the Nervous Original, rather than in the Brain or in its middle or marrowie Part. For it seems, that during Sleep, the Pores and Passages in the globous frame of the Brain, are stuffed up so, that the Spirits there, like to water frozen, are thrust in hard together; in the mean time, the Substance within the Medullar Processes of the Brain, and the Oblong Marrow, which lead towards the Nervous Original, is more loose, and possessed less with an adventitious Humour; that the Spirits there being ready for Motion, easily make way for themselves to go forth, and entring the little heads of the Nerves, produce local Motions, of which the Common Sense, and the Superior Facuities of the Soul are utterly ignorant. For such a Disposition of the Brain and its Appendix, which inclines to wandring by Night, as if it depended upon a certain peculiar Conformation of the Organ, is proper to some Men from their Birth; nor does it indifferently happen to all Men, or is ever contracted by the reason of inordinate Living. I have known in a certain Family, where both the Father, and all his Children were obnoxious to this Affection, the Brothers would often run up and down in the Night, in their Sleep, sometimes meet and lay hold upon one another, and so awake one another. But others, who had not this Evil impress'd upon them from their Birth, have fallen into this Distemper, without any fore-warning or manifest Occasion.

Thus much concerning Sleep, and by the by of Dreams: we have largely handled thus the Nature of it, because this Speculation very much Conduces to the illustrating the Affections of the Brain, and the Nervous Stock. It behoves us next, that we consider of the *Aurora* of Sleep, to wit, Waking; but this may be considered under a twofold respect; either First, for as much as it succeeds Sleep, it is its bound; or Secondly, according to its proper Essence. As to the former, we Awake, or Sleep is shaken off, either because it ends of its own accord, or because it is interrupted. That it may end of its own accord, two things are requisite, to wit, that the Animal Spirits, being enough refreshed, rise up of their own accord, and return to their wonted watches; which indeed, they for the most part do, at a set-time, unless hinder'd: Secondly, That what ever is superfluous of the serous Humor, by whose Embraces the Spirits are bound, be evaporated: for after Banquetting, or often Drinking, by which a greater plenty of the serous and spirituous *Latex* is carried to the Brain, we Sleep longer; so that there is need that Sleep be longer protracted, that it may suffice to spew forth the untamed Wine. But Rest is very much interrupted by a violent Sensation; to wit, some Spirits dwelling about the Extremities of the Nerves, being awakned by the impulse of some strong object, awake others in the Common Sensory, whereby Sensation is performed, and then the stroke being further continued, all, being, as it were at a Sign given, called to Arms, awake suddenly, and fall to their watches. This kind of troublesom Sensation, which awakes the Animal Spirits from Sleep, is not only brought in from an outward sensible thing, as when a great sound, or stroke made on the Flesh, shakes off Sleep; but sometimes the Nervous Parts are pulled by a sharp Humor, Physick, Worms, and other Internal Distempers, and so a Convulsion or Pain arising, the Spirits are compelled into Motion, and for that reason,

Of Waking.
A double Consideration of it.
1. As it follows upon Sleep.
Waking is either Natural or Violent.

son, we are excited from Sleep. As often as Sleep is broken off sooner than it ought, often yawning, and reatching, for the most part follows: the reason of which is, because the Spirits being awakned, strive by contracting and extending those Parts, to shake off the Dewie Humor, not sufficiently evaporated from the Brain and Nervous Parts. Further, If we are forced to awake, before the Spirits are refreshed with their wonted Provision, they from thence become dull and heavy, and less ready for the exercise of the Animal Function.

The Essence or formal Reason of Waking. As to the Essence or formal Reason of Waking, it consists in the liberty and expansion of the Animal Spirits, in the Brain, and the whole Nervous Stock. For these, like standing Souldiers, desire to watch, both to meet the sensible Object, also by reason of their obedience towards the Superior Powers of the Soul, so long as they are fit for this work: But that the Animal Spirits may be able to perform their watches in a just time, and with their whole strength it is required, that they should be free without any Impediments; to wit, that they be not irritated with any gross, or otherways Excrementitious Humor, nor drowned with a serous heap, but that being free from all burthen, they might remain ready, and still nimble for the swiftest Motions. Then Secondly, That the Spirits may rightly perform their watches, there is need, that they should be only intangled in moderate Affairs. Being fitted by these Kind of defences, they lively accomplish their Task, and daily for so many hours, continue their Motion, like the Wheels of a Clock, and then, the time being expired, they go to Rest of their own accord.

The End of the First Part.

THE SECOND PART PATHOLOGICAL:

OR

Of the DISEASES which belong to the Corporeal Soul and its Subjects, *viz.*

The Brain and the Nervous Stock.

CHAP. I.

Of the Headach.

THE pain of the Head is wont to be accounted the chiefest of the Diseases of the Head, and as it were to lead the troops of the other Affections of that part; for that it is the most common and most frequent symptom, to which indeed there is none but is sometimes obnoxious, so that it is become a Proverb, as a sign of a more rare and admirable thing, *That his Head did never ake.* *The Pain of the Head the chiefest and most common affection among Diseases.*

The Headach, though it be a most frequent Distemper, hath so various, uncertain, and often a contrary original, that it seems most difficult to deliver an exact *Theorie* of its appearance, containing the solutions of so manifold, and often opposite things. This Disease being constant to no temperament, constitution, or manner of living, nor to no kind of evident or adjoyning causes; ordinarily falls upon cold and hot, sober and intemperate, the empty and the full bellied, the fat and the lean, the young and old, yea upon Men and Women of every age, state, or condition. Hence, because they cannot satisfie any one sick with this Distemper, with the causes of it, most commonly they say, they all proceed from Vapours. Further, the Cure of this Disease is more happily instituted, not so much by certain Indications, as by trying various things, and at length, by collecting an Extempory method of Healing, from things helping and hurting. Wherefore, if I should go about to untye this hard knot, by drawing forth the matter more deeply and more accurately, I must ask for pardon, if I am carried, by a long compass, thorow the various Series and Complication of Causes: and if at length, by any means, the *Ætiology* or the Reason of this Disease may be fully detected, a more certain way to its Cure may be opened. *The Causes of it manifold, and very diverse, that they can hardly be methodically recited.*
Hence it is, that its Cure is often instituted Empirically.

Therefore, that we may go on more fully to institute this *Pathology*, or shewing the Causes or *symptoms* of this Disease, we ought first of all to unfold the Subject, and the formal reason of this Disease, together with the Causes and differences; then to subjoyn the Curatory method, and to illustrate it with some more rare Cases and Observations. *what things belong to its Pathology.*

As to the former, as all pain is a hurt or violated Action, or a troublesome sension or feeling, depending on a Convulsion, or a Corrugation of the Nerves, the Subject of the Headach are the most nervous parts of the Head, that is, the Nerves themselves, as also the Fibres and Membranes, and such as are more and most sensible, seated both without and within the skull. But the parts of this kind, which are affected with pain, are first the two *Meninges*, and their various processes, the Coats of *The Subject of this Disease.*

Of the Headach.

the Nerves, the *Pericranium* (or skin compassing the skull) and other thin skinny Membranes, the fleshy Panicle of the Muscle, and lastly the skin it self. As to the Brain and Cerebel, and their Medullary dependences, we affirm, That these Bodies are free from pains, because they want sensible Fibres, apt to be wrinkled and distended: the same, for the like reason, may be said of the Skull.

The formal Reason of it.

2. But whensoever pain is excited any where about the nervous parts of the Head, its formal reason consists in this, That the Animal Spirits being drawn one from another, and put to flight, cause the containing Bodies to be pulled together and wrinkled, and so stir up a troublesome sension or feeling: But that which so distracts the Spirits, that from thence a troublesome feeling arises, is some improportionate thing, rushing upon the Spirits themselves, or on the Bodies containing them, which entring the Pores of, and spaces between, the Fibres, pulls them one from another, and so drives the spirits dwelling there into disorder.

The differences and kinds. Pain is either without, or within the Skull;

3. As to the differences of the Headach, the common distinction is, That the pain of the Head is either without the Skull, or within its cavity: The former is a more rare and a more gentle disease, because the parts above the Skull are not so sensible as the interior *Meninges*; nor are they watered with so plentiful a flood of Blood, that by its sudden and vehement incursion, they may be easily distended, or inflamed above measure. Secondly, The other kind of Headach, to wit, within the Skull, is more frequent, and much more cruel, because the Membranes, cloathing the Brain, are very sensible, and the Blood is poured upon them by a manifold passage, and by many and greater Arteries. Further, because the Blood or its Serum, sometimes passing thorow all the Arteries at once, both the *Carotides* and the *Vertebrals*, and sometimes apart, thorow these or those, on the one side or the opposite, bring hurt to the *Meninges*, hence the pain is caused that is interior; which is either universal, infesting the whole Head or its greatest part; or particular, which is limited to some private region; and sometimes produces a Meagrim on the side, sometimes in the forepart, and sometimes in the hinder part of the Head.

Or universal, or particular.
This either before, behind, or on the side.

Many other differences of it noted;

There are many other differences of this Disease, to wit, That the Pain is either light or vehement, sharp or dull, short or of continuance, continual or intermitting; its approaches sometimes periodical and exact, sometimes wandring and uncertain. Also by reason of the Conjunct Cause, which (as shall be declared by and by) sometimes is the Blood, sometimes certain excrements of it, as either the Serum, or nourishing juice, or vapours, or wind; sometimes it is the nervous liquor, sometimes a congression or striving of it with the bloody liquor: The Headach may be called, either bloody, and that either simple, or else serous, vaporous, or otherways excrementitious; or else Convulsive, from the humor watering the nervous Fibres, and irritating them into painful Corrugations.

Of which the chiefest is, that it is either occasional, or habitual.

Concerning these, that we may proceed methodically, we shall rehearse in a certain order, the various kinds of this Disease, with their Causes; and it seems good, that we distinguish the Pain of the Head to be either accidental, or occasional and habitual: The former is wont to be excited without any foregoing cause, or previous disposition, by the solitary evident cause, as when an Headach happens almost to all men after the drinking of Wine, Surfetting, lying in the Sun, or vehement exercise, also in the fitts of Feavours; to wit, forasmuch as the Blood being incited, more than it was wont, and boiling up immoderately, very much blows up and distends the Membranes it passes thorow; yea the Serum and Vapors, copiously sent forth, from it, then growing hot, and rushing on the Membranes, pull and provoke the nervous Fibres.

The reason of the former unfolded.

The habitual Pain of the Head hath always a more remote Cause, besides the evident Cause.

Secondly, The habitual pain of the Head, hath some *procatartick* or more remote Cause fixed somewhere, by reason of which it is troubled, either constantly or often; so that though it sometimes intermits, yet it often returns of its own accord, and is excited also upon every light occasion: but this, whether it be continual or intermitting, hath neither always, nor only, the Suffusions or too great Evaporations of the Blood or Serum, for the Conjunct Cause, (although these are often present, where notwithstanding they are rather instead of the Evident Cause, than the Conjunct) but beside, an evil *procatarxis*, or a certain predisposition, is always affixed to the part affected, or wont to be distemper'd; by reason of which, the aforesaid Causes, also the inordinations of the Nervous Liquor, and the meeting and growing hot of it with the bloody Serum, or the Nutritious Juice, raise up the fits of pains.

The evils, or the weak Constitution of the affected part, and the easie flowing in of the morbific matter, concur to this more remote cause.

The Parts of the Head predisposed, and their vices, viz. an evil or weak conformation are noted.

Although the more remote Cause of the Headach be manifold and diverse, so that its several kinds can scarcely be number'd, yet for the constituting it, these two, to wit, either one or both of them, do chiefly or for the most part lead the way, viz. First, The evil or weak Constitution of the affected part. Secondly, Then, because of the more easie and ready heaping up of the Morbific matter in it.

As

Of the Headach.

As to the former, the parts of the Head obnoxious to pains, are the Nervous Fibres, belonging to the Membranes, Tendons, the Musculous flesh, and other sensible Bodies; the Morbid provision of which consists in their evil conformation or debility.

Of these, that the former is sometimes innate and hereditary, appears from hence, *The former often* because the Disease is often delivered from the Parents to the Children: and seems to *times is innate* be done chiefly by this means: because the covering of the Head being made more *and hereditary;* thick, or more close than it ought, neither the humors, nor the vapours do easily pass thorow; wherefore being by these restrained, and hindred in their Motion, and so heaped up, the *Meninges, Pericranium,* and other sensible parts, being too much stuffed, or inflated, or hauled, receive pains: to which happens, that sometimes, by reason of the original intemperance of the Brain, the Humors or Vapours about the parts, hanging like an arch over it, are variously heaped up together.

2. But it more often comes to pass, that the Vices of an evil Conformation, by *But more often* which these or those parts of the Head are disposed to the Headach, are contracted a- *is contracted a-* new, and that by a various kind of production: for sometimes by Cold taken, by rea- *new:* son of the Northern winds, Snow, or Rain, the Pores of the skin in some region of the Head, yea and the nervous Fibres themselves, are so closed up, or otherwise perverted or weakned, that they are not able to bear the outward air, nor the agita- *And chiefly* tions of the Blood or Humors, but presently the Headach arises. *from Cold,*

Nor is the predisposition of the Headach less rarely produced, in the disorderly use- *Also by reason of* ing the six not natural things. For the Blood being stirred up above measure, upon *the inordinati-* any cause whatsoever, impresses by its boyling up, or by the insinuation of the Serum *ons in the six* or Vapours, a breaking of the unity in some nervous parts, or some other sort of hurt, *non naturals.* for which reason, as there is a present Headach, by and by stirred up, so afterwards there is a disposition to the same, upon every light occasion. But oftentimes *By accident.* a disposition to the Headach not easily blotted out, is induced by a vehement Passion, Surfeit, Drunkenness, also by a blow, wound, or contusion of the Head: so that either the proper or excrementitious humors being heaped up, and standing in those parts, being afterwards moved of themselves, or growing hot with other inflowing *From internal* juices, stir up inflations, or painful haulings or pullings. Yea, I have known Inflamma- *Concretions.* tions, Imposthumes, Whelks, *Scirrhous* tumors growing to the *Meninges* with the Skull, and other Diseases of an evil conformation, excited in the Membranes of the Brain; by which, at first for a long time, frequent Headaches, and most cruel, and then afterwards a sleepy and deadly distemper hath been induced; the cause of the Disease not detected, but after death by *Anatomy*; and indeed it is to be suspected, that inveterate and pertinacious pains in the Head, which return, and dayly become more tormentive, in spight of all Remedies, depend upon some such invincible cause.

2. Not only an evil conformation, or the breach of unity, but also sometimes a *2. The debility* meer weakness or enervation, renders some parts of the Head obnoxious to the Head- *of the distem-* ach; for when as the Fibres are somewhere so infirm, that they are neither able of *per'd part is al-* themselves to rule the proper humor, nor to resist the incursions of a strange humor; *so a more remote* the part so disposed, by reason of any light occasion, is moved into painful wrinklings: *cause of the* These kind of debilities of the Fibres, sometimes external accidents, as the excess of *Which outward* cold or heat; sometimes also errors in Dyet or living, as Surfeit, Drunkenness, and *accidents and* especially sleeping at noon; moreover great *Catarrhs,* and a long lodging of a sharp *errours in feed-* Serum are wont to bring in. *ing and other*

So much for the primary more remote cause of the Headach, which is also fixed *wont to produce.* and rooted: The other cause of it, secondary and moveable, consists in a ready and *The other part of* easie heaping up of the Morbific matter about the predisposed parts, from which *the more remote* come the fits of pains, and their approaches: But as the matter is manifold, it is *and moveable,* wont to be heaped up after a diverse manner, and to excite pains which affect after a *consisting in the,* diverse sort: This, as we have said, is either the Blood, or its Serum, or the nourish- *flowing in of the* ing Juice, or the nervous Liquor. Every of these being variously disposed, or imbued *morbific mat-* with feculences or dregs, are by degrees heaped up about the predisposed parts of the *This matter is ei-* Head, sometimes before the fit; and sometimes, that coming, they are plentifully *ther the Blood,* cast down. But sometimes one only humour with its plenitude and acrimony, distends *or its serum, or* or provokes the sensible Fibres; sometimes more meeting together, by their mutual *the nutritious, or* growing hot, pull or haule the Fibres, and so stir up painful Convulsions. We shall *nervous Juice.* briefly take notice of the several kinds of these, with their signs, and the manner of their *Which some-* being made. When therefore a part of the Head, as chiefly the *Meninges,* or some re- *sometimes meet-* gion of the *Pericranium,* is predisposed, by reason of an evil conformation or debility, *ing together,* to the Headach; the approaches or fits of the Disease are wont to be excited, by rea- *irritate the pre-*
disposed parts.

B 2 son

son of the various incursions or coming together of the following humors, sometimes of this, sometimes of that humor, and sometimes of many together.

How the Blood excites the Headach.

1. Sometimes the Blood it self being incited into a more rapid motion, and boiling up into the Head, is straitned or stopp'd in its passage about the predisposed places, and from thence, being by and by heaped up there, distends the Vessels, greatly blows up the Membranes, and pulls the nervous Fibres one from another, and so brings to them painful corrugations or wrinklings. For this reason those obnoxious to the Headach, are forced to shun all occasions by which the Blood should grow hot above measure, as drinking of Wine, Exercise, Baths, &c

2 How the Serum.

2. The Serum being more copiously heaped up in the bloody Mass, oftentimes conceives a sudden Flux, either of its own accord through meer fulness, or stirred up by an evident cause, and so presently running forth from the Blood doth not only rush into the Lungs, but very often into the Head, and being poured upon its Membranes or Muscles, is copiously heaped up about the parts predisposed to the Headach, and there induces painful Corrugations and Inflations. Further, the Serum carries with it infestous Recrements, as sulphureous, saline, sharp, acid, bilious, or melancholic, or of some other kind, and fixes them to the nervous Fibres, which cause an acute or dull, a shorter or a longer pain. The Headaches arising by reason of this kind of remote cause, infest more grievously in the Winter time, in a moist Air, and in a Southern Wind: Moreover, *Catarrhs* of the Face, Mouth, *Larynx*, and of other parts, oftentimes accompany this Disease.

3 How the nutritious Juice.

3. The nourishing Juice, or fresh *Chyme*, being carried from the Blood to the solid parts, and laid upon them, by reason it becomes improportionate to some parts of the Head evilly disposed, is wont to excite periodical fits of the Headach. For this provision being laid up near some nervous Fibres, because it cannot be assimilated, begins to trouble them or burthen them, after some stay, and at length provokes them into wrinklings to expulse that which troubles them. An Headach proceeding from such a cause, as I have observed in many, doth dayly come at so many hours after eating, and continues a like space of time; yea the times alter according to the manner of taking their repast, both as to the quality and quantity, and so also the fits of the pains are wont to vary.

4 How the nervous Liquor is a cause of this Disease.

4. The nervous Liquor, is a cause of pains, by its inordination, as oftentimes in other parts, so also not seldom in the Head; for this either degenerating from its temper, or being imbued with dregs or filthiness, does not pass thorow so freely the nervous Fibers, but is apt to stagnate, and be heaped up in them to an irritative fulness: and that chiefly within the Fibres made weak beforehand, or of an evil conformation (such as are sometimes the Membranes of the Head) because in these predisposed, the watering Liquor being hindred in Motion, easily arises to an aggravating or provoking fulness; so that the Fibres being so filled, like the stomach too much crammed, enter into Convulsions and painful wrinklings, for the putting away their contents, nor do they cease from them, till they are freed of their burthen; which notwithstanding, afterwards being heaped up again, sometimes sooner and sometimes later, cause from thence others, and so again other fits of pains. The Headach arising from such a cause, springs oftentimes without any notable turgescency of the Blood, and gently and as it were of its own accord, without any errors in dyet or living; yet sometimes it may sooner arise by reason of disorders in the non-naturals, and other accidents: This is wont to come more often in the Morning, and after long sleeping, when the nervous Fibres have drunk in this humor more largely.

The Headach arising from the fault of the nervous Liquor infests chiefly in the Morning.

5 How many humors meeting together, and mutually growing hot, stir up Headaches.

In the aforesaid Headaches, the Morbifick matter is made up for the most part of one singular humor, and so the fits of the pains are something more gentle, and oftentimes sooner pass over. But there is another Cause of this Disease, when two humors (like divers kinds of Salts) meet together, and grow mutually hot, and so from the strife of dissimilar particles, the Fibres are very much pulled, and moved into very acute and cutting pains, and are most commonly longer infested with them. In this case one of the champions is always the nervous liquor, but the other, either the serous water or the nourishing juice. We exempt the Blood, because it only washes the passages of the Nerves, and does not enter them deeply; but the nervous humor, by reason of the vices but now recited, sometimes of it self, pulls the containing Fibres, and provokes them into painful Convulsions. If that another humor, either the Nutritious or Serous, (for both of them are wont to be guilty) being little of kin, be plentifully poured upon this so predisposed, and copiously heaped up within the Fibres; presently all the particles being raised up, strive among themselves, and so by a mutual effervency, notably distend and haule the Fibres, that from hence from their being long and greatly wrinkled, most sharp and long remaining pains are induced. Whether it be

this

Of the Headach.

this or that humor, meeting with the nervous juice, that causes the Headach, may be easily known from the proper irregularities, above described, of either peccant humor by it self.

By what means, and for what more remote causes, the humors, either Nutritious or Serous, offend, as often as meeting with the Nervous humour, contained within the Fibres, move the fits of pains, shall be declared anon: in the mean time, I think it sufficiently appears, that the more frequent and habitual Headaches are produced chiefly by the fault of the nervous liquor, because this is most intimate both with the Fibres themselves, which are wrinkled, and the Spirits which are moved into painful distractions; also because the pains of the Head sometimes arise without any disorder or tumult of the Blood, Serum, or nourishing Juice, and these being emptied or allayed, after what manner soever, oftentimes the Headach most pertinaciously continues. *The habitual Headach depends chiefly upon the fault of the nervous humor.*

But concerning the nervous Liquor, when it is the cause of the Headach, we observe that its fault is sometimes universal, and sometimes private: for sometimes it doth acquire its evil from the distempered part: to wit, forasmuch as being constrained to subsist or stagnate within the Fibres, hurt by their conformation, it is so perverted that at length being infested, fermenting either by it self, or with some other humor, it irritates them into painful Corrugations: Yet sometimes, and especially in the more grievous Headaches, we may suppose that the whole Mass of the nervous Liquor is in fault, but the nervous parts of the Head partake of its evil, before any others in the whole Body; because these are the chief and nearest springs of the nervous Liquor, and are also highly sensible: wherefore, the nervous Liquor, when ever it is vicious, either swelling up of its own accord, or growing hot by another humour being poured unto it, within the *Meninges* and other Membranes of the Head, more than in the other parts of the Body, becomes painful. The thing appears to be so, because a long and grievous Headach is wont to be Cured, not so much by Remedies applyed or proper for the Head, as by those which restore the *Crasis* or Constitution of the nervous Juice, and the bloody Mass; and such are *Chalybeats*, or Steel Medicines, and *Antiscorbuticks*, or Medicines against the Scurvy. Which certainly argues that the nervous Liquor, where-ever it is in fault thorow the whole Body, chiefly punishes the parts of the Head. *The fault of the nervous liquor is either universal, or particular, proper to the place distempered.*

Thus much for the causes of the Headach, both the procatartick or foregoing, and the Conjunct: there yet remain others more remote, called Evident, which raise up the former, and provoke them into act, or the painful means of affecting. But they are of a various kind, and of a divers operation: to wit, Whatever things are apt, first, to transfer the Morbifick matter from another place into the part affected; or secondly, to move it before lodging in it; or thirdly, and lastly, which impress on the Fibres themselves, predisposed to painful Convulsions, this Distemper, by the consent of the other parts afar off, they belong to this rank. *The more remote or evident Causes of the Headach are noted.*

As to the former, the Blood and its inmate humors, to wit, the Serous and nutritious; also the bilous, acid, and otherwise vicious recrements, are apt to be moved from various Causes, and to be transferred into the Membranes of the Head, viz. many accidents from without ordinarily effect this, as great and sudden mutations of the Air, or the season of the year, excess of heat or cold, or of moisture, plentiful feeding, drinking of Wine, Bathing, immoderate Venus, violent passions; yea many other occasions sufficiently known, and to be avoided by all subject to Headaches. Further, these humors sometimes swell up of their own accord, and without any external Cause, or other ways evident, being moved, drive themselves forward into the Head: in which place, when they come, and settle upon the Fibres before indisposed, though they constitute a part of the Conjunct Cause, yet they, when they are first in motion or flux, become the means of the Evident Cause. Wherefore, when we have first unfolded, by what means the Blood, with its contents, being carried to the distempered Membranes, stir up Headaches; we shall then shew by what means, and upon what occasions, the same humors are wont to be moved, and to be snatched into the Membranes. *Of which sort are, first, those which move the morbifick matter flowing from another place, to wit, either the Blood, or Serum, or nourishing juice, and stir it up within the places affected of the Head. The Blood and its contents, in Headaches are sometimes the means of the Conjunct, sometimes of the Evident Cause.*

And first the Blood growing hot of its own accord, and by reason of the strife, and intestine motions of its particles, imparts its trouble to the Head: Its frequent and wandring turgency or boiling up, happens not only in the fits of Feavours, but also without any cause or suspicion of disease, which in others scarce perceiveable, those obnoxious to the Headach sufficiently take notice of and feel; neither doth the blood only bestow the hurt to the Head, from its own proper provision, but receiving it elsewhere, sends it thither. Oftentimes the Blood receives the incongruous matter from the Stomach, Spleen, Mesentery, Liver, and other parts, or Inwards, infestous to it self or nervous Stock; which growing hot a little time after, *For what Causes the Blood is wont to be moved, and to bring hurt to the distempered Head.*

that

The Blood deli-
vers to the head
the morbifick
matter received
from any other
part. that it might extrude or thrust it forth; it pours it upon the Membranes of the Head, and so produces the Headach, commonly called Sympathetick, *viz.* by a consent excited in other parts; which kind of Distemper being transmitted from other parts to the Head, sometimes also it happens after another manner, as shall be by and by declared.

A Flux of the
Serum sometimes
from meer full-
ness. When the Mass of Blood abounds with Serum, it is sometimes excited to the putting it off by meer fulness, wherefore it conceives a flux, or as it were a certain melting, to wit, by which the thin and watery part may be separated from the thick and bloody. Then, because the Blood becomes more diluted in its swelling up, and passes more swiftly and more copiously thorow the Arteries, than can be carried back by the Veins, almost all that is serous is sent away by the spaces between the Vessels, being poured sometimes on these parts, and sometimes on those, as falling down in many places, it causes tumors or Catharrs, so lying on the Membranes of the Head, it stirs up fits of pains.

Sometimes from
other Causes. But the serous heap, from many other causes sweating forth from the Blood suffering a flux, rushes on the Meninges and the Pericranium, and causes in them most troublesome Headaches. A sudden Constipation or closing of the Pores by Cold or Wet, almost constantly produces such a Distemper in most, obnoxious to this Disease. Sharp and thin Wines, Cyder, yea and Beer, that by reason of its sourenefs is apt to ferment, because they fuse the Blood, and precipitate its serosities, are forbid to those troubled with Headaches, as so much poyson: And lastly, whatever is wont to cause a Flux in those troubled with the Gout, the same also for the like reason causes it in these, for the rising Serum, in either, flows to the distemper'd part, where it oftentimes grows hot with the nervous humor.

Sometimes the
watry humor
suffering a flux
offends the Head. Further, not only the meer and simple Serum of the Blood, dropping forth upon the Membranes of the Head, stirs up pains, but sometimes other humors joyning together, and by this passage being admitted to the distemper'd part, encrease the tragedy of the Disease; it often happens, that a thin and watery humor doth suddenly flow forth from the Lymphic Vessels, the Glandula's, and perhaps from the Passages and Pores of the solid parts (in which it is gathered together) and is poured forth into the Blood in the Veins; from whence presently passing thorow the bosom of the Heart, and being confused with the Arterious Blood, and by that soon separated, is cast back by any way it can find; therefore, being partly sent away by the Reins, it

Hence in those
that have the
Headach, as in
Convulsive Dis-
eases, there is of-
ten a clear and
copious Urine. causes a flowing down of a clear and copious Urine, also sometimes partly redounding on the Brain or Nervous Originals, produces Sleepy or Convulsive Distempers, as we have elsewhere shown. Yea sometimes, a certain part of the same limpid humor, being snatched with the Serum into the Membranes of the Head, raises up fits of a most cruel Headach: For indeed, I have observed in many, a watry and very plentiful Urine, either to precede or accompany the fits of this Disease.

The recrements
of other parts,
often carried
violently to the
head with the
Serum. But we may believe other manner of recrements, of the other parts, *viz.* bile from the Liver, black bilary feculencies from the Spleen, and perhaps incongruous humors from the Stomach, Reins, Pancrace, *&c.* are supped up by the Serum of the Blood, and deeply boiled with it, by which, whilst it is infested, it more readily conceives Effervescencies, and so rushing impetuously into the Cephalick Vessels, and there fermenting with the nervous Liquor, brings forth Convulsions, and painful and very troublesome pullings or haulings.

The evacuation
of the Serum
thorow its right
ways, being
suppressed,
brings its flux
to the Head. The serous heap, whether it be simple, or as we have shown, complicated, is sufficiently infestous to the Head, whenever its usual evacuation, thorow its due and accustomed ways, is hindred: *viz.* whether if the Pores being bound up, transpiration be inhibited, or by reason of the evil distemper of the Reins, an Evacuation by Urine is not copiously performed; either defect greatly punishes those subject to Headaches. Further, the Membranes of the Head are oppressed, by reason of the passages of the Blood being obstructed in other places: for if the lower or middle parts of the Belly, and especially the Liver and Lungs, are troubled with an obstruction, so that the Blood can scarce pass thorow in those places, its more full torrent is directed into other parts, and especially towards the Head; so that for this Cause, I have known to have followed, not only Headaches, but also soporiferors or sleepy, and sometimes deadly distempers.

3. The nutriti-
ous juice some-
times the cause
of the Headach,
either,
1. Because it is
carried with
the Blood into
the Head. 3. As the Serum in the bosom of the Blood, so the nourishing Juice, that is the fresh Chyme made out of the Aliments, lodges there too, and is circulated with it, and forced to follow its inexorbitances, being as it were in the current of the same River. Wherefore, when the Blood, presently after eating, is carried impetuously or inordinately to the Head, and the nourishing Juice being half Concocted or depraved, is fixed there to the Membranaceous Fibres, it causes painful pullings or haulings to follow;

for

Of the Headach.   111

for hence it is, that exercise, bathing, violent passions, reading, or any serious intention of the Mind, upon a full stomach, hurt those troubled with Headaches.

Sometimes the nutritious Juice is not presently or easily mixed with the Blood, but being carried fresh to it, by and by stirs up a turgency, so that many, constantly after eating, are troubled with an high Colour, and oftentimes also with an Headach. This commonly, but amiss, is imputed to the obstruction of the Liver, when indeed it proceeds from an evil disposition of the Blood, hardly bearing the mixture of the fresh Chyme. Wherefore, such a distemper, follows for the most part dangerous Feavours, and especially the Small Pox, and sometimes great Surfeits. *2. Because not being agreeable to the blood, it stirs up its effervescency.*

4. There yet remains another sort of Evident Causes, (to wit, by which the leading Causes, or predispositions to the Headach are actuated) plainly different from the former irregularities of the Blood, Serum, and nourishing juice; to wit, when Headaches are very often most terrible, follow, by reason of Convulsions, begun in other parts, and from them continued to the Head. 'Tis an usual thing for a certain sense, or feeling, of a Formication, or little pricking, to creep forward from the *Hypochondria*, as also from the region of the Stomach, Mesentery, Womb, yea sometimes from the Members or outward parts, to the Head, and by and by sometime after to excite a pain that will last for a good while. This kind of Distemper, which is wont oftentimes to be the forerunner of the *Vertigo*, also of the *Epilepsie*, or the *Apoplexie*, is commonly believed to be the ascent of Vapours; when indeed it is only a Convulsion, begun in the extremity of some Nerve, which creeping upward towards its original, and then coming to the Skull, for as much as it either is communicated to the parts within the Head, or to the *Meninges*, either one or both of them, it stirs up Convulsions or pains. Which passions notwithstanding, follow this Formication or tingling, brought from elsewhere, sometimes as a sign, and sometimes as the cause. We have in another place largely enough unfolded the reason of the former, to wit, it being shown, that when the Morbifick matter possesses the beginnings of the Nerves, or the nearest parts to them in the Head, a Convulsion oftentimes beginning from the ends of the same Nerves, being carried thence upwards towards the places first distemper'd, ascends as it were by a creeping forward: wherefore not only upon the Vertigo, but upon the Headach, a Vomiting comes very frequently. *Sometimes the evident causes of the Headach are Convulsions somewhere begun and continued by the passage of the nerves, into the Head.*

Convulsions beginning afar off, are sometimes signs of an Headach shortly to follow.

But further, an Irritation in some distant Member or Viscera, is sometimes the occasion, and in a sort the cause of the Headach; to wit, when the Morbifick matter is heaped up, even to a fulness of Turgency in the part of the Head already disaffected, there is need only of a light Vellication or pulling of the Containing Fibres, that this matter being stirred, should cause a fit of the Disease; to which movement, it often suffices, that by an intimate concent of some distant Inward, as the Ventricle, Spleen, or Womb, with the Head, the nervous Fibres should be pulled or hauled; for presently from thence, the trouble being communicated by the Nerves, some Membranaceous Fibres of the Head, being evilly disposed, and burthened with the Morbific Matter, begin to be strained and wrinkled, and so when the Mine of the Disease is moved from its moved Particles, the Fibres are urged into grievous and continual Corrugations. *Sometimes also the cause of it.*

Headaches that seem to begin after this manner from the Viscera, and commonly called Sympathetic, are wont to be ascribed to Vapors, *viz.* by supposing a Mine of the noxious humor to lye hid in some Inward, from which being moved, whilst the Effluvia ascend into the Head, and there sharply pierce thorow and pull the nervous Fibres, pains are excited. We have already so plainly refuted this doctrine, that there is no need here to bring any other reasons to oppose it. But in the mean time, let us inquire whether pains of the Head do not arise also by other means, besides a Convulsive communication thorow the Nerves, by reason of the Morbific Cause lodging in the Stomach, Spleen, and other places. *Convulsive Headaches seem to arise so from the Viscera, not from Vapours.*

Concerning this, we may suppose, that Matter oftentimes degenerate, is heaped up in remote parts, which carries its hurt to the Head, by the passage or Circulation of the Blood. 'Tis a usual thing for Corrupt humors, *viz.* sometimes sharp, sometimes acid or austere, to be heaped up in the Ventricle; Bile in the Liver, atrabilary or melancholic dregs about the Spleen, yea and other sort of degenerate Matter about the Mesentery, Womb, or other parts: from which being heaped up to a fulness of swelling up, a Fermentative *Miasm* or Infection is fixed to the Blood; from which, that, being as it were imbued with rage, impetuously grows hot, and partly by its swelling up, and partly by transferring what is incongruous into the Membranes of the Head, stirs up fierce and cruel fits of pains. *But this sympathetick Distemper perhaps proceeds elsewhere, by reason of an evil ferment, communicated to the blood.*

As to the Ventricle, that it is so, some obnoxious to this Disease have plain experience. Because some of them, after the Bile or Choler flowing in the Stomach, and *So sometimes it seems to be carried from the Ventricle.*

Of the Headach.

and others after a noted sourenefs, and ravenous hunger, most certainly expect a fit of the Headach. The reason of which seems partly to be, that those contents of the Ventricle being supped up by the Blood, make it hot, and stir up in the same a Cephalic Turgency or swelling up; moreover, from this kind of sharp Vitriolick, or otherways infestous matter, being heaped up and moved within the Stomach, a Convulsion, or Corrugation very troublesome, is impressed on the Fibres and the extremities of the Nerves there inserted, which immediately being continued into the Head, by the passages of the same Nerves of the eighth pair, and of the Intercostal, is communicated to the Membranes, and the nervous Fibres, predisposed to painful wrinklings.

The Head and the Stomach intimately conspire, and mutually affect one another.

By reason of the same Reciprocal Communication, between the Stomach and the Head, a nauseousness and Vomiting, as we said but now, follows upon the Headach, viz. the Membranes being stirred up into painful wrinklings, by the Morbifick matter (even as is wont by a blow or wound) and transferring the evil by the passage of the Nerves to the Ventricle, guiltless of it self, a vain endeavour of Vomiting sometimes arises, nothing remaining within the Ventricle, that should be cast forth: yet sometimes, from a cruel shaking of the Inwards, in striving to Vomit, the Gallish or Pancreatick humor, either one or both of them, being thrust forth into the *Duodenum*, and cast forth by Vomit, is ignorantly taken for the Cephalick matter.

2. How the Head-ach seems to arise from the Spleen.

2. The pains of the Head are wont to be imputed no less to the Spleen, than the Ventricle; and indeed 'tis ordinarily observed in Hypochondriacks, obnoxious also to this Disease, when a Pain, Inflation, a Rumbling, or some other Perturbation of the distemper'd Spleen, happens in the left-side, that the Headach, as if raised up by it, by and by frequently succeeds; hence, presently 'tis the voice of the people, that these Vapours being sent forth from the disturbed Spleen, stir up the pain of the Head: But indeed, we may grant that the Headach arises sometimes from the default of the Spleen, yet reject this opinion, that it ought for this cause to be imputed to Vapors, but indeed either to an evil Ferment, transmitted into the Blood from the Spleen, or from a Convulsion, from thence communicated to the Head, by the Nerves: because in the Spleen evilly affected, the Melancholic humor being degenerate, sometimes into a Vitriolic Nature, sometimes a biting, sometimes a sharp, or otherways infestous, is oftentimes heaped up, which of its own accord being shaken forth, by reason of plenitude, or occasionally by reason of some perturbation, and being confused with the Blood, impresses a Fermentation upon it, by which its Liquor rushing by it self on the Membranes of the Head, or growing hot with the nervous Liquor, causes painful pullings or haulings. Further, it is no less probable, that sometimes a Convulsion being excited in the nervous Fibres, which are very much disposed about the Spleen, brought thence by the passages of the Nerves of the wandring and Intercostal pair, and continued to the Head, impresses the like Distemper to the Membranes predisposed to it.

The like reason is for this Disease, arising from the Liver, Mesentery, or Womb.

3. A reason may be also rendred, according to the same *Pathology*, to wit, either from an evil Transmission of the Ferment, or a continuation of the Convulsion, for Headaches which are said to be raised up by consent, from the Liver, Mesentery, the Womb, and other parts.

The kinds of habitual Headach are noted. It is either, Continual,

The habitual Headach, the *Æsiology*, or the Reason of which, we have already sufficiently handled, is yet divided into certain kinds, to wit, it is either Continual, or Intermitting; but the periods of this are sometimes determined to a certain time, and are sometimes wandring and uncertain: we shall speak briefly of each of these.

1. Sometimes therefore it happens, that some are afflicted with a Continual pain of the Head, to wit, for many days or months, little intermitting, unless when sleep helps; in which case we suppose, that there is not only present a Procatartick or leading cause, but also a Conjunct, somewhere fixed and constant. For besides that the parts affected, or that are wont to be affected, are weak, and their watering liquor much depraved, is apt to stagnate, or to grow hot with other humors; there is moreover oftentimes excited in them, a breaking of the unity, to wit, an Inflammation, a red and painful swelling, a Scirrhous tumor, or Imposthum, or of some such kind; about which, whilst the humors of divers kinds do meet together, and are heaped up, there arise almost perpetual pains, by reason of the nervous Fibres being continually pulled or hauled. These kinds of Headaches, do not rarely end in sleepy distempers, and at length deadly; for when I have opened the Heads of many dead of these Diseases, the signs or footsteps, declaring the aforesaid kinds of Morbific causes, have appeared; some examples of these shall be added hereafter.

or Intermitting.

2. The habitual Headach, is for the most part Intermitting, whose fits, as they are certain and Periodical, or coming at a set period of time, are wont often to return in the space of half a day and night, or once in twelve hours. Some more rare cases I have known, which exactly repeating the Fits, came every other day, yea once in a week

week, or a month. It is an ufual thing, for Headaches, that feem to be driven away, to return again about the Equinoxes or Solſtices; to wit, becauſe at theſe times, the Blood and Humors conceive greater Turgences or riſings up, than are wont, and therefore are more apt to grow hot with the watering Liquor of the nervous parts of the Head, and to renew the wonted fits of pains. But when about theſe times of the year, Headaches return, they are not prorogued by a longer acceſſion for a great while, but for the moſt part, having gotten ſubordinate periods, they are wont to infeſt at ſome certain ſtanding hours, for the ſpace of twelve hours. *The Fits of the intermitting, either periodical, or certain;*

When therefore a Periodical Headach hath its daily fits, for the moſt part the reaſon of theſe, as of Intermitting Feavors, ought to be ſought from the fault of the Morbifick Matter, ariſing to a plenitude at a ſet time, and then growing hot. For it may be ſuppoſed, that the proper Liquor is perverted ſomewhere about the Membranes of the Head, and the nervous Fibres evilly diſpoſed, or doth not well paſs thorow them; wherefore, when the nouriſhing Juice, placed alſo on the ſame parts from the Blood, is not preſently aſſimilated, nor doth well agree with the other humor; at length, from both of them heaped up together and diſagreeing, a mutual growing hot ariſes, and from thence a painful pulling of the Fibres: but for that the fits of the pains, are not always at the ſame diſtance after Eating, but ariſe in ſome ſooner, and in others later, and ſometimes before ſleep, and ſometimes after; the cauſe is, that partly the offices of Concoction, and diſtribution of the Aliments, are performed ſometime ſooner, ſometimes later; and partly, becauſe in theſe the nervous Liquor, and in thoſe the nutritions Juice, is moſt in fault: wherefore, as the fulneſs of this happens ſooner, and of that later, ſo the times of the fit vary: we ſhall illuſtrate theſe afterwards, with obſervations made concerning the caſes of ſick perſons.

3. When the fits of the intermitting Headach are wandring and uncertain, the Procatarxis or foregoing cauſe of the Diſeaſe, is neither great nor conſtant, nor is the Evident Cauſe continual: Wherefore, when that either cauſe is oftentimes abſent, and one of them often wanting, the fits of the Diſeaſe are not tyed to certain times, but in ſome, they are as it were by chance and accidental, in others, in whom a prediſpoſition to this Diſtemper is a little more firmly rooted: the pains of the Head more frequently moleſt, and are ordinarily excited, by reaſon of various occaſions, yea and for ſome, they are wont to be moſt certainly expected. The reaſons of the fits ſo variouſly happening appear clearly above, from the *Ætiology* delivered of this Diſeaſe; beſides, the whole buſineſs ſhall be illuſtrated anon, by examples. *or incertain, and wandring.*

CHAP. II.

The Prognoſtick and Cure of the Headach.

SO much for the Cauſes of the Headach, which being ſo various and diverſe, and their Series ſo perplex'd and intricate, it will not ſeem eaſie to keep one Method concerning all caſes of the Sick, whereby we may be led preſently to the true knowledge and Cure of this Diſeaſe; nor is there leſs difficulty concerning its Prognoſtick: But common experience affords ſome obſervations, from which it may be gathered, that the Cure of this Sickneſs is ſometimes eaſie, ſometimes difficult, or ſcarce poſſible; ſo that from thence it may be lawful to declare the event of the Diſeaſe, either ſafe, or very dangerous, or wholely uncertain. *The prognoſtick of the Headach, ſhews it eaſie or difficult to be cured; alſo, the event of the Diſeaſe ſafe or dangerous.*

Truly, if any one enjoying formerly a perfect Health, ſhould fall into ſomething a cruel Headach, and of ſome long ſtanding, by reaſon of a more ſtrong Evident Cauſe, as drinking of Wine, Surfeit, Venus, immoderate Exerciſe, or ſuch like; foraſmuch as the fore leading Morbid Cauſe is not as yet firmly laid, we may pronounce ſuch a Diſtemper to be ſafe enough, and not pertinacious *By what ſigns we may pronounce it ſafe, and eaſie to be cured.*

But if the Morbific diſpoſition ſhould be inveterate, ſo that for many years the fits repeat often of their own accord, and upon every light occaſion, this, though not dangerouſly ſick, yet we predict it not eaſie to be Cured. Further, the Cure will be yet more difficult, if Hypochondriack or Hyſterical Diſtempers, oftentimes troubleſome, are oft wont to excite the Headach at every turn, or if the taint of an inveterate Venereal Diſeaſe be rooted in any diſtemper'd part. *By what difficult.*

If that the pain of the Head ſhall be not only inveterate, but almoſt continual, that we might ſuſpect it to ariſe from an Inflammation, or a Scirrhous Tumour, an hot Swelling, *By what ſcarce poſſible.*

ling, an Impoſthum, or Worms, there is none or very little hope of Cure; eſpecially becauſe the ſick will refuſe great remedies, as Salivation, or opening the Skull; which if they be made uſe of perhaps at any time with any fruit or ſucceſs, yet the former and this two for the moſt part are wont to be tedious to the ſick, before they can effect any thing worth the trouble and expectation.

By what, dangerous.
The pain of the Head either Continual or Periodical, if it be great, and hath joyned with it a Vertigo, Vomitting, or other Convulſive or Soporiferous Diſtempers, ſhews a ſuſpicion of great danger: even which often paſſes into a deadly *Apoplexie*, and not ſeldom into an *Epilepſie*, Palſie, Blindneſs, Deafneſs, and other funeſtous and incurable Diſeaſes.

The Curatory method of the Headach comprehends many Indications, and thoſe of a various kind, according to the manifold Species, Cauſes, and differences of this Diſeaſe, which will not be an eaſie thing here to ſet down, and rehearſe in order.

Accidental Headach eaſily cured.
The accidental Pain of the Head, with the remote Evident Cauſe, and its conſequences, ceaſes for the moſt part of its own accord, or at leaſt is taken away by letting of Blood, Reſt, and Sweat.

The habitual affords more indications.
The habitual Pain, by reaſon of the diverſity of Cauſes, *viz.* both the *Procatartick* and alſo the Conjunct, ſuggeſts alſo different intentions of Healing; we ſhall here briefly touch upon the chief of theſe, and to which all the reſt may be placed.

Two chief ſcopes of Cure.
In every habitual Headach, whether Continual or Intermitting, there are two chief ſcopes or intentions of Cure to be met with; to which all the other Curatory intentions ought to be aimed, and by which we ſhould provide againſt either Cauſe of the Morbid *Procatarxis*.

1. To cut in two the Bed or Root of the Diſeaſe.
1. To wit, in the firſt place, that all the Tinder or inkindling of the Diſeaſe be cut off, you muſt endeavour, that both the matter flowing to the diſtempered places of the Head, or thoſe evilly diſpoſed, or apt from thence to flow to them, be ſuppreſt, or called from thence to another place; then moreover, that Convulſions in other places excited, and that are wont to be propagated from thence into the Head, be prevented.

2. To root out the Conjunct Cauſe.
2. Then ſecondly, it muſt be indeavoured (if it may be done) that the Diſeaſe it ſelf, or its Conjunct Cauſe may be rooted out, that the places of the Head prediſpoſed to Headaches, (whether they be only enfeebled or hurt in their Conformation) whilſt they are defended from the frequent Excurſions of the infeſtous matter, may recover their former ſtate and vigour. Which kind of Indication, though it be very ſeldom ſuddenly or wholely performed, yet ſometimes the Cure is by degrees laboured out, by diligence and care, however fixed and rooted the Morbid matter be.

The Neſt or Tinder of the Diſeaſe, the blood, ſerum, nouriſhing juice, nervous Liquor, and the Recrements carried thorow the Blood.
As to what appertains to the firſt ſcope of healing, which is firſt and eſpecially to be regarded; we ſaid, that the Matter or Humours, which are wont to be gathered together about the parts of the Head prediſpoſed to the Headach, and to excite the fits of the Diſeaſe, are either the Blood or the Serum, or the nouriſhing or nervous Juice, or Liquor. Moreover, with every one of theſe Vapours and Effluvia's, as alſo Recrements, ſometimes Bilous, ſometimes Melancholic, ſometimes Acid, Salt, Sulphureous, and of ſome others of a various kind, taken into the Blood, from the Viſcera, ſometimes from thoſe, and ſometimes from theſe, we have ſhewed to be transferred by its paſſages into the Head: againſt the force and incurſion of all theſe, Medicinal fortifications are to be inſtituted.

How the inordinations of the Blood may be taken away and prevented.
1. And in the firſt place, if the leading cauſe to pains, or a diſpoſition thereto, lye about the Membranes of the Head, for that the Blood being hot, and apt to riſe up, ruſhes by heaps into the Membranes of the Head, and when it cannot eaſily paſs thorow them, diſtending the Veſſels above meaſure, and pulling the nervous Fibres, excites the fits of this Diſeaſe (whoſe ſigns are a Sanguine temperament, heat, and a fluſhing or redneſs about the head and face, alſo an high pulſe, and ſhaking, with veins diſtended with Blood) preſently it muſt be endeavoured, both that the Blood be made more ſedate, that it may not be ſo readily moved into rage or ſwelling up; as alſo that it be not incited, and boiling up may not be carried with a greater tendency or inclination into the Head, than into other parts, nor in like manner be compelled to ſtagnate, by reaſon of the boſomes of the *Meninges* being too full. Wherefore, if the fit inſeſts long, let blood in the Arm, or the Jugular Vein: out of the fit, ſometimes it is expedient to take Blood from the Sedal Veins, with Leeches; to wit, by this means, that the Blood by chance boiling up, may be brought down towards that place, to which it often tends of its own accord. Let there be Medicines of Vinegar, Roſecakes, and Nutmeg, or ſome other *Epithems* or Medicines of the ſame nature applyed to the Head: Alſo give to drink *Juleps, Emulſions*, or *Decoctions*, which allay the fervour or madneſs of the Blood. Let the Belly be cooled and kept ſoluble by the uſe of Clyſters.

Clysters. Moreover, for prevention, use at times Whey, or Spaw-waters; also drinking of Water, a thin and a cooling diet help; the shunning of Wine, spiced Meats, Baths, Venus, violent motions of the mind or body, yea and of all hot things is to be ordered. Then for the fixing of the Blood, its Effervescencies or growing hot must be prevented, for which, Distilled Waters, Juices of Herbs, or Decoctions, Electuaries, Powders, and especially *Crystal Mineral*, are in frequent use. There is no need here to add a method or particular forms of Medicines, when in this case, almost every body labouring, is wont to be his own Physician, being taught by frequent experience, from things hurting or helping.

2. It is rarely, that the Blood alone or only by it self is in the fault; more often other humors, being carried by its passage to the Head, and there disposed, cause the hurt: Therefore, when ever the Serous Colluvies, or heap, goes out from the Blood (as was shown but now) it causes Headaches frequently, (the signs of which are *Catarrhs* about other parts, *viz.* the Nose, Mouth, or Throat, being infested with them) then abstinency and rest is to be ordered, and that the belly be emptied by a Clyster, for the allaying the flux of the Serum, and that the matter be suffered to evaporate from the Membranes of the Head; if these do not succeed, and that the Headach ceases not quickly, and of its own accord, oftentimes in a more hot Constitution, Phlebotomy is convenient; to wit, because the Vessels being emptied of Blood, sup up the extravasated Serum: But in frigid tempers, Vesicatories or Blisters are of notable use, applied to the hinder-part of the Head, or nigh the Ears. Then after the Belly is emptied by a Clyster, the Flux may be allayed, by the use of *Anodynes*, or more gentle opiats: that being allayed it may be convenient to exhibit a gentle Purge, then Medicines, which either move by Urine or Sweat, or by both together, that so they may gently evacuate the superfluous Serosities.

The pain of the Head from the serous heap, how to be cured.

Phlebotomy.

Purges.

Medicines fit for this purpose may be every where found in Books: which notwithstanding are not to be made use of by *Empericks* rashly, and without distinction; but ought to be designed according to the judgment and skill of a prudent Physician, always having a respect to the Constitution, the temperament, and proper disposition of the Patient, and to other accidents and circumstances, and to be compounded or altered according as the matter requires; yea sometimes to be prescribed extempore. Wherefore, since it will be altogether needless, here to heap up many Receipts, and a great pile of Medicines, it shall be sufficient to propose in this place, one or two forms only, of every sort of Medicines, respecting the chief intentions.

Take *Pills of Amber half a dram, Resine of Jalap four grains, of Peruvian Balsam what will suffice to make four Pills, let three be taken when the Patient goes to sleep, and the other in the morning, if they work not enough.*

Pills.

Or Take *of sulphurated Scammony half a scruple, of the Ceruse of Antimony fifteen grains, of the Cream of Tartar eight grains; make a Powder, to be taken in a spoonful of Grewel, early in the morning.*

Purging Powders.

Take *of the Sulphur of Antimony four grains, of the Resine of Jalap five grains, of the Cream of Tartar six grains, bruise them together, and with what will suffice of the Conserve of Violets, make a Bolus, to be taken early in the morning with care, or by government.*

An imetick Powder.

Take *of the Roots of Butchers-Broom, Burdocks, Cherefoil, Avens, each one ounce; of preserv'd Eryngo an ounce and an half, of the Florentine Iris three drams, of the lesser Galangal a dram and an half, of the Seeds of Burdock three drams, of the dryed leaves of Betony, Sage, Vervine, female Betony, each half an handful; of Raisins of the Sun stoned two ounces; boil these in four pints of fair water, till a third part be consumed, then add to it of white Wine half a pound, strain it, and sweeten it (if need be) with syrup of the Five Roots two ounces; take of this six ounces warm, twice or thrice in a day, a good while after meals.*

An Apozem.

For such as are indued with a more Cold and Phlegmatick Constitution, the like Decoction of the Wood of Guaicum, Sasafrass, Sarsaparilla, with the addition of the aforesaid Ingredients, make an Apozem, of which take six or eight Ounces, twice or thrice in a day warm.

A decoction of Woods.

For the poor, and oftentimes with good success for the rich, I was wont to prescribe a Decoction of the dry'd leaves sometimes of Sage or Betony, Vervine, or Rosemary, made of Spring-water, and impregnated with the tincture of the Powder of the Berries of Coffee, taken warm twice a day, about six or eight Ounces.

A Cephalick Decoction impregnated with the Tincture of Coffee.

3. If that with the running out Serum, Saline, Acid, Bilous, or otherways Infestous particles, received either wholely from the Mass of Blood, or by its means from the

The Headach from other humors mixt with the serum, how to be cured.

the Viscera, are carried into the Membranes of the Head, and being there fixed, bring forth great, acute, and continual pains, then it will be convenient to iterate spareingly, the taking away of Blood, yea and sometime a gentle Purge, to apply cooling Medicines, *Anodynes*, and sweetners to the distemper'd places; so oftentimes also to exhibit more gentle *Hypnoticks*, or Medicines causing sleep, at every turn; also *Apozems*, and the Juices of Herbs pressed forth, which allay the fervour of Choler, carry it forth gently by Stool or Urine, and are of known use: but in the mean time more sharp Medicines, or the more strong, whether they be purgative, working by Sweat or Urine, helping it, for that they too much fuse and shake the Blood and Humors, are carefully to be shunned. I have frequently observed in those labouring with an acute and pertinacious pain in the Head, the Serum swimming in the Blood being let forth, to be dyed with a yellowness, or Bilous Recrements being boiled in it; also in this case, let Phlebotomy be sparingly but often celebrated, and the drinking Whey, or Spaw-waters plentifully, have helped before any thing else.

The Headach arising from any Inward, how to be cured.

4. Further, by the fault of any Inward, as the Stomach, Liver, Spleen, or Womb, or of any other (by reason of the transmission of an evil Ferment) the parts of the Head suffer, then in the Cure of the Disease, Remedies for the Spleen are to be given, with *Cephalicks*, or such as are proper to the Head: Hence the Stomach being also in the fault, these often times are helpful to such as are troubled with Headaches, *Elixir Proprietatis*, the *Elixir* of *Vitriol* of *Mynsich*, the sacred Tincture, *Vitriol* of Steel, the Powder of *Aron* Compound, and others ordinarily had for the Stomach; for others whose heads partake of the evils of the Spleen, *Chalybeats*, or Medicines made of Steel often yield help. Some Women troubled with Headaches have felt ease from *Hysterical* Remedies. In like manner, when the vices of other parts contribute to the Headach, let there be joyned with the former shown you, things to be taken for those parts.

Rais'd up from the fault of the nourishing Juice, how to be handled.

5. Sometimes the nourishing Juice (as we showed already) is the cause of the periodical Headach, viz. forasmuch as this being poured on the Blood, and not rightly assimilated, by reason of disagreeing particles, causes a swelling up in it, so that the Blood boiling up into the Head, carries its leavings or superfluities into the *Meninges*, or into some of their predisposed parts, and by this means stir up the Fibres into painful Convulsions. I have known many for this cause, to have been obnoxious to dayly Headaches, whose Mass of Blood hath been vitiated after the Small Pox, Measiels, and other Feavours, and sicknesses: viz. so many hours after eating, sometimes sooner and sometimes later, first a flushing of redness in the Face, then a fullness in the Head, and a pain would infest them, and especially after drinking of Wine, or eating of Meats apt to swell up, they would be more vexed. The coming of the Disease is wont to keep its distance, according as Meats are taken more or less, as the *Chyme* begins to swell up, either a little after its first entring into the Blood, or after a little stay in it.

Frequently follows the Small Pox and Measles.

Easily cured.

This Distemper is free from danger, and for the most part is easily enough Cured. After a provision of the whole, a gentle Purge, and sometimes Blood-letting being ordered, Remedies profit most which restore the Complexion of the Blood, such chiefly are *Antiscorbuticks* and *Chalybeates*.

An Electuary.

Take *of the Conserve of Fumitory, of Tansie, and Wood-Sorrel, each two ounces; of the Powder of Aron Compound three drams, of Ivory, Crabs-Eyes, Coral prepared, each one dram; Powder of yellow Saunders, and Lignum Aloes, each half a dram; of the Vitriol of Steel one dram, of the Salt of Wormwood a dram and a half, of the Syrup of the Five Roots what will suffice to make an Electuary. Take of it in the morning, and at five a clock in the afternoon the quantity of a Chesnut, drinking after it three ounces of the following liquor.*

A Julep.

Ta'e *of the water of the leaves of Aron, of Vervine, of Elderflowers, each six ounces, of the Water of Snails, and the Magisterial of Earth-worms, each two ounces; of Sugar one ounce: Mingle them.*

Antiscorbutick Remedies good for it.

Hither may be brought various Remedies, that are wont to be made use of against the Scorbutick Dyscrasie, or evil disposition of the Blood, and may be given with good success: For Headaches, which are so familiar in the Scurvy, oftentimes proceed from the vice of the Blood perverting the nutritious Humor, and carrying its Recrements to the Membranes of the Head: Wherefore Remedies against that Distemper, in another place noted by me, may be used here.

The Headach raised up from the vice of the

6. There yet remains another humor, to wit, the nervous Liquor, which being heaped up within the Fibres of the Meninges, and of other parts of the Head, sometimes

times becomes improportionate, by its proper incongruity, to the Fibres, because *nervous humor,* sharp or otherways degenerate, sometimes pulls the containing parts, and provokes *how to be cured.* them into painful Convulsions, or Distentions, because it grows hot with some other Humor flowing thither, to wit, the Nutritious or the Serous.

The Nervous Humor, when it is so Morbific or faulty in its whole Mass, carries its *Its fault either* evil to the predisposed Head, or if of it self innocent, is perverted within the distem- *private or par-* per'd Fibres, and so secondarily becomes Morbific or Diseased; then the Cure of it *ticular,* depends upon the restitution of the containing parts; to wit, if the Debilities, or the hurt Conformation of the Fibres may be mended, presently the Humor watering them will be free from fault. We shall tell you by and by, by what Remedies the vices of the parts predisposed to Headaches may be taken away.

In the mean time, if the nervous humor, being degenerate in the whole Mass, im- *Or universal;* parts its evil to the Head prepared for pain, those kind of Medicines, and method *and then letting* are to be made use of, by which it being reduced to its due Constitution, passing thorow *of blood, or* those Fibres, it little or nothing provokes them. For which end, neither letting of *stronger Purges,* Blood, nor yet strong Purges are at all convenient, because those things which shake *are not conve-* the Blood and Humors, and lessen strength, impress by that means a greater sharp- *nient.* ness and rage to the faulty Nerve. But gentle Solutives, and a sparing taking of Blood, sometimes may be useful, whereby the Inwards may be cleansed, and the bloody Mass somewhat purged, and a way made for other Medicines, that may better succeed.

But Medicines, which render the nervous Liquor more friendly and benigne to the *Remedies called* Membranes of the Head, that are wont to be troubled by it, are of that sort commonly *Cephalicks pro-* called *Cephalicks*, whose particles being active, thin, and subtil, pass thorow the *per here.* Blood without trouble or tumult; then insinuating themselves with the nervous Liquor, gently move it, and so cause the nervous passages to be unfolded, so that the Animal Spirits, more freely beam forth thorow all the Bodies, both sensible and mo- *Of which sort* tive, and inspire them without any lessening, Convulsions, or irregular distenti- *are these,* ons.

These kind of Remedies, although they are not always effectual, yet they often- *which are con-* times take away some Headaches not much inveterate, and in some, help sometimes *venient in Dis-* how pertinacious soever they be. Further, the same which are prescribed with good *eases of the* success for the pains of the Head, are also for the distempers of the Brain and Ner- *Brain, and in* vous Stock; and so on the contrary, what are used for these, also for those; to wit, *these kind of* the virtues of those being unfolded within the Head, against the Apoplexy, Palsie, *Headaches.* Lethargy, and other Diseases a-kin to them, help also within the moving Fibres, against Convulsions and Convulsive Motions; besides, putting forth their virtues within the sensible Fibres, they often give help to pains.

A very large field of these Medicines are opened in physical Books, yet so, that *A great many* the poorness of them, and their abundance, bring confusion to the Method of heal- *of these every* ing; for oftentimes among so many various and different Remedies, heaped up to- *where to be* gether, lye hid or obscured, what may be of great use, but even as Wheat among *found in Physi-* Chaff, harder to be separated than that to be thorowly sifted out from the husks. *cal Books.*

Therefore in this case, a provision of the whole being made, and applyed, and things given which by Dyet or Medicine, restrain the Inordinations of the Blood, and immediately allay them; Medicines called Cephalicks, or such as take away the disorders of the nervous Juice, are prescribed to be carefully taken. I shall add some few forms of these.

 Take *of the Conserve of the Flowers of Betony, of Clove-gilliflowers, each three ounces;* *An Electuary.*
 of the Powder of the Root of the male Pæony half an ounce, of Cretick Dittanny one
 dram; of the wood Aloes, and yellow Sanders, each one dram; of red Coral pre-
 pared, of Pearl, of Ivory, each one dram and a half; of the Salt of Vervine one
 dram and a half, of the Syrup of the Flowers of Pæony, what will suffice: make an
 Opiat, take of it to the quantity of a Chesnut, drinking after it of the following
 Julep three ounces.
 Take *of simple black Cherry water, and of Walnuts, and of Vervine, each four* *Julep.*
 ounces; of Cowslip Flowers three ounces, of Pæony Compound two ounces, of Sugar-
 Candy six drams.
 Take *of the Flowers of Vervine, Misleto Berries, each ten handfuls; of the male* *A distilled wa-*
 Pæony Roots two pound, of Mace and Nutmegs, each half an ounce; of Coriander *ter.*
 Seeds one ounce, cut and bruise them and put to them eight pints of new-milk (or else
 seven pints of Milk and one pint of Malago) Distil them in a common Still, and
 mix all the liquor together: Take of it three ounces at a time.

Take

Tablets. Take *of the Powder of the Root of the male Pæony half an ounce, of red Coral prepared two drams, of Ivory and Pearls prepared, each one dram; make of them all a very fine Powder, add to it of Sugar what will suffice; boil them to the consistence of Tablets with six ounces of black Cherry-water, of the Tincture of Coral one dram; make of them Tablets according to Art, to the weight of half a dram: Eat three or four in the Morning, and at five of the Clock in the Afternoon, drinking after them a draught of Tea.*

Tinctures. Or Take *of the Tincture of Coral one ounce; take of it from fifteen to twenty drops twice in a day, in a little draught of Julep, or of the distilled water.*

Spirits. They who are of a Phlegmatick or more Cold temper may take a Dose twice a day, either of the Tincture of Antimony, or of the Spirits of Armoniac, impregnated with Amber or Coral, or of Spirits of Harts horn, or of Sut, in a proper Vehicle.

The use of millepedes notably helps. We ought not to omit, or postpone the use of Millepedes or Woodlice, for that the Juice of them, wrung forth, with the distilled Water, also a Powder of them prepared, oftentimes bring notable help, for the Curing of old and pertinacious Headaches. I might here propose divers other kinds of Medicines; yea all those which I have formerly heaped up, against Convulsive Distempers, may be brought hither. But yet the most difficult knot of the Cure of the Headach, remains to be untied, to wit, how the conjunct Cause of this Disease, and fixed, consisting in the weakness, or hurt Conformation of the Fibres, may be healed or taken away

The other part of the conjunct Cause, consisting in the weakness or evil conformation of the distempered part, how to be handled. We are not to despair of the Cure. Although this is sometimes incurable, to wit, when as a *Scirrhous*, or *Callous* Tumor, or some other old and fixed swelling, has possest the *Meninges*; yet, for that the knowledge of this is uncertain, and that the leading Cause, how cruel soever it seems, is sometimes overcome by a long course of Physick; therefore in every Headach, so long as the Patient will admit of Remedies, let it not seem troublesome to the Physician, to prescribe those things which seem most convenient.

Here those Medicines are only profitable, that cut off the inkindling or root of the Disease. Chyrurgical Remedies chiefly help here; of which are, Therefore, first of all, which we hinted before, you must carefully endeavour that the nest, or feeding of the Disease be cut off or intercepted, and that the frequent coming of the fits be hindred; for so the indisposed Fibres, so long as they are no more affected only by the means of Nature, will recover health.

In this case the helps of the Medical Art, are rather to be sought from the Chirurgical part, than from Physick: for whatsoever is taken at the mouth, going about by long turnings and windings, spends all the vertue before it comes to the Membranes of the Head.

1. Plasters. Among Chirurgical Remedies, first Topicks are met with, and among these, Plasters are of most profitable use, and oftentimes give the greatest benefit: Let not these be very hot, which may rather draw the humors to the distemper'd place, but moderately discussing and strengthening. I was wont to prescribe Plasters of Red-Lead, and of Sope, with double of the proportion of the Plaster of *Paracelsus*, to be applied to the part, it being first shaven, and to be let remain there for some time The Antients frequently administred Plasters made of Mustard, and such as raised wheals or

Medicines raising Wheals and Blisters. whelks over the parts, and it is a daily practice to apply sometimes to all the hinder part of the Head, and sometimes to the former, Vesicatories or blistering Plasters, against most cruel Headaches: when ease is got from these more hot *Topicks*, it is because by these administrations, plenty of the more sharp Serum is drawn away from the disaffected part.

Liniments, Fomentations and Bathings, help not. Liniments of Oyls and Oyntments, though often made use of, effect little; because (as I think) if they should penetrate deeply into the tones of the Fibres, they would loosen them more; so that they would more easily lye open to the Incursions of the Morbifick matter: Further, they stop up the Pores of the skin, whereby the Effluvia's do less evaporate. Almost for the same reason, as hot stupes or Fomentations made of boiled Spices, or other Cephalicks, oftner hurt than profit; forasmuch as they draw the humors towards the distemper'd parts, and also open the Pores and passages,

An Embrocation, or a dipping of the head in cold water, oftentimes helps. whereby they are more readily admitted; it is that a Bathing of the Head, or an Embrocation or washing of the Head, at the pumps in hot Baths, is used with no better success for Headaches: When on the contrary, it hath been beneficial to many, to pour cold water every Morning and Evening on the temples, forehead, and forepart of the Head: yea to wash or pump the whole Head, every Morning with cold water, or at least to dip it into a Bucket or Pit of water.

Issues. Another Chirurgical help, especially for an inveterate and cruel Headach, and much cry'd up, is wont to be the burning or cutting of Issues, in several parts of the Body. It is without doubt, that these being made in the Arms or Legs, are both less troublesome, and do bring something of help because they draw away the feeding of the

Disease

The Cure of the Headach.

Difeafe in part, and call it away far from the diftemper'd part. Befides, Iffues in the nape of the Neck, and a Seaton in the hinder part of the Neck, behind the Ear, or near it; alfo a piece of the root of wild Hellebore, being put into an hole made in the Ear, becaufe they evacuate much ferofity, and draw it to other Emunctuaries, to wit, the Glandulas, are oftentimes adminiftred with benefit. But indeed, there hath been a talk, and much expectation from Cauteries, made on the grieved place, or near it, and fo large Iffues have been made on the top of the Head, or nigh to the joyning of the Sutures. If we fhould meafure this practice by the fruit or fuccefs, it will appear to be rarely beneficial, but more often unlucky. For I never knew any healed, but many troubled with Headaches, to be much the worfe for it. And truly, reafon plainly tells us, that where a Fontinel is made, thither the Serous Humor flows, from the whole bloody Mafs, and by confequence from the whole body, and oftentimes is there heaped up more copioufly than can conftantly be put forth by that Emiffary: wherefore, there ordinarily arife about Iffues, a red fwelling, puftles, and various humors. Why fhould I not then believe, that a Cautery made nigh to the grieved part of the Head, fhould rather caufe the Morbific matter to be there heaped up?

Iffues made upon or near the diftemper'd place, help little.

There is yet another Chirurgical operation cry'd up by many for a pertinacious Headach, but by none (that I know of) yet attempted, to wit, an opening of the Skull, near the grieved place, with a *Trypaning* Iron. This our moft ingenious *Harvey* endeavoured to perfuade a Noble Lady, labouring with a moft grievous and inveterate Headach, promifing a Cure from thence; but neither fhe, nor any other would admit that adminiftration. Indeed, it did not appear to me, that there could be any thing of certainty expected from the opening of the Skull where it was pained; if an Impofthum lay hid there, this had been the only way of Cure; but that would rather have caufed fleepy diftempers, or deadly Convulfions than the Headach. If that a red fwelling, or puftles, or a burning boil, fhould be in the enfoldings of the Head, I know not if thofe Tumors, expofed to the open Air, would more eafily evaporate, or whether Remedies applyed to thofe naked places, would effect any thing or not; becaufe, if the pains arife by reafon of the *Meninges* being befet with little whelks, a Scirrhous or a Callous Tumor, I think the opening of the Skull will profit little or nothing.

The opening of the Skull cry'd up by many, but rarely or never attempted.

But letting this alone till it is practifed, we fhall pafs over to other things; and now in the next place, we fhall confider, whether Salivation for the Curing old and confirmed Headaches is to be adminiftred. Indeed, if the pains of the Head arife from the Venereal Difeafe, no doubt but that evil Remedy ought to be applyed to that evil Diftemper: But having tryed that kind of remedy in Headaches arifing from other Caufes, I found not the harveft worth the pains, and I confefs fome examples in thofe kind of cafes, have terrified me from that method. A certain noble Lady (whofe ficknefs is below defcribed) for the Curing of a cruel and continual Headach, underwent a plentiful Salivation three times, *viz.* the firft by a Mercurial Oyntment, by the counfel of Sir *Theodore Mayern*, and afterwards twice by taking the lately famous Powder of *Charles Huis*, without any help, I wifh not with fome detriment: for afterwards for many years, even to this day, the difeafe being by degrees increafed, fhe fuffer'd under its heavy tyranny. It happened fomewhat worfe, fo that noted man Doctor *G. D* to whom a Mercurial Oyntment was applied for his akeing Head, for the Cure of an old Headach, by which a Salivation being excited, and the Difeafe not Cured, he fell into blindnefs. Indeed thefe kind of effects from Quickfilver, rafhly given, every one, rightly weighing its operation on an humane body, ought to fear. For the Mercury, I fhall not fay is malignant or wholely venomous, becaufe it brings little or no hurt, its particles being united, fo that oftentimes a great quantity may be taken fafely enough; yet the Mercurial little bodies, being divided and feparated one from another, (whether it be done by Chymical Salts, as in the Mercury fublimate, and precipitate, or by ftraining thorow the Pores of the Skin when they are anointed) immediately become fierce and untameable, and ftir up, before any other Medicines, great perturbations in the humane body: They fometimes bring trouble, firft to the nervous parts, whereby oftentimes happen, (by reafon of the Fibres of the Ventricle, Inteftines, and other Vifcera's, being pulled or hauled) Torments, horrid Vomitings, fharp and frequently Bloody-ftools, Heart-burnings, Swoonings, and other moft terrible Diftempers, a little after the Medicine is given. Yet fometimes the particles of the Mercury, when they are not prefently diffolved, go forth without any great hurt to the Bowels, and before their ftrength be deduced into the bloody Mafs. Therefore they eafily enter into this, being highly active, and unfolding themfelves on every fide, and immediately infecting the whole,

Whether falivation in inveterate Headaches, without any fufpicion of the Venereal Difeafe, ought to be adminiftred.

The means and manner of falivation by Mercury, unfolded.

fhake

shake it, and frequently (when fully diſſolved) ſtir it up into a great burning. Then the Blood, that it might put away from it ſelf, the incongruous little bodies, Fermenting, delivers the ſame which way it can, and boils it with the humors, contained within its boſom, to wit, the Scrum and the nouriſhing Juice, and ſo endeavours, with thoſe imbued with that preternatural mixture, to put it off. But this ſucceeds not plentifully enough by Urine and Sweat, becauſe the meltings of the Blood, by the particles of the Mercury boiled in it, like the ladder of a Waſh-Ball, become more clammy and thick, ſo that they cannot paſs thorow the fine ſtrainers of the Reins and the Skin, but oftentimes breaking forth (unleſs hindred) into the *Cæliac* Arteries, go forth, by exciting a *Diarrhœa* or *Dyſentery*; but by that the intent of Salivation is hindred or fruſtrated: but more often, the Liquor imbued with the *Mercury*, remaining within the Blood, in a manner alſo infected, is carried about with it, hither and thither, impetuouſly thorow the Arteries and Veins, and is ſeparated into various parts, and either breaks forth what way it can, or is forced upon the Bowels, Membranes, and other parts, oftentimes with great hurt. Alſo it is ſeen that ſome Mercurial particles do penetrate the Brain, and inſinuating themſelves into the nervous Juice, are diffuſed, not only into the whole Head, but into all the nervous parts, and ſo in ſome meaſure ferment the nervous Liquor.

But in the mean time the Mercurial Seroſities, reſiding in the Blood, are laid up for the greateſt part into the Glandula's, which are the neareſt Emunctuaries of the Arteries: wherefore, when the Glandula's about the parts of the Mouth (by which great plenty of Scrum is deſtinated for ſpittle) being both many and great, are there placed, and that from theſe paſſages lye open, by the Excretory Veſſels, into the cavity of the Mouth; ſurely by this moſt certain way, the invenom'd liquor of the Blood, finds a paſſage forth, when it cannot eaſily elſewhere. Wherefore, a ſpitting at the Mouth being excited, the Blood long Fermenting, caſts forth whatſoever is extraneous, and not agreeable, either that lyes in its boſom, or that it licks up elſewhere from the Bowels, or receives from the ſolid parts, or from other humors, like working Ale or Wine, thorow the Salival paſſages, and innumerable pipes opening every where into the Mouth. Further, it is moſt likely, as the purgings of the Blood, ſo alſo of the liquor watering the Head, and the nervous Appendix, being excited by the Mercury entering therein, are alſo put forth by this way, to wit, by the Salival paſſages.

Therefore, a Salivation induced by Mercury, if by chance it ſucceeds rightly, it ſometimes takes away difficult and untameable Diſeaſes, not to be dealt with by any other Remedies; becauſe this operation thorowly purges the Blood and nervous Juice, and other humors, by a long purgation, deſtroys all exotick Ferments, overcomes the enormities of the Salts and Sulphures; yea, and ſhakes, and oftentimes carries forth the Morbific matter, where-ever remaining or impacted.

Salivation not always ſafe, wherefore to be ſuſpected in Headaches.

But this Medicine is not without danger, foraſmuch as the Mercury becoming enormous, and carrying with it abundance of moſt ſharp, and as it were poiſonous Serum, ruſhing on the noble parts, and eſpecially the Head, with the Medullary and nervous appendixes, or on the Lungs, and parts about the Heart, brings to them an incurable and ſometimes a deadly evil. Wherefore in a more grievous and old Headach, there is danger leſt the indiſpoſed Fibres ſhould be more irritated, by the Mercury going thorow them, with much, and corroſive Serum, and ſhould move them into more painful Convulſions and wrinklings; further, leſt it ſhould invade the Brain, by a great falling of the Humors upon the Head, by which means, as it often happens to the Brain, ſleepy and Convulſive diſtempers are cauſed. I ſhould have ſaid many things more concerning this, but that we expect ſhortly to be made publick, by the Learned Phyſician Doctor *Needham*, an exact method of Salivation, and a full account of it, as to its meaſures and effects, and its benefits and hurt.

What the cutting of the Artery may profit in this Diſeaſe.

There is yet a celebrated Remedy remaining among Chirurgical helps, *viz.* a cutting or opening an Artery. This was of great eſteem among the Ancients, and ſome of the Moderns make uſe of it, and very much cry it up. But it appears to our obſervation, that this ſo cry'd up ſucceſs moſt often fails. Nor no wonder, becauſe reaſon holds not at all, on which the Ancients depended, that the Arterious Blood was different from the Venous, or that of the Veins, and was in greater fault and more rageing, and therefore to be let forth. Nor indeed is there any reaſon wherefore the Blood being drawn from the Artery, rather than from the Vein, near the pained place, ſhould bring eaſe; but rather on the contrary, more help ought to be expected from opening of the Vein; becauſe, the Artery being emptied, receives and draws nothing from the diſtemper'd part; but the Vein being opened, draws from the

the place of the effused Blood, and from its whole neighbourhood, and oftentimes sups back, and renders to a Circulation the Blood, and other Humors, heaped up and stagnating near the nest of the Disease. But however, that we may not recede too much from the practice of the Ancients, we shall grant, that sometimes it may be helpful, though attributing nothing to the section of the Artery, and not immediately, yet causally, and only by consequence and by accident: to wit, forasmuch as the *Nevertheless in* ends of the Artery being cut, grow fast together, so that the passage of the Blood by *this Distemper* that way is shut up for the future; from hence when as a lesser provision of Blood is *it is often helpful, and* carried by the Artery towards the place: and the like still carried away from it by *by what means,* the Veins, it therefore sometimes happens, that the nest of the Morbific Matter some- *is shewn.* times lessened, and its mine is by degrees consumed. For this reason, this administration oftentimes succeeds happily in diseases of the Eyes. Further, Farriers make use *Farriers use the* of the like practice for the Curing of evil tumors in the Legs of Horses; to wit, they *like practice.* take and bind the Artery, by which the Matter flows to the distemper'd part, and in the mean time, that which was impacted, partly evaporates, and is partly supped up by the Vein. And I have heard, that the same has been try'd by our *Harvey,* and not without success, for the Curing also of *Strumous* and *Scirrhous* Tumors in the *And perhaps it* humane body. I might here subjoyn many other kinds of Remedies, yea also the pre- *may be conveni-* scriptions and forms of Medicines, which are wont to be administer'd for the Curing *ent for the cu-* of Headaches, both by *Physicians* and by *Empericks*: but enough of these are to be had *ring of strumous* in Physical Books. It will be to our purpose, that after the delivering the *Ætiology,* *mours, such as* or the reason of this Disease so confusedly shown, and its *Therapeutic* or Curatory part *the Kings Evil.* sufficiently shadowed, for the more clear illustrating of these things, that we add some more rare cases of sick persons, and examples of a continual and most grievous Headach, which also for an invincible cause was oftentimes deadly.

A Woman of about fifty years of age, after she had labour'd for about six months *The History of a* with a most grievous pain in the Head, troubling her almost perpetually, under the *continual and a* *Sagittal* Suture (or the seam that goes thorow the length of the Skull, dividing it in- *ach.* to two parts) yielding to no Medicines, or method, at length fell into a *Lethargy,* with a partial resolution of her members; from which notwithstanding, being shortly recovered by timely Remedies, she awaked with the Headach, as cruel as before; moreover, within two or three weeks after, relapsing into the sleepy distemper, she de- *A continual* parted this life. Her skull being opened, there grew from the side of the third bosom, *and inveterate* to the Membranes, a *Scirrhous* Tumor three fingers broad, by the coming between of *Headach passing* which, both the *Dura mater* for a little space was grown to the *Pia mater,* and the *into a Lethargy.* sanguiferous Vessels, which should open there into the cavity of the bosom, were stopped up. Further, the cranklings or turnings in of the Brain, both the exterior and the inward cavity, was filled with a clear water. From these things being observed, the invincible and at length deadly cause most clearly appeared: to wit, the most sensible Fibres of the *Meninges* being continually pulled and torn, partly by reason of the breaking of the unity, and partly from the humor belonging to the Nerves, being there heaped up and stagnating, together with others flowing thither, and growing hot with it, were provoked into Convulsions perpetually, or painful Distentions: Afterwards, when the Blood being for a long time hindred in its circulation, by reason of that Tumor, or that at least it could not pass thorow it, by any means, sent copiously away from it self the Serous Water (as its manner is wherecover it finds an hindrance) and at length a *Dropsie* in the Brain was raised, which was the cause of the deadly *Lethargy.* I remember I have seen the like case in another, whom I have opened. Further, as I think, the disease in many troubled with Headaches, doth depend on the like invincible cause; I will however describe one example yet living, of this kind of Distemper.

Some years since, I was sent for to visit a most noble Lady, for above twenty years *A second Histo-* sick with almost a continual Headach, at first intermitting: She was of a most beau- *ry of an incu-* tiful form, and a great wit, so that she was skilled in the Liberal Arts, and in all *rable Headach,* sorts of Literature, beyond the condition of her sex; and as if it were thought too *in a most noble* much by Nature, for her to enjoy so great endowments, without some detriment, she *Lady labouring* was extreamly punished with this Disease. Growing well of a Feavour before she was *twenty years.* twelve years old, she became obnoxious to pains in the Head, which were wont to arise, sometimes of their own accord, and more often upon every light occasion. This sickness being limited to no one place of the Head, troubled her sometimes on one side, sometimes on the other, and often thorow the whole compass of the Head. During the fit (which rarely ended under a day and a nights space, and often held for two, three, or four days) she was impatient of light, speaking, noise, or of any motion, sitting upright in her Bed, the Chamber made dark, she would talk to no body, nor take

take any sleep, or sustenance. At length about the declination of the fit, she was wont to lye down with an heavy and disturbed sleep, from which awaking, she found her self better, and so by degrees grew well, and continued indifferently well till the time of the intermission. Formerly, the fits came not but occasionally, and seldom under twenty days or a month, but afterwards they came more often: and lately, she was seldom free. Moreover, upon sundry occasions, or evident causes (such as the change of the Air, or the year, the great Aspects of the Sun and Moon, violent passions, and errors in diet) she was more cruelly tormented with them. But although this Distemper most grievously afflicting this noble Lady, above twenty years (when I saw her) having pitched its tents near the confines of the Brain, had so long besieged its regal tower, yet it had not taken it: for the sick Lady, being free from a Vertigo, swimming in the Head, Convulsive Distempers, and any Soporiferous symptom, found the chief faculties of her soul sound enough.

Remeasts of every kind for the curing this Headach, try'd in vain.

For the obtaining a Cure, or rather for a tryal, very many Remedies were administred, thorow the whole progress of the Disease, by the most skilful Physicians, both of our own Nation, and the prescriptions of others beyond Seas, without any success or ease; also great Remedies of every kind and form she tryed, but still in vain. Some years before, she had endured from an oyntment of Quicksilver, a long and troublesome Salivation, so that she ran the hazard of her life. Afterwards twice a Cure was attempted (though in vain) by a Flux at the Mouth, from a Mercurial Powder, which she took from the noted Emperick *Charles Hues* ordinarily gave: with the like success with the rest she tryed the Baths, and the Spaw-waters, almost of every kind and nature: she admitted of frequent Blood-letting, and also once the opening of an Artery; she had also made about her several Issues, sometimes in the hinder part of her Head, and sometimes in the forepart, and in other parts. She also took the Air of several Countries besides her own native Air, she went into *Ireland* and into *France:* There was no kind of Medicines both *Cephalicks, Antiscorbuticks, Hysterical*, all famous *Specificks*, which she took not, both from the Learned and the unlearned, from *Quacks*, and old Women; and yet notwithstanding she professed, that she had received from no Remedy, or method of Curing, any thing of Cure or Ease, but that the contumacious and rebellious Disease, refused to be tamed, being deaf to the charms of every Medicine. Further, this so long possessing the out-parts of the Head, though it could not invade the cloysters of the Brain; yet, when I visited her, unfolding its ends in some other parts of the nervous kind, it had begun to stir up most cruel pains in her members, and also in her Loins, and bottom of her Belly, as is wont to be in the *Rheumatism*, and in the *Scorbutick Colick*.

Conjectures concerning the reason of this cruel Disease.

If we should inquire into the *Ætiology* or the Causes of this inveterate Disease, we can suspect nothing less than that the *Meninges* of the Brain, being from the beginning more lightly touched, had afterwards contracted an habitual and indelible vice. It appears by the History, that the distemper at first arose from a Morbific matter, which was translated into the Head, after an ill cured Feavour. Then perchance, by reason of some hurt brought to the Membranes, the tone of the Fibres was so much endamaged, that afterwards, the Humors flowing in them, both the nervous and others, being heaped up to a fulness, or growing hot by mere aggravation, raised up the fits of the Headach. But at length the diseased cause growing worse, by reason of the frequent fits, it seems that the unity of those Fibres, were so much broken, that from thence little Tumors, or *Scirrhous* knots or swellings, being raised up in all the exterior *Meninge*, or in a great part of it, produced pains almost continual, and those apt to be made worse or imbitter'd upon every light occasion: Certainly it seems most likely, that the invincible and permanent cause of so long, and yet not deadly Headach, proceeds from some such thing, viz. a *Scirrhous* Distemper of the *Dura mater*, the *Pia mater* being in the mean time safe. For from any other cause, if there had been a conflict of Nature and Medicine with the Disease, either a quick death or a joyful victory had far sooner been obtained.

A third History of a deadly continual Headach.

A noted Gentleman of about forty years of Age, strong and healthy, going a journey for a whole day in a continual rain, the wet beating on the hinder part of his Head, caught cold, and the next day he began to feel a pain in that part; which in a short time after becoming very bitter, afflicted him night and day, and kept him almost continually without sleep. For the Cure of this Distemper, Phlebotomy, Purging, Glisters, Blisterings, and Remedies to cause rest; yea and many others of every kind, though diligently applyed, by the Counsel also of many Physicians, helpt little or nothing. When the Disease notwithstanding these, grew every day worse, after a fortnights time, preternatural swell'd kernels and painful arose all about his Neck, the pain in his Head nothing remitting: Further, the Tendons of his Neck

being

being very much diftended and ftiff, became very troublefome to him; to which, in a fhort time, fucceeded Convulfive motions, and a fudden leaping of the Tendons, in feveral parts, with a delirium, and at length, the fick perfon worn out with pains and watching, yielded to death.

Though we had not leave for the diffecting the dead body, yet it may be fufpected, *A conjecture concerning the reafon of the Difeafe.* that both the *Pericranium*, and the *Meninges* in the hinder part of the Head, cloathing the *Cerebel*, where they are more thick and very nappy, were firft affected; and then from thence the evil was afterwards communicated to the whole Head, and wandered into all the nervous ftock: whenas in thofe Membranes, tranfpiration was hindred, from the cold and the wet, and alfo the tone of the Fibres very much hurt, it is probable, that the nervous Liquor watering them, being then hindred in its motion, and ftagnating, did burthen the containing bodies; then that being depraved in its Complexion, grew hot with other humors flowing thither, and being at length coagulated with them, grew together into *Scirrhous* and *Strumous* Tumors, and fo laid the copious feed-plot of a moft grievous Headach: Then afterwards, when through watching and perpetual pains, a great inordination of the Spirits, and a great *Difcrafie* of the Juice watering the Head, were produced; for that reafon, the knotty Concretions in the Neck, the ftifnefs of the Tendons, and at length Convulfions and Convulfive Motions followed in the Brain, and in the whole nervous Stock: and fo, when as ths animal œconomy or regiment was much decayed, and that the motion of the Præcordia could not be continued, the vital flame expired.

Sometimes deadly and incurable Headaches are no lefs raifed up from a fiery fwelling and Impofthum, than from thefe kind of knots, and little pimples of the *Meninges*. *A fourth Hiftory of an Headach, excited from a fiery Swelling, or an Inflammation of the Meninges.* Sometime fince, a young man of the Univerfity, whenas he had complained for a fortnight of a moft grievous pain in the Head, inceffantly afflicting him; it was at length increafed by a Feavour, and afterwads, waking, Convulfive motions, and talking idly followed; at which time a Phyfician being fent for, letting blood, Clyfters, Plafters, Revulfives, Bliftrings, alfo internal Remedies which call away the Flux of the Blood and Humors from the Head, being carefully adminiftred, profited nothing; fo that death foon followed. His Skull being opened, the Veffels leading to the *Meninges* were full of Blood, and very much diftended, as if the whole Mafs of Blood had flowed thither, fo that the bofoms being diffected and opened, the Blood prefently rufhing forth, flow'd to the weight of feveral ounces above half a pint: Further, the Membranes themfelves being diftemper'd thorow the whole, with a fiery Tumor, appeared difcoloured: Thefe coverings being taken away, all the infoldings of the Brain, and of its Ventricle, were full of a clear water, and its fubftance being too much watred, was wet, and not firm. Without doubt in this cafe, the incurfion of the heated blood into the *Meninges*, and the heaping of it up there, exciting the *Phlegmon* or fiery fwelling, was the caufe of the Headach, and of the following *Delirium*: Then the Blood being accumulated there, when it could not circulate, flung from it felf plenty of *Serum*, by which the whole inward part of the Head was over-flowed; fo that the Difeafe, at firft perhaps curable by Phlebotomy, from thence afterwards became mortal.

I remember another *Academick*, who after a long Headach, under the temporal *An Hiftory of an Headach raifed up from an Impofthume in the Meuinges.* Suture, tormenting him perpetually for three weeks together, immediately fell into a deadly *Apoplexie*. His Head being opened, a fiery fwelling had grown in the *Meninges*, near the place where the pain was, from which, being ripened and broke, the filthy bloody matter falling on the Brain, had diftemper'd its fubftance with a rottennefs and blacknefs. Befides, thefe invincible caufes, detected by *Anatomy*, I obferved more chances after the fame manner, as of other fick people; by which we may conclude its *Ætiology*, to be the fame, or very near of kin, with the figns and fymptoms of the like nature, and but now defcribed.

But although a continual Headach (efpecially if it be without intermiffions for many weeks) is not without danger: yet we ought not therefore to defpair of its Cure, *A continual Headach, not always to be accounted incurable.* becaufe the caufe of this, how fixed and immoveable foever it feem, oftentimes by the long ufe of Medicines, and fometimes without them, is helped by Nature and time: however, in a cafe almoft defperate, there is need of fome Medicines, left the prefent Diftemper fhould pafs into a worfe, to wit, a Soporiferous or Convulfive. Thus much for a Continual Headach: it now remains, that we fhould propofe fome more rare examples and inftances of the *Intermitting*.

Therefore, that we may let alone here, the Headaches, whofe fits being wandring *An intermitting Headach, whofe Fits are uncertain, are fo frequent that we need fhew no inftances of it.* and uncertain, proceed from the Blood or Serum rufhing on the diftemper'd places, as cafes very well known, and commonly feen; we fhall now fhew you now fome felect Obfervations of this Difeafe, either periodical, or caufed by the confent of fome Inward:

Inward: As to the first, we have shown the periodical fits of the pains of the Head, to be produced by the nutritious Humor, or by the nervous Juice: we shall now shew you Examples of either.

The sixth History of a periodical intermitting Headach.

A venerable Matron of about forty five years of Age, of a lean habit of Body, and indued with a Cholerick Temper, after she had lived for a long time obnoxious to Headaches, wont to be caused occasionally, she began about the beginning of Autumn, to be troubled with a periodical pain of the Head: This Distemper invading her about four of the Clock in the Afternoon, was wont to continue till midnight, when being wearied with pain and watching, she was compelled to sleep; then afterwards awaking out of a profound sleep, she found her self well again. She being sick after this manner for three weeks, suffered the daily fits of this Disease, and forbore to take any Medicine, which she greatly abhorr'd; but at length her Appetite being lost, and her strength worn out, being forced to seek for Cure; after letting blood and a gentle Purge, she took twice a day for a week or two, the quantity of a Chestnut of the following *Electuary*, and grew perfectly well.

The Cure of the same.

Take of the Conserve of the Flowers of Succory and Fumitory, each three ounces; of the Powder of the Root of Aron Compound two drams and a half, of Ivory one dram and a half, of yellow Sanders, and of Lignum Aloes, each half a dram of the Salt of Wormwood one dram and a half, of Vitrial of Steel one dram, of the Syrup of the Five Roots what will suffice to make an Electuary.

The reason of this Case unfolded.

In this Case, that after a disposition to the Headach, the fits of the Disease became at length periodical, after the manner of intermitting Feavours, the cause without doubt was, the assimilation of the *Chyme*, or nourishing Humor, into Blood, being hindred: because, when its provision being received into the Mass of Blood, could not be overcome, it was wont after a little stay to disagree, and with its particles, to grow hot; therefore presently the Blood swelling up, that it might shake off the incongruous mixture, laid aside its recrements, as in other parts, so especially and with a greater sense of trouble into the before weak Fibres of the *Meninges*, or hurt in their conformation: This Matter being poured on the Head, or rushing of it self thorow the sensible Fibres, or growing hot with the Juice watering them, raised up the fit of the pain but now described; which continued until the heterogeneous particles growing hot, with their mutual coming together, were either subdued or exhaled.

The seventh History of the same Distemper, excited by the default of the nervous Liquor.

A very comely Woman, tall and slender, being for a long time grievously obnoxious to distempers of the Head, was wont sometimes to be troubled for many days, yea weeks, every day as soon as she awaked in the Morning, with a most Cruel Headach, afflicting her for three or four hours and in the mean time, she was vexed with a weight of her whole Head, a numness of her sences, and a dulness of mind: which kind of Distemper, together with the pain, like disculsed Clouds, vanished before noon, and left her quiet and calm. Then again the next morning, it possessed her Head like a dark Cloud. For the Curing of it I prescribed the use of Purging Pills, Phlebotomy sparingly, besides a Blistering, and Spirits of Harts-horn, or of Sut, with *Cephalic* Juleps or Waters.

The Cure of it.

The reason of the Case unfolded.

That in this Lady, otherways than in the other sick Lady, the pains of the Head rather followed after sleep, than were healed by it, the reason seems to be, because in this morning Headach, the Morbifick Matter resided in the nervous Juice, whose more notable crudity, and fuller aggestion about the Head, happen immediately after sleep, as we have elsewhere shown at large: But the other Evening fits of this Disease, depended upon the fulness and swelling up of the nourishing Liquor within the bloody Mass, and therefore happening so many hours after dinner, was not allayed but by sleep, which quiets the disorders of the Blood.

An Instance of an intermitting Headach, which seem'd to be excited from the Womb.

It doth no less clearly appear, that the fits of the Headach do arise, sometimes by consent from other parts, *viz.* the Womb, Spleen, Stomach, *&c.* and though the complaints, and the experience of the sick, declare it to arise from Vapors, yet from the Histories of them, and their appearances rightly weighed, 'tis most clear, that this proceeds from another reason, than from Vapors carried to the Head from the distempered Inward. And in the first place, as to the pains of the Head, that seem to arise from the Womb, there is nothing more frequent than that upon the suppression of the Monthly Flowers, or the *Lochia* after being brought to bed, or (as they call it) the flooding, for cruel Headaches to succeed. Further, although the Terms do rightly flow, yet some at the instant of its flowing, others at the stopping of the same, are wont to be troubled with a cruel pain of the Head. But indeed, though

though at the same time, as the Head, the Womb also is distemper'd: however it doth not follow, that the evil is transferred from hence, thither immediately: but the Blood it self, which fixes the Morbific Matter to the Head, carries it, sometimes begotten in its proper bosom, and destinated to the Womb, wrongfully into the *Meninges* of the Brain; and sometimes snatching it from the parts of the Womb, delivers it with greater malice to the Head. This same reason may also serve for the Headach, commonly attributed to the Stomach, Spleen, and other parts.

A beautiful and young Woman, indued with a slender habit of body, and an hot Blood, being obnoxious to an hereditary Headach, was wont to be afflicted with frequent and wandring fits of it, to wit, some upon every light occasion, and some of their own accord; that is, arising without any evident cause. On the day before the coming of the spontaneous fit of this Disease, growing very hungry in the Evening, she eat a most plentiful Supper, with an hungry, I may say greedy appetite; presaging by this sign, that the pain of the Head would most certainly follow the next Morning; and the event never failed this Augury. For as soon as she awaked, being afflicted by a most sharp torment, thorow the whole forepart of her Head, she was troubled also with Vomiting, sometimes of an Acid, and as it were a Vitriolick, Humor, and sometimes of a Cholerick and highly bitterish: hence according to this sign, this Headach is thought to arise from the vice of the Stomach. *The eighth History of an intermitting Headach, seeming to arise from the Stomach.*

That I may render a reason of this, first it appears, that a Vomiting will succeed a hurt upon the Head, to wit, after a blow, or wound, or a fall; yet a pain of the Head rarely or never follows, upon Vomiting, the pain of the Heart, or the Stomach, any otherways labouring, unless the Blood comes between. Wherefore in the aforesaid case of the sick person, as it appears plainly that the *Meninges* of the Brain were before disposed to Headaches, its fits were stirred up by every agitation of the Blood; hence it is obvious to be conceived, when the heterogeneous particles are heaped up together to a fulness, in the bloody Mass, by reason of the vice of the Chyle, presently a flux of it arising, for the expulsion of the trouble, those being but evilly match'd, being separated by the Blood, and partly poured forth out of the Arteries into the Ventricle, do raise up its Ferment, and so produce hunger; and partly rushing into the predisposed *Meninges* of the Head do there dispose the tinder, or rather incentive of the Headach about to follow. This sick Gentlewoman, averse to all Physick, when she would undergo no method of Medicine, at length became obnoxious also to Paralytick, and Convulsive distempers. Out of these it will be easie to design the reason of every other Headach, *viz.* of the *Hypochondriac, Hepatic,* or otherways *Sympathetical,* so that there need not here to be added any more Histories or Observations. *A reason of this Case delivered.*

The like reason is for other Headaches, seeming to arise from the Spleen, Liver, Mesentery, &c.

CHAP. III.

Of the Lethargy.

THUS far we have described, by what Disease chiefly, and after what sort, the out-skirts of the Head, or the coverings of that enclosed within the Skull, are wont to be affected; and now descending to its more internal part, and which lyes next to the Cortical or shelly substance, we shall see to what distempers this part is found to be chiefly obnoxious. We have shew'd at large in another place, that the *Cortex* or shelly part of the Brain is the seat of the Memory, and the porch of sleep: wherefore, we rightly referr the Disease, which is wont to cause an excess of sleep, and an eclipse or defect of memory, to wit, the *Lethargy,* to that Cortical part of the Brain. *The Seat of the Lethargy is the same with that of Sleep and Memory; to wit, about the Shell of the Brain.*

The word *Lethargy* is wont to signifie two sorts of Distempers, which are as it were the act and the disposition of this Disease; for those who are said to labour with this Disease, or are sick of its great assaults, are overwhelmed with so great sleepiness, that they can scarce be excited by any impression of a sensible object, yea if by chance being prick't or pinch't, they open their Eyes, or move their members, presently they let them fall again, and become insensible; and oftentimes when left to themselves indulging a perpetual sleep, by an easie transition, they pass into death it self, whose type this Disease is; which kind of fits, have often a Feavour joyned with them, which when the sick awake, and return perfectly to themselves, for the most part *By this name both the Fits of the Lethargy are called.*

And also the so-poriferous disposition, or Sleepiness;

part ceases of its own accord. Or secondly, they are accounted *Lethargical*, who being oppressed with an immoderate torpor or numness of the senses, are found to be almost ever prone to sleep; so that in the midst of a journey, yea at dinner, or though busied about any thing, they presently fall into a drousiness. But as there are di-

Of which there are various kinds: The continual Sleepiness, the Coma, &c.

verse degrees, and various manners of this sleepy distemper, so also they constitute the various kinds of this *Lethargick* disposition. We shall for the present speak first of the former *Lethargy*, and properly so called, and afterwards of continual Sleepiness, also of the *Coma, Caro*, and other soporiferous Diseases akin to it, and likewise of Continual Waking.

In every Lethargick Distemper there is an excess of Sleep, and a defect of Memory.

In the mean time, it is to be noted, that almost in every kind of Lethargy, there is always as its *Pathognomick* sign, a Torpor or Sleepiness, and oblivion or forgetfulness. Those who suffer the more grievous fits of this Disease, if they are awakened by any force in their declination, forget all things, nor are they able to remember their own, nor the names of their Friends: also, those who have drunk more sparingly of this forgetful cup, as much as they are proclive to Sleep, so much are they deficient in Memory; so that they forget late actions, and oftentimes repeat things done, and very often ask the same questions: As to the other faculties, as Reason, Phantasie, the sensitive and loco-motive powers, the failings or defects of them, are proportionate according to the enormities of Sleep and Memory. Wherefore, that the formal reason, and the causes of the *Lethargy*, may be the beter known, we should here first of all discourse concerning sleep and oblivion, and for what causes they are excited.

The essence and causes of natural and non-natural Sleep, rehearsed.

But having already discoursed concerning the former of these, we shewed that the essence of Sleep did consist in the corporeal souls withdrawing it self by little and little, and contracting the sphere of its irradiation, left destitute and as it were shut forth of doors, the outmost compass of the Brain, or its shelly part, and so the exterior, and all the organs of sense and motion, from the emanation of the spirits; so that they for refreshment sake, being called inward, lye down and give themselves to rest; in the mean time, the Pores and passages of the outward part of the Brain, being free and empty from the excursions of the spirits, are prepared for the coming of the nervous Liquor, stilled forth from the Blood, for a new provision of Spirits. In accustomed and natural Sleep, these two causes conspire and happen together, as it were out of a certain mutual compact of Nature; *viz.* at the same time, the Spirits give place, the nervous Humor enters: but in unnatural sleep, or that which is extraordinary, sometimes this cause, and sometimes that is the former; for the Spirits being wearied or called away, first withdraw themselves, and so offer an entrance to the nervous humor heaped up before the doors; or else the nervous humor driving to those places more plentifully, and as it were making its way by force, repels the Spirits, and entring into their passages, does as it were drown them: we have particularly assigned the various occasions of either of these, and after what manner they come to pass. Concerning the eclipse or defect of the Memory, we need not speak much here, because it is wholely from the same cause, as immoderate Sleep, to wit, the exclusion, and an interdiction for a time, of the passing up and down of the Animal Spirits, from the exterior passages of the Brain, full of some humor.

The causes of preternatural Sleep are,

Preternatural Sleep, or an insatiable sleepiness (which is the chief *symptom* in the *Lethargy*, and sleepy Diseases) seems to arise wholely from the same causes as non-natural Sleep, carried forth only with greater force or energy; to wit, either the Animal Spirits, being first distemper'd, leave the outward compass of the Brain, and

An insarion or obstruction of the outward part of the Brain, and a recess of the Spirits from thence: Sometimes this, sometimes that, is the cause.

give an entrance, not only to the nervous, but to the serous, and some other vicious Humor; or else, the superfluous and excrementitious humors, together with the nervous, break thorow the cortical doors of the Brain, and as it were overflowing its Pores and passages, drive thence and repel the Spirits; sometimes this is chiefly the cause, sometimes the former, and sometimes both together. We shall first speak of that which is the more frequent cause of the *Lethargy*, to wit, the eruption of either too much, or too incongruous humor, upon the confines of the Brain, and then afterwards of the departure of the Spirits from the affected part.

The Lethargy oftentimes from the serous heap overflowing the outward part of the Brain: And sometimes from a Dropsie of the whole Brain.

I have often found by Anatomical observation, that the *Lethargy* doth arise from the Serous heap rushing into the outward infoldings of the Brain, and entering into its Pores and Cortical passages; for in many dead of this Disease, I found the spaces between the foldings of the Brain, full of clear water, yea and its outmost substance soft and infirm, from too much wet; moreover in some I found the interior cavities swelled with water, and the whole frame of the Brain overflowed with a Dropsie, or rather a flood. When therefore in a great and mortal *Lethargy*, it hath appeared that it has been after this manner, we may well suspect in a lesser and cureable sleepiness,

Of the Lethargy.

ness, that the out-borders of the Brain, are at least too much watered with humor, and the tracts of the Spirits overflowed; especially if there appear any signs of water or of Serum, abounding about other parts of the Head.

A grievous sleepiness is wont to be excited, not only from the Serum being too much, or from the over plenty of any other Morbific humor, but sometimes from its malignity: for it often happens, that a certain infestous and virulent matter is instilled from the Flood into the Brain, which entering the Pores of the Cortical substance, profligates the Spirits, and either extinguishing them, or driving them away inwards, so that this region being left destitute of them, a sleepiness and forgetfulness succeeds. There is none almost who hath not taken notice, that this often happens in malignant and ill handled Feavours: also in the *Scorbutick Cachexie*, the *Yellow Jaundice*, and certain other *Chronical* Diseases, oftentimes a sluggish and vapid or tasteless water is sent in, instead of the subtil and spirituous nervous Juice, that is the parent of forgetfulness, and of sleepiness. *Not only a plenty of humours, but the malignity, often causes this Disease.*

This Conjunct Cause of the *Lethargy*, to wit, the heaping up of too much Humor, or too incongruous, within the shelly part of the Brain, depends upon other Causes, to wit, more remote leading causes, and also evident causes. As to the former, they are wont to be in fault, both when the Blood supplies the distemper'd part with Morbific matter, and also because that the Brain it self too easily admits it. *The procatartick causes of the Lethargy. In what respect they are in fault;*

For indeed, the Blood transfers to the Head in some, a great quantity of a watery humor, and in others of a salt or scorbutical humor, also again in others excrementitious humors, and deadly to the animal government, sometimes taken from these bowels, and sometimes from those; and as occasion serves, instills them together with the nervous Juice, out of the Arteries on the outer borders of the Brain, and there by little and little insinuating this kind of Morbific Matter, by a long congestion, causes a dark cloud, or else by a sudden transportation of it, overflows at once all the outward part of the Brain, and drives away the inhabiting Spirits, like a Sea breaking in, and compels them to run more inwardly. *Both the Blood breeding evil humours, and sending them to the Brain;*

But indeed the Morbific Matter, how copiously or infestous soever it be, and poured on the Head, doth not induce the *Lethargic* Distemper, unless the very weak or vicious constitution of the Brain be also in fault: for if this be strong and of good temper, it easily resists the assaults of all those; yea it bears, without hurt, the errors and enormities in the six non-naturals. Those who have this part too humid, or too cold, as Children and old Men; also, those distempered with *Cacochymical* Humors, the *Dropsie*, *Scurvy*, or Humors gathered about the mouth of the Stomach, are very prone to sleep, and sometimes fall from a stronger Evident Cause, into a continual drowsiness. Besides, those who have a weak Brain, and their Pores too lax or open, that by that means the feculencies obtruded from the Blood find a more easie passage, often become obnoxious to sleepiness, yea and to the *Lethargy*: for such as are given to Surfeiting and Drunkenness, are wont presently after to fall asleep, which weakens the tone of the Brain, and fill, and too much open its Pores, with a crude and filthy Juice; so that when it hath been for a long time accustomed, by reason of these occasions, to admit into them the Serous superfluities, it afterwards refuses nothing brought to it, but that its passages, like a course or wide strainer, suffers all the grosser particles, both Saline, watery, and earthy, easily to pass thorow them. *and the Brain too easily receiving them. Upon what occasions the Brain is prone to the Lethargy.*

Besides these more remote leading causes (which become the act of the stirred up Morbific) there are more strong Evident Causes, for so great danger does not hang over the Brain, as that its whole compass should be invaded, from every morbid provision, nor upon every light occasion, But there are many and diverse occasions, by which the sleepy assaults are seen to be incited: the chief of these are great Surfeits, Drunkenness, especially of Wine, or the Drinking immoderately of Strongwaters, then after such excess to lye all night, or sleep in the open Air: further, an evacuation of the Serum, by other ways, after having been long suppressed; also if Spaw-waters being drunk in a larger quantity, and not again render'd presently by Urine, threaten a *Lethargy*. And so also do recrements of other Diseases, either not well or not at all Cured, being translated to the Head; so as a continual sleepiness often happens after acute Feavours, or such as continue long, and other *Chronical* Diseases, and especially the Headach, Frensie, *Empyema*, or collection of gross Humors upon the Lungs and the *Colick*. *The evident causes of this Disease.*

Thus much of the *Lethargy*, whose assault proceeds from the *Cortex* or shelly part of the Brain, being affected; to which succeed either an eclipse or an exclusion of the Spirits there inhabiting, with a sleepiness and oblivion. But as non-natural sleep, so sometimes what is preternatural, begins from the Spirits being first dejected; and which is usual to succeed another Cause. It is obvious to any one, that this ordinarily *Another conjunct cause of the Lethargy consistsin the afflicting the Spirits with some narcotick.*

ordinarily happens from more strong Opiates, without any previous flood or stopping of the cortical part of the Brain: for it is not probable that Narcoticks stir up the Humors, and send them to the Brain, when it plainly appears, that all the effervescences and flowings of these, are allayed by them. But if it should be asked after what manner, and by what means, Opiates cause sleep, and sometimes a deadly Torpor or sleepiness, we say; That this Medicine is a certain kind of poison, beating down or extinguishing the Animal Spirits, by its blasting; the Blood and solid parts in the mean time being almost untouch'd: Wherefore, when the Animal Spirits become raging, and as it were struck with madness, running hither and thither, and will not be quieted and allayed, Opiates being administer'd, like water flung upon a flame, destroy some of the outmost bands of them, so that the rest being lessened, and flying inwards, quietly lye down. We have at large discoursed of these things in a particular Tract, *Of the Operations of Medicines on the Humane Body*: For the present we shall note (which is to the purpose) that *Narcoticks* (or Medicines causing rest) being taken at the mouth, do put forth their powers partly in the Ventricle, and indeed immediately, and partly in the Brain, both that and the Mass of Blood mediating. By what means *Narcoticks* do operate, whilst in the Ventricle, and provoke sleep, we have shewn, *Chap. XV.* When they are moderate, in either province, they gently intoxicate some unquiet Spirits, and so immediately quiet the rest; but if any one takes Opiates in too large a Dose, he shall presently feel hurt both in the Ventricle and in the Brain, and a little after being insensible, shall suffer a greater evil in either: to wit, a mighty heaviness, and as it were an immoveable weight in the Stomach, which seems to opress both it and the neighbouring parts; indeed by this sign, the Fibres of this place (the Spirits which before actuated them being broken) become without life, and as it were dead; then by reason of the Opiate, particles being carried about with the Blood, to the frame or compass of the Brain, and instilled into its Cortical or shelly part, the Spirits being driven away from thence or extinguished, an irresistable, and oftentimes a deadly sleep follows: yea, I have sometimes known, from a more grievous hurt inflicted on the Ventricle, only by the use of a more strong *Narcotic*, Death it self to have followed before sleep could creep upon them, coming by a long way about. A strong man vexed with a most cruel *Colick*, for ease sake (whilst a *Physician* was sent for) took rashly a great quantity of Opium; a little after he had taken it, he complained of a great burthen oppressing, and mightily weighing down the Ventricle: His Friends and the by-standers gave him Cordial waters, Wine, and Strong-waters, but without any ease: This oppression creeping wider about the Precordia, raised up pains and swoonings; but still being awake, and constant in mind, he cryed out, that his spirits more and more failed him; till about three hours after, complaining that his sight was gone, he presently dyed.

But that we may return to the *Lethargy*, as it is a Disease and not the effects of *Opium*, whence we digressed; concerning which we are yet to enquire, whether it may arise from a Narcotick Humor begotten in us, as some *Chymists* assert? We shall tell you our conjecture, that we think this 'tis sufficiently plain, that there are other sorts of Morbifick particles produced in our Bodies, than those commonly called Elementary and Humoral, and that they do affect after a various manner, *viz.* besides the Watery, Earthly, Bilous, Phlegmatick, or Melancholic, we may find others *Vitriolick, Nitro-sulphureous*, and others participating of enormous Sulphurs and Salts, and active to our evil. The Convulsive *Pathology* can by no other means be delivered and explained, unless by supposing that some extraneous little bodies, and as it were *Nitro-sulphureous*, which sticking to the Spirits, and at last cast off by them, stir up the Explosive, that is Convulsive force: In like manner we may think, that others of another nature may perhaps be begotten, such as are of a *Sulphureous, Vitriolick,* or Narcotick nature, which when they creep into the Brain and nervous Stock, fall upon some Animal Spirits, which they by chance do meet, with extinguishing and fixing them, ordinarily induce their losses and eclipses, such as happen in the *Vertigo, Apoplexy,* or *Palsie,* as we shall more fully shew hereafter. In like manner, in a great fit of the *Lethargy*, though it be improbable, that these kind of *Narcotick* particles should be in heaps derived from the Blood into the Brain, in so great a quantity, that they should at once overturn the spirits dwelling in its whole precincts, and fix them; yet we may believe, that this may be some part of the Cause. Wherefore, in every long sleepiness, or *Lethargick* disposition, we do suspect the Animal Spirits, to be burthened with such a *Lethaan Copula*, and that we should direct the darts of every Medicine against it.

Thus

Of the Lethargy.

Thus much concerning the formal reason, subject, and causes of the *Lethargy*, properly so called, the summ of all which is, That the Animal Spirits, the inhabitants of the exterior Brain, being hindred from their wonted motion and emanation, lye down in a profound and inextricable sleep: but they are hindred either by the proper vice of themselves, because having taken or being distemper'd by some Narcotick, they are as it were coagulated and become immoveable; or because their exterior tracts or paths in the Brain, are obstructed and possessed by some strange guest, so that there is no fit space granted them for their expansion. *{What things belong to the Theory of the Lethargy.}*

The symptoms of this Disease, which now come in order to be explained, the chief are Sleep, and forgetfulness, or a cessation of every other knowing or spontaneous function, unequal and slow breathing, a Feavour, and oftentimes, the distemper growing worse, Convulsions, a leaping of the Tendons, and at length universal and deadly Cramps or Convulsions. *{Its symptoms.}*

As to the too former of these, we mentioned before, that Memory is deficient altogether for the same reason, as Sleep exceeds; to wit, forasmuch as the Spirits inhabiting the outward part of the Brain, being either bound up or expulsed from their tracts, do not irradiate or beam forth from the Callous Body, into the Cortex or shelly part of the Brain, by which imagination or waking is made; nor do they, being carried inwards, and repeating their former footsteps, represent the Ideas or Images of things before acted. Indeed, Sleep, Watching, and Memory, are affections of the same parts and places: of which it is no light sign, and which vulgarly appears by experience, that *Opiate* Medicines, by which Sleep is provoked, being often given, hurt the Memory. Yea I my self knew one, having taken a strong *Hypnotick*, or Medicine to cause sleep, after being sick with a Feavour, lived many nights and days without sleep, and almost wholely lost his Memory, especially as to any thing long past. *{The chief of which are, a sleepiness, and oblivion.}*

As to what respects the other faculties of the Corporeal Soul, to wit, the Imagination, Appetite or desire, Sense and Motion, although no *Narcotick* or sleepy chains are cast upon the Spirits destinated to these offices, and that the Pores and passages of the interior Brain, within which they are wont to expatiate, are seen to be open enough, yet these Spirits, because during the fit, they are denied their commerce with the others bound up, of themselves lye down, and are overcome by Sleep. For as a continual sleepiness beginning about the root of the sensitive Soul, to wit, the Cortex or shelly part of the Brain, immediately its whole province is obscured, as it were with a veil, to wit, the knowing, desiring, and self-moving part of the Soul, and also the intellect it self, its windows being every where shut up, hardly speculates, or beholds any thing. *{By what means the other faculties of the Soul, to wit, the knowing, desiring and locomotive, are affected.}*

Further, the power or force of this Disease, is seen to be extended to the other part of the sensitive Soul, presiding o're the Cerebel and its Regiment; wherefore, during the fit of the *Lethargy*, the respiration and Pulse are altered: for that becomes unequal and slow, sometimes drawing the breath deep and long, sometimes short, repeated, and as it were double: and this being great and swift, diffuseth a feavourish heat thorow the whole body. *{The evil of the Disease reaches also to the Cerebel.}*

The reason of the former, if I am not deceived, is this, to wit, that the same Morbifick Cause, which infects the outward part of the Brain, and its inhabitants, infects also in part the *Cerebel*, and the Spirits there serving for the motions of the *Precordia*; which being by that means disturbed and hindred, though they omit not thir tasks, yet they perform them difficultly, and with interruption; hence the *Diaphragma* and Muscles of the *Thorax*, do not so easily and swiftly as before, perform their *Systoles*, but laboriously and with a longer straining or endeavour, and sometimes with repeated tryals or forces. This kind of unequal, long, and difficult breathing, frequently happens also in a Phrensie; wherefore, some judge the cause both of this and that, to be from the inflammation of the Midriff or *Diaphragma*, but amiss, because the *symptom* in both these *Cephalick* Diseases depends on the *Cerebel*, participating the hurt of the Brain, grievously distemper'd. *{Hence breathing is often hurt, or altered.} {This proceeds not from the Inflammation of the Midriff.}*

As to the Feavour of one troubled with a *Lethargy*, to be known by the great and quick Pulse, hot breathing, with a burning of the Tongue and Mouth, without any heat in the extream parts, some deduce this from the same cause as the *Lethargy*, to wit, either from Phlegm putrefying in the Brain, or from a cold inflammation of the Brain. Others on the contrary, affirm the Feavour to be the primary effect, and thence the Morbifick Matter to be carried into the Head, from the burning Blood. *{From whence the Lethargick Feavers}*

Concerning these, we grant, that a *Lethargy* comes often after a Feavour, but we can say nothing of the Phlegm putrefying in the Brain, or of its frigid Inflammation, which is as much as to say, icy fire; for if this be malignant, or of evil custom, happening *{Not from Phlegm putrifying in the Brain.}*

S pening

Of the Lethargy.

pening also to Children, old Men, and other Phlegmatick, Scorbutick, or very *Cacochymical* persons, or such as are full of ill humors, about the height of a Disease, not well Cured, oftentimes in the place of a *Crisis*, the feavourish matter being snatch'd into the Head, induces a cruel and oftentimes a deadly Torpor or sleepiness; which notwithstanding ought not to be esteemed the symptom of the Disease, but of that Feavour. After this manner I have often observed, and elsewhere have particularly described, that Soporiferous Feavours, and as it were marked with a certain sleepiness, have raged and become *Epidemical*, at sometimes, by reason of the evil constitution of the year.

Nor is the former always the cause of it in the Lethargy. Lib. de Morb. Convulf. Cap. vij. p. 96.

But it is no less usual when a *Lethargy* is the principal distemper, for a Feavour to follow, and to owe to it as much its original, as its Cure; for a Feavour beginning after a continual sleepiness, that being shaken off or discussed, ceases soon of it self; such a Feavour we think to arise, not from the Blood growing hot by reason of the strife of intestine particles, but because of the impulse of the containing and neighbouring bodies, variously altering and disturbing its course. For indeed the right temper of the Blood very much depends, not only on its particles being truly mixt and overcome, but also upon the motion impressed on the Heart and the Vessels, or the Organical Circulation; to wit, that its Liquor may every where flow with an equal and alike flowing and ebbing; which, if finding any where a stop or Remora, it be retarded, its motion is made more impetuous, and with a Feavourish tumult in the whole channel besides. This manifestly appears in violent passions, acute pains, a breaking of the unity, in all which the Blood being obstructed in one place, or straitned, it is snatched more vehemently in others, and conceives a Feavourish heat; for this cause, to wit, lest the thread of its circulation should be broken, on which life necessarily depends; wherefore as the Proverb says, *None dyes without a Feavour*: For how poor or deficient soever the Blood is, and that the strength of all the moving parts are weak, yet in the instant agony of Death, by the mere impulse of Nature, they either pursue their functions, or the nervous Fibres every where erect themselves, and put forth their utmost endeavours, that they might drive forward the Blood flowing in them, and Circulate it with a rapid motion. I once visited an illustrious Lady, who for some time had been miserably afflicted with *Colick* and Convulsive distempers, and quite worn out, and at length fell suddenly into a deadly *Lethargy*. When I perceived her Pulse to beat strongly, I prescribed that four ounces of Blood should be taken out of the jugular Vein, which immediately leap'd from the opened Vessel, with such force that, I believe, if it had been suffered, the whole Mass of Blood would have flowed thence: for the next day after, her dead body being opened, I found scarce four ounces more of Blood in her whole Body, and yet she dyed thus in a Feavour. The reason of the *Lethargick* Feavour is wholely the same, which is seen to arise only from the Vital Organs, being very much incited by labouring Nature, and therefore vehemently driving about the Blood.

More often the effect of this Disease

proceeds from the Organical Circulation of the Blood, being hindred or altered.

How none dyes without a Feaver.

The *prognostick* of the *Lethargy* is shut within a strait limit; for the fit of the Disease being for the most part acute, is soon terminated either in Death or health, and for the most part it is wont to give more of fear, than of hope. If it comes upon a malignant Feavour or hard to be cured, or if it comes upon other *Cephalick* or Convulsive Diseases, as the Headach, Phrensie, Madness, Epilepsie, or also upon a long and grievous Colick, or Gout, the *Physician* can predict nothing but evil: nor is it less to be feared if it happen in a Body full of evil Humors, or one long sick, or in an old Man.

The Prognostick of the Lethargy.

When the Disease is desperate.

In like manner it is an evil omen, if the sick, being presently overwhelmed with a great Torpor or stupidness, and almost *Apoplectick*, cannot be awakened, and if he breaths unequally, and slowly, or with a great snorting, then the Disease increasing, and the sick troubled with tremblings, Cramps, leapings of the Tendons, and at length with Convulsive Motions, it is to be esteemed desperate or without hope.

When it is only so.

But if the Distemper be excited, without any great foregoing Cause, with an only Evident Cause, as a Surfeit, Drunkenness, or by the use of Narcoticks, a blow on the Head, or some not deadly stroke, we may expect the event to be less deadly or mortal.

When some hope may be conceived.

Then if the Distemper, arising from such occasions, happens to a Body before whole and strong; if it does not wholly take away the Sense and Memory at the first assault, and after a short time the *symptoms* begin to remit a little, of such a sick person you ought not to despair.

From whence more hope may be had.

In every *Lethargy*, if any Cause of the Disease is seen to be cut off and removed, so that if by the help of Medicines, or the instinct of Nature, copious and helpful evacuations by Sweat, Urine, or by Stool do follow, with ease or help, or if by applying

Whence more of hope than of fear.

Of the Lethargy.

plying of Blistering Plasters a great deal of water flows forth, if a swelling or great whelks or pustles break out behind the Ears, or in the Neck, if frequent sneezing happens, or water flow from the Eyes or Nose, thence a certain hope of health may be expected.

Hippocrates l. Coac. c. 145. mentions a Cure of the *Lethargy*, to be often made by the distemper of the *Thorax*; saying, *That many Lethargicks that are stuffed with Phlegm have recovered:* Which words are wonderfully wrested by Interpreters. *Mercurialis* understands by suppuration, the putrified matter of the Disease, to be evacuated by the Ears and Nostrils. *Prosper Martianus* will have *Hippocrates* to be understood in the word *Lethargy*, not the disease of the Head, but of the Breast. But wherefore are all these subterfuges? when it often happens that the Morbific matter, at first fixed in the Head, and stirring up a continual sleepiness, or *Lethargy*; the same being thence supped up by the Blood, and deposited in the breast, doth produce an *Empyema*, or a spitting like those whose Lungs are wasted. In the description of a Soporiferous Epidemical Feavour, which raged in the year 1661. we noted the same to have happened to many. *A red Swelling coming upon a Lethargy sometimes cures it. Lib. 9. of Convulsive Diseases.*

Concerning the Cure of this Disease, for that it has no respite or truces, it is not to be deliberated on: after a sharp Clyster being given, let a Vein be opened presently, for the Vessels being emptied of Blood, they are more apt to sup up the Serum, or other Humors deposited in the Brain. Further, in this case, I advise rather to open the Vein in the Neck, than that in the Arm. Because by this means, the Blood being very much heaped up, within the bosoms of the Head, and perhaps standing still, is more easily reduced to an equal Circulation. *The Cure of the Lethargy. Phlebotomy almost always necessary.*

Letting blood being performed, immediately other remedies of every kind are to be made use of: Let Vesicatories or blistering Plasters be applied largely to the Neck and Legs; anoint the Temples and Face with Oyl of Amber, or *Cephalick* Balsoms; lay over all the Feet a *Cataplasm* or Poultis, made of Rue, Crowfoot, and Pepperwort, with black Sope and Bay-salt; use hard frictions or rubbings to the Members, frequently apply to the Nostrils Salt of Urine, or Spirits of *Sal Armoniac*. *Outward Administrations.*

Then let there be administred Cephalick Remedies. *Internal Remedies.*

Take *of the Water of Pæony Flowers, of black Cherries, Rue, and of Walnuts, simple, each three ounces; of the Water of Pæony Compound two ounces, of Castor tyed up in a rag and hung in the glass two drams, of Sugar three drams; mix them and make a Julep, let it be given about four or five sponfuls every three or four hours;* also with every Dose of this, give twelve or fifteen drops of the Spirits *of Amber, or of Sal Armoniac, or a paper of the following Powder.* *Julep. Spirits.*

Take *of the Powder of the Root of Pæony the male, of a Mans Skull, of the Root of Virginian Serpentworth or Snakeweed, of Contrayerva, each one dram; Bezoar, and of Pearl, each half a dram; of Coral prepared one dram, make a Powder, and divide it into twelve parts.* *A Powder.*

Further, here it is to be considered, whether an evacuation, either by Vomit or Stool, should not be made. I know that this is variously controverted among Authors, and I have also known it performed with various success: which being weighed and laid together, I shall briefly propose my opinion. *A Vomit or Purge.*

If the *Lethargy* should arise upon a Surfeit, or a late Drinking, or if from taking some disagreeable things, or *Narcoticks*; presently let a Vomit be given; wherefore, you may give Salt of *Vitriol*, with Wine and *Oxymel* of Squills; or in strong bodies an Infusion of *Crocus Metallorum*, or of *Mercurius Vitæ*, with black Cherry water. Let it be given, and if it doth not work of it self, provoke Vomiting with a Feather thrust down the Throat. *How they are indicated.*

But if the fit of the Disease comes upon a Feavour, or any other Cephalick Distempers, or if it be raised up primarily, or of it self, by reason of some foregoing cause before lying in the Blood or Brain, then a Vomit or Purge being given at the beginning, when the matter is flowing, doth oftentimes more hurt than good; because the Humors whilst in motion, are more shaken and agitated, and when they cannot be subdued and brought away, they drive them into the distempered part. *When to be avoided.*

On the second day, if the numness doth not remit, let Phlebotomy be repeated, if the Pulse shew it fitting; or else instead thereof, take forth blood from the Shoulders, after Scarification by Cupping Glasses; then a little after (if nothing hinders) let a Vomit or Purge be administred. *Scarification.*

S 2 Take

Of the Lethargy.

Catharticks. Take *of the Sulphur of Antimony five grains, of Scammony sulphurated eight grains, of the Cream of Tartar six grains; mingle them, make a Powder; let it be given in a spoonful of the afore prescribed Julep.*
Or Take *of Scammony sulphurated twelve grains, of the Cream of Tartar fifteen grains, of Castor three grains; make a Powder, and let it be given after the same manner. In the mean time, let altering Medicines, or such as derive the matter from the place, the same or such like, be still continued.*

Errhines, Sneezing Powders, and Apophlegmatisms, &c. On the third day, and afterwards ought to be applied such things, which are forbid at the beginning of the Disease, for fear of a new Fluxion, *viz. Errhines*, or things that Purge the Head at the Nose, Sneezing Medicines or Powders, *Apophlegmatisms*, or Medicines which draw the Humors from the head by the mouth. Further, it is then sometimes expedient to apply the warm intrails of some animal new killed, to the forepart of the Head, after the hair is clipped or shaven off, and often changed: also sometimes to foment those places with a Discussing and *Cephalick* Decoction, or Fomentation: but before all other *Topicks*, I have known great help brought from a large *Vesicatory* or Blistering, with many running sores made all over the compass of the Head. I saw two sick with the *Lethargy*, after the Disease held long, and that not only the Memory, but almost all knowledge was lost, Cured chiefly by this Remedy: for in both of them, the fleyed places, when they could not be easily covered, poured forth great plenty of thin matter, about half a pint every day. It will not be needful to set down any more Medicines of this nature, being commonly and every where to be had; it now remains, that we illustrate what we have said, with some Histories of sick people, which I shall here add.

A Blistering applyed to the Forepart of the Head very much helps.

The first History. A Country-man about thirty years old, of a Phlegmatick Complexion, something inclining to Sanguine, being a long time obnoxious to frequent Headaches, about the beginning of Winter, became sleepy and very stupid; and one day, whilst he was following the Plow in the Fields, lying down on the ground, he fell into a profound sleep, and when he could not be awakened by his servant and others calling him, he was carried home and put to bed; his Friends in the mean time expecting that after he had finished his sleep, he would awake of himself. After the space of twelve hours being past, when he could not be awakened by pulling, thumping, noise, and other means, they sent for me; as soon as I came, I applied Blistering Plasters, large ones, all about the hinder part of the Neck, then taking from him about sixteen ounces of Blood, I caused him to take a strong Clyster, and his Face and Temples to be anointed with Oyl of Amber, and Frictions and painful Ligatures to be applied to his Legs. Also I prescribed him to take oftentimes in a day, Spirit of Sut, with a *Cephalick* Julep. Notwithstanding he lay all that day stupid, without any sense; and if being provoked by some strong or hard pulling, he lifted up himself a little, and opened his Eyes, presently falling down again, and shutting them, he fell into his continual sleep again. About Evening I took care to have Cupping Glasses, with a great flame to be applied to his shoulders, which done, he began a little to awake; and about that time he had a great stool, and very much Serum flowed forth from the Blisters, the Plasters being taken off, then we had great hopes of his health. And therefore at every turn, remedies being applied that night; awaking in the morning following he knew his Friends, and answered aptly to those who interrogated him: But as yet the whole cloud was not vanished, but that being sleepy, he remained several days oblivious, till at length, being purged twice, he perfectly grew well.

The reason of this. This case has the exact type of the *Lethargy*, properly so called, where for the conjunct Cause, it had an heaping up of abundance of Serum about the compass of the Brain, and then a breaking in of it into its infoldings: and when by a timely use of Remedies, the flowing in of new matter was hindered, and that which lay upon the part was partly supped up into the Blood, and partly being rarified into Vapours and Effluvia's, was shaken off, the Cure of the Disease quickly and wholly followed.

A second History. An *Oxford* Gardiner being sick of a Feavour, about the height of the Disease, instead of a *Crisis* he fell into a continual Sleep, and lay drowned in it for three or four days, so that he could not be awakened by the use of any Remedies: But at length, his Head being shaven, Blistering Plasters were applied all over his Head, and many running sores left open, and awakening he recovered the use of his senses a little: But his Memory being almost wholely lost, he became so stupid, that he remembered the name of no Man, nor their words, and remained like a Bruit. When he had thus remained foolish for the space of almost two months, and still very sleepy, the cloud

cloud began a little to be difpelled : and at length, he returning to his wonted labour, was in indifferent good health ; but he never had afterwards the fame vigor of mind and wit, as he had before this Difeafe. In this cafe you have an example of a *Lethargy* coming upon an ill Cured Feavour, in which the Morbific Matter, by a fudden tranflation of it into the outward part of the Brain, had for a little while filled, not only all the Pores and paffages, but alfo had fo hurt their Conformation, that the Spirits being for fome time excluded, and at length freed, they could not recover their former paths, or wonted tracts, till of a long time after.

I remember very well, the example of a *Lethargy*, arifing from the ufe of Opiates, in a Country Village where I lodged by chance one night, by reafon of the foulnefs of the weather. For being about to go to bed, mine Hoft asked me if I would vifit two poor people his Neighbours, diftemper'd after a wonderful and miferable manner. When I fhewed my felf ready to do the office, not only out of Charity, but led alfo by curiofity, I was carried willingly into a fmall and poor Cottage, where I found the Father an old Man, and his Son, both of them in two Beds in one and the fame Chamber, overwhelmed with a moft profound Sleep, which had oppreffed them the day before, after they had eaten fome roots, which they had dug up in the Garden, being it feems Henbane, which they took for Parfnips. *The third Hiftory.*

After they had both Oyl and *Oxymel* poured down their throats, and a Feather thruft down a great way, that made them vomit, I prefcribed for them tincture of *Caftor*, with a fpoonful of *Treacle*-water (which Remedies I had then about me) to be given them at every turn all night: befides, that they fhould anoint their Noftrils and Temples with the fame Tincture; and if it might be done, that a ftrong Clyfter fhould be given them: the following day the old Man firft, and afterwards the Son awaking, returned to themfelves, the fleepinefs being almoft wholely fhaken off. In thefe diftemper'd, after the reliques of the *Narcotick* were caft out by Vomit, left they fhould do further hurt, there was only need, that by fit Medicines (among which *Caftor* defervedly is efteemed to be contrary to the venom of *Opiates*) the Spirits being excited, fhould be fet free from the fleepy poifon afflicting them. *The Cure defcribed.*

CHAP. IV.

Of fome other fleepy Diftempers, viz. a continual Somnolency, *the* Coma, *or heavy Sleeping* ; *and the* Caros, *or a deprivation of the Senfes.*

IN the former Chapter, we have fully fhown what doth belong to the knowledge, *prognoftick*, and Cure of the *Lethargy*, properly fo called. But we did not only therefore affirm, that the feat of this Difeafe was in the unequal compafs, the cranklings, or infoldings of the outward part of the Brain, becaufe we had there affigned the repofitory of the Memory, and the porch of Sleep, (although we might from hence conclude it;) but befides, becaufe it hath appeared fo to me from *Anatomical* obfervations very often, that the *Lethargy* does not arife (as is commonly thought) from the interior Ventricles of the Brain being diftemper'd : for we have known, thefe to be frequently overflown with water, and fometimes diftended with extravafated Blood, and yet the fick whilft they lived, were free from the *Coma*, or any great ftupidity. I muft confefs, that fometimes the Dropfie of the whole Brain caufes the continual fleepinefs : but in this cafe not only the internal Cavity, but alfo the *Interftitia*, or the fpaces between the outward Infoldings, are filled with a flood of waters. *Sleepy Difeafes do not arife by reafon of the Ventricles of the Brain being filled with waters.*

The *Lethargy* therefore being confined to the outmoft borders of the Brain, we fo conftitute its limits, that thofe circlings about, being almoft wholely poffeffed, together with the interfperfed Marrow, perpetual and inexplicable Sleep, or hard to be rid of, with oblivion or forgetfulnefs, is induced; in the mean time, the middle part of the Brain, or the *Callous* body, from whence the Animal Spirits irradiate, or beam forth, into all parts both fenfible and motional, being almoft unhurt; for the total eclipfe of this caufes the *Apoplexy*, as fhall be fhewed hereafter. But indeed on either fides of thefe ends or limits, other foporiferous diftempers are ordinarily found, which though of kin to the *Lethargy*, yet fome of them are leffer than it, as *Somnolency* or continual fleeping, and the *Coma*; only one is greater, as the *Caros*. Therefore *The ends or limits of the Lethargy, as to the places diftempered, are conftituted. Some fleepy Diftempers leffer than that, viz. Sleepinefs, and the Coma: The Caros is greater than it.*

fore we shall now, and in order, speak briefly of every one of these, as also of some opposite passions, *viz.* thorow waking, and the waking *Coma*: and first of Continual Sleepiness.

Continual Sleepiness described. Most Authors call this not a Disease, but an evil habit, or a sleepy disposition, for the distemper'd, as to other things, are well enough; they eat and drink well, go abroad, take care well enough of their domestick affairs, yet whilst talking, or walking, or eating, yea their mouths being full of meat, they shall nod, and unless rouzed up by others, fall fast asleep: and thus they sleep continually almost, not only some days or months, but (as it is said of *Epemenides*) many years; wherefore we ought to believe this a Disease, and worthy of Cure, which defrauds one of more than half his life.

Its Seat assigned. The seat of *sleepiness*, as that of the *Lethargy*, is to be placed in the outward part of the Brain; but with this difference; that the material or conjunct Cause of this Distemper, though it vexes, or troubles always without doors, yet it penetrates less deeply than the *Lethargy*; yea it disturbs or affects almost the whole superficies of the Brain, or the mere *Cortical* substances of the infoldings, the included marrow being almost untouch'd:

In what respect it differs both from the Lethargy and the Coma. in which respect, it differs not only from the *Lethargy*, but the *Coma* also; for in the Distempers which we described, though continual sleep presses on them, yet 'tis easily broken off; then besides, being fully awakened they remember many things, and converse with their Friends, though immediately prone again to sleep: whence it appears, that the cause of this Disease sticks only in the outer border of the Brain, nor does it enter deep into its compass, as other sleepy distempers do.

The conjunct cause of Sleepiness. But indeed it may be suspected, that while the Blood every where washing the border of the Brain, with thick rivulets, and instils every where into it a subtil water, for the matter of Spirits, oftentimes a great plenty of water flowing thither with it, and entering together the *Cortex*, and remaining there, mightily fills it, and (like an *Anasarca* in the Body) swells it up: But this *Cortical* or shelly part being swelled up after this manner, and as it were dropical, so presses the Medullary infoldings, every where lying under it, that the expansion of the Spirits being hindred,

That the deluge or Anasarca of the Cortical part of the Brain is. by reason of the Pores of the exterior part of the Brain being something bound up, sleepiness is induced; to which it happens, that the Blood, that by reason of the *Cortex* of the Brain being intumefied with water, as it were between the Skin, Circulates less expeditiously, thorow all the neighbouring parts, and so is apt to fill the Vessels and bosoms, and to stagnate in them;

To which happen an heaping up, or as it were a stagnation of the Blood, about the compass of the Brain. by which means it comes to pass, that the exterior border is yet more compressed, and so the spaces requisite for the emanation of the Spirits, are also more streightned. Indeed this appears to be part of the cause, from hence, because this kind of sleepiness, by reason of the Blood not freely circulating in the Head, and therefore apt to stagnate, is wont to make red the Face, with a certain blueness and blackness: Further, whilst the subtil Liquor, which is for the matter of Spirits, passing thorow this pond or deluge heaped together in the *Cortex* of the Brain, goes forward into the Marrow lying under, it is probable, that with it do creep thorow some extraneous, and as it were very small

Also a Torpor or Sleepiness of the Spirits. *Narcotick* particles, which growing to the Spirits immediately render them torpid or stupid, and prone to sloth of their own accord.

This Distemper, as I have observed in many, is not very dangerous, for as it often happens, it is wholely Cured, or at least remaining for many years, without the *Carus* or *Apoplexy* (which is wont to be feared) it doth not become mortal or terrible. The Cure of this Disease often happens, the seat of it being changed, to wit, when clearing the Brain, the Morbific Matter is transferred to the *Cerebel*, which coming thither, produces tremblings of the Heart, the *Asthma*, loss of Spirits, and other troublesome *Symptoms*, commonly taken for *Hypochondriacal*,

The Cure of Somnolency. The Curatory Method suggests chiefly these intentions, to wit, that after a provision or foresight of the whole, that (where it is convenient) Phlebotomy be performed, and a Purge given; then those Remedies to be diligently administred, by which the Blood and the Brain may be freed from the watery deluge, and this latter may be strengthened, whereby it may for the future receive and retain the Serous superfluities. For those ends, once or twice a week, may be given Pills of Amber, or of *Cochia*, with the Resine of *Jalap*; at other times, let there be taken daily Morning and Evening, a Dose of a *Cephalick Electuary*, or Spirits of Tincture of *Sal Armoniack*, Amber, Sut, with a *Cephalick* Julep: the forms of which may be picked out of those above described. At eight of the Clock in the Morning, and at five in the Afternoon, let them drink a draught of *Coffee*, or the Liquor prepared of that Berry, first boiling in it, the leaves of *Sage* or *Rosemary*, till it has got a
greenish

greenish Tincture. Let them drink for their ordinary drink, a Decoction of *Lignum Sanctum*, adding towards the end, the leaves of *Sage* or *Betony*, or other *Cephalicks*. Further, it is expedient that two large Issues be made between the Shoulders, and also frequent Blistering Plasters be applied about the Neck. The hair being cut off, let a quilted thing of *Cephalicks* and Spices be worn under the Cap. Let them also hold their noise often over a Vessel fill'd with Salt of Urine, or the Spirit of *Sal Armoniack*; let care be taken that they keep to an exact order of diet, and that those attending the sick, do not only rouse them from sleep, but daily at some set hours keep them waking.

A certain Gentleman of a Sanguine Complexion, and when he was young, of a sharp and cunning wit, but afterwards growing aged, being given to idleness and drunkenness, became dull and stupid, and also Dropsical, with a great paunch, and his thighs and legs swelled. Yet from these Diseases (which he frequently fell into) when he abstained at any time from drinking, and took Physick, he oftentimes quickly grew well. But at length, though he was freed from the Dropsie, he was oppressed with so heavy a sleepiness, and that almost perpetually, that in what place soever he was, or what ever he was doing he would sleep; then being awakened by his Servants or Friends, his mind appeared well enough, and for a few minutes he would discourse of any thing well enough, then immediately fall again to sleep. To this man I prescribed, after he had taken in vain several Medicines, that every Morning and Evening he should take of the Powder of the Leaves of Betony dryed in the Sun, and kept in a Glass, a spoonful in a draught of the distilled water of Lavender Flowers. By which Remedy finding ease, after a few days, he was perfectly Cured within a month, and enjoyed perfect health for four years after: Afterwards by reason of his evil manner of living, the same returned again, but the same Remedy found not the same success; yea there was need of other Medicines besides; sometimes he took the Spirits of Harts-horn, or of Sut, with an appropriate Julep; sometimes *Cephalick* Conserves and Powders, to which sometimes Steel was added. When he would indulge himself by Drinking, instead of Wine or Beer, he drunk Coffee; but for his ordinary drink, he had sometimes Ale, with the leaves of Scurvigrass, Sage, and Spices infused in it; and sometimes with Woods, Spices, and *Cephalick* Herbs boiled with it: He lived thus for many years after, almost always intemperate, and full of gross humors, yet free from the *Lethargy*; at length a *Cachexy* or evil state of Body invading him, and wasting with a Cough and *Asthma*, by degrees, he dyed.

An History.

The Cure of the Sick described.

The next sleepy Distemper before spoken of, greater than this last, and yet lesser than the *Lethargy*, is that which is commonly called the sleepy *Coma*. Those troubled with this, are for the most part oppressed with an heavy sleep, which they almost still indulge, and lye with their mouth gaping, and their lower Jaw fallen down, more like dead than living persons; being rouzed up by some strong pulling or pinching, they look about, speak to those standing by, answer their questions, but immediately sleeping again; they are much troubled to be hinderd or disturbed from sleep so pleasingly creeping on them. And thus indisposed after this manner, they continue for many days, yea sometimes months, sleeping without any Feavour accompanying, or following it, nor have their breathing hurt, and not very forgetful, in which it differs from the *Lethargy*: Again, they differ from those sick of the Distemper but now described no less; because, those sick of this *Coma*, are for the most part fixed to their Bed or Chair, and walk not abroad as the others, nor take any care of their houshould affairs. They answer to any short questions properly, but they cannot discourse, or deliberate about doing any business.

The sleepy Coma.

Without doubt, the Cause of this is of the same nature as the former, but of a middle degree between those two but now described; for indeed, it may be well suspected in this Distemper, that the Morbific Matter doth penetrate the Brain a little larger than in a Continual Sleepiness: to wit, the turning cranklings, or Cortical infoldings, together with the small Rivulets of the included Marrow are invaded: But yet they reach not to the greater bosoms of the Marrow, within the Callous Body, that are wont to be possessed in the *Lethargy*.

The reason of it.

The *Coma* sometimes beginning first and of it self, like the *Lethargy*, proceeds either from a Serous deluge poured forth from the Blood into the *Cortex* of the Brain; or else from a *Narcosis*, or a sleepy stupidness inflicted on the spirits dwelling there; and then, by how much this Distemper is lesser than the *Lethargy*, by so much it is esteemed less dangerous. But this Disease more frequently comes upon other Chronical or acute Diseases, to wit, the Headach, Convulsions, and frequently ill-judged Feavours, especially in Children, old Men and Women, and Phlegmatick people. Some time since, I observed in the Epidemical Feavour of the Nerves, (which have elsewhere

The Coma is either a primary Disease, or it comes after other Distempers.

136   *Of the Caros.*

The Cure of it when it is a Disease of it self.

where described) as some were *Lethargical*, so many were troubled with this Sleepy *Coma*; of whom many grew well, the Morbific matter being translated from the Head into the Breast. Further, in other cases, this Distemper of a doubtful event, between hope and fear, requires the careful pains of a prudent Physician.

In the primary *Coma*, the Curatory Method suggests almost the same intentions of healing as in the *Lethargy*: as to the Morbific Matter, indeavour must be had, both that a new flowing into the Brain may be prevented; and also that what is already impacted, may be discussed or taken away. Further, the Animal Spirits ought to be rouzed up, or excited, and all sleepiness or stupidity shaken from them. For this end, ought to be applied Purging, Blood-letting, Cupping-glasses, Blistering Plasters, repelling and discussing Topicks, and *Cephalick* Medicines to be given, and chiefly such as are impregnated with a Volatile Salt, and many other means of administrations already recited.

The Cure of the Coma as it is the symptom of another Disease.

But if this Disease coming upon other Distempers, happens to a person, whose Body is already much worn out, the Blood vitiated, or greatly depauperated, you must seriously deliberate before taking away of Blood, or Purging: yea, also abstain very much from them. Yet sometimes that the Conjunct Cause, or matter of the Disease impacted in the Brain, may be put into motion, it may be expedient, to take away Blood moderately, either from the Forehead or Temples, by Leeches, or from between the Shoulders by Cupping-glasses and Scarification. Here Blistering Plasters are in chief esteem, to be applied not only to the hinder part of the Neck, or Head, but to the Legs and Arms, and other parts of the body, by turns. Further, let there be given frequently the Spirits of Harts-horn, of Sut, of *Sal Armoniack*, Amber, or a Mans Scull, Coral, and others, impregnated with other *Cephalicks*, with a *Julep*, or any other proper Liquor. The forms or Receipts of these,

In Lib. Of Convulsive Diseases Chap. viii.

and of other Remedies, used in these cases, together with the Histories of the sick, and examples of Cures, are extant in the description of the aforesaid soporiferous Feavor; so that there is no need to inculcate here again, the same, or such like.

3. Of the Caros.

There yet remains an other sleepy Distemper, or kind of Lethargy or continual sleeping, commonly called *Carus*, which is greater than the *Lethargy*, and somewhat lesser than the *Apoplexy*, and is so near akin to this, that it often passes into it; but yet it is wont to be differenced from either: For those sick with the *Carus*, breath well for the most part, and when they are strongly pulled, they move their Members, sometimes lift themselves up, open their Eyes, and often speak, which *Apople-*

How it differs from the Lethargy and the Apoplexy.

ctical persons do not; yet the same, though excited or moved, do scarcely understand any thing, or plainly discern, in which respect they are distinguished from such as have the *Lethargy*.

The Seat of the Caros is a little deeper in the Brain than that of the Lethargy.

From these it appears, that the Conjunct Cause of the *Carus*, doth penetrate deeper towards the middle part of the Brain, and hath its seat in the outmost border at least of the *Callous* Body; wherefore the Animal Spirits, being restrained from their wonted expansion, within this *Emporium*, the acts of the Imagination and Memory cease, and although the Species being impressed from a more strong sensible, is directed inwards, and oftentimes the local motion is retorted to it, yet because this impression reaches not to the *Callous* Body, by reason the Spirits are there amazed or stupefied, the sick know nothing what they feel or do.

Its Conjunct Cause.

The Conjunct Cause of this Disease therefore, is very often the same, but somewhat more strong, than that of the *Somnolency*, *Coma*, and *Lethargy:* The Morbific Matter is seen to possess both the *Cortex* of the Brain, and the Marrow lying under, and being carried forward, some greater bosoms of the middle part, and the upper borders of the *Callous* body; yea sometimes, as this matter is partly carried forward by degrees, these Diseases arise, and every next is but the augmentation of the former.

The Caros is either a primary Disease, or it comes upon other Distempers.

But sometimes the Morbific Cause, without any gradual progress thorow these parts, affects the middle part of the Brain at the first assault, and there (as it is more lightly or more deeply placed) causes the *Carus* or the *Apoplexy*. In which case, it is not to be thought, that the whole compass of the Callous Body, like the Cortical part of the Brain, should be possessed by the soporiferous matter: because it is sufficient, this matter rushing into any one place, and invading some part of the middle Marrow, that presently for that reason, an Eclipse, or at least a beating down of the Spirits follows, in all that region. After this manner it is wont to be, when the *Carus* comes upon a malignant or ill handled Feavour, or upon the Headach, or some Convulsive Distempers, or when it is excited by a blow on the Head, or by a fall, or by reason of an Imposthum broken in the *Meninges:* for by reason of these accidents, the interior Marrow of the Brain is wont to be so pressed together, shaken,

or

or otherways altered, that presently the tracts or paths of the Spirits are obliterated or blotted out.

The prognostick of the *Carus* for the most part is but evil, especially if this Disease comes upon a malignant, or a long continued, a gentle and not Cured Feavour, or on a Woman in Childbed, no less danger is also threatned, if it follows after other *Cephalick* Diseases, or is excited by reason of a Wound in the Head: but yet in these cases, all hope of Cure is not presently to be cast off; for I my self have observed, some sick after this manner, and esteemed desperate or past all hope, to have recovered. *The Prognostick of the Carus.*

The event of this Disease is wont to be various, either in Death or in health. The *Carus* passes not rarely into a soon killing Apoplexy, that after first the animadvertive faculty being lost, with a short breathing, and without motion, then by reason of the evil being transmitted to the Cerebel, there follow alterations of breathing and the Pulse, and quickly death it self. *The event of this Disease is various, sometimes it passes into an Apoplexy:*

But sometimes the Morbific Matter setling more deeply, and falling from the Callous Body, into the streaked Body, one or both together, the Brain clears up a little, so that the sick look about them, talk, and know things, yet in the whole body besides, a Palsie, or Dead-Palsie on one side follows: but so, that life is not out of danger: for oftentimes, when the Brain begins to be restored, the *Cerebel* grows worse, that for that cause the Spirits there being evilly disposed or affected, which perform the offices of the vital function, and merely natural, either Convulsions are stirred up in the Bowels, and Precordia, or deadly impediments of the Pulse and respiration; yet sometimes when the Morbific matter is not so plentiful, nor very malignant, it is partly supped up into the Blood, and partly shook off, so that the sick grow perfectly well again. *Sometimes into the Palsie.*

The Curatory Method suggests the same intentions of Healing, and requires wholly the same Remedies, as those which are wont to be administred in the *Lethargy* and the *Apoplexy*. Wherefore, there will be no need to add here a company of Indications, nor to heap together a great pile of Medicines. But what seems more to the purpose, that I give you one or two Histories of sick people, of which I have many by me. *Its Cure is the same with the Lethargy and the Apoplexy.*

A known person of about forty years of Age, who having through Intempernace lost his health, took I know not what Medicines, prescribed by an *Emperick*, and fell into the *Carus*; perchance it was because the Morbific Matter being moved and agitated by the Medicine, it rushed into the Head. Visiting this Man on the second day, I found him buried in a profound sleep, and almost insensible; for although he opened his Eyes, moved his Members, when prick'd or strongly pull'd, yet presently sleeping again, he perceived nothing of what he did or suffer'd. Though in this case, I could prognosticate nothing but what was sad, however I did not desist from giving him my Medicinal help: abstaining from letting of blood, his strength being worn out, and his Blood depauperated, I took care for a large Blistering Plaster to be applied to the hinder part of the Neck, and a strong Clyster as soon as I could, to be given him, made of a Decoction of *Briony* Roots, with *Carminative* Flowers and Seeds, adding thereto of the Species of *Hiera* two drams: his Nose and Temples were anointed with Balsoms. *Cataplasms* of Rue, and the Roots of *Bryony* were laid all over his Feet. Besides, every other, or every third hour, I order'd him to drink a Dose of the Spirits of Harts-horn, with a *Cephalick Julep*; yea, and I took care to have administred several other administrations, used in this case. By which, when the Disease did not wholly give place on the following day, I prescribed a Purge of prepared *Scammony* to be taken in a spoonful of Broth; by which, when he had gone often and plentifully to Stool, he began to open his Eyes, speak to, and to know those standing about him, and a little after returning to himself, he fully awaked. This Disease therefore (as I think) was easily and quickly Cured beyond hope, because that cloud, being by chance sent into the Brain by Physick, might the better be deduced thence by the help of other Physick. *The first History.*

A noble person about fifty, fat in body, and in time past obnoxious to the *Vertigo*, and to *Asthmatical* Distempers, using for two years Physick every spring and fall, having also a large Issue between his shoulders, lived in indifferent health: The Summer coming on, and he living in the Country, neglected his Issue for several weeks, so that the recrements there, flowed much less than they were wont; yet he was still well, till about the *Solstice* (or middle of *June*) when one morning chearfully talking with his Friends, sitting in the Porch of his House, rising suddenly he complained, that he was not well; and going into the House, sitting down in a Chair, immediately leaning backward, fell into a profound sleep, and lay so buried in it, that all that day *Another History.*

T

day he could not be awakened. Coming to him in the Evening, I took care to have *Phlebotomy* administred, and also a *Clyster*, a *Vesicatory*, and many other Remedies, proper in such a Case. On the next day, his Brain began a little to grow clear, so that he looked about him, and spake a few words; he seem'd to know his Friends, but could not utter the name of any; but by reason of this matter sinking down more deeply into the Brain, a Pallie seized his whole right side. Further, when as yet his great sleepiness continued, that day Blood was taken out of the other Arm, and also other Remedies as the former, were continued: On the third day, being less stupid, he knew many, and could tell the names of some of them, he perceived then his own sickness, and began to be careful for the taking of Remedis. But indeed, whilst his Brain grew better, the evil spread it self on the *Cerebel*, and the nervous Stock; for on the fourth day, his breathing became unequal, and more laborious, his Pulse weaker, and his whole body troubled with a stifness, and Convulsive shakings: On the fifty day, more cruel Convulsions and Cramps did more often infest him; then his Pulse by degrees lessening; on the sixth day, though more freed from his sleeping, he dyed. In this case, and in others like it, 'tis probable that the Morbific matter did at once invade the Brain and the *Cerebel*, but whilst it stuck in the *Cortex* of this latter (contrary to what happens in the Brain) it caused no sensible hurt, because this part, which was hurt, was neither the seat of Sleep nor of the Memory; but afterwards, perhaps on the fourth or fifth day, the matter sinking down from thence, to the middle parts of the *Cerebel*, whilst as to the other Distemper the sick grew better, the vital function, by reason of the spirits destinated to it being oppressed in their fountain, began to faint, and afterwards suddenly declining, took away unexpectedly all hope of recovery, which before seemed favourable.

CHAP. V.

Of thorow or long Waking, and of the Waking Coma.

EVEN as Light and Darkness, so Sleep and Waking, being placed nigh together, best illustrate the natures of one another; so that it will be to the purpose, after the Sleepy Distempers, to discourse here of preternatural Watching, or Waking; to wit, forasmuch as it exceeding its limits, and hurting some functions, is both a Disease, and requires Cure. In this rank there are commonly two Distempers, to wit, thorow or long Waking, and the Waking Coma; of both which we will now speak in order.

Long Waking is either the symptom of other Diseases, or else is a Disease of it self.
Concerning thorow Waking, we must here first distinguish, to wit, that it is a symptom coming upon some other Disease, as a Feavour, Phrensie, Madness, the Colick, Gout, or such like; then the Cure and consideration of it belongs to that distemper, whose issue it is: or else immoderate Waking, arising of it self, without any notable sickness, is seen to be a Disease almost solitary or alone of it self. So I have known some, free from any Feavour or pain, well in their Stomach, and fit enough for their business, being in Bed, could take no more Sleep than the Dragon of the *Hesperides*. Some troubled with this kind of Waking, though destitute of Sleep, scarce seem to want it it; for their Spirits appear neither sluggish, or weary, or exhausted: but others hardly bearing watching, become from thence languishing, and without Appetite, and are forced to fly to *Opiates*, which sometimes they use daily, and in a large Dose unhurt.

The cause of natural Waking consists in the restlesness of the Spirits, and the openness of the Cortical part of the Brain
We have before hinted, that the Cause of Natural Waking, which is interlaced with Sleep, consists in these two things, either in one of them, or both together; to wit, first that the Animal Spirits being sufficiently refreshed, and freed from the stocks of the nervous Liquor, do come forth lively, and are on every side streamed forth, and chiefly from the middle part of the Brain into its circumference; then secondly, although they obtain every where an open space, and especially in the exterior compass of the Brain, then freed from the incursions of the nervous Juice, yet lest this expansion of Spirits (which is waking) should be protracted to their loss, longer than is fit, the Spirits by it being wearied, become faint, and as it were lye down of their own accord, and at the same time, the nervous Liquor being poured into the *Cortex* of the Brain, stops or shuts up their passages. Hence it follows, that preternatural

Of Long Waking.   139

ternatural Waking, or that which is immoderate depends upon these two, either on one or both together; for either they being grown too outragious, and as it were struck with a fury, will not lye down of themselves, or the nervous Liquor doth not so fill and stop up the Pores of the outward part of the Brain, that from thence the Spirits may be compelled inward to rest: Examples of both of these are ordinarily to be met withal. *In like manner also preternatural watching depends upon one or both.*

And first of all we shall take notice, that the Animal Spirits, sometimes becoming outrageous and so *Elastick* or shooting forth, or otherways enormous, that they will not only not lye down and be quieted, but scarce be contained within the proper sphere of their emanation; wherefore, being spread abroad in continual waking, so fill the Brain, and keep it extended, that the nervous Juice though it lyes heaped up at their doors, cannot be admitted; but if it enters of it self, and the Spirits are called back inwards, from the Cortex of the Brain, presently they being forced thither, or tumultuating within the middle part of the Brain, raise up many, and often most horrid phantasies, whereby sleep is driven away; or directing thence their declination further, into the nervous Stock, there stir up great disorders, which continually drive away, and break off Sleep, though it seems ready to creep upon them. *The former means described, by shewing how many ways the unquiet or elastick Spirits stir up long waking.*

As to the former of these, I have often observed, that some being disturbed with waking, were afraid to sleep, though desiredly coming upon them; for as soon as they shut their eyes to sleep, presently leaping up, they would cry out they should grow mad, with a multitude of confused phantasms, so that they were necessitated to abstain from sleep. *First, Because being recalled for Sleep into the middle part of the Brain, they grow tumultuous.*

Secondly, whilst the Spirits become more outrageous, and are for sleep sake recalled towards the interior compass of the Brain, sometimes they convert their rage into the nervous Stock, and then tumultuarily rushing in upon the Nerves, destinated for the Precordia, or the Inwards, raise up inordinations in the respective parts: hence in those thus distemper'd, as often as they shut their eyes to invite sleep, either tremblings, leapings, and binding up of the heart, with loss of Spirits, and breathing stopped, or inflations, and rising up of the Bowels, with a sense of choaking, and other symptoms commonly called or taken to be *Hysterical*, follow: or else secondly, the Spirits being recalled from their watches, and turning on the nervous Stock, transfer their rage sometimes on the spinal Marrow, and the Nerves reaching from thence into all the exterior Members: Wherefore, in some, whilst they would indulge sleep, in their beds, immediately follow leapings up of the Tendons, in their Arms and Legs, with Cramps, and such unquietness and flying about of their members, that the sick can no more sleep, than those on the Rack. Once I was consulted with for a noble Woman, who was in the day-time cruelly tormented with the pain about the heart, and Vomiting, but in the night she was hindred from sleep, though it seemed to approach, by reason of these kind of Convulsive Distempers invading her, with it; nor indeed could she sleep all the night, unless she had before taken a large Dose of *Laudanum*; wherefore, this Medicine at first being permitted her, only twice a week, afterwards she took it daily for three whole months, contracting by it no hurt, either in her Brain, or about any other function; and when in the mean time, by the use of other Remedies, the *Dyscrasies* of the Blood and the nervous Juice were amended, and the Animal Spirits were made more benign and gentle, she having after that wholly left off her Opium, could sleep indifferently well. *Secondly, Because being called back into the nervous Stock, they impetuously leap forth. And so, either into the interior Nerves, serving the Præcordia and Viscera; Or, into the Spinal Marrow, and the exterior Nerves.*

These kind of sleep-destroying Distempers, stirred up either within the middle part of the Brain, or within the nervous Stock, either more inward or more outward, do depend wholly on the evil constitution of the Animal Spirits: for those who ought to be gentle, clear, and bright, and to actuate gently the containing bodies, and to influence them with a benign influence, become sharp and fierce, and like Effluvia's sent from *Stygian* Waters, unable to be restrained, do distend them too much, and refuse to be governed by the command of the will, and to be quieted by sleep; yea being restrained in one place, they immediately grow tumultuous in another. Such a constitution of the Animal Spirits proceeds from the acid, and oftentimes as it were Vitriolick Dyscrasies of the Blood begetting it, and of the nervous Juice cherishing and increasing it: as shall be more fully shewed hereafter, when we speak of madness. *The causes of the aforesaid Distempers assigned.*

In the mean time, as to what belongs to the Cure of thorow or long waking, (which we but now described) because it cannot be long tolerated, therefore those things, which may bring present ease, ought first to be administred; for this end, those things which sooth the Spirits, and gently moderate their disorders, are convenient, as those commonly called *Anodynes*, viz. Distilled Waters, Decoctions, Syrups, and Conserves of the Flowers of Water-Lilies, Cowslips, Mallows, Violets, Hearts-ease, *The Cure of them declared.*

T 2

Hearts-ease, of the leaves of Willow, Lettice, Purslain, also Emulsions, or Juicy expressions. If that the unquiet Spirits will not be allayed by gentle flatteries, you must compel them into quietness, as it were with bouds and strokes: plenty of them ought to be diminished, and the places also to be inlarged, in which they may expand themselves in freedom, and without tumult, and quitted from the intanglements of other Humors, to wit, of the Blood and Serum: For which ends, sometimes the opening of a Vein is convenient, and Blisterings are always to be made use of ; also *Diacodium*, and *Laudanum*, if it be convenient, are frequently given ; and in the mean time, whilst that *Opiates* give some truce to the Disease, the cause of it ought carefully to be rooted out by the use of other Remedies, as much as may be; wherefore, such as take away the sharpness of the Blood and nervous Juice, and render a sweetness to them, are to be administred, day after day, in Physical hours: In which rank are shelly Powders, *Apozems*, and Distilled Waters ; Alterers, made out of temperate Antiscorbuticks; the more gentle prepared *Chalybeats*, Spirits of Harts-horn, and of Sut, and almost before all other things, the Tincture of *Antimony* is much esteemed.

The second sort of thorow or long waking, arising both from the too much openness of the Brain, and from the unquietness of the Spirits;

There remains another sort of thorow or long Waking, the cause of which in some, if not in the greatest part, consists in almost a continual openness, or too much gaping of the Pores, or passages in the *Cortex* of the Brain. For besides, that the Animal Spirits becoming sharp, and somewhat outragious, refuse to lye down of their own accord, and to indulge rest; moreover, no stop or yoke is imposed upon them from the nervous Liquor, entring into the Pores of the Brain, but being free and quitted of all burthens, they are also expanded within the exterior spaces of the Brain, every where open: wherefore, for this cause, those troubled with long Waking, feel no sleepiness or heaviness in the fore part of their head, no desire or approach of Sleep. I have known some distemper'd after this manner, who, when they had lived for many nights continually without Sleep, seemed still chearful, active, strong in their stomach, and ready for business, and not to want Sleep. The cause of this without

its foreleading Cause.

doubt is, because the burnt and melancholy Blood, supplies the exterior part of the Brain with a nervous Juice, that is not soft and favourable, but too much parched, and stuffed with adust particles, which, for that reason, is apt neither to stay long within the Pores of the Brain, nor gently to embrace and hold the Animal Spirits. Further, the Spirits themselves, procreated out of it, become of their own nature too *Elastick*, and unquiet, so that they are not easily setled, or are prone of their own accord to Sleep: But these more fixed, do not readily fly away, nor being wearied, do suddenly grow faint, but indure for a long time, without any great refection, and yet remain lively. Concerning this waking disposition of the Animal Spirits, as it is

Which also causes waking in Melancholick People.
For the same reason Coffee causes waking

the same in *Melancholicks*, we shall have an opportunity of speaking of it more largely hereafter. We may also here take notice, that for the same reason (to wit, that the adust Particles of the Melancholick and torrid Blood, being poured into the Brain, together with the nervous Juice, causes waking) the drinking of *Coffee* also, (in use formerly among the *Arabians* and *Turks*) which is drunk by our Country Men, either Physically or out of wantonness, all sleepiness being driven away, doth produce unwonted waking, and an unwearied exercise of the Animal faculty; that some having a necessity to study late in the night, or presently after drinking, or a full meal, by drinking a due quantity of this Liquor become still waking, and perform any hard task of the mind, without sleepiness. Surely the cause of this is, because this drink insinuates adust particles (of which it is full, as may be perceived both by the smell and taste) immediately into the Blood, and then into the nervous Juice; which still detain the pores of the Brain open, by their agility and inquietude, and add to the Spirits, all sleepiness being shaken off, certain provocatives, and madness, by which they are excited to a longer performance of their offices. Further, we shall deliver afterwards, where we speak of Melancholy, those things which belong to the preventive Cure of this long waking, or the removing of the Morbific cause: In the mean time, for the taking away immediately this *symptom*, as often as it is grievously troublesome, we noted that *Opiates* were little profitable ; for a bare Dose being given, doth rarely cause sleep, and render the sick more weak and languishing: It often better succeeds, if they go to bed, and take some soft and pleasing Liquor, as our own Ale, clear and mild, or Posset-drink with Cowslip Flowers boiled in it, or an Emulsion of Melon Seeds, and Almonds in a great quantity, to wit, two or three pints.

An History shewing an example of this Disease.

I was some times past consulted with about an old *Hypochondriacal* person, who besides other *Symptoms* usual in that case, was for many years obnoxious to frequent, very troublesome, and noisie belchings: he was wont every day, two or three times, for about two hours, continually to belch, with such a noise, that he might be heard far and near, at a great distance: But sometimes for a week or two, and sometimes

for

Of the Waking Coma.

for a month, this belching would be changed into a long waking, for having that Distemper much remitted, this Gentleman was kept without sleep almost whole nights; and when he had thus been for three days, and sometimes more, perfectly waking, he seemed not to want sleep, and complained not of sleepiness, dulness, or languor of spirits. And when *Narcoticks* rarely brought to him any help, he took sometimes in the evening a Posset made of Ale and Canary Wine; and night coming on, he sometimes drunk Distilled Waters, by the use of which, oftentimes he got some sleep; then afterwards, his waking perfectly vanishing by degrees; his belching returned: Hence it appears, there was but one cause for either, to wit, the adust particles, and irritative, being poured forth from the bloody Mass, sometimes into the coats of the Ventricle, and sometimes into the Cortical part of the Brain.

Secondly, besides these distinct Distempers of Sleep and Waking, or their inordinations, there remain other conjunct, or complicated irregularities of them, in which, the acts of either function are prevaricated together. Which indeed is observable in that Distemper or affection called the Waking *Coma*; of which we shall now speak briefly.

Those sick with the Waking *Coma*, although they are continually prone to Sleep, yet they can scarce sleep at all, but after the manner of *Tantalus*, up to the chin in the *Lethaean* River, to tast which as soon as he stoops down, the water slides away from him and sinks lower. For they feel a cruel heaviness in their Heads, with a sleepiness or numness of all their senses, and faculties, that they hardly endure to turn themselves in their Bed, or to be disturbed by the by-standers with talking, and expect they shall presently fall into a sweet sleep; but when they would indulge it, and endeavour strongly to embrace it, various phantasms rolling about in their mind, keep them still waking; neither are they suffered to take any sleep at all, which seems to them to be still at hand. Upon this, not seldom follows a *Delirium*, that whilst the sick lye with their eyes shut, they perpetually talk absurd and senseless things, and fling about hither and thither their Arms and Legs excessively, and being raised up, they look about them doggedly. It is an usual thing for those sick of Feavours, to remain a whole night as it were drowned in sleep; and in the mean time are scarce silent a minute of an hour, but murmur various things to themselves; also sometimes cry out, houl, and leap out of Bed. If the reason of these be inquired after, we may say, that the Pores and passages in the Brain, which are the walking places of the Spirits, are very much possessed with a thick and soperiferous matter, poured forth from the Mass of the Blood, that the Spirits being very much hindred from their wonted expansion, and mutual commerce, an heavy and invincible sleep seems to hang over them; but because some sharp and highly active particles, like so many goads, cleave to these Spirits, they are perpetually incited into motion; and so some of them break thorow the ways, howsoever fast shut and stopped with mounds, and run forth either directly or obliquely as they can; and thus such motions of theirs, however confused and diverted, by reason of impediments, and not able to exercise compleatly the Animal function, yet they easily drive away or hinder its cessation and rest; for this reason indeed, such who are distemper'd with this Disease, are like those living under the Pole, who only see (when the Sun is in the *Equinox*) the light on the *Horizon*, and have neither perfect night, nor perfect day; so these only enjoy a kind of twilight betwixt sleep and waking.

The Waking *Coma* is rarely a Disease of it self, but for the most part it is a symptom coming upon other Diseases, as the Feavour, Phrensie, Lethargy, and the like; wherefore it requires not a Curatory Method peculiarly, but there is only need, that to the Remedies prescribed for the first or primary Disease, there should be added other *Cephalicks*, which may dispel these clouds and meteors of the Brain; or if both will not be expelled together, the same Medicine which cherishes the parts of the one, getting the better, will immediately overcome the other: so in the Waking *Somnolency*, it is convenient to procure either perfect sleep, or perfect waking, and in this case I have often given *Narcoticks* with good success.

A description of the waking Coma.

The cause of this Distemper shewn.

It is more often a symptom of other Distempers than a Disease of it self.

CHAP.

CHAP. VI.

Of the Incubus, or Night-Mare.

<small>The Seat of the Incubus is in the Cerebel.</small>

THUS much concerning the morbid exorbitancies of irregular sleep and waking; which are almost proper, and as it were of the region of the Brain. and affect not the *Cerebel* but rarely, and that secondarily and collaterally, as hath been shown. But there remains a distemper, commonly called the Night-Mare, in Latine the *Incubus*, which is both peculiar to this Region, and also seems in some measure analogical to the sleepy diseases; forasmuch as its fits arise, for the most part from sleep, by reason of the Animal Spirits being bound in the Cerebel or suppressed; their eclipse or interruption (though short) about the exercise of the vital function, is induced.

<small>A Description of it.</small>

That the subject, nature, and causes of this Disease may be the better known, we shall first consider its *Phænomena*, or the appearance of it. The fits of the *Incubus*, or Night-Mare, for the most part, and indeed only falling on one in sleep, are used to be excited mostly after the stomach is loaded with undigested meats, and lying on the back in Bed. They who labour with it, seem to feel the hurt chiefly in the Breast, and about the *Præcordia*, for respiration being suppressed, and very much hindred, they think that a certain weight lying heavily upon their Breast, doth oppress them, which weight mocks their imaginations with the Image of some spectre or other; and this, whilst they think to shake off, or put away, by the moving of their Body or members, they are not able to stir themselves any way: But after a long space, and sometimes till they are almost dead, they at last awake with a strugling about their heart, and being more fully rouzed from sleep, the imaginary weight suddenly vanishes, and the motive force of the body is restored, but for the most part a trembling of the heart remains, and frequently a swift and violent beating of the *Diaphragma*. Then the fit being over, the deception of the phantasie, conceiving the horrid image of the *Incubus* or spectre, is perceived.

<small>It most often proceeds from natural causes.</small>

The common people superstitiously believe, that this passion is indeed caused by the Devil, and that the evil spirits lying on them, procures that weight and oppression upon their heart. Though indeed we do grant, such a thing may be, but we suppose that this *symptom* proceeds oftenest from meer natural causes; though what they are, and in what place the Morbific matter doth subsist, is not agreed on among Authors, nor indeed is it easily to be assigned.

<small>The Seat of this is falsly placed in the Brain.</small>

Because the imagination is deceived, and the error being propagated further into the senses themselves, so imposes on the sight and feeling, that they believe they plainly see and feel a monster of this or that shape or figure lying upon them; and for that the loco-motive faculty of the whole body is hindred, in the mean time; some have placed the seat of this Disease wholly in the Brain, and would have the oppression of the breast to be merely phantastical: But although we grant the monstrous shape of the *Incubus* (which is conceived) to be a mere dream; the Precordia to be truly affected, is apparent, and the motion of the Pulse and breathing is suppressed or hindred; for that the heavy weight of the breast is plainly felt by most, in their waking, yea, and when thorowly fresh awaken, and when that is removed, the tremblings of the Heart and *Diaphragma*, and inordinate motions follow: whence it follows that these parts labour and suffer a real hurt.

<small>The Præcordia truly labour.</small>

<small>The cause doth not stick partly in the Brain, and partly in the Breast.</small>

Wherefore others, that they might the more easily unloose this knot, dividing the Morbific Cause, assign a portion of it to the Brain, and another to the Breast; for they say, that the motion of the Lungs are hindred, by a viscous and very gross humor impacted about them, and that doth excite as it were the oppression of a bulk lying on them, with want of breathing; then Vapors being raised to the Head, do fill the principal Nerves, and so hinder the loco-motive force: which opinion (no more likely than the conceptions of those troubled with the Night-Mare) deserves not to be assented to; because there are not any signs of this humor heaped up about the *Præcordia*, which appear before or after the fit, yea when this region is very much burthened, as in the *Phthisis*, *Asthma*, or Dropsie of the Breast, the *Incubus* does not therefore infest more frequently or more grievously: Further it appears not, how the matter heaped up in the *Præcordia*, should be only troublesome in sleep, or by what passage or way, the Vapours from thence so suddenly inducing want of motion, should

be

Of the Incubus or Night-Mare. 143

be elevated to the Head. Wherefore, the Reason or *Ætiology* of this Distemper, I think to be taken or judged of far otherwise.

Therefore this heavy weight or load lying on the breast, seems indeed to be left, because the motion of the Heart, and the organs serving for breathing, is hindred; for from the motion of the heart ceasing, or being hardly performed, the Blood in its bosoms, and in the breathing or *Pneumonick* Vessels stagnating, and being there very much streightned, a sense of as it were a weight opresses the region of the breast: which also seems therefore the more grievous, because the Lungs, *Diaphragma*, and Muscles of the *Thorax*, being hindred in their motions, and as it were bound together, at the same time with the heart, do labour with a great endeavour, to exercise or to put forth themselves. But the most hard question yet is, concerning the Cause, by reason of which the motion or action of the Præcordia is suppressed, or hindred. This seems impossible to be done by matter impacted in the organs themselves, of which indeed, there must be a very great deal, to suffice for the hindrance of so many parts, and some signs of it at least would appear somewhat out of the fit; wherefore, it seems that we may rather say, that the action of those parts are hindred, because the influx of the animal spirits are hindred or suppressed. This is frequently done in Convulsive Distempers, as we have elsewhere declared, and have clearly shewed by *Anatomical* Experiment, to wit, by tying the trunk of the Nerves of the eighth pair, in a living Dog: But in those distemper'd by the *Incubus* or Night-Mare, the obstruction of the Spirits, seems to be excited neither in the organs themselves, nor in their Nerves; for such a cause happening to those awake as well as to those sleeping, doth not become presently moveable, but is fixed and permanent.

The next cause of this is, the hindrance of the inflowing of the Spirits to the Præcordia.

This not in the Parts affected:

Not in the Nerves themselves:

Wherefore, we think the fit of the Night-Mare to be induced, for that in sleeping, a certain incongruous matter is instilled into the Cerebel, together with the nervous Juice, which causing a certain torpor or benummedness in the first spring of the spirits, compells them immediately, by little and little, to cease from the offices of their functions; so that as it were another Lethargy being excited within the Cerebel, the vital actions suffer a short eclipse; during which, partly from a strife of the obstructed or bound together *Præcordia*, and partly from the blood very much heaped up and stagnating in them, that weight, or a sense as it were of a great bulk lying on them, is caused; then, because all the rest of the faculties depend upon the motion of the heart, therefore this being suppressed and hindred, presently those eclipses or disorders of them follow; but especially because the flowing of the Blood into the Brain, for the making of Animal Spirits, is interrupted, therefore immediately the flowing forth of these into the nervous *System* is suppressed, so that the sick, whilst they endeavour to shake off the imaginary load of the breast, are not able to move their Body, or any member; to wit, because the irradiation of the Spirits, (whilst they are destitute of the flowing in of the Blood) is kept from the moving parts. In the mean time, those which reside in the Brain, being spread abroad here and there, conceive confused phantasms, and from the trouble impressed from the *Præcordia*, horrid dreams of spectres.

But happens in the Cerebel, where the first Spring of the Spirits is.

From whence the sense of the weight proceeds.

Whence loss of motion proceeds.

The fit of the *Incubus* is soon ended, because the matter, rarely or never entring deeply into the Cerebel, is easily shaken off, or is supt back again into the Blood: for after the spirits became free from its embrace, and having got the liberty of motion within their wonted spaces, they repeat the exercises of their functions: wherefore, the afflux of the Blood then presently returning to the Brain, immediately the afflux or flowing forth, and emanation of the Spirits, are restored, like a light new kindled, both in its middle or marrowy part, and also in the nervous Stock: whence the being awakened, the motive force returns, and the error of the imagination is perceived. But that there follow in the Heart and *Diaphragma* tremblings and most swift beatings, the reason is, because these Bodies, so long as they were hindred from their motions labouring with an endeavour of exercising, or putting forth themselves, are not able to contain themselves within their just limits, as soon as they are restored, but putting forth at once all their strength, and being too active, exceed the due performance of their duty: even as a wand, being held a while bent, being afterwards let go, recovering it self with a certain force, enters into a motion of trembling or shaking.

Wherefore the fit being so grievous, is so soon ended, without leaving any evil.

Whence after the Fit, the tremblings of the Heart and the Præcordia.

After this manner, the fit of the Night-Mare, because it immediately stops the vital function, as it were the first moving wheel in the animal Machine, compels forthwith all the other faculties to cease, yea the whole corporeal soul (more than the more grievous fits of the *Apoplexy* or the *Lethargy*) to shake, and as it were to suffer an eclipse. Notwithstanding, little danger is threatned from this Distemper, because the Morbific matter being poured forth from the Blood, into the compass of the

The Incubus of it self rarely dangerous.

Cerebel,

Cerebel, is not suffer'd to penetrate deeply; because the Spirits of that province, being always in a readiness and watchful, most swiftly run to meet the enemy, and oppose his entrance strongly, though the offices of the vital function be omitted in the mean time; further, the Animal Spirits which are in the region of the Brain, being awakened, fly presently to assist those of the labouring Cerebel: For those sick of the *Incubus*, if by chance they be awakened by any one lying with them, they sooner come out of the fit.

The Prognostick of the Incubus. But although it is rare, that any one dyes of this Disease only; yet those often obnoxious to it, if they are taken with other *Cephalick* Distempers, as the *Lethargy, Carus, Apoplexy*, or the *Epilepsie*, are in far greater danger: because the Morbifick matter, being poured forth from the Blood into the Brain, easily invades the Cerebel so predisposed; so that the sick therefore suffering at once an eclipse of the vital and the animal function, are brought into greater danger of their Life. Hence 'tis a vulgar observation, that those who frequently are troubled with the *Night-Mare*, fall into the *Apoplexy*.

The Event of it is shewn. There is wont to be another event of the *Incubus*, less dangerous, that leads often into the *Cardiack* passion, and other affections, commonly taken to be *Hypochondriack*: I knew several while young, grievously afflicted with the *Night-Mare*, who being freed from it in their riper Age, were troubled with the trembling and palpitation of the Heart, and other pains about the *Præcordia*, and *Hypochondria*; and also with Convulsions in those parts. We think the cause of this morbid commutation to be, because the Morbifick matter, after it was wont so often to besiege the region of the Cerebel, at length an impression being made, it did penetrate more deeply into some private place, and passing thorow its frame, became impacted on the Nerves destinated to the *Præcordia*.

Its Cure. As to the Cure of this Disease, there needs no help for the fits, because they pass away quickly of themselves. The method of Cure after a considering the whole, suggests Blood-letting, (where it is convenient) and a gentle Purge, and chiefly the use of Remedies, which are commonly called *Cephalicks*. Therefore, here Powders of *Amber, Coral*, and *Pearls*, with the Roots of the *Male Pæony, Cretick Dittany, Contrayerva*; also *Electuaries, Tablets*, and *Distilled Waters, Tinctures, Elixirs*, and other things that are wont to be prescribed in the *Lethargy* and *Apoplexy*, have the chief place; but especially a right course of dyet being ordered, let gross and ill digested meats be shunned, Pulse and Summer-fruits; nor let sleep, study, or reading be presently yielded to after eating: late and large Suppers, and lying on the back, are to be forbidden.

Infants and Boys obnoxious to this Disease, how they ought to be handled. Because Children and Youths, are often sick of this Disease (the sign of which is, that they are shaken in their sleeping, and waking cruelly cry out) and more often suffer its fits, which oftentimes bring them to Convulsive passions, therefore a method of healing them ought to be administred, as soon as they are seen to be distemper'd: you ought to inquire into the milk they suck, whether it be of it self pure and laudable, and truly convenient for the Stomach: let them not sleep presently after they have sucked their fill: The Nurse using a good dyet, let her take also Morning and Evening a Dose of *Cephalick* Powder, or *Electuary*, drinking after it a draught of Posset drink, with the leaves of Sage or Betony, or the Roots or Seeds of *Pæony* boiled in it: Let the Infant take twice a day, a spoonful of proper Distilled Water. Let him have an Issue made in the nape of the Neck, and let it lye sometimes on one side, and sometimes on the other, and rarely or never on its back. If a Neck-lace of Coral, or little balls of the Seeds or Roots of the *male Pæony* be worn about the Neck, or at the pit of the Stomach, it is not altogether useless; if that in sleep being often and grievously shaken, they are seen to be more dangerously troubled with this Distemper, let Blisters be raised in the hinder part of the Neck, or behind the Ears, also Evening and Morning let there be daily given a Dose of the Powder of *Ammoniacum*, or other proper Dose, in a spoonful of Distilled Water or *Julep*.

CHAP.

CHAP. VII.

Of the Vertigo, or a turning round in the Head.

HAving viewed the exterior compass of either part of the Head, and detected the Diseases which beset the sensitive soul, about the first beginnings, and last springs of the Animal Spirits; we shall next descend to the middle part of the Brain, where the phantasie and common sense reside, and behold what kind of passions these parts are obnoxious to. Concerning this in the first place we shall note, that sometimes troops or rather mighty armies of Spirits, inhabiting these places, are affected, and sometimes also small handfuls or bands: then again many of them are affected together, or else only a few at a time; or they become Elastick from an heterogeneous *Copula*, and so are compelled into inordinate motions, or as it were explosive or shooting off, as in the *Epileptick* fit; or suffering an *eclipse*, as in the *Apoplexy*, are deprived of all motion. Concerning the former disposition of the Spirits, we have formerly treated largely enough, and the astonishing Disease we shall handle afterwards. But in this place, we shall speak of a certain Passion or distemper belonging to these parts, *viz.* the *Vertigo*, in which a certain band or handful of the Spirits are affected, and their motions are seen to be partly perverted, and partly suppressed. *The Seat of the Vertigo.*

Being but little solicitous about the names by which the *Vertigo* is wont to be known, we shall describe the nature, or formal reason of it after this manner, *viz.* "The *Vertigo* is an Affection or Distemper, in which the visible objects seem to turn "round, and the sick feel a perturbation, or confusion of the Animal Spirits in the "Brain that they do not rightly flow into the Nerves: Wherefore the visive, and "the loco-motive faculties, do often in some measure fail, that those labouring with "it fall, and oftentimes are covered with darkness. *A Description of it.*

In this fit it is observed, that the imagination and the common sense are in a manner deceived, whilst they believe, the quiet objects to be moved, but the rational judgment remains; for we understand our error, and we presently ascribe this fallacy to the inordination of the Animal Spirits; for that we plainly know that the spirits flowing within the Brain do decline from their wonted irradiation or beaming forth, and do not rightly perform the offices of motion and sensation, during the fit.

That we may find out the Morbifick Cause, and the preternatural manner of the *Vertigo*, we shall inquire after what manner this same affection or Distemper, how extempory or sudden soever it be, is wont to be excited from non-natural things; for men ordinarily become Vertiginous (or have a turning in their head) with a long turning round of the body, looking down from an high place, passing over Bridges, Sailing, and by Drunkenness, and many other ways. It will be worth our while to consider a little further, the means of affecting, by which these exterior actions stir up this turning or rolling about, from whence it will the better appear, what kind of intrinsick causes may be able to excite this passion. In the first place therefore, when men are for some time turned about, both in that motion all things seem to be turned about, and also they ceasing from turning about, that still continues in the phantasie; so that the affected oftentimes fall to the ground; further, though they shut their eyes, they still perceive as it were a turning round, like the turning about of a Mill, in the Brain. *The Causes and the Manner of the non-natural Vertigo.*

The reason of these is not, that the deception of the sight is first brought to the eyes, and afterwards continued for some time; because this affection is caused by the turning round of the body, whether they look with, or shut their eyes: But indeed the cause of this apparition wholly depends upon the fluid substance of the animal spirits. For that the spirits flowing within the Brain, are even like to water, or a thick heap of Vapors, included in a Phial, which being shaken round about, together with the Vessel, and made so to turn about, continues for a time that motion, though the Vessel stands still; in like manner also, when the body of a man is turned round about, the spirits inhabiting the Brain, from that turning about of the Head, like the containing Vessel, are agitated into spiral or round motions; and when therefore they cannot irradiate the Nerves with their wonted influx and direct beams, from hence oftentimes a *Scotomy* or dizzness, and a failing of the feet, together with a rotation or whirling about of visible objects, are induced. The visible Hemisphere seems to turn round, because as the sensible impression *The Reasons of them shewn.*

V

146 *Of the Vertigo.*

sion is received by the means of the recipient, so the objects, as the spirits, seem to be moved round about.

Why looking down from on high, and passing over Bridges, cause a turning round in the Head.

Secondly, looking from on high, and passing over Bridges, stir up a *Vertigo* or giddiness in the Head, for that there is a terror cast on the imagination from unaccustomed objects, as also from the site of the body, or going in danger, whence that being very solicitous, how it should rightly order and more firmly direct the spirits into the bodies of the Nerves, calls them back into the middle part of the Brain, and so perverts them from their wonted afflux and irradiation; and whilst it indeavours to set their battel in better array, and to direct them more surely, by too great a care, drives them into a certain confusion and irregular motion. Wherefore 'tis observed, that drunken men, and very bold, because they are not careful or solicitous concerning the guiding of the animal spirits, suffer no such thing. Sailing, or riding in a Coach, causes a turning in the Head by the like reason, as the turning round of the Body; because, the very fluid spirits being too much agitated, like water shaken in a Glass, leap hither and thither disorderly. Further, it is wholly for the same reason, why many going by Ship, or by Coach, are subject also to cruel Vomiting; to wit, because the spirits being snatched into disorder, by too great a motion, and confused fluctuation, run inordinately into the heads of the Nerves of the wandring pair, and for that reason stir up Convulsions and Convulsive motions in the Bowels.

How Drunkenness.

Thirdly, 'Tis observed, that the *Vertigo* comes upon Drunkenness, as a known *symptom*; and that to those unaccustomed, the drinking, though moderately, of Wine or strong Ale, also the taking of *Tabaco*, easily induces the same affection; the reason of which is, because from the Liquor, or vapour so taken, certain fierce particles, and untameable, are carried into the Brain, by the passages of the Blood and nervous Juice; which being improportionate, and incongruous to the Animal Spirits, drive them hither and thither from their wonted tracks of flowing and reflowing or ebbing, and so move them into whirlings, and turnings about;

A perturbation of the Spirits in the Brain, and a revocation of them from their flowing into the Nerves, depend mutually on one another.

These are the chief occasions, or solitary evident causes, which do use to bring the *Vertigo*, or turning round in the Head to some men, how sound of constitution soever they be: which kind of effect, these occasions produce, forasmuch as the Animal Spirits, being disturbed beyond their set courses, and orders, are moved inordinately, fluctuating here and there, both within the passages of the Brain, and also some of them, like a thred broken off, from their wonted irradiation, into the nervous Stock. For these being always reciprocal, depend mutually one of another, to wit, a perturbation of the Spirits within the middle part of the Brain, and their flowing forth into the nervous Stock being hindered; for from what ever cause either effect is induced, the other immediately follows. A turning round of the body, going in a Coach, or in a Boat or Ship, also Drunkenness, and the unaccustomed fume of *Tabaco*, compel the spirits in the Brain to fluctuate and shake disorderly, which, for that cause, are presently inhibited from their wonted flowing into the Nerves, that those so affected, can hardly go or stand; in like manner, on the contrary, looking from on high, passing over Bridges, a languishment or *syncope* falling on them, recal the spirits from their wonted emanation, who, for that cause tumultuating within the Brain, or being moved inordinately, cause a *Scotomy* or dizziness, or a turning round of the objects.

From what causes the preternatural Vertigo is wont to be excited.

These things being thus premised, concerning the *Vertigo*, raised up by reason of an outward accident, or from a solitary evident and non-natural cause; we shall next inquire, how and by what means, it is wont to be induced, from an intrinsick and preternatural cause.

Concerning these take notice, that the *Vertigo* is sometimes a symptom depending upon some other Distemper, placed sometimes within the Brain, and sometimes without it: but sometimes this is a Disease of it self, which being raised up within the middle part of the Brain, becomes very troublesome, and often terrible, and very hard to be Cured.

Sometimes the Vertigo is a symptom of other Cephalick Diseases.

As to the former, many *Cephalick* Diseases (or such as belong to the Head) *viz.* Acute pain, the *Lethargy, Epilepsie, Carus, Apoplexy*, with many others, do often accompany the *Vertigo*; to wit, because the equal expansion of the Spirits in the Brain, and therefore their irradiation into the nervous Stock, from such like various Morbific causes, are easily hindred or disturbed; as shall hereafter appear, when we deliver the *Ætiology* or reason of the *Vertigo*, as it is a Disease of the Brain.

Sometimes it is excited by reason of the Distemper of other

But sometimes this *symptom* is wont to be produced, by reason of other Distempers, placed a long way from the Brain, and that chiefly by two ways or means. For first it is usual for a dizziness to arise, by reason of the flowing of the Blood being suddenly

Of the Vertigo.

denly called away from the Brain, as in a *Syncope* or Swooning, great want coming near it, wicked hard labour great *Hæmorrhagies* or expence of blood, long fasting, in passions of violent sadness and fear; yea by reason of other occasions, when the motion of the blood is deficient or fails in the heart; so that the affected are proclive to faintings and swooning away; presently, because the tribute of the vital liquor is withdrawn, the animal Spirits growing deficient in the Brain, withdraw their radiation from the nervous Stock; for when their spring is cut off, those that remain, leaping back from their emanation, wander about confusedly in the Brain, and very often stir up the Vertiginous Distemper. *distant parts, viz. from the Stomach, Spleen, &c. and so by two means: 1. Either by reason of the Flood of the Blood being kept back.*

Secondly, an inordinate recourse or flowing back of the Animal Spirits, from some inward, or from some outward member, often causes the *Vertigo*: forasmuch as the Spirits being disturbed from the affected part, by a long series, thorow the passages of the Nerves, at length disturb others inhabiting the middle part of the Brain, and drive them into the like disorders; for this cause it is, that sharp humors gnawing or pulling the Fibres of the Ventricle, because the infestous and irritative matter being moved in the Spleen, *Pancreas*, or Intestines, causes light dizzinesses in the Brain. I have known from an accute pain, an Ulcer, or a mortified Inflammation in the Foot or Arm, frequent tremblings and failings, though short, in the Brain, to have been induced. Whilst that the conceived inordination of the spirits, is transferred from the distemper'd part, thorow the Nerves into the Brain, a certain Formication or tingling, or as it were the ascent of a cold air, is seen and perceived; wherefore the cause of this Distemper is commonly ascribed to Vapours, arising up to the Head: which error we have elsewhere sufficiently confuted. Further, many are wont, when they have fasted, or stayed long beyond their hour of dining, to have a dimness before their eyes, and their heads to have a turning, and then afterwards those clouds vanish, having eaten a little; this does not so happen (according to the vogue of the people) for that wind or vapours ascend to the Head, from the empty Stomach, which the aliments being taken in, do immediately suppress; but because the Fibres of the Ventricle, and the nervous Filaments or little strings, being destitute of the nervous Juice, with which they desire to be watered, are wont to enter into corrugations or wrinklings, and light Convulsions, which kind of Convulsions and disorders of Spirits, for that they are continued thorow the passages of the Nerves, into the Brain, produce the Vertiginous Distemper; which, as soon as the Fibres of the Stomach remit their wrinklings, ceases of its own accord. For this reason I have known some, by a Vomit being given, tearing the coats of the Ventricle, have been taken with a cruel *Vertigo*: yea I do suspect, that this Distemper does sometimes arise from meats of ill digestion, and ungrateful to the stomach. *2. Or by reason of an inordinate recourse, or flowing back of the Spirits towards the Brain.*

Not by reason of vapours, elevated from these parts as it is excited.

But the *Vertigo* is not only a *symptom*, but sometimes a primary Disease of it self; whose nature, that we may the better search into, we ought to inquire into its subject, the formal reasons, and causes of it; and then these being found out, and truly unfolded, we will proceed to its prognostick and Cure.

Without doubt the immediate subject of the *Vertigo* are the Animal Spirits, which every one labouring with this Disease finds to be greatly disturbed, and wandring up and down; but the mediate subject are those parts of the Brain, in which the Imagination and common sense reside, and whence the next way lies into the nervous Stock. These are the Callous and streaked bodies. *The immediate Subject of the Vertigo is the Animal Spirits.*

For indeed, the Animal Spirits love to expatiate themselves, and to be expanded or stretched forth on every side, within these medullary places, as in a most ample Field, and pleasant Garden; wherefore like beams of light, with a full and streight ray, they pass thorow all the Pores and most chick passages of the marrow: hence it is, that whilst they gently flow in one line, from the outmost border of the Callous body (to wit, from the streaked bodies, and turnings and windings of the Brain) towards its middle part, they represent pleasant imaginations and phantasies; and whilst in another line they flow forth, perhaps thorow other passages from the middle of the Callous body, into the infoldings or windings about of the Brain, they transferr thither signets or marks of notions for the Memory; and then, whilst they tend into the streaked bodies, and the beginnings of the Nerves, they actuate all the moving parts, and carry to them, as often as there is occasion, the instincts of the motions they are to perform. *The mediate the Callous Body.*

But in the *Vertigo*, these equal emanations of the Spirits, as it were rays of light, seem to be intercepted, and diversly perverted in various places; because some bands or handfuls of the Spirits are obscured, others are bended another way, and moved hither and thither into turnings round and whirling about, and oftentimes snatched transverse, or cross one another. Wherefore, confused phantasms, wandring and inconstant *Its formal reason.*

Of the Vertigo.

stant images, or actions of sensible things are represented, in the Brain, by reason of the Spirits so disturbed: Then forasmuch as the irradiation into the nervous stock is lessened or hindred, a dizziness and failing of the motive function follows.

If that we should yet further inquire into what hinders or obstructs the ways, whereby the Spirits are compelled thus to go aside, or tumultuate within the Brain; it seems probable, that these inordinations of theirs do depend upon a two fold cause, *viz.* first, that certain fierce and extraneous Particles, being entred deeply into the Brain, together with the nervous Juice, stick close to the spirits, and move them into enormous motions; but this, as appears from common experience, happens to every one, on the immoderate drinking of Wine or Strong-waters, or the unaccustomed taking of *Tobacco*, by the eating of some Vegetables, or being anointed with *Mercury*; for that some Heterogeneous bodies and infestous to the Spirits, follow them, and are snatched with them, even to the middle part of the Brain: why may not such kind of Morbific particles and Vertiginous be supplied from the Blood, and other humors very much vitiated, and insinuated into the inmost conclave of the Brain? Then secondly, we may suspect, that when the serous foulness doth by degrees creep forward with the nervous Juice, and at length penetrated deeply, that it doth contaminate these pure marrows, and greatly stuff up its Pores, so that the Animal Spirits do not shine or beam forth with a clear and full light, but with a weak, broken, and as it were with many shadows mingled or interspersed with it.

Its Conjunct Cause.

1. From the perturbation of the Spirits.

2. From their ways or passages being obstructed.

In an habitual *Vertigo*, and inveterate, it seems to be plain, that the Conjunct Cause doth contain both these, from the proof, and that not light, taken from things that are hurtful and helpful: For I have observed in many, that this affection or Distemper hath been altered, much for the worse or for the better, upon two occasions; for whatsoever things being inwardly taken, that beget turgid particles, and apt to grow too hot and rageing, as Wine, Strong-waters, spiced, pepper'd, and flatulous or windy food, always hurt those troubled with the *Vertigo*: and for the same occasions, no less hurtful are those things, by which the brain is filled, and more stuffed, as Surfeits, sleeping at Noon, or overlong in the Morning, the Southern wind, a cloudy, thick, and moist air, a low and watry habitation; on the contrary, the same persons are much helped, as they easily perceive, by a slender and light dyet, also by a clear air, and an open soil, where the wind has a thorow passage.

This is seen by things helpful and hurtful.

Thus much concerning the subject, the formal reason, and the conjunct cause of the *Vertigo*; now in the next place, let us inquire into its *Procatartick*, or more remote leading cause; by reason of whose morbid provision or predisposition, these two evils are wont to be induced on the spirits inhabiting the middle part of the Brain: But here we apprehend both the Brain it self, with the watering Liquor, and also the Blood with its infected humors to be in fault.

The more remote foregoing cause of the Vertigo consists both in the vice of the Blood, and of the Brain.

The vice of this is most often, that it turns from its right temper, into a sour, acid, and otherways vicious disposition, and being degenerate, perverts the nourishing Juice; and also gathers in its bosom a Serum, and filthiness of diverse kinds, which it is ready to pour forth into the Head. But there are many evident causes, to wit, an evil dyet, and errors in the non-naturals, also the Scurvy, a long or malignant Feavour, and other Diseases going before, by reason of which the Blood becomes so full of ill humors, and so hurtful to the Head.

The Reason of the former explained.

In the mean time, the crime of the Brain is, for that its temper is humid and weak, its frame loose and infirm, with its Pores too much open and gapeing, more than they ought, so that all the heterogeneous, strange, and elastick Particles, together with the serous, or otherways diseased recrements, being poured forth from the Blood into the Head, are easily admitted into the Brain, together with the nervous Juice; and because of its more open Pores, fall down without any let or stop into the middle part, *viz.* the Callous and streaked Bodies. This kind of too dissolute or loose habit of the brain, is in some innate and originally; further, those who are of a tender constitution, to wit, delicate, soft, and luxurious Men and Women, whose spirits are not able to suffer any thing strongly, easily contract a Vertiginous Distemper, or rather increase it; to wit, because when the spirits of the Brain cannot resist the incursions of strangers, they give way to every matter that is drove to them: but in others, though strong, inordinate feeding, a sedentary life, frequent surfeiting, also intemperate sleep, and study, an inveterate Scurvey, evil gross humors, a long Feavour, and other diseases of the Head, do very often cause this kind of evil disposition of the Brain.

The vices of the Brain noted.

The differences of this Disease.

From what hath been said, the differences of this Disease are easily gathered; for that I may pass by what we but now mentioned, that it was either a primary Distemper

Of the Vertigo.

stemper of it self, or secondary arising or depending upon others: further we noted, that the primary *Vertigo*, so it were light and not deeply rooted, was only troublesome with fits excited from an evident cause; so that oftentimes the distemper'd are well enough, but by reason of their evil manner of living, or other accidents they become *Vertiginous*; but sometimes this Distemper becoming habitual, they are found to be obnoxious to it almost at all times. Secondly, As to the seat of this Disease there is a notable difference; for this is sometimes more outward as is seen happening in the Callous body, and hath almost only the tumults and failings of the Spirits, and the wandring, inconstant, and often confused acts of notions and sense, in the forepart of the Head; but sometimes the Morbific matter falling down more backward, about the streaked bodies, stirs up the *Scotomy*, or turning of the Head, and a loss or failing of the motive function, that oftentimes the Eyes are darkened, and they reel or stumble, and their Legs fail them.

As to the *prognostick* of this Disease, the *symptomatick* or accidental *Vertigo*, yea almost all the others, while fresh, are free from much danger, and are easily to be Cured. *Its Prognostick.*

But the habitual, and almost continual, although great danger and suddenly to fall is rarely threatned; yet because it admits of only a difficult and long Cure, it so tires out both the Patient and the Physician, that before the Disease can be Cured, they both become weary of one another.

The primary *Vertigo* being placed before, or more outward, which hath scarce a darkness or falling accompanying it, is more safe, and healable, but is often changed into an inveterate Headach, and sometimes also it is cured of it self, by an *Hæmorrhage*, or bleeding at the nose, or by a flowing down of the *Hæmorrhoids*; it is also oftentimes taken away by Medicine.

The *Vertiginous* Distemper, arising behind, and intercepting the beamings forth of the Spirits into the Nerves, is far more dangerous, and oftentimes passes into an *Apoplexy*, or a *Palsie*, or into Convulsive Diseases.

There does not properly belong to the *symptomatick Vertigo* any Curatory Method. There it is only needful to joyn some *Cephalick* Remedies, discussing the clouds of the Brain, and quieting the disorders of the Spirits, to those other primary indications; or rather that we may speak to the capacity of the vulgar (which ought to be done sometimes, though feignedly) let some Medicines contrary to Vapors be added. *The Cure of the Vertigo.*

The accidental *Vertigo*, or any other fresh or newly taken, may be healed with *Phlebotomy*, and a gentle Purge, and sometimes iterated: but that the Disease may be more certainly extirpated, let there be besides administer'd carefully *Cephalick* Remedies, such as are anon described.

For the Cure of an habitual *Vertigo*, and become inveterate, there ought to be instituted almost the like method, as is against most other *Cephalick* Diseases, which suggests these three chief intentions of healing, *viz.* in the first place must be endeavoured that the root or nest of the Disease may be cut off, and that the brain may remain free from any new flowings in of the Morbific matter; for which end a right order of dyet being commanded, sometimes letting of blood, and most often a gentle Purge in the intervals are convenient. Let a dry and open air be chosen, let immoderate and untimely sleep and study be shunned, let morning and evening draughts be wholly abstained from; in the place of the former, let a draught of *Tea* or *Coffee*, with Sage leaves boiled in it, be given. Let an Issue be made in the Leg or Arm, and sometimes let the *Hemorrhoidal* Vessels be kept open with Leeches; let the distemper'd rise early in the morning, and wash every day the fore-part of his Head with water, and also his Temples, and rub them with a course cloth. *There are three chief intentions of healing. 1. To take away the root or feeding of the Disease.*

Secondly, The second curatory intention is, to take away the *Procatartick* or more remote foregoing causes; wherefore, endeavour that both the *Dyscrasie* or evil disposition of the Blood may be removed, and also that the weak and too loose constitution of the Brain may be mended: For the former, altering remedies chiefly are convenient, as temperate *Antiscorbuticks*, and sometimes *Spaw* Waters, or Whey. To which always may be added for the latter indication, *Cephalick* Medicines, to wit, such as are prepared of Coral, Amber, humane Skull, the root of the *male Pæony*, Misleto, the dung of a Peacock, and the like, the forms of which we shall shew you by and by. *2. To remove the procatartick causes.*

The third Intention, which is properly curatory, endeavours to take away the Conjunct Cause of this Disease; which however the Procatartick Causes being removed, for the most part ceases of it self: for if the coming of every extraneous Matter into the Brain be cut off, there will remain nothing but pure and clear Spirits, and they having gotten open and free spaces, within the Callous Body, will from thence *3. To take away the Conjunct Cause.*

thence flow forth on every side: However, for the scope of healing this, you must prosecute it with the former; with Medicines indued with a volatile salt, whose particles being very subtil and active, do refresh the Animal Spirits, of which sort are chiefly Spirits of Harts-Horn, Sut, of *Sal Armoniack, &c.* impregnated with Amber, and humane Skull, Tinctures of Coral, Amber, Antimony, Elixir of *Pæony*, &c.

The Curatory Method is shewn.

These things being premised, concerning the *Vertigo* in general, it will seem to the purpose, to draw or shadow forth the Curatory Method particularly, and as it were to direct you by a thred: and in the first place is shewn what is to be done for the Cure in the fit, and what out of it, for prevention.

1. As to the first, although the invasion of the *Vertigo* seem cruel, it is for the most part without danger, and easily passes over of its own accord; In such a case, if the Pulse shews it, let Phlebotomy be made use of, after having given a Glyster; but because the sick think themselves dying, and expect medicinal help, in that case let there be Blisters made in the Neck, and stinking things held to the Nose, as *Castor*, the Spirits or Salt of Harts-horn, or Urine, or of *Sal Armoniack*. Further, let these Spirits be given twice or thrice a day with a convenient Dose of *Cephalick Julep*: going to sleep, let them take a *Bolus* of *Mithridate*, with the Powder of *Castor*: let them take the next day, if the Distemper doth not yet vanish, a light Purge, or if the sick be prone or easie to Vomit, an *Emetick*, than which a better Remedy can scarce be taken.

Take *Pills of Amber twenty five grains, of the Resine of Jalap six grains, of Tartar Vitriolated seven grains, of the Balsom of Peru what will suffice to make four Pills, to be taken going to bed, or early in the morning.*

Or Take *of the Sulphur of Antimony five grains, of the Cream of Tartar half a scruple, of Castor seven grains; make a Powder: Let it be taken with care, expecting to Vomit.*

why vomiting Medicines are so much noted in this, and other Diseases of the Head.

That Vomiting Medicines do oftenest help in the *Vertigo*, besides the testimony of Authors, appears plain enough also from common observation; and besides, since those troubled with the *Vertigo* do often Vomit of their own accord, many have been of the opinion, that the cause of this Disease most commonly lyes hid in the stomach; but it is much otherways, and as we have elsewhere shewed; Vomiting frequently follows upon the Spirits being disturbed in the Brain: But that Vomits help much in this Disease, the reason is, because this kind of Physick causes a great revulsion of the humors from the Brain, and very much restrains the Spirits tumultuating in it. When the Membranes and Fibres of the Ventricle, and Viscera planted nigh them, are pulled; various humors, *viz.* the *nervous, serous, watery, pancratick,* and *cholerick* are drawn into those parts, and so squeesed forth, so that the Head being freed from their flowing to it, doth easily shake off from it many impacted there before: then as to the Animal Spirits, we have shewed somewhere, that there is a most intimate commerce, and agreement between those inhabiting the stomach, and those dwelling in the Brain; to wit, that therefore the grateful or ingrateful affection of the Ventricle, from things taken into it, might bring rejoycing or dejection to the Spirits dwelling in the Brain. *Opiates* whilst they lye in the stomach cause sleep; in like manner, it doth not a little help in the *Vertigo*, and other *Cephalick* Diseases, whereby the Spirits of the Brain wandring up and down, and agitated enormously may be repressed, and returned into order; if their Companions or Kindred be striken down, by the working of the Medicine; because whilst many are called forth from the Brain, to their assistance; the others remaining, remitting their disorders, resume their wonted offices or functions: without doubt it is for this reason chiefly, *Emeticks* bring so often help in the Distemper of madness; so that *Empericks* do almost only use them.

What is to be done out of the Fit, for prevention sake.

2. But to return from our digression, let us consider what is to be done for the Curing of an inveterate and almost continual *Vertigo*, out of the fit. Therefore, first a method being instituted concerning bleeding, and purging, according to the constitution and strength of the Patient, and after rest, to be repeated; let a Vomit also, by my advice, be taken once a month (if nothing to the contrary hinders it) for which end let there be given to the weaker, after the stomach is filled with slippery Meats, Wine, and *Oxymel* of Squils, to about two or three ounces, and after it let a great quantity of Posset-drink be drunk, with *Carduus* boiled in it, that the Patient may vomit of himself, or by provocation. To others may be given an Emetick of the Salt of *Vitriol*, or the Sulphur of *Antimony*, or of the infusion of *Crocus Metallorum*:

Of the Vertigo. 151

lorum: as concerning Issues, Blisterings, the bleeding at the *Hemorrhoidal* Veins, Plasters, or quilted Caps to be worn upon the Head, or other Topicks to be applied to the soals of the Feet, or to the wrists, for revulsion or derivation sake, let the Physician deliberate.

Take of the Conserve of the Flowers of the male Pæony six ounces, of the Powder of its Root one ounce, of the Seeds of Pæony powder'd two drams, of Amber, Coral, Pearls powder'd, of each two drams and a half; of the Salt of Coral one dram, of the Syrup of Coral, what will suffice to make an Electuary: the Dose is one dram and an half, or two drams, Evening and Morning; drinking after it of the following distilled water three ounces. *Electuary.*

Take of the fresh leaves of Misleto six handfuls, of the root of the male Pæony, and of Angellico, each one pound and an half; of the whitest dung of the Peacock two pound, of Cardamoms bruised two ounces, of Castor three drams; all being cut small and mixt together, pour to them eight pints either of White Wine, or Whey, made of it: Let them be distilled in fit Stills, and the whole liquor mixed together. *A distilled Water.*

Take of the Powder of the Root of the male Pæony half an ounce, of red Coral prepared, of Species Diambræ, each one dram and a half; of the Powder of the Flowers of the male Pæony fresh bruised and dryed in the Sun, one dram; make a Powder, to which add of the whitest Sugar, dissolved in the water of Pæony, and boiled to the consistence of Tablets ten ounces: of this make Lozenges according to art, each weighing half a dram; eat one or two of them often in a day. *Tablets.*

Because all things are not convenient to all Men, and that the *Physician* ought to try diverse Medicines, and institute various methods, and to try now this, now that, therefore we shall here add some other forms of another kind.

Take of our Syrup of Steel six ounces, and drink a spoonful of it in the Morning, and at five in the Evening, with the distilled water, but now described, or any other Cephalick, to the quantity of three ounces; or take of our Tincture of Steel, from fifteen to twenty drops, in a draught of the same distilled water, twice in a day. I have known this to have given notable help to many. *Chalybeats or Steel-Medicines*

Let there be given daily after the same manner, Doses, sometimes of the Spirit of Sut, Harts-horn, or of Sal Armoniack, impregnated with Coral, Amber, or the Skull of a Man: or of the Tincture of Antimony, Amber or Coral. *Spirits.*

Take of the Powder of the Root of the male Pæony one ounce and an half, of the Seeds of Pæony, Coral prepared, and of the whitest Amber, each three drams; of Pearls prepared, of the Powder of the Flowers of the male Pæony, fresh bruised and dryed in the Sun, of each two drams; of Sugar-Candy one ounce: make a Powder, and take one dram twice in a day with a draught of Tea or Coffee, or a Decoction of Sage or Rosemary. *Powders.*

For poor people may be prescribed, Powder of the leaves of the Apple-tree, Misleto, dryed in the Sun, and powder'd, to the quantity of a dram, to be taken twice in a day. Or take of the whitest Peacocks dung six ounces, of the Powder of the Flowers of the male Pæony one ounce, of Sugar two ounces: make a Powder, of which let them take a spoonful twice in a day, in some convenient liquor.

Let those troubled with the *Vertigo* drink for their ordinary drink, small Ale, with leaves of the Orchard Misleto boiled in it instead of Hops, and in the Vessel holding about four gallons, let a little bag be hanged, in which put half a pint of Peacocks dung, and three drams of Cloves bruised.

Examples of those labouring with the *Vertigo* are so frequently met withal and almost daily, that there seems no need to add here any; but however, that the image or type of this Disease may be known, I shall only mention some few and more rare cases. *Cases and Examples of the Sick.*

A Divine about sixty years of age, after he had been troubled for about three months with a light *Vertigo*, or as it were a frequent coruscation or brandishing of the Spirits, in the fore part of the Head, at length the Disease growing worse, he became ready to fall, and with a darkness before his eyes; in so much, that in walking he sometimes would fall flat on the ground. Being sent for to Cure him, I prescribed *Phlebotomy*, with a gentle Purge, and after a little respite, to be repeated again; further, I took care to have the *Electuary*, and mixtures given him, such as we noted above, with Blistering Plasters, and other administrations not to be neglected: A fortnight after, no ease following from these, I gave him a Vomit of the Salt of *Vitriol*, and the infusion of *Crocus Metallorum*, by which when he had easily vomited ten times, he began to find himself better, and by using further altering *Cephalicks*, for about *The first History.*

about a fortnight more, he became perfectly well, and from that time, for six years, he took yearly spring and fall a Vomit, with some other Medicines; though he continued in perfect health.

The second History. A certain Gentleman about sixty six years of Age, when he had lived for a long time obnoxious to a light *Vertigo*, and that was wont to be excited only occasionally, about the end of the last *Autumn*, labouring more grievously with this Distemper, he also became forgetful. Being sent for to visit this Man, after he had been sick about three weeks, I found him very much changed in his looks and countenance, the vigor of both being diminished. Seeing that he was daily distemper'd towards evening with a small Feavour, his Pulse beating high and vehemently: I first caused blood to be taken out of his Arm, and after six or seven days, out of the *Hæmorrhoidal* Veins; and then I took care for Blisters to be made behind the Ears and hind part of the Neck, and two large Issues between the shoulders: Inwardly, at physical hours, he took daily *Cephalick* Medicines, almost of every kind. Within a months space he seem'd to recover, and began to walk abroad, and to take care of his houshold affairs, and other businesses: but in the beginning of the Winter, taking cold by going daily abroad, he fell into a little Feavour, with a greater perturbation of the spirits within his Head: for becoming every evening delirous, he hardly knew what he said or did. But within seven or eight days, blood being taken away, and a slender dyet used, the Feavour vanished, but the distemper of the Brain was changed from its former state. For the *Vertigo* wholly ceasing, he became very forgetful, and *Paralytick*, in all his right side. As to his Head, being asked, whether it was clear, and free from the dizziness and confused Phantasms; he answered, that as to those things, he never was better in his life: For he well understood his infirmity, knew his Friends and Relations, and others who came to visit him, but could hardly remember the names of any of them; and when he began to talk of any thing, he wanted words to express his mind: Then as to his Distemper in his side, in his right Arm and Leg; there was not only a loosning wholly, and a want of motion, but in either there grew a great white waterish Tumor, in so much that not only the Cure, but his life was despaired of, to be long prolonged; yea, the Magistracy and Offices which he held, were sought for by others.

However I did not desist from my curatory work, the most skilful Physician Doctor *Wharton* being called to my assistance. Carefully administring to the sick by our joint counsels, we prescribed solutive Pills to be taken at times, and in Medicinal hours on other days *Cephalick*, *Antiscorbutick*, and *Antiparalytick* Remedies: His head being shaven, we ordered a Plaster of Gumms and Balsoms to be laid upon it, and the loosened parts to be anointed with Oyls and Balsoms, and to be strongly rubbed. Whilst these things were doing, with some success as to the greater clearness of his intellect, I know not from what cause, he fell into a Feavour, in the midst of the Winter, so that for several days and nights, he grew extreamly hot, with burning, great thirst, and interrupted sleep; his tongue being scorch'd, and having a white scurf, his Pulse was high, his Urine red, and full of contents. We abstained from *Phlebotomy*, by reason of his Age and *Palsie*, and especially because of the Dropsie begun in the distemper'd side: but with a slender dyet prepared of Barly Broths, and Grewel, we order'd him day by day *Juleps*, *Apozems*, and other Remedies moving Sweat and Urine; and when about this time the Issues between his shoulders flowed very much, the sick man began to grow better as to his Memory, and Palsie, and from thence profiting daily, and by degrees growing well, of both his distempers, together with his Feavour, he was restored to perfect health within a fortnight, and is still living in health.

The Reason of the Case described. In this sick man there was a notable motion, and a various change or translation of the Morbifick matter; for what was at first in the middle part of the Brain, *viz.* sitting on the Callous Body, stirred up the cruel *Vertigo*; the same afterwards increased, and (as it is probable) being further diffused into the infoldings of the Brain, brought forgetfulness or oblivion to the former Distemper: Then forasmuch as the same matter being moved by the Feavour, and a little discussed, falling partly on one of the streaked bodies, brought the Palsie of one side, and being partly expulsed into the compass of the Brain, almost took away the Memory, the *Callous* Body in the mean time obtaining a clearness; and lastly, it was not without the help of the other Feavour, that the Morbifick matter being discussed from these two last nests, was wholly carried away, the sick being restored to health.

The third History. Lately being tired out with the continual complaints of a certain man, troubled with the *Vertigo*, after many other Remedies tried in vain, I prescribed at length, that for the space of a month, he should take daily, twice a day, about a spoonful of
the

the following Powder, drinking after it a draught of the Decoction of Sage or Rosemary, impregnated with the Tincture of Coffee.

Take *of the Powder of the Roots of the male Pæony two ounces, of the Flowers of the same bruised and dryed in the Sun one ounce, of the whitest dung of the Peacock half a pound, of white Suger two ounces; make a Powder.*

It is scarce credible how much help he received from this Remedy; visiting me after a month, he seem'd a new and another man; being freed of the *Vertigo*, he not only confidently walked about, but was able to take care of his houshold affairs, and to meddle with any hard business, which he was not able to do before.

CHAP. VIII.

Of the Apoplexy.

AS the seat of the *Vertigo*, so also of the *Apoplexy*, seems to be within the same more inward cloyster of the Brain, *viz.* the *Callous* Body; to wit, because in either Distemper, although in a far different degree, the imagination and the common sense are affected, *viz.* in the first, the irradiation of the Spirits is wont to be obscured in some places, and as it were broken with intersperfed shades; but in the latter, the same is wholly darkened, and suffers a full eclipse. *The Seat of the Apoplexy.*

The word *Apoplexy* denotes percussion, and by reason of the stupendous nature of the Disease, containing as it were something divine, it is called a *Sideration* or Blasting; for those taken with it, being as it were Planet struck, or with an invisible *Numen*, fall suddenly to the ground, and being deprived of sense and motion, and tho whole animal function ceasing (unless that they breath) they lye a long time as if dead, and sometimes yield to death; But if they revive, oftentimes they are taken with an universal Palsie, or else of one side. *A Description of the Disease.*

The immediate subject of the *Apoplexy*, and the nearest, are the Animal Spirits inhabiting that region of the Brain where the principle faculties of the knowing or understanding soul reside; to wit, the *Callous* Body: but we conclude the mediate subject, to be the middle part of the Brain; because from hence, the instincts of all spontaneous motions proceed, and in this, the perceptions of all sensible things are terminated: by what means the *Cerebel* and *Præcordia*, and all the other parts both Animal and Vital, are secundarily affected, we shall shew anon, when the *symptoms* of this Disease and their reasons are delivered. Upon the coming of the *Apoplectick* fit, all the acts of every spontaneous and knowing function (to wit, which depend upon the brain it self) are forthwith hindred and cease; the reason of which is, because the Animal Spirits being suppressed in their chief place of meeting, to wit, the *Callous* Body, both their next motion of expansion in that place, as also their flowing forth into the nervous appendix, is wholly defective: For therefore, by reason of such an eclipse of them in that place, an immediate and an universal darkness is caused in the whole animal region, which is under this government: yet in the mean time, the Pulse and respiration, as also the motion of the Ventricle and Intestines, are after a sort performed, either perfectly and freely, or at least interruptedly and with pain; forasmuch as their actions proceed wholly from the *Cerebel*, which is not at all, or but little hurt by the Morbifick matter. *Its Subject. The spontaneous Functions only deficient in the Apoplexy.*

But it will seem difficult to be explained, after what manner, and from what causes, the Animal Spirits are so suddenly, and all at once suppressed, and as it were extinguished, about their first spring of emanation; so that all sense and motion depending thereon ceases every where. Concerning this, there are many and diverse opinions of Authors; whilst some place the cause of the *Apoplexy* in the Heart, and others in the Brain; then some lay the fault on the intemperance of that, and others on the evil conformation of this. Further, the obstruction of the Brain is said by some to cause the *Apoplexy* in the greater Ventricles, by others in its Pores or lesser passages: then the obstruction being taken for the cause of the Disease, and wholly binding up the lesser Pores of the Brain, is said to excite the fit, either because the afflux of the blood, for the begetting of Spirits is hindred from those parts; or because *The opinions of others concerning this Disease.*

X

cause, the flowing forth or emanation from thence, of the Animal spirits is kept back. It would be a tedious thing to examine the opinions of every one, and to consider the weight of their reasons.

The Theory of this Disease is best shewn by the famous Dr. Webfer.

The *Theory* of this Disease seems to be very exactly delivered by the famous *Webferus*; for in the first place, for the finding out of its so abstruse and hidden causes, he brings Histories or *Anatomical* observations, in which the *Phænomena* are declared in many dead Carcases of those dying of this Disease; to wit, in three struck or blasted, he had found the blood extravasated or out of the Vessels here and there in great clodders, and had largely marked the substance of the Brain; in another the Serous Colluvies had overflowed the whole head, both without and within the Skull. From these footsteps of this most hidden Disease thus detected, the Author concludes, " That the principal places affected are not the greater Ventricles, but the middle mar-" rowy substance of the Brain and Cerebel, which is every where porous, and indued with " very small passages, both that the vital spirits may flow in thither from the blood, and " that the animal may flow forth: But indeed he affirms, That the whole cause of every " *Apoplexy* doth consist in these two, *viz.* either in one of them, or both of them toge-" ther: to wit, either because the flowing of the blood thorow the Arteries to the Brain " is deny'd, or else by reason that the flowing forth of the Animal Spirit from the Brain " and Cerebel, thorow the Nerves and Spinal Marrow, is prohibited; or for both these " causes together. As to the former, he proposes a threefold means, whereby the " blood may be hindred; *viz.* First, Either by reason of the obstruction of the inner " *Carotid* Arteries, and of the *Vertebrals*, to wit, which happens in the greater Vessels, " and chiefly about the ascent of the Brain, from the blood concreted into cloddery " pieces; or in the lesser Vessels, which pass thorow the brain from a Viscous Mat-" ter planted in them: Or, Secondly, the flowing in of the blood is detained from the " brain, by reason of the compression of those Vessels, which sometimes happens, be-" cause the *Paristhmia*, or Kirnels of the hinder part of the Neck, do so swell up, from " a Serous heap of watry Humors, that by pressing together the Arteries passing " thorow, shuts forth the passage of blood to the Head. Or, Thirdly, The bloody " flood may be hindred, because a Vessel being preternaturally opened within the " Skull, great quantity of blood is poured forth, which should otherways go to the " benefit of the brain. As to the other cause of the astonishing Disease, *viz.* from " the flowing forth of the Spirits being hindred, he affirms that may be caused by " two ways; to wit, either by reason of the obstruction of the beginning of all the " Nerves, caused by a serous inundation, or by a sudden compression of the same; " which is caused either by an heaping up of too much blood in the *Meninges*, or in " some parts of the brain it self, or in its Ventricles; or else by a disposition of " the *Phlegmonodes*.

Another Reason given by the Author.

These most ingenious reasons indeed seem to challenge our assent, for that more probable or more likely are not easily to be brought; but because we think some of these are to be altered, and others to be added, therefore we shall here institute, though not a different, yet somewhat another reason of this Disease.

The Exclusion of the Blood from the Brain doth not easily happen;

And in the first place, though we grant that the flowing in of the blood, may be sometimes denyed to the Brain; yet we do not believe, that it only happens after the aforesaid ways, nor that, for that reason, the *Apoplexy* doth arise. We have elsewhere shewed, that the *Cephalick* Arteries, *viz.* the *Carotides*, and the *Vertebrals*, do so communicate one with another, and all of them in several places, are so ingraffed one in another mutually, that if it happen, that many of them should be stopped or pressed together at once, yet the blood being admitted to the Head, by the passage of one Artery only, either the *Carotid* or the *Vertebral*, it would presently pass thorow all those parts both exterior and interior: which indeed we have sufficiently proved by an experiment, for that Ink being squirted in the trunk of one Vessel, quickly filled all the sanguiferous passages, and every where stained the Brain it self. I once o-

Because all the Arteries communicate one with another, and some of them supply the defects of the others.

pened the dead carcase of one wasted away, in which the right Arteries, both the *Carotid* and the *Vertebral*, within the Skull, were become bony and impervious, and did shut forth the blood from that side, notwithstanding the sick person was not troubled with the astonishing Disease; wherefore, it may be doubted, whether the blood excluded from the Brain, by reason of some Arteries being obstructed or compressed, doth bring forth this Disease. Certainly there is more of danger, that the cause of the *Apoplexy*, should be from its too great incursion and extravasation within the Brain, as it was in the three *Apoplectick* people, cited by the Author; and that not only, because the marrowie substance of the Brain was deprived of the Blood coming to its use, (for such a defect might have been supplied by the other Vessels, extending their branches every where) but rather, because by the extravasated Blood, and not

Of the Apoplexy.

not seldom being concreted into an hard and mighty bulk, the marrow of the Brain is pressed together, the passages of the Spirits being by that means shut up.

But indeed, though we deny this to the afflux of the blood into the Brain, being hindred in any part only, yet it may be granted to its total exclusion, for therefore we have often noted, a want of all motion to be caused: which Distemper however hath been rarely taken for the astonishing disease, but rather is wont to be called a *Syncopy*, or Swooning away, or the *Hysterical* Passion: If at any time the motion of the Heart be wholly suppressed, presently, the Blood being retained without the Brain, the Animal Spirits fall down, even as the light vanishes when the flame is put out. *A total Exclusion of the blood from the Brain sometimes happening, causes a terrible Syncopy.*

The action of the Heart is stopped or hindred, either by reason of the improportionate flowing in of the Blood, as in the violent passions of fear or sadness, or by reason of the Animal Spirits, which serve for its motion, being denyed by the Cerebel. This we think to happen sometimes, because the *Cardiack* Nerves being Distemper'd with a Convulsion, or otherways bound together, after which manner it is usual in Convulsive and *Hysterical* Passions; sometimes for the outward parts, as the Arms and Legs, and sometimes the Inward, to wit, the Præcordia and Viscera, one after another to be affected: but a want of motion follows the inordinations of these, in which the sick lie for some time without motion or sense, with a small or seldom beating Pulse as if dead. Which indeed so seems to come to pass, by reason of the Cardiack Nerves being contracted at that time, and so the Spirits which were about to flow being suspended; though we believe such a want of motion sometimes to be produced by the mere contusion of the Spirits within the Brain, but in this case, the heart it self is lively enough moved, and the Pulse is also strong and laudable. *This depends oftenest on the motion of the heart, being hindred, and so either because of the Cardiack Nerves being bound together;*

But besides, it seems most likely, that the motion of the Heart is ofen suppressed or inhibited, by reason of the Animal Spirits, destinated to the vital function, being suppressed in the fountain it self; to wit, within the Cerebel. We have mentioned this to be done in the Distemper of the *Incubus*: but without doubt it ought to be attributed to this cause, for that I have observed in some, a failing of the Spirits, with a sudden privation of all the Animal functions to follow, upon a great weight in the hinder-part of the Head, in which the sick become senseless and immoveable, with the Pulse and breathing very much lessened, and scarce perceivable, and lye quite cold for many hours; yea oftentimes, a day or two, more like dead than living persons. I have known sometimes those distemper'd, to be stiff and cold, Pulse and breathing to be thought quite gone, and to be indeed esteemed quite dead, and put into their Coffin, yet after two or three days to have reviv'd again: but whoever awakes out of this fit, whether it be of short or long continuance, does not for that reason fall into a Palsie, or half Palsie of one side, as those for the most part do, who are distemper'd with the *Apoplexy*. Further, no doubt but that many die from such a Morbific cause, whose death wrongfully hath been ascribed, either to the mortal *Syncopy*, or to the *Apoplexy* properly so called. Truly the case afterwards described, can only have the like reason given for it. Wherefore, though it may seem a *Paradox*, yet it is not incongruous to reason, that we affirm, that there is a twofold *Apoplexy*, one in the *Cerebel*, which we but now described; the other seated in the middle of the Brain, into the causes of which, and the manner of it, we shall now inquire. *Or, By reason of the Spirits in the Cerebel, being hindred from their flowing into the Nerves.*

Hence there is a twofold Apoplexy, one in the Brain, the other proper to the Cerebel.

But here in the first place we must distinguish concerning the various assault or fit of this Disease, to wit, forasmuch as sometimes being excited, without any previous disposition, or *Procatarxis*, from a sudden and solitary cause, it is often invincible, and for the most part mortal; against this there can be no preventive method of healing, or preservatories instituted; and the Curatory method which is wont to be taken, proves very oft ineffectual. Or, Secondly, the *Apoplectick* fit having an antecedent cause, or previous *Procatarxis*, is brought into act by reason of various occasions, or evident causes. *The Theory of the former delivered.* *This Disease either accidental, or habitual.*

As to what belongs to the blasting, or being stricken, of the former kind, to wit, suddenly and unthought of, its conjunct or next cause is, either a great solution or breach of the unity, happening some where within or near the middle of the Brain, by reason of which its Pores and passages being obstructed or pressed together, the whole emanation of the Spirits is suppressed: or else it is an huge and sudden profligation of the Spirits, or an extinction of those dwelling in the Brain. We shall shew the formal reasons of both of them particularly, and the several ways of their being affected. *The cause of the former is, either a great breach of the unity in or near the middle of the Brain;*

Or a sudden stupefaction or extinction of the Spirits.

Extravasated Blood, the breaking of an Imposthum, and a great flood of Serous humor plentifully flowing forth, are wont to effect the greater breach of the unity within the Brain.

X 2 From

Of the Apoplexy.

1. A Solution of the unity, either from blood let forth of the Vessels; Or,

From Blood effused or extravasated within the Brain, and there either growing together in clodders, or striking on the affected places, doth often times cause mortal *Apoplectick* fits, as I my self have proved by *Anatomical* inspection in some others, besides the instances brought by the famous *Webfer*; but such Morbifick extravasations of the Blood within the Brain, proceed either from an external cause, as a fall from on high, or by a blow on the Head, or by hitting it against some hard thing, and the like; or from an inward cause, to wit, for that the Blood being sharp and thin, and the little mouths of the Vessels, and the places between being too loose, it growing more than ordinarily hot, either of its own accord or occasionally, and flowing forth thorow these, easily breaks into the soft and yielding substance of the Brain. Further, although we have assigned the seat of this Disease in the *Callous* Body, yet the blood, because effused somewhere nigh or above it; because it compresses the underlying Marrow, by intumifying the distemper'd places, causes the *Apoplectick* fit.

2. From an Imposthume, or the breaking of an Ulcer; Or,

Secondly, An Imposthum or Ulcer is rarely wont to be excited within the Brain, but often in the *Meninges*, and almost for the same occasions, by which the extravasation of the blood happens: while it is ripening, it causes only an Headach or heaviness, but when it is broke, the filthy stuff flowing from it, into the shelly part of the Brain, gnaws and putrefies it, and then by degrees instilling its putrid particles, and very infestous to the Spirits, into the middle or marrowie part of the Brain, raises up at last the fit of the astonishing disease.

3. From a Deluge of the Serum.

Thirdly, The Serous heap or deluge being poured forth from the blood, into the Head, though rarely or never of it self, yet sometimes by reason of more strong evident causes, runs so suddenly into the Brain, that filling and stuffing soon all its Marrowie Pores, causes astonishment or deprivation of sense and motion: And this I have known to happen to some, from drinking of sharp thin Wine, or *Spaw-*waters, and sleeping upon it; and I have observed the like effect, from a long and total suppression of Urine, also in *Hæmorrhages* (or fluxes of blood) being suddenly stopped: And lastly, the Serous Recrements in malignant Feavours, being translated to the Head, by a critical transposition, often causes a mortal senselessness, or becoming speechless.

An extinction of the Spirits from Opiates, or from immoderate Drinking of hot Waters.

Another kind of evident causes, from which sudden blasting or being smitten is wont to be caused, consists in the sudden profligation or extinction of the Spirits, which indeed doth not seldom or rarely happen, from strong *Narcoticks*, or Medicines causing sleep, and also from the immoderate drinking of hot waters.

The operation of Opiates, as it is assigned by the famous Webfer.

Though we have already discoursed concerning the use and effects of *Opiates*, I cannot however pass over their way of affecting, assigned by that most famous Doctor *Webfer*. This Learned Man affirms, That *Narcoticks* only do too much open and dilate the Pores and passages of the Brain, and as it were open the doors of it, before fast shut, whereby every extraneous and incongruous thing is admitted into the Chamber or sleeping place of the Spirits, together with the subtil liquor poured forth from the blood; and so by a violent incursion, dissipates their ranks and orders. But indeed it appears from what hath been above said, that *Narcoticks* do not only or always operate so; for we have shewn that whilst they are yet within the Ventricle, they often cause sleep, and sometimes death it self: Besides, it should follow from thence, that *Opiates* being often given should bring still a greater evil, because by dilating more and more the Pores of the Brain, they cause a much more easie entrance to all manner of impurities; but truly it is clear enough, that *Narcoticks* are most hurtful at the first time being taken, and afterwards being often taken do little hurt, so that some accustomed to *Opium*, will devour a great quantity of it without hurt; which is certainly a sign, that this doth not so much alter the conformation of the Brain as that it doth immediately agitate or work upon the Animal Spirits; whom at first (because so very improportionate to them) it slays with a mere blast; then afterwards there being a certain familiarity between them, and this Medicine, it disturbs them not.

The formal reason of the habitual Apoplexy.

Thus much concerning the causes of the accidental and sudden *Apoplexy*, which falls indifferently upon all men, though not at all predisposed: for which also there can be no preventive Medicines instituted, and it is rarely that it is cured. But besides, we observe, that this Disease is sometimes habitual, and that it remains as a constant disposition in some men, by reason of which, at first they are exercised only with light skirmishes, but after some time they become more grievous, and of which at last for the most part they dye. Concerning this therefore, we shall inquire, 1. what the Conjunct Cause of this Disease may be, and the formal reason of it. 2. In what the *Apoplectick* Disposition or *Procatarxis* of the Disease consists: Then 3. What Evident Causes it hath.

1. As

Of the Apoplexy. 157

1. As to the first, we may suppose, upon the coming of the *Apoplectick* fit, that a certain matter before heaped up, and dispersed in the compass of the Brain, at length doth descend into its middle or marrowie part, and there doth assault all the Spirits, and suppress and beat them down in the very fountain of their emanation: Although it doth not plainly appear, whether they effect it either by stuffing only the Pores of the Marrow, or by driving away the Spirits themselves, or by inflicting on them a numness; notwithstanding it is likely, that it may be done by either of the ways. And indeed we say the medullary Pores of the Brain, may be somewhat stopped or obstructed, because the same matter, which at first setling on the *Callous* Body, caused senselesness, being sliden down from thence lower into the *Callous* Body, and then stuffing its Pores, is wont to excite the Palsie of one side. But yet we may not conclude, that the sideration or being struck, doth arise only from the Pores of the Brain being stopped, because then the fit would oftentimes creep on them gently, and by little and little; forasmuch as all the Pores cannot be possessed by the inflowing matter at once, but successively, and some after others: But when as this Distemper leaps upon one suddenly, and like lightning, what can we conceive less, than that the Spirits are struck down as it were by a blast, from the malignant contact of the matter rushing upon them? For it seems, that its particles descending on every side from the compass of the Brain, into its middle part or the *Callous* Body, and entring it from every part, do presently fill the passages how strait so ever they be, and drive to flight hither and thither the Spirits, and compel them into a close place, who being then beset and reduced to a strait corner, when they can neither resist long, nor are able to penetrate into other Pores possessed by the Morbifick matter, at length are struck flat down, letting go every function of the knowing soul; but then they do not easily nor quickly rise up again, because they are not able to quit themselves from the embraces, or bonds of the malignant matter, nor pass any where into empty or open places; wherefore, they lie long suppressed, till at length sometimes perhaps that matter, though leasurely, is dissipated, or supped up into the Blood, or issuing forth from the little Pores of the Marrow, slides forward into the Ventricles of the Brain; or at length, that matter sliding a little lower, and being impacted on the Streaked Bodies, either one or both of them, causes the *Hemiplegia*, or half Palsie, or the Palsie: In the mean time, as the Spirits, within the *Callous* Body grow free, and getting wider spaces, they resume their wonted offices; which they indeed execute, until new matter springing again in the compass of the Brain, and being by degrees increased, descending into the *Callous* Body, brings on another fit; out of which, if the Spirits get not, by either of the aforesaid ways, being wholly discomfited, they perish by degrees.

1. What its Conjunct Cause is.

It consists in the Pores of the callous Body, being suddenly stop'd, and the Spirits being driven away, by the contact of malignant matter.

If you should ask after the nature or disposition of this Morbific matter; it may be suspected, that the Animal Spirits in the *Apoplexy* are plainly affected after another manner, than in Convulsive passions; to wit, those obnoxious to this blasting obtain a *Copula* contrary to the explosive, that is, *Vitriolick*, rather than *Nitro-sulphureous*; and so by it their spiritous-saline particles are wholly fixed, and are hindred from entring into any motions or explosions, even as when the *Vitriolick* particles being beaten and combined with the fulminating gold, they quite take away its explosive or letting off virtue, and congeal and render immoveable all other active particles, like the blowing of a freezing air. The Animal Spirits seem to be not unlike the same, and their *Copula*'s have divers sorts of adjuncts, some of which induce an *Elastick* and very *explosive* virtue, as in the Convulsive Distempers, and others a stupor, numness, or immobility, as in the sleepy Diseases, and also in the *Apoplexy* and *Palsie*.

What the nature or disposition of the morbifick matter is.

Thus much concerning the Conjunct Cause, and formal reason of the *Apoplexy*; as to its *Procatartick* or fore-leading Causes, they are much after the same manner as in most other *Cephalick* Distempers; to wit, both the Blood is in fault, for that it affords to the Head extraneous particles, and very contrary, or as it were destructive to the Texture or constitution of the Animal Spirits, either begotten in it self, or taken from some other place: and then the Brain is in fault, for that being weak in its disposition, and so its Pores and passages too dissolute and lax, so that it always and easily admits without impediment, the Morbific matter poured forth from the Blood. There is no need that we should here reherse or unfold particularly the peculiar reasons of either, and the various ways by which it is done; but we shall rather referr you to what we have already said very largely, concerning the foreleading causes of the inveterate Headach, and also of the *Lethargy*. Further, the like or the same evident causes, which were noted in those Distempers, and in other sleepy Diseases, ought here to be taken notice of, to be shunned carefully by *Apoplectick* people.

The procatartick Cause of the habitual Apoplexy.

From

The differences of this Difeafe.

From what hath been faid, the differences of this Difeafe may be eafily known: 1. What we mentioned but now; The *Apoplexy* is either accidental, which is fuddenly, and at once excited, without any foregoing caufe, and almoft indifferently in all, from fome ftrong evident caufe; or it is wont to be efteemed habitual, which depending upon a previous difpofition, hath frequent fits, by reafon of feveral occafions: 2. From the reafon of the fubject, this Difeafe is faid to be proper, either to the Brain or Cerebel, or common to both: previous and frequent *Scotomies* or dizzinefs with mifts before the eyes, and the Diftemper of the *Vertigo*, denote the Brain more obnoxious to this Difeafe: A frequent Night-Mare, intermitting Pulfe, often Swooning and failing of the Spirits, argue the *Cerebel* to be evilly difpofed.

3. In refpect of magnitude, it is either univerfal, every function, both merely natural and the fpontaneous ceafing; or it is partial, this or that part being affected by it felf, then for that the faculties of either, now all, now many only, yet none excepted fuffer an *eclipfe*; for in either regiment, the morbific matter defcending to the middle or marrowie part, poffeffes fometimes all its whole fubftance, fometimes part of it, to wit, the fore part, hinder, or middle part. 4. In refpect of the antecedent caufe, the *Apoplectical* difpofition is either hereditary or innate; or acquired by means of an evil dyet, or other accidents.

Its Prognofticks

The *prognoftick* or fore-iudging of this Difeafe is always denounced deadly or dubious; for the *Apoplexy* is never without prefent or future danger. But it is worft of all, in which, befides the abolition of all the fpontaneous functions, the Pulfe and breathing alfo are either deficient, or are performed laborioufly; and then for the moft part it happens, with a foam at the mouth, and fnorting; upon which comes a fweat, which is often like melted greace, and indicates a very fudden death to be at hand.

Thofe who are blafted or ftrucken, and are prefently deprived of Pulfe and breathing, and a little after growing cold, and feem dead or without any life, are not prefently to be had from bed, or left deftitute of Medicinal helps: further, though there be no hopes of life, they ought not to be buried under three or four days; becaufe fuch do fometimes revive again, either of their own accord, or by the ufe of Remedies: which certainly comes to pafs, not becaufe a vital heat is at laft ftirred up in the heart (for it is not there extinguifhed altogether;) but becaufe the Morbific matter being difcuffed, or evaporated from the *Cerebel*, the motion of the heart is reftored, like a Clock when the weights are put on.

In the *Apoplectical* fit, if any help follows upon letting of Blood, there is hope of health. But if after this and other Remedies, the Diftemper continues without intermiffion, above the fpace of a night or a day, or grows worfe, the cafe is defparate.

If after the firft fpeechlefs fit being over, the fick perfon becomes more nummed and duller, and diftemper'd with a *Scotomy*, and frequent *Vertigo*, it is a fign that he will be obnoxious to more fits of this aftonifhing Difeafe: for the aforefaid diftempers proceed from the Morbific matter, already laid up in the compafs of the Brain, and there flowing fprinklingly, and thence defcending thorow the very fmall Pores only, into the middle part: which matter whether *Vitriolick* or *Narcotick*, growing to a greater fulnefs, calls on this blafting or being fuddenly fmitten.

The Curatory Method.

The *Therapeutick* Method, is either Curatory, for the taking away the fit, when it is upon one; or prefervatory to prevent it, that it may not return: the former belongs to every *Apoplexy*, the other only to the habitual.

What is to be done in the Fit.

The affault or fit of this Difeafe being come, (if it proceeds not from fome outward or vehement hurt of the head) although it is not known, whether it be excited or no from an invincible caufe, fuch as the Blood being let forth of the Veffels, or the breaking of an Impofthum in the Brain, yet we ought carefully to endeavour the Cure of it. And becaufe the blood being too hot or fwelling up, is wont fometimes to bring in the Morbific caufe, or at leaft to increafe it, and the fame finking down, and becoming more fetled, fometimes carries it away; therefore in the firft place, you ought to deliberate, concerning the moderating its courfe. And here a queftion arifes, concerning the placing of the Patient, to wit, whether he ought prefently to be put to bed, or to be detained out of it for fome time: fome religioufly

In what pofition the Sick ought to be kept.

obferve the latter, and that not without reafon; to wit, becaufe in Bed there is a greater propenfity to fleep, and the blood growing hot, and flaming forth more plentifully, by reafon of the heat of the Bed-cloaths, pours forth ftill more recrementitious matter into the diftemper'd Brain: on the contrary, whilft the fick is thinly cloathed, and placed in a Chair, the blood flows more flowly, and the finking Veffels feem more apt rather to fup back the humors out of the Head, than to fend them thither.

Wherefore,

Wherefore, if the Patient be strong enough, it will be expedient perhaps to let him stay out of bed for six or eight hours, till the flux of the Morbific Matter passes over, and the course of the Blood be made more quiet by *Phlebotomy*, and other Remedies carefully administred: but the weak, and who are of a tender constitution, let them be put to bed as soon as they are smitten. But let not the sick, whether in bed or up, lye upon his back, but with his head somewhat upright, and inclining either to one side or the other.

Phlebotomy, necessary almost in all *Apoplectical* persons, is not to be deferred: but the Blood is copiously drawn back by a strong *Clyster*. In the *Clyster* may be dissolved the *Species* of *Hiera Diacolycinthia*, and a troubled Infusion of *Crocus Metallorum*. Let a large Blistering Plaster be applied to the hinder part of the Head, and other drawing *Cataplasms* to the Legs and Feet: Let the Temples and Nostrils be anointed with proper *Oyls* and *Balsoms*, and let painful rubbings be used almost to the whole Body: In the mean time, let things that stir up the Animal Spirits, and help them out of their bonds be given them; *viz.* Spirits of Harts-horn, Sut, and the like, with a *Cephalick Julep*. *Phlebotomy. Other ways of Administration noted.*

After this the sick being placed in the bed (if he be able and doth easily Vomit) let an *Emetick* be given him, of the Salt of *Vitriol*, *Oxymel* of *Squills*, or an Infusion of *Crocus Metallorum*, and then with a Feather put down the throat, provoke vomiting four or five times, drinking between whiles Posset-drink. *Vomiting Medicines.*

Vomiting being over, let there be given Comforters, as the *Elixir Vitæ* of *Quercitan*, Spirits of *Lavender*, or *Camphorated Treacle*, *Tincture* of *Pæony*, or of *Amber*, or of *Coral*, with *Apoplectical* Water, or other appropriate Waters in a convenient Dose, and repeated as the business requires. *Comforters.*

On the second day, the same Remedies being still continued, let dry Cupping-Glasses, or with Scarification, be applied between the shoulders, or to the hinder part of the Neck; or if more blood ought to be taken away, let the jugular Vein be opened; the *Clyster* repeated; apply to the Nose Spirit of *Sal Armoniack*, or a fume of *Galbanum* boiled in strong Vinegar. Besides, let *Errhines* or Sneezing Powders, and things to chew in the mouth to draw away Rheum be used. Then in the Evening let a Purge be ordered of *Pil. Rudii*, or a Solutive Electuary of Roses, dissolved in some liquor. *Cupping-glasses.*

None of these things helping, though there be small or no hope, the top of the Head being shaven, let glowing Iron be held over it, or a large Blister made upon it; and let the other part, especially the Forehead, and forepart of the Head, be bathed with *Bezoardick* Vinegar; let Leeches be set to the Temples, or behind the Ears; let also a large Dose of Spirits of Harts-horn, or of Sut, be often poured down the throat; these and other the like administrations, are to be used till you see death at hand; which (as *Celsus* saith) these sort of Remedies only defer, but some times hasten life. *Hot or glowing Iron.*

The *Prophylactick* or preventive Method, respects both those who have been troubled with one or more fits, and also those who are seen to be prone to it, as those who are born of *Apoplectick* Parents, or are frequently obnoxious to the *Vertigo*, the *Incubus*, or Swooning away; also such who have short and brawny Necks. *The preservatory Method.*

Let Purging and Bleeding be ordered Spring and Fall, where it is convenient; as to the former, those who are easie to vomit, let them first take an *Emetick*, of the infusion of *Crocus Metallorum*, with the Salt of *Vitriol*, or of the *Sulphur of Antimony*; and then after three or four days, let there be given a Dose of *Pil. Rudii*, or of *Amber*; and after a due distance between, let it be repeated three or four times: Let two large Issues be made between the shoulders; or if that place doth not please some, let them be made, in one of the Arms, and in the opposite Leg. *Purging and Bleeding Spring and Fall.*

On other days, free from purging, let altering and *Cephalick* Medicines be taken twice a day. *Cephalick Remedies.*

Take *of the Conserves of the Flowers of the Lilies of the valley (or of the male Pæony) six ounces, of the Powder of the Root of the male Pæony half an ounce, of humane Skull prepared three drams, of the Seeds and the Flowers of the male Pæony powdered, each two drams; of red Coral prepared, of Pearls, and of the whitest Amber, each one dram; of the Salt of Coral four scruples, of the Syrup of the Flowers of the male Pæony, what will suffice to make an Electuary: The Dose two drams morning and evening, drinking after it two or three ounces of the following Water.* *An Electuary.*

Take *of the Roots of the male Pæony, of Imperatorian Angelica, each half a pound; of the Root of Zedoary, of the lesser Galangal, each one ounce; of the leaves of the Orchard Misleto, of Rue, Sage, and Betony, each four handfuls; of the outer rind* *A distilled Water.*

of

of ten *Orenges*, and eight *Lemons*, of *Cardomums, Cloves, Nutmegs*, each half an ounce; all being cut and bruised, pour to them of white *Wine* (in which two pints of the dung of the *Peacok* hath been infused for a day) ten pints: let them infuse, close shut for three days; then distil it according to art, and let the whole liquor be mixed together.

Lozenges. Take of the Species of *Diambræ* two drams, of the Powder of the Root of the male *Pæony*, of *Zedoary* picked, each one dram and a half; of Pearl one dram, of the Oyl of the purest *Amber* half a dram, of the whitest Sugar half a dram, being dissolved in six ounces of the water of *Pæony*, and boiled up to a consistence: make Lozenges according to art, each weighing half a dram: Let the Patients eat one or two often in a day, at his pleasure.

Spirits and Tinctures. Within the fifteenth or twentieth day, that the Remedies may not be irksome, and may profit the better, let them be changed: therefore, instead of the *Electuary* let there be substituted for two or three weeks, sometimes the Spirit of *Sal Armoniack*, with Amber or Coral, or else impregnated with humane Skull or *Castor*; sometimes *Elixir* of *Pæony*, or *Tincture* of *Amber* or *Coral*, or *Elixir Vitæ* of *Quercitan*, or the simple mixture: also instead of it, may be drunk compounded Waters, or Water of black Cherries, or Walnuts; or the simple Waters of Rosemary, or Lavender; sometimes a draught of Posset-drink, with Flowers of the *male Pæony* or

Tea, Coffee, and Chocalate prepared, how the *Lilies* of the valley boiled in it; or a draught of *Tea* or *Coffee* in the morning, (let the water of which it is prepared have such ingredients first boiled in it) or let *Chocalate* be prepared after this same manner.

to be made and taken. Take of the Powder of the Root of the male *Pæony*, of humane *Skull* prepared, each half an ounce; of the Species of *Diambræ* two drams, make a Powder; to every paper add of the Kirnels of the *Cocoa Nuts* one pound, of Sugar what will suffice; of this make Chocalate: take of it half an ounce or six drams every Morning in a draught of the Decoction of Sage, or of the Flowers of Pæony, or such like.

A Powder. Take of the Powder of the Root of the male *Pæony*, of humane Skull prepared, each one ounce and a half; of the pick'd Root of *Zedoary*, *Cretick Dittany*, *Angelica*, *Contrayerva*, each two drams; make a fine Powder of them all, add to it of the yellow of *Orenges* and *Lemons* Candied, each two ounces; let all be beaten to a Powder: take about half a dram, or a dram an hour before and after meals.

For ordinary drink, let a *Vessel* of four gallons be filled with ordinary *Ale*, in which six handfuls of white *Horehound* dryed had been boiled, of *Anacardine* and *Cardomums* cut and beaten, each one ounce and a half; of it make a bag to hang in it.

Medical Air. First of all, a very strict dyet ought to be ordered; let a temperate, dry and open air be chosen; let good and wholesome meats be eaten, and slender meals. Let suppers be sparingly taken, or none at all: Let noon-sleeps, drinking bouts, and other customary things about the non-naturals be shunned.

Examples. I could here propose many Histories of *Apoplectical* persons, to wit, of some who were once or twice touch'd, and yet living; and of others who have dyed at the first assault, or in the second or third fit. The most Reverend Father in God the Lord *Gilbert* Archbishop of *Canterbury*, recovered of a grievous *Apoplectical* Fit, six years ago, (God prospering our medicinal help, to whom we render eternal thanks) and from that time, though he sometimes suffer'd some light skirmishes of the Disease, yet he never fell, or became speechless or senseless. But we shall not stay upon this or other examples to unfold them largely, because there is nothing in them very rare, that may illustrate the *Ætiology* of this Disease. Some of their dead Carcases I have dissected, but only of such as the cause of death was from some former great hurt of the head, as some blow, or by means of some blast; in all which the extravasated Blood, or an Imposthum was the cause of their death: We have been prohibited often by their Friends, from opening those dying of an habitual *Apoplexy*, who expecting to have them revive again, held it as a deadly thing, and so wholly forbid *Anatomy*: But I shall here relate a notable *Anatomical* observation taken about five years since at *Oxford*.

A very rare History. An ancient Divine, an honest and a godly Man, indued with a fat body, a short and brawny Neck, being long unhealthy, and living a sedentary life, contracted a very *Scorbutick* evil disposition: being troubled with a difficult and laborious breathing, with an heaviness of the Head, and unwonted numness, was scarce able to endure any thing of labour or exercise, more than that he daily went and came from his Chamber to the Chapel and Hall: one Morning he came to the Chapel a little before Prayers begun, and while he was on his knees, he was suddenly struck, and immediately

ately became speechless and senseless, and fell on the ground; but being carried thence, and his cloaths taken off, he was put into a warm Bed. I and other Physicians being presently sent for, and coming as soon as we could possibly, we found him not only without Pulse, sense, and breathing, but all his Body cold and quite stiff; nor could he be recalled to life or heat, by any Remedies or ways of administrations, though used for some time: by which we suspected, that the Pulse of his heart was wholly hindred at the first stroke, and that its flame being put out, presently all motion of the Blood was suppressed.

The next day, seeing the Carcase dead enough, and stiff, we opened it, nothing doubting but that the Distemper so suddenly mortal, would shew clear marks of it within the Head. But there, or in any other part, was not the least shadow of this most cruel Disease: The Vessels watering the *Meninges* were moderately filled with Blood, without any Inflammation or Extravasation: The Brain, the Cerebel, and the oblong Marrow, with all their processes and prominences, appeared every where thoroughout firm, and well coloured, both without and within: nor was there any Serum or Blood poured forth any where, within the Pores or passages, nor yet within the greater Ventricles, nor heaped up; yea the *Choroeidal* Infoldings placed both within the cavity of the Brain, and behind the Cerebel, seem'd free from all fault; so that the Morbifick matter, equally thin and subtil like the Animal Spirits, whom it affected, remained wholly invisible, and we could only argue its presence by the effect. *An Anatomical Observation.*

But lest this should lye hid some where without the Head, after the contents of the head were diligently inspected, we came to the Breast: where the discoloured Lungs being through the whole stuffed with a frothy matter, manifestly shewed the cause of the short and difficult breathing. But the Heart was sound and firm enough, free from any obstruction or fleshy Concretions. Further, neither in the neighbouring parts, or in others about the Viscera, was found any Imposthum or Ulcer, by whose contact or stink, the Heart could be suddenly oppressed, or the Vital Spirits (if this be possible) might be choaked.

Wherefore in this case, nothing could be suspected else, but that the Animal Spirits implanted within the middle of the Cerebel, were put to flight, and as it were extinguished suddenly, by some malignant, or *narcotick*, or otherways deadly Particles, so that the motion of the Heart presently failing, like the first moving wheel in a Clock or Watch, immediately all the other functions, their impulses being taken away, wholly ceased.

CHAP. IX.

Of the Palsie.

THE middle of the Brain, or the *Callous* Body, to which we have assigned the seat of the *Vertigo* and *Apoplexy*, seems also to be the primary distemper'd place in the *Epilepsie*: Concerning which, as also concerning Convulsive Diseases, since we have elsewhere largely treated, we shall therefore here pass over purposely in this part of the Diseases belonging to the Head, and according to our wonted method, descend yet lower, to the other regions of the Brain, and its dependences; and now we shall endeavour next to describe the Distempers which belong to the Streaked Bodies, Oblong Marrow, and also to the Nerves, and nervous Fibres. *The middle of the Brain, which is the Seat of the Apoplexy is also the Seat of the Epilepsy.*

We have formerly shewed, that these parts do perform all the functions belonging to motion and sense; wherefore, the failing or the enormities of these, are the affections of those Bodies, or of the Spirits inhabiting them. But indeed sense and motion are hurt chiefly after two manner of ways: to wit, either is wont to be perverted or hindred; when Motion is perverted, Cramps and Convulsions; when Sense, pain arises; when either function or both together is hindred or abolished, the Distemper is thence stirred up called the *Palsie*; which we are at present about to handle. Concerning Convulsion and Pain we have already treated. *The streaked Bodies, the Medullar Trunks, and the Nerves, are the Seat of the Palsy.*

The *Palsie* is described after this manner, to wit, *That it is a resolution, loosening, or relaxation of the nervous parts, from their due tensity or stiffness; by which means Motion* *What the Palsie is.*

V

:lon and Sense, to wit, either one only, or both together, in the whole Body, or in some parts, cannot be exercised after their due manner.

Its Conjunct Causes are, Obstruction of the passages, and the Impotency of the Spirits.
The nervous parts are loosened, because the Animal Spirits do not sufficiently irradiate them, not blow them up, nor actuate them with vigor. The cause of which defect is, either an obstruction of the ways, by which their trajection or passage is hindred; or the impotency of the Animal Spirits, for that they are distemper'd with a numness, or that being but few in number they do not lively enough unfold themselves. By reason of these various means of being affected, there arise diverse kinds of *Palsies*. For in the first place, as to motion by it self, this spontaneous faculty (which is chiefly and almost only lyable to the *Palsie*) is sometimes taken away in the whole, or altogether in some parts; but sometimes this, being only hindred, is lessened or depraved.

In the Palsie either motion, or sense only, or both together, is hurt.
Secondly, in like manner also one sense only by it self, or more together, is sometimes wholly taken away, and sometimes only much diminished or vitiated. Thirdly, Sometimes it happens that both powers are hurt at once. We shall speak of each of these in their order; and first of the *Palsie*, in which spontaneous motion is abolished; which we say is excited from two causes chiefly; to wit, the ways being obstructed, and the Animal Spirits being touched with a numness, or as it were with a certain malignant blast.

Spontaneous motion is abolished by reason of the ways being obstructed, either in their beginnings, or the middle passages, or about the ends.
As to the former, an interception of the Spirits from the loosned parts, by reason of their passages being obstructed, that always existing above them, is wont to be caused in various places, and for divers causes; but chiefly it happens in the first *sensory, viz.* in the Streaked Bodies, or some where about the Medullar Trunks, or lastly in the Nerves themselves, and so, either in their beginnings, or middle processes, or in their extreme ends, (*i. e.*) the nervous Fibres. When the evil or hurt is brought to the Streaked Bodies, or the oblong, or spinal Marrow, it either obstructs the whole Medullar thread or rope, from whence arises an universal Palsie below the distemper'd part; or one moiety of it, whence comes the *Hemiplegia* or Palsie of one side; or it affects in one side, or in both at once, the little heads of some Nerves, whence loosnings or resolutions are caused in this or that member apart from the others.

The ways are obstructed by Impletion, or Compression, or by a breaking of the Unity.
There are many means whereby the ways or passages of the Animal Spirits are obstructed in the aforesaid bodies. First, Either their passages are filled by an extraneous matter impacted in them: Or, Secondly, They are pressed together by Blood flowing out of the Vessels, a Serous deluge, or some Tumor lying upon them: Or, Thirdly and lastly, the unity or continuity is broken, as by a stroke, or wound, or bruise, also by excess of cold or heat. According as these several places are distemper'd, and the several means of their being affected, we shall run thorow the chief cases of the *Palsie*, together with the *Ætiology*, or reason thereof, with the manifold appearances of *Symptoms* in them; and in the first place we will speak of the *Palsie* arising from an hurt brought to the common *Sensory*, to wit, the Streaked Bodies.

An obstruction in the streaked Bodies causes the Universal Palsie, or the Palsie of one side.
And indeed, that it so comes to pass, I have proved by ocular inspection, and shall be plainly demonstrated anon by *Anatomical* observation. Further, as often as an universal or an half *Palsie* follows, (as it is often wont to do) upon a *Lethargy* the *Carus*, or *Apoplexy*, any one may conceive, that such a change of the Disease, happens from a translation of the Morbific matter; for that this at length going out of the Pores and passages of the *Callous* Body, which it at first possest, and sinking down a little lower, runs into the Medullary tracts of one of the Streaked Bodies or perhaps both of them. And so, when the Animal Spirits are hindred from their wonted out-flowing, or irradiation into the nervous Stock, the motive faculty only, or (if the obstruction be very great) both this, together with the sensitive, is hindred.

I have sometimes observed in a *Palsie*, coming after a grievous fit of some other Disease, that all the moving parts, of either side, have been loosened after a more light manner: For though they were not able to perform the more strong motive endeavours, yet for the most part they could extend, bend, yea and move their members hither and thither, to wit, because the Morbific matter being diffused abroad, thorow both the Streaked Bodies, had not so closely filled every where all the passages: Moreover, on the contrary, I have known in a *Palsie* of one side, so suddenly excited, that there has been a far greater resolution so that they so struck, were not able to move any way hand or foot, nor any other member on the distemper'd side. Further, sometimes it happens, from the Morbific matter being copiously taken down, and obstructing closely all the Medullary tracts of one of the Streaked Bodies, that all the respective parts, have not only been destitute of motion, but some of

them

them also of sense; so that some members felt not any painful impression, how vehement so ever it was. Such a Distemper happening in a lesser degree, is wont to excite a sense of numness, or pricking or tingling, such as in members lean'd or lain upon.

If it be demanded, why sense is not always hindred as well as motion in every *Palsie*, since as it seems either is performed by the same Nerves and Fibres, within the same Medullary tracts, so that one faculty is only the inversion of the other? as to this we may say, that as light beams thorow glass, when wind is excluded, so also sense being safe, oftentimes motion is lost. Besides, sense is only a passion, and a sensible impression, which is propagated from the organ, by a continuity of the nervous process, to the common sensory, without any endeavour or labour of the Spirits; which may be done, though the common sensory be in some measure obstructed, and the Spirits inhabiting it benummed: But motion is a difficult and laborious action, to which is required, that the Spirits expand or stretch out themselves lively, and not only put forth as it were explosive endeavours in the moving organs, but chiefly about the parts, where the beginning of the motion and its first force is, and from thence, in the whole passage thorow the nervous parts. Wherefore, as but a few Spirits and bound, suffice for sense; many, free, and expeditious as to their expansions, are required for motion. *Why sense is not hindred as well as motion in every Palsie.*

But that the Morbifick matter being slid down into the Streaked Body, the Muscles of the Eyes, Mouth, and Face, do still retain their motions; it is because that some of them, about the beginning of the Spinal Marrow, below all the Nerves, arising from the oblong Marrow, have their place of obstruction, I say, that it is so, because the Nerves destinated to the aforesaid Muscles, (the motions of which are stirred up by natural instincts) and brought from the fifth and sixth pair, even as the Nerves serving the Præcordia and Viscera, derive chiefly the influences of the Animal Spirits from the Cerebel; whose regiment, though the Streaked Body be distemper'd, remains often unhurt. *In an universal Palsie why all the Muscles of the Eyes and Face are not loosned.*

Not only an obstruction of the Streaked Body, but also a compression sometimes causes the *Palsie*, as shall be shewed by and by from *Anatomical* observation; to wit, when the blood is extravasated, and growing cloddery within the inferior cavity of the Brain (and perhaps a Serous deluge is there heaped up) and doth lie heavily upon the Streaked Body, and press it together, so that for that reason, the Medullary tracts being bound together, are hindred from the Spirits flowing into them. *A Compression of the Streaked Body sometimes stirs up the Palsie.*

Next after the Streaked Bodies, the seat of the Morbifick Cause is in the oblong and spinal Marrow; also sometimes in these, though rarely an obstruction, but more often a compression, or a solution of the unity, excite the *Palsie*. *A Paralytick obstruction doth sometimes happen in the Oblong and Spinal Marrow.*

As to the former, it is not probable, that great plenty of Morbifick matter should be sent from the Brain, into this or that part together and in heaps; for such a great and sudden flux hardly happens beyond the Streaked Bodies. But it may be suspected, that *Narcotick* or otherways deadly Particles, being forthwith poured forth into the Brain, and from thence thrust forth into its appendix, doth at first stick within the more narrow spaces of the Medullary Trunk, and then by degrees being heaped up, causes the *Paralytick* obstruction, whilst these Particles are carried in the Brain here and there, in the *Callous* or Streaked Bodies they stir up frequent *Vertigoes*, and mists before the eyes, and sometimes in the motive parts short numnesses; but these being by degrees heaped up together within the Trunk of the oblong Marrow, or the spinal, forasmuch as they possess all or part of its passage, and by that means either obstruct all the Pores of the Spirits at once, or some ranks or orders of them, they bring forth either an half Palsie, or a loosening of some members, sometimes the superior, sometimes the inferior.

I have observed in many, that when, the Brain being first indisposed, they have been distemper'd with a dullness of mind, and forgetfulness, and afterwards with a stupidity and foolishness, after that, have fallen into a Palsie, which I often did predict; to wit, the Morbifick matter being by degrees fallen down, and at length being heaped up some where within the Medullar Trunk, (where the Marrowy Tracts are more straitned than in the Streaked Body) to a stopping fulness. For according as the places obstructed are more or less large, so either an universal *Palsie*, or an half *Palsie* of one side, or else some partial resolutions of members happen. *A Palsie often succeeds stupidity, or becoming foolish.*

But in either Marrow, and especially the Spinal, an interception or inhibition of the Spirits, creating a *Palsie*, most often happens from a compression, or a breaking of the unity: The extravasated Blood, or the Corruption flowing from the broken Imposthum, and perhaps a Serous deluge being deposited within the hollowness of the Back-bone; yea also an hard Tumor, being risen somewhere in it, by pressing together *A Palsie sometimes from the pressing together of the Marrowy Cord.*

Y 2

Of the Palsie.

together the marrowy rope, shuts up the ways of the Spirits. Further, either a stroke, wound, or bruise of the Head, or *spine*; yea and a distortion of this latter, do often pervert or break off the Marrowy Tracts; yea an excess of cold taken in Frost and Snow, straitens and stops up the passages of the Spirits. Those kind of cases, and instances, being obvious enough to common observation, there will not be any need here to speak of them particularly, or to unfold them more largely.

Sometimes from the unity being broke.

Thirdly, The Morbific cause being sometimes planted lower, possesses either the greater Trunks, or the lesser shoots of the Nerves themselves; and that likewise is either an obstruction or a compression, or a breaking of the unity, by reason of any of these ways, and according to the like means of affecting, within the nervous passages, as in the marrowy, it is wont to be excited.

The State of the Palsie sometimes in the Nerves themselves, which are either obstructed, or compressed, or the unity broken.
1. An Obstruction.

The oppilative or stopping Particles being fallen down, from the Brain, and carried forward into the oblong Marrow, enter into the Nerves, destinated to the Muscles of some parts of the Face, and by obstructing the ways of the Spirits in them, bring forth the *Palsie* in the Tongue, and sometimes a loosening in these or those Muscles of the Eyes, Eye-lids, Lips, and of other parts; and then by reason of the contrary Muscles being contracted beyond measure, they stir up a Cramp or Convulsion in the opposite part.

Sometimes in the beginning of the Nerves.

Nor is it less usual, for the same Particles, for that they are fewer, to be carried yet further, without any great hurt into the Spinal Marrow; and lastly going forth from it, to run sometimes into the several Trunks of the Nerves, and sometimes into some handfuls of them; and for that reason, to induce the Palsie to the several Muscles or members, or in some of them only. As often as for this cause, the Muscles of one side of the Neck are resolved, or loosened, the other opposite being too much contracted, render the Neck twisted or awry. It ordinarily happens, by reason of some private Nerves being so obstructed, for some Fingers of the Hand, or Toes of the Feet to be loosened. But if many handfuls of Nerves together happen to be stopped, a *Palsie* follows, oftentimes in the whole Arm or Thigh. It would be too tedious to mention every case here, by which the Nerves are wont to be stopped, about their beginnings, middle processes, or utmost ends, to wit, the Membranaceous or Musculous Fibres, by reason of compression, or breaking of the continuity, and so deny the exercise of the moving faculty to the respective parts: The reasons of these kind of Distempers are so clear and manifest, and so commonly known, that it would be superfluous to insist on the opening them any longer. But we shall rather pass to the other conjunct cause of the *Palsie*, which more immediately affecting the Animal Spirits, and sometimes striking down, and as it were extinguishing them, by mere contact, or as it were by a malignant blast, brings in a resolution or loosening in the respective parts.

2. Sometimes in the middle.
3. Or in their utmost processes.
The other conjunct cause of the Palsie, to wit, the impotency of the Spirits;

What we before affirmed in the *Apoplexy*, we now again do the same in the *Palsie*, that there are deadly Particles, not only oppilative or stopping, but sometimes *Narcotick* or *Stupefactive*, and as it were extinguishers of the Spirits; which kind of affection, if it be strong, causes sometime *Paralytick* Symptoms, without any great obstruction of the ways. The breath or steams of *Antimony*, *Mercury*, or *Auripigment*, often causes weaknesses, tremblings, and loosening of the Members, in such as are long conversant among the Furnaces of *Chymists*, and of Metals. We may in like manner believe, that in some *Scorbutick* and very *Cacochymical* people, heterogeneous Particles, and as it seems of a *Vitriolick* nature (passing thorow the Brain, and its marrowy appendix) do enter into the nervous passages, together with their watering Juice, and cast down some handfuls of the Spirits in them, or suppress their motion. Hence suddenly arise stupors, numness, or loosenes in the Members, or Muscles, sometimes in these, sometimes in those, and soon after vanishing in one place, presently spring up again in another: But at length, when these sort of Particles being abundantly poured forth into the Nerves, and laid up in heaps, they become variously fixed here and there; and moreover, shut up the ways of the Spirits, and so cause a fixed and permanant *Palsie*. And indeed, in every *Palsie*, made by obstruction, the Morbific matter is not thick and cold Phlegm, (as *Galen* and many other Physicians have asserted) for such doth not pass thorow the Brain, much less the nervous passages; but it seems to consist of most subtil and very active Particles, though Infestous or deadly to the animal regiment: But indeed the *Palsie* happens in Men, no otherwise than the blasting, or burning, or withering in Trees; because some winds being indued with very frigid or cold blasts, to wit, with a Nitrous or a *Vitriolick* Spirit, when they blow upon the green and tender sprigs of trees, cause them suddenly to wither, for that the tender stalks like Nerves every where inter-woven with the sprigs and leaves, are bound together by the blast of the malignant air so fully, that

Often arises from narcotick or vitriolick Particles, by which the Spirits are put to flight.

In every Palsie the matter is not so thick or cold, as it is vitriolick or otheir ways infestious to the Spirits.

The blasting or withering in Trees like the Palsie.

Of the Palsie.

that they receive not any more the Juice sent from the Trunk or Root, by reason of which defect they wither. Much after the same manner, extraneous Particles, and as it were *Vitriolick*, being admitted within the organs of sense and motion, for that they at once bind up the Pores, or cast down or suppress from motion the Animal Spirits, cause in the respective parts, as it were a withering or drying up. But this is not so caused by mere Phlegm, or a Serous flood, as plainly appears, because those indued with a moist and cold Brain, have always their Nose and Eyes moist, with the distillation of a snotty or watry humor; yea those who are troubled with a Dropsical Brain, in which the Brain, and the tops of either Marrow do as it were swim in water, are not for that reason disposed to the *Palsie*, unless by the pressing together of the Marrow.

We have hitherto described the various cases of the *Palsie*, and the means by which it is caused, together with their several formal reasons, and conjunct causes. As to what belongs to the other causes of this Disease we must first distinguish, that it is either accidental or habitual: The former happens to some, from a solitary evident cause, such as a stroke, wound, bruise, and excess of either heat or cold, without any previous disposition; and besides this, and the conjunct cause, which for the most part is a compression, or breach of the unity, it hath none: The habitual Palsie depends upon a *Procatartick* cause, which is always an extraneous, and as it were a *Vitriolick* matter begotten somewhere before, and heaped up, which being from thence suffused into the organs of sense and motion, for that it stops up the marrowy or nervous Tracts or sometimes profligates the Spirits by mere contact, or effects both together, brings forth loosenings in the respective parts, by reason of the influence of the Spirits being deny'd them.

The more remote foregoing causes of the Palsy, which are two:

This kind of *Procatarxis* or foregoing Cause, depends upon a twofold antecedent or secret leading cause, to wit, one remote, which is a vicious Blood, carrying to the Head a Morbific matter, either begotten in it self, or taken from the Bowels, or some other place; and the other more near, which is an indisposed Brain, to wit, weak, and too lax or loose, or otherways evilly made, and so easily admitting heterogeneous, or strange and deadly Particles.

1. More remote, to wit, a vicious Blood, and for that reason pouring forth a deadly matter upon the head.

The Morbific matter being brought to the Brain, sometimes induces the *Palsie* primarily, but more often secondarily, and not but after other Diseases first excited.

2. Nearer, to wit, a weak and loose Brain, admitting the evil Particles.

The reason of the former, (to wit, that the habitual *Palsie* be a primary Disease, and by it self) requires these two things, *viz.* That the heterogeneous Particles be disposed chiefly for the causing or stirring up the *Palsie*; then that they be admitted by degrees, and but in small quantity, for if they enter in great heaps, they would first cause the *Carus* or *Apoplexy*: and if they be not of a plain *Vitriolick* nature or quality, when having passed thorow the Brain, they come to enter into the organs of Sense and Motion, they would first occasion in them Convulsive and painful Distempers, yea sometimes the *Colick*, *Gout*, or *Scurvy* first, and then at length, the *Palsie*.

The Palsy is either a primary Distemper, and a Disease of it self;

2. The secondary *Palsie* often succeeds Distempers for the most part *Chronical*, after the natural and vital faculties being by them very much hurt: a slow and long *Feavour*, strength being at length worn out, causes oftentimes enervations or resolutions of the whole Body, or of some Members. Long and immoderate sadness, a Consumption, a *Scorbutick Atrophy* or wasting, being long fixed in Bed, unhealthy old Age; yea and many other passions, after a notable evil first brought to the Brain, and nervous Stock, at length brings on the *Palsie*. But indeed this Disease more frequently comes upon some other Distempers, either of the Brain, as chiefly the *Carus* and *Apoplexy*, or of the nervous stock, and such chiefly are the *Scurvy*, *Convulsions*, *Colick*, and *Gout*. By what means it succeeds *Cephalick* Diseases, we have already shewed in this; and how the Scurvy, in another tract: we shall now inquire how it is often the off-spring of the other three.

Or secondarily, viz. Coming upon or succeeding other Diseases.

3. We have shewn already, that the *Spasme* or Cramp or Convulsion, doth sometimes bring in the *Palsie*, to wit, when from contrary or opposite Muscles, being one of them loosened and the other pulled together: Further, it is an usual thing, for those who are long obnoxious to Convulsive Distempers, to suffer at length debilities in some members, and at length resolutions or want of motion. I have known many *Epileptical* persons, and others troubled with Convulsions, by reason of the motive function being abolished or inhibited, in this or that part, to become at first lame, and then Bed-rid; the reason of which seems to be, because the Morbific matter, being continually admitted within the tracts of the Brain and its appendix, both medullar and nervous, and often thrust forth, doth at length so debilitate and dilate

Wherefore the Palsie often succeeds Convulsive Diseases.

dilate them, so that it gives an open passage besides to other kind of Particles, either *Narcotick* or *Vitriolick*; by reason of which, the *Palsie* comes after the Convulsion. Further, I have often observed, by reason of the diverse mingling of the Morbifick matter, (like as when Rain and Snow happen together) that the sick have at once been infested both with Convulsive motions, and the *Palsie*. A notable example of this, with the reason of it, we have fully described in our Tract of Convulsive Diseases, Chap. IX. p. 115.

Wherefore the Distemper of the Colick.

2. They who are frequently and grievously obnoxious to the *Colick,* at length become also *Paralytick.* The case is so frequent here, that the succession of this Disease is accounted among its *prognosticks*; for those who are wont to suffer cruel fits of torments in the Belly, returning by intervals, or are troubled with pains about the Viscera of the *Abdomen*, cruel and almost continual, at length have wandring pains in their Body and Members, and then afterwards stupors or numness, and lastly resolutions or want of motion. The cause of these effects proceeds, both from the seat of the Disease, and the Morbifick matter being changed, to wit, this, which being very small but sharp and irritative, runs only into the *Sphlanchnick* Nerves, and so by reason of the Fibres of the *Viscera* being pulled, did stir up in them Cramps and pains; afterwards becoming more copious, and also duller and *Narcotick*, pours down thorow the *Spinal* Marrow, and entering into the Nerves destinated to these or those Members or Muscles, brings forth resolutions in the respective parts. We shall more largely shew the reason of this, when we treat of the *Colick*.

3. Wherefore the Gout.

It is a very ordinary observation, that the *Palsie* comes upon the *Gout* frequently, in the Members obnoxious to it; the reason of it is easily known, forasmuch as in this sickness the Morbifick matter is twofold, and doth depose salt and as it were lixivial Particles thorow the Arteries, and as we suppose others sourish or acetosous to come to them by the Nerves; (as shall be more largely shown hereafter) it is no wonder, if that at length, other sorts of Particles become companions to them, by other beaten ways, and at length either by filling or by compressing, obstruct the very small passages of the Spirits.

The evident Causes of the habitual Palsie.

As to what belongs to the evident causes of the *Palsie*, to wit, for what fore-causes or occasions those disposed to this Disease contract it the sooner, or that having been taken with it already, are yet wont to be more grievously tormented; I say, whatsoever doth more vitiate the Blood, also those things that stop up the Brain and its nervous appendix, or stir up suffusions of the Morbifick matter in it, also what do inflict a *Narcosis* or stupefaction to the Spirits, or lessen their numbers, may be brought hither. In this rank first occur the disorders in the six non-naturals, an evil manner of living, drinking thin clear Wine, or strong hot liquors, too much sleep, or too untimely, an idle and sedentary life, immoderate *Venus*, too much loss of blood, a moist Air or Marshie dwelling, an House new Plastered, Metalick fumes and vapors, frequent use of Narcoticks, or stupefying Medicines, or too much taking Tobacco, excess of cold, heat, or moisture, vehement and long passions of sadness or fear, with many others, all which we have not here leasure to recite.

Want or paucity of Spirits oftentimes the Cause of the Spurious or Bastard Palsy.

Thus much concerning the *Palsie*, in which the loco-motive faculty is abolished or lost, or very much hindered; by reason of the ways of the Spirits being obstructed, and themselves affected with a certain stupefaction, in the whole, or in the respective parts. There follows another kind of this Disease, depending upon the want and fewness of Spirits, in which, although motion be not deficient in any part or member wholly, yet it is not performed by any but weakly and depravedly only. For though the distemper'd are free from want of motion, they are not able however to move their members strongly, or to bear any weight; moreover, in every motive indeavour, they labour with a trembling of their limbs, which is only a defect of debility, and of a broken strength in the motive power. For when strength is wanting for the lifting up of any member firmly, and at one essay or endeavour, Nature flagging, acts with a more often repeated tryal or endeavour, and so the part being in motion, is compelled as it were to shake and tremble. To which happens, that when the nervous Fibres flagging or growing weak, they are not able to sustain the Tonick endeavour, or the stiffness in the Animal regiment, and these endeavouring or striving to exert or put forth their utmost power, enter into motions as it were Convulsive, and reiterate them perpetually. Wherefore, in some *Paralyticks*, there is always a trembling and shaking in all the limbs.

Those who thus become *Paralytick*, by the paucity or want of Spirits, and so from their small or diminished dispensation into the nervous *System*, are made obnoxious to such a Distemper, by reason of various causes and occasions.

First,

Of the Palsie.

First, Extream or unhealthy old age, or immoderate loss of blood, or the genital humor, induce this kind of *Paralytick* disposition in many men; to wit, because from the wasted blood and almost liveless, there is stilled forth into the Brain but a very small stock or provision of Animal Spirits. *For this Reason Old Men are obnoxious to this Disease.*

Secondly, Almost for the same reason, the loco-motive faculty grows weak or fails in persons greatly *Scorbutick*, and such as are full of indigested juice; for such not being fit for any strong exercise, go infirmly and weakly, and are very much tired by any long or swift walking; further, by any more heavy endeavour, they suffer oftentimes a numness in their limbs, with an impotency of moving them. For indeed, the bloody Mass is in these very watry, and stuft with impurities, and for that the Brain being weak and loose, as to its Pores, admits easily all sorts of filthinesses into it self; wherefore, fewer Animal Spirits being only created, and those not clear and subtil, but dull and hindred, by the adhesion of a more thick matter (although there is not always an obstruction of the ways, or a *Narcotick* disposition) they are not able to unfold themselves into motive endeavours. *2. Also Scorbutical Persons, and such as are full of ill humours.*

Thirdly, Not only *Scorbutical* persons, but also many others, hardly and long growing well from some *Chronical* Disease, are distemper'd with Members very much loosened from their due vigor and strength, and with a languishing of their Limbs; that though they are well in their stomach, and have a good and laudable Pulse and Urine, yet they are as if they were enervated, and cannot stand upright, and dare scarce enter upon local motions, or if they do, cannot perform them long: yea, some without any notable sickness, are for a long time fixed in their Bed, as if they were every day about to dye; whilst they lye undisturbed, talk with their Friends, and are chearful, but they will not, nor dare not move or walk; yea they shun all motion, as a most horrid thing. Without doubt in these, although the Animal Spirits do after a manner actuate and irradiate the whole nervous Stock, yet their numbers are so small, and in so few heaps, that when as many spirits ought to be heaped together somewhere in it for motion, there is great danger lest presently in the neighbouring parts, their continuity should be broken. Wherefore, when the spirits inhabiting the Brain, are conscious of the debility of others disposed in the Members, they themselves refuse local motions, for that it would be too difficult a task to impose on their companions; wherefore, the sick are scarce brought by any perswasion, to try whether they can go or not; Nevertheless, those labouring with a want of Spirits, who will exercise local motions, as well as they can, in the morning are able to walk firmly, to fling about their Arms hither and thither, or to take up any heavy thing; before noon the stock of the Spirits being spent, which had flowed into the Muscles, they are scarce able to move Hand or Foot. At this time I have under my charge a prudent and an honest Woman, who for many years hath been obnoxious to this sort of spurious *Palsie*, not only in her Members, but also in her tongue; she for some time can speak freely and readily enough, but after she has spoke long, or hastily, or eagerly, she is not able to speak a word, but becomes as mute as a Fish, nor can she recover the use of her voice under an hour or two. *3. Also others long sick.* *Hence some dare not venture on local motion.* *Others endeavouring, cannot bear them long.*

In this kind of spurious *Palsie*, arising from the defect, or rather the weakness of the Animal Spirits, than from their obstruction, it may be suspected, that not only the Spirits themselves, as to their first numbers of them, and particular originals, are in fault; but besides, that sometimes the imbecillity and impotency of local motion, doth in some measure also depend upon the fault of the explosive Copula, suffused every where from the blood, into the moving Fibres. For indeed, from a very *Cacochymical* blood, or full of juice, and for that cause vappid, and liveless; as the Animal Spirits are but few, that are instilled into the Brain, so it is probable, that those themselves derived from the Brain, into the Nerves, being disposed at length within the muscular Fibres, do meet with other Nitro-sulphureous Particles (which we have somewhere shown to be necessarily required to the Muscular motion) from the so vitious blood that are but dull, and degenerate, from the Elastick power; wherefore indeed the Spirits being concreted so evilly within the Muscles, even as Gunpowder being full of more thick seculences, rarely and weakly perform the acts of explosions. *The Impotency of the Spirits proceeds in some measure from the default of the explosive Copula.*

As to what belongs to the other species of the *Palsie*, in which the sensitive faculty is also affected, we say, that this is hurt either by it self, or together with the motive; and such an hurt of both together, doth almost only happen, forasmuch as the passages and ways of the Spirits are more firmly shut up, so that whether they tend forward or backward all their irradiation is intercepted: That sometimes happens, though rarely from the Morbific matter fallen down from the Brain into the oblong Marrow, but more often by reason of a grievous hurt of the Spine or Back-bone, *2. The kind of Palsy, in which Motion and Sense are hurt at once.*

as from a fall from on high, stroke, or wound inflicted on them: For from such occasions, by compressing the marrowy cord, or by too much distending or writhing it, all the tracts of the Spirits are blotted out.

3. Kind, in which sense only is affected.

Sometimes the sensitive faculty is hurt by it self, the motive being still safe; this is sufficiently obvious, and the reason very clear, of the organs, whose Nerves are only sensible, to wit, as of the sight, hearing, tast, and smell. But indeed, that in the extream habit of the body or members, the touch or feeling sometimes perishes, the loco-motive power being unhurt; as is ordinarily discerned in Lepers, those distemper'd with the *Elephantiasis*, and some Mad-men, who are wont to go naked, and lye on the ground, whose skin and musculous flesh are so benumned, that they feel not the gashes made in their flesh with a Pen-knife, nor Needles any where thrust into them; this I say seems very hard to be unfolded. But as to this it may be said, that perhaps the same Nerves, carry the instincts of motions, and the impressions of sensible things forward and backward, or to and fro, but that the same Fibres, which are loco-motive, are not altogether or chiefly sensible. We have elsewhere shewed, that its power is performed by the tendinous and musculous Fibres; but the sensible Species, is almost only received by the membranaceous Fibres; wherefore, the outer skin is the primary organ of feeling; after this, the Membranes covering the Muscles, and lastly those constituting the Viscera, are somewhat affected by the Tangible object. Wherefore, the loss or hurt of feeling arises, by reason of an hurt, brought to the exterior Membranes; to wit, when the Fibres of these are obstructed by a *Vitriolick* matter, or are benummed very much by excess of cold; so that the Animal Spirits, which ought to receive their impressions, are excluded from their organs. And indeed, from hence it appears, that these inhabiting the exterior Membranes, are only affected, because sense being lost, the members wither not, as when deprived of motion, but remain full and round; which is a sign that the Animal Spirits entring still the Nerves, and fleshy Fibres, do contribute their virtue to the office of nourishment; after what manner we have already shewn; but when motion is lost, the Spirits are almost wholly banished from those parts, and the flesh consumes, because the nourishing matter, though carried thorow the Arteries, is not assimilated. We have largely discoursed of this in our Treatise of the Nerves.

Wherefore feeling is sometimes lost, and motion fast.

What is the proper Organ of feeling.

The Prognostick of the Palsy.

The Theory of this many-form'd Disease being now at length finished, its kinds and differences, all, or at least the most and chiefest of it, together with the reasons of each of them, being rehearsed in order, we shall shew next those things which belong to its prognosticks and Cure.

1 Every *Palsie*, whether accidental or habitual, and either of them, whether universal or partial, or whether suddenly excited or by degrees, if it happens that the knowing and vital faculty be unhurt, it ought not to be accounted an acute Disease; but being free from sudden danger, admits a long Cure, or at least an endeavour of it.

2. This Disease coming from a solitary evident cause, as from a stroke, a fall, wound, *&c.* or coming upon the *Apoplexy, Carus, Convulsion,* the *Colick,* or other Distempers of the Brain, or nervous *System,* if it be not in a short time altered for the better, or gives not place to Medicines, it remains for the most part incureable.

3. If that a total resolution follows, from a total obstruction in the beginning of the oblong Marrow, or from the Back-bone being vehemently hurt, and that sense and motion are both taken away, the Distemper is hardly, or scarce at all to be Cured.

4. Those who are once cured of a *Palsie,* arising from an evident solitary cause, do not so easily relapse into the same, as when the Disease depends upon a *procatartick* cause

5. A *Palsie,* happening to men of years, to *Cacochymical,* very *Scorbutical,* and intemperate persons, although the Distemper be not very great, is difficultly Cured.

Its Cure.

Three means of healing, according to which this Disease is, 1. Either accidental; 2. The off-spring of another Disease; 3. Habitual.

As the *Palsies* are manifold, and are from diverse causes, so the Cure is not to be instituted always after one manner, but after a various method, to wit, appropriate to every kind of this Disease. For the most part there are these three kinds of it, or rather there are three means of healing; of which there ought to be had concerning the Cure of this Disease, now this, now that, or now another; to wit, because resolution (whatever, or in what place soever it be) is either caused, 1. from an external accident, as a stroke, a fall, a wound, excess of cold, or the like, suddenly: Or 2. It succeeds to some other Distemper, as the *Apoplexy, Carus, Colick,* or a long Feavour: Or, 3. It is primary and a Disease by it self, by degrees excited, and depending upon a *procatartick* cause, or a previous provision. Concerning each of these, we shall speak particularly.

1. Therefore

1. Therefore, when the *Palsie* is caused, by reason of some accident, with a vehement hurt, there are not many intentions of healing; but only that the part hurt may recover its pristine conformation. And first of all, that the Blood and other humors flowing to it, being weak and distemper'd, and staying there, might not increase the hurt, *Phlebotomy* is most requisite in this case, and presently to be celebrated; then the belly being made slippery by the use of Clysters, and a slender dyet, if the matter requires it, let there be instituted either easily digested meats, or moderate *Hydroticks*, or water meats; to wit, that whilst the sick is kept in bed, he may continue in a gentle sweat, that all the superfluities may copiously exhale from the hurt part, and that the Spirits being gently agitated, may repeat their former ways and tracts, within those Pores and passages, so unlocked by the warm Effluvia's.

1. The Cure of the former.

For this end, the Powder *ad Casum*, described in the *Augustan Pharmacopœa*, or as it is in ours, is of common use; let there be given of *Irish* Slate, to the quantity of about a dram, in a draught of white Wine warm'd, or of Posset-drink made of it; and repeated every six or eight hours. Besides, if there be at hand the *Decoctum Traumaticum*, let it be taken ever now and then, frequently in Posset-drink, or a Decoction of the Roots of Madder, or of Butter-bur, or of St. *Johns-wort* Flowers.

A Powder for a Fall.

Further, in the mean time, let the distemper'd part be carefully lookt to, which may be easily known, partly from the hurt inflicted, and partly from the loosened members. If there be any thing dislocated in it, you must take care that as soon as it can, it may be put again in its place; if a Tumor, Contusion, or a wound be excited, they are to be succour'd by *Balsams*, *Liniments*, Stuphes or Fomentations, or Pultesses: But if nothing preternatural appears outwardly, let a Plaster of *Oxycrocium* and of Red-lead, each alike, what will suffice, be laid upon it, and let the sick be kept quiet, and in a moderate heat, for three or four days. If the resolution remains confirmed, and the afflux of new matter be not feared, let more resolving and discussing Remedies be applied to the distemper'd places; wherefore, make use of Fomentations, and hotter Oyntments, yea natural Baths, if they are at hand, or at least artificial. Sometimes it may be expedient for the distemper'd Members to be wrapped in Horse-dung, or in warm grains, and to be kept so for some time; and lastly, between whiles, besides the use of these, to add Clysters and gentle Purges. But if no help follows these administrations, the sick ought then to be handled with the like long method, and with the same Remedies, as those that have an habitual *Palsie*, or any other coming upon other Diseases and confirmed; which means of Cure, for every common *Palsie* more deeply rooted, shall be shewed anon.

Topicks to be applied to the Distempered part.

2. When the *Palsie* coming upon a *Feavour*, *Apoplexy*, *Carus*, or other *Cephalick* or Convulsive Diseases, is greatly and suddenly excited, first the Physician ought to endeavour the taking away of the conjunct cause, which hath almost ever its seat in the oblong or spinal Marrow. Wherefore, at the beginning of the Disease, Blood-letting, and Purging (if nothing shews the contrary) Clysters, Vesicatories, Cupping-glasses, Sneezing Powders, Oyntments, and other administrations used in *Cephalick* Diseases, to wit, which by any means may shake off, or pull away the deadly matter, fixed to the Medullary Trunk, or to the little heads of the Nerves coming from it, are to be made use of. If that at first, the force of Medicine effects nothing within fifteen or twenty days, for that the Distemper is radicated, and become habitual, it must be expunged by a long method, and equally by preservatory as well as curatory Indications; of which we shall speak anon.

2. How the Palsie coming upon another Disease is to be cured.

3. The habitual *Palsie*, depending upon a *procatartick* cause, whether it be in *fieri* or in disposition, or whether it be made, or in the nest or bird, either requires a peculiar means of healing

The Cure of the habitual Palsie.

There are two chief causes of the former, in both which the Curatory Method, respecting only the fore-leading Causes, is designed after the like manner, to wit, whether any falling dangerously ill of the *Palsie*, or growing well of it, relapses into danger, the same Remedies almost are to be insisted on.

Whilst it is in fieri, or doing.

The intentions therefore of healing are, First, That the offices of *Chilification*, and of making of Blood, be rightly performed, and matter for the procreating the Animal Spirits be supplied, both laudable and sufficient to the Head; then, Secondly, That the Brain being still firm and well made, the heterogeneous Particles being excluded, it may admit all that are fitting, and rightly exalt then into Animal Spirits. For these ends, I think convenient to propose the following method, which ought to be varied, according to the various constitutions of the sick,

The Intentions of healing respect the Blood and the Brain.

In Spring and Fall, that they enter into the ordinary course of Physick, yea the whole year besides, some Remedis are in constant use. Blood-letting is not always convenient to all men: But though we forbid this, it is not for the same reason with the

the Ancients, supposing the *Palsie* to be a cold Disease, but because the Animal Spirits, are both procreated out of the Blood, and become also Elastick in the motional Fibres, by reason of the bloody *Copula*; therefore, if plenty of this be taken away, they grow weak and deficient. Which thing indeed I have observed in many, and for the most part languishings and tremblings to have been begun in the Arm, out of which the *Bloodletting.* blood had been taken. However in some, indued with a sharp and hot blood, and apt to flame forth too much, though disposed to the *Palsie*, it is sometimes convenient to let blood a little and sparingly.

A Purge. About the Æquinox, a Purge ought to be instituted, and after due times between, to be iterated three or four times. But first, if nothing oppose, let a Vomit be given, of the Salt of *Vitriol*, *Sulphur* of *Antimony*, or an Infusion of *Crocus Metallorum*, or of *Mercurius Vitæ*; then let there be taken Pills of *Amber*, or of *Aloephanginæ*, by it self, or with the *Resine* of *Jalap*, every seventh or eighth day. At other times we *Cephalick Remedies.* prescribe *Cephalick* Remedies, such as in the sleepy Diseases: viz. *Electuaries*, *Powders*, *Spirits*, and *Volatile Salts*, *Tinctures*, *Elixirs*, with distilled Waters and *Apozems*, sometimes these, sometimes those, or others. Let Issues be made in the Arm or Leg, yea in fat people, and such as are full of ill humors, in both together, or between the shoulders. Let them drink all the year medicated Beer of Sage, Betony, Stechades, Sassafrass Wood, and Winterines Bark. Wine and Women ought to be forbidden, or but moderately to be used.

2. How the Disease in habit is to be cured. If that the *Palsie* be excited, after a previous disposition, either of one side, or in some members, and that it still continues, notwithstanding the first attempt of Medicine, a long and complicated method is always requisite, and oftentimes doth not suffice; for not only the Disease, or its conjunct cause, or its foregoing severally, but *Bloodletting and Purging cautiously and rarely to be admitted.* all together ought to be opposed: for which ends *Phlebotomy* being for the most part interdicted, only a gentle Purge and rarely is convenient. Besides, some chief *Cephalick* Medicines, and *Antiscorbuticks* are wont to help against the foregoing cause of this Disease. But all of this sort, are not convenient to all; yea as we have observed in the Scurvy, according to the various Constitutions of the Sick, there are also Re*Altering Medicines ought to be given with choice.* medies of a diverse kind and virtue. For to *Cholerick Paralyticks*, to wit, in whose sharp and hot Blood there is much of *Salt* and *Sulphur*, and very little of *Serum*, the more hot Medicines and indued with very active Particles, are not agreeable, yea are often hurtful; which things notwithstanding are very profitable to Phlegmatick persons, whose Blood is colder, and contains much of *Serum*, and but few active Elements. Wherefore, for this twofold state or condition of sick persons, it seems convenient that we institute here a double Method of Cure, and two classes of Medicines, of which these may be given to cold *Parlyticks*, and those to the hot.

How the Palsy is to be healed in a cold temperament. In the former case, for the taking away the *Procatartick* cause, after Vomiting and Purging being rightly instituted, I was wont to prescribe according to these following forms.

Electuary. Take *of the Conserves of the leaves of the Garden Scurvy-grass, of Rocket, made with an equal part of Sugar, each three ounces; of Ginger Candied in India half an ounce, of the rinds of Oranges and Lemons Candied, each six drams; of the Powder of the Claws and Eyes of Crabs, each four scruples; of the Species of Diambre two drams, of Winterene Bark one dram and a half, of the Roots of Zedoary, the lesser Galingal, of Cubebs, the Seeds of Water-Cresses, Rocket, each one dram; of the Spirits of Scurvy-grass, Lavender, each two drams; of the Syrup of Candied Ginger, what will suffice to make an Electuary. Take of it about the quantity of a Walnut, at eight of the Clock in the Morning, and at five in the Afternoon, drinking after it a pint of* *Coffee.* *the following Decoction, warm, or Coffee, with the leaves of Sage boiled in it six ounces, or of Viper Wine three ounces.*

A Decoction. Take *of the shavings of Lignum Sanctum six ounces, of Sarsaparilla, and of Sassaphras, each four ounces; of white and yellow Sanders, of the shavings of Ivory, of Hartshorn, each half an ounce, infuse them according to art, and boil them in sixteen pints of Spring water, till half be consumed, adding of Crude Antimony in Powder, and tyed in a rag four ounces, of the Root of the Aromatick Reed, of the lesser Galingal, each half an ounce; of the Florentine Iris one ounce, of Cardamums six drams, of Coriander Seeds half an ounce, six Dates, make a Decoction to be used for ordinary drink.*

Spirits. Going to sleep, and first in the morning, *let a Dose of the Spirits of Sut, or Hartshorn, or of Armoniacal Amber, or of Blood, &c. be taken, with three ounces of the following distilled water.*

A Distilled Water. Take *of the leaves or roots of Aron one pound, of the leaves of Garden Scurvy-grass,*

Of the Palsie.

of the greater Rocket, of Rosemary, Sage, Savory, Thyme, four handfuls; of the Flowers of Lavender three handfuls, the outer rinds of ten Oranges, and six Lemons, of Winterans Bark three ounces, of the roots of the lesser Galingal, of Calamus Aromaticus, the Florentine Iris, each two ounces; of Cubebs, Cloves, Nutmegs, each two ounces; all being cut and bruised, pour to them of white Wine, and of Brunswick Beer or Mum, each four pints: distil it in common Stills, and let all the liquor be mixed together.

Sometimes in the place of the Electuary may be taken for fifteen or twenty days a Dose of the *Tincture* of *Sulphur* Turpentined, of the *Tincture* of *Antimony*, or of *Amber*: Also sometimes *Elixir Proprietatis*, or of *Pæony*; let them be taken in a spoonful of distilled Water, drinking after it three ounces of the same: Also sometimes the following Powders or Lozenges may be taken by turns, in the medical course. *Tinctures and Elixirs.*

Take of the Powder of Vipers flesh of *Monpillier* prepared one ounce, of the hearts and livers of the same half an ounce, of Species Diambre two ounces; make a Powder, take one dram once or twice a day with the distilled Water three ounces, or with Viper Wine, with a Decoction of the leaves of Sage, of the root and seeds of the Burdock, and the Candied roots of Eringo, made of Spring-water, what will suffice, and boiled to one moiety; six or eight ounces in the Morning warm, expecting to sweat after it.

Take of *Bezoartick Mineral Solar* half an ounce, of Cloves powdered two drams, mingle them, make a Powder and divide it into twelve parts, let one be taken after the same manner, twice in a day; between these kind of Remedies, gentle purging may be often used. *Powders.*

Take of the Powder of the picked roots of Zedoary, the lesser Galingal, each half a dram; of Species Diambre one dram, of the Powder of the seeds of Mustard, Rocket, Scurvygrass, Water-Cresses, each half a dram; make of them all a fine Powder, add to it of the Oyl of the purest Amber half a dram, and with white Sugar dissolved in the compounded Pæony water, and boiled up to the consistency of Lozenges six ounces: make Lozenges according to art, weighing each half a dram: Eat of them three or four twice in a day, drinking after every Dose, of the liquors before mentioned. *Lozenges.*

Take of the Powder of Virginian Snakeweed two drams, of the lesser Galingal one dram, of the gummed extract of the remains of the distillation of the Elixir Vitæ of Quercitan two drams, of the Flowers of Sal Armoniack, (or the most pure Volatile Salt of Sut or Harts-horn) one dram, of the Balsom of Peru one scruple, of the Balsom of Capivus what will suffice to make a mass; let it be made into small Pills involved in the Species Diambre. The Dose is half a dram evening or morning. *Pills.*

Take of the Resine or Gum of Guaicum three drams, of the Species Diambre one dram, of the Chymical Oyl of Guaicum rightly rectified one dram and a half, of liquid Amber what will suffice to make a mass: let it be formed into Pills, to be taken after the same manner.

If that the Palsie happens in a Cholerick temper, or to a young Man, it admits only of milder Medicines, and all the more hot things, and *Elastick*, do but imbitter the Disease: The following forms are in use, for the taking away of its foregoing cause. *How the Cholerick or hot Palsie is to be cured.*

Take of the Conserves of the Flowers of Betony, of Fumitory, of Primroses, each two ounces; of the Species Diambre one dram, of Ivory, Crabs Eyes, and Claws, each four scruples; of the Powder of the Flowers of Pæony two drams, of Lignum Aloes, of yellow Sanders, each one dram; of the Salt of Wormwood one dram and a half, and with the Syrup of the Flowers of Pæony what will suffice, make an Electuary. The Dose is two drams twice in a day, drinking after it, either the simple water of the Flowers of Aron, or of the following Compounded Water three ounces, or of the Decoction of Sage, with the leaves of Tea infused in it four or six ounces. *An Electuary.*

Take of the Roots of Aron or Cuckopint, of the male Pæony, Angelica, Imperatoria, each half a pound; of the Flowers of Sage, Rosemary, Marjoram, Brooklime, Water-Cresses, each four handfuls; of the rinds of six Oranges, and four Lemons, of Primroses, Cowslips, Marigold flowers, each three handfuls; let them be all bruised and cut, and pour to them of new Milk six pints, of Malaga Wine one quart; distil them in common Stils, and let the whole liquor be mixed together. *A Distilled Water.*

Sometimes instead of the Electuary may be taken between whiles, for fourteen or fifteen days, of the Syrup of Steel, of which let one spoonful be taken in three ounces of the distilled Water: It may be made after this manner. *Chalybeats or Steeled Medicines.*

Take

Of the Palsie.

Take of the whitest Sugar dissolved in black Cherry Water, and boil'd up to a consistency, eight ounces, adding to it of our Steel in Powder three drams; let them be stirred together over the fire, and then by degrees pour to it of the Water of Rosemary warm twelve ounces; let it boil gently for a quarter of an hour, scumming it, and pouring it forth warm thorow an hair sieve or strainer.

There may be also made steeled Lozenges after this manner, to wit, with Sugar sufficiently boiled with Steel, adding of the Chymical Oyl of Amber or of Rosemary half a dram, and presently let it be poured forth that it may flow into a consistency of Lozenges: The Dose is two drams twice in a day, drinking after it of distilled Water, or of the following Apozem six ounces.

A Decoction. Take of *China* Root one ounce, of the shavings of *Ivory*, *Harts-horn*, each half an ounce; of white and yellow *Sanders*, of the Wood of the *Mastick-tree*, each half an ounce; let them be infused in warm water and close stopt for a whole night, six pints; in the morning add to them of the Roots of *Chervil*, of sweet smelling *Avens*, of *Broom*, and *Parsley*, each one ounce and a half; of the dryed leaves of ground *Ivy*, *Sage*, *Germander*, *Betony*, each one handful, of Coriander seeds three drams; let them be boiled till half is consumed, then add to it of white *Wine* half a pint, and strain it into a jugg, upon the leaves of *Water-Cresses* bruised two handful: Let it infuse warm and close shut, for two hours, strain it again, and keep it in a close *Vessel* well stopt.

In the Scorbutick *Palsie*, the Juices and expressions of Herbs, do often bring notable help.

The juice and expressions of Herbs. Take of the leaves of *Brooklime*, *Water-Cresses*, and *Plantan* fresh gathered, each four handfuls, bruise them together, and pour to them of the distilled Water but now described eight ounces, squeese the juice strangly forth, and keep it in a glass, and take of it twice or thrice in a day three or four ounces.

At the extream Physical hours, *viz.* Morning and Evening, may be taken these following Pills.

Pills. Take of *Millipedes* prepared three drams and a half, of Pearls one dram and a half, of the Root of the *Cretick Dittany* one dram, *Venice Turpentine* what will suffice to make a mass: let it be formed into small Pills, the Dose is half a dram, drinking after it a draught of the distilled Water.

For ordinary drink, let there be prescribed, either a Bochet of Sarse, China, yellow Sanders, &c. or small Ale, with the dryed leaves of ground Ivy, boiled in it; and of Sage, with the Wood of Sassafras, infused therein.

2. Whilst these things are doing, for the taking away the foregoing cause of the Disease, there is no less a curatory care required, for its conjunct cause; to wit, that all obstructed places being opened, they might admit the Animal Spirits, free from stupefaction, and that they may pass freely thorow.

Topick and particular Remedies. There are two chief kinds of Remedies, which conduce to those ends, *viz.* one particular and private, to be applied to the distemper'd places: to wit, that by Fomentations, Oyntments, Plasters, and such like outward applications, the sleepy Spirits might be awakned, and their passages opened: the other universal, to wit, that the Blood and Spirits, and the other humors (and the active Particles flowing in the whole Body) being very much agitated, and put into a rapid motion, like a torrent, they might cast down and remove all impacted heaps or stays, by which the Spirits are obstructed.

The administrations used to the distempered parts are so ordinarily and commonly known, that it were superfluous to insist here on the describing them more largely. First *Liniments*, made out of Oyls, Oyntments, and Balsoms, are to be applied according to the temper of the Patient, more or less hot, and with frictions or strong rubbing twice a day. Sometimes, before these are made use of, Fomentations made of *Cephalick* Herbs, or spices boiled in Spring Water, adding to it sometimes Strong Waters, Wine, or Bear or their Lees. Further, oftentimes it is convenient to make about the distemper'd places Blisters, and to use Cupping-glasses, and Medicines to take away the hairs, and to raise pimples. Little Bags and Plasters often help. Moreover, if the business will admit it, let the *Paralytick* members be covered over with hot

Of the Palsie.

hot grains, or with the refuse of the Grapes when flung out of the Wine-press; or let them be thrust into the belly of a Beast new slain, or bathed in an artificial Bath, or in the natural Baths, and be kept for a long while in any of these.

But if these help not, you must then come to universal Remedies, or great Remedies; of which sort, in the first place, are *Diaphoreticks* or sweating Medicines, *Mercurial* Medicines stirring up Salivation; and strong Vomiting Medicines: of each of which we shall speak briefly. *Universal Remedies.*

In the Cure of the *Palsie*, sometimes *Diaphoreticks*, or Medicines causing sweats, do very much help; and that they sometimes are hurtful, the common people do ordinarily observe. Wherefore it is very requisite, that we should unfold the reasons of this so different effect; and that so indications may be taken as to the use or rejection of them. *1. Diaphoreticks.*

Therefore, a plentiful sweating is wont to be helpful sometimes to *Paralyticks*, chiefly for two reasons; to wit, for that it doth thrust forth or exterminate in a great measure the impurities of the Blood, and the nervous juice, being apt to breath forth; so that the Morbific matter doth not flow any more to the Brain, and the distemper'd parts; and that whatever hath already flowed forth from them, is partly conveyed forth of doors. Then, Secondly, Because the Effluvia's of heat falling away from the boiling blood, do very much open the nervous Passages before obstructed, whilst in evaporating they pass thorow them, and make an open way for the Spirits. Wherefore this administration is chiefly and almost only convenient for those, whose Blood is not stuffed with fixed Salt and Sulphur, but is diluted with a limpid and saltless Serum. For on the contrary, *Paralyticks* whose blood and humors are full of fierce, Exotick, and fixed Particles of enormous Salts and Sulphur, and unfit to be exhaled, do often receive great harm by a violent and forced sweating. Of this kind of effect we have assigned these two causes, to wit, because that the Morbific Particles, by reason of agitation being too much exalted, become more outragious; then secondly, because these being more plentifully brought to the Brain and nervous Stock, they oftentimes increase the old obstructions, and not rarely produce new. *They are not to be administred indifferently to all.* *They often hurt the Cholerick.*

That a plentiful sweating or *Diaphoresis* may be easily provoked, both internal Medicines, and outward administrations are wont to be made use of. The former stir up either the Blood or Serum into an heat, or provoke the heart into more swift motions; and for that cause (whether one or both be done) when the bloody liquor is rapidly circulated thorow the Heart and Vessels, and is wrought into a frothy swelling up, there is a necessity, that very many Effluvia's, which are the matter of sweat, should go away from it. For this end, Medicines of a various kind are commended to *Paralyticks*, of which the most noted are, a Decoction of *Guaicum, Sarsaparilla, &c.* Spirits and Oyl of *Guaicum*, the simple mixture, Flowers and Spirits of *Sal Armoniack*, *Aurum Diaphoreticum*, the Salt of *Vipers*, as also the Powder and Wine of the same: the solar *Bezoartick minerale*, Tincture of *Antimony, &c.* *Sweating Medicines.*

External administrations move sweat, because they hold in, and stir up the moderate heat in the whole body; and so the blood being made hot, is compelled to move more swiftly, and to evaporate more, and at the same time, the Pores of the skin, being unlocked, readily let forth all the Particles that are apt to exhale. For this use, besides the Bed-cloaths (which only hold in the Effluvia's of heat sent from the body, about it still) there are little sweating Chairs, or Stoves, made hot with Coals or with the Spirits of Wine: also Hot-houses and Baths of various kinds and forms, and our natural Baths, are wont to be made use of: But of all of them, our natural Baths of the *Bath* (if they agree with the temper of the sick) are thought to be the best Remedy; which the many Crutches, hung up as so many trophies of this Disease being overcome, belonging to many Cured of the Palsie, do sufficiently shew. *Stoves, Baths, Natural Baths.*

But as the best Medicines, if they prove not a Remedy to the Disease, often pass into poisons; so the use of *Baths*, when it cures not some *Paralyticks*, renders them much worse; so that when as the sick had before many members distemper'd and resolved or loosened, there was no other occasion for them of leaving behind them there their Crutches, unless it were because they could use them no longer. We have above shewed the cause of this; to wit, because bathing, shaking, or moving the blood, and all the humors, more exalts all the Morbific and extraneous particles, and they becoming more outragious, drives them from the Viscera into the bloody mass; from whence (when they cannot easily evaporate) entring into the Brain and nervous Stock, increase the *Paralytick* Distemper, and very often adds to it the Convulsive. For this reason Bathing sometimes actuates or stirs up the *Nephritick*, and the Gouty disposition; and further, in many where there was not a disposition, it causes a spitting of blood, the *Asthma*, or Consumption. Wherefore Baths ought not to be tryed *When the use of Baths is hurtful in the Palsie.*

without

Of the Palsie.

without the advice of a *Physician*, and then having tryed them, if they seem not agreeable, they are to be soon left.

Salivation. I have by my own experience sufficiently try'd, and known also by that of several other *Physicians*, that some *Paralyticks* have been cured by Salivation excited by *Mercury*. But I think this kind of Remedy, is only to be used to the habitual *Palsie*, to wit, which hath its foregoing cause in the Blood and Brain, easily moveable, and its conjunct cause, in the nervous appendix, not very fixed. But when this Distemper is caused from an outward and great hurt, or follows upon the *Carus, Apoplexy*, or *Convulsions*, a Salivation or spitting is attempted in vain, and sometimes not without great hurt. But whoever are indued with a weak and too loose a Brain, and are obnoxious to frequent Convulsive motions, are not rashly to make use of *Mercury*. Yet sometimes a Salivation in an habitual *Palsie*, and not very fixed, hath highly profited, forasmuch as by taking away the impurities of the blood, it cuts off all the nourishment of the Disease; also, because some *Mercurial* Particles, whilst passing thorow the Brain, and entring the nervous passages, divide the Morbific matter impacted in them, and drawing its parts one from another, variously disperse some forward, and others backwards; when oftentimes it is the fault of other Medicines, that they only urge forward the heap obstructing the ways of the Spirits, so that if they pull it not to pieces, they drive it more firmly into the obstructed places.

Vomitories. In some measure it is for this reason also, that Vomits do frequently yield notable help in the Cure of the *Palsie*, to wit, because they draw away the nourishment of the conjunct cause, yea and do not always drive forward, but pull back the matter impacted in the Nerves, do greatly shake, and often break it in bits; so that when the continuity of the heap is broken, the Animal Spirits themselves easily dissipate the Particles of the Morbific matter, loosened one from another. We have before mentioned another reason of the help of *Emeticks* in the Sleepy Disease, which also may have a place in the *Palsie*.

Histories and Examples of Paralyticks. Instances and examples of *Paralyticks* are so ordinarily and almost daily met with, that their various Types and Histories would fill a Volume, if they should be described. Wherefore I shall only add here some few and more rare ones, to wit, one or two, by which the chief kinds of this Disease may be illustrated. For as it will be little to the purpose, to describe the resolutions of members, excited by outward accident, as from a fall, wound, or stroke; I shall insist only on those cases, where the *Palsie* either arises by its self, after a previous disposition, or comes upon some other Disease.

The Example of the Palsie habitual excited of it self. The first History. Some time since, a certain Gentleman, strong, and well flesh'd, and beyond the tenth lustre of his age, almost ever healthful; at length being given to a sedentary and idle life, and from thence becoming more dull and heavy than usual, refused any exercise, and more hard motion of the body: moreover he was wont to be melancholick and sad, upon any light occasion, yea sometimes to break forth into weeping and tears, without any manifest occasion. This man a little after (which I also observed in many others) was distemper'd with an imbecillity and trembling of all his members, and then with a resolution of the lower parts; to which Disease (for that he was melancholick, and soon weary of Medicines) he gave himself up as overcome, and by degrees being made more weak and languishing, he dyed within six months.

I remember many others, but especially two committed to our Cure, who were highly ingenious and very learned, in the former part of their life; but afterwards in their declining age, partly through the evil disposition of the body, and partly through the perturbation of the mind, became dull and forgetful, and after that (notwithstanding the use of the Remedies in the beginning of the Disease) *Paralytick*.

The Reason of it. In these kind of cases, first the Brain it self, as to its temper and make, seems to be so weakened, that the Spirits inhabiting it, becoming torpid, and wandring out of their tracts, did not rightly perform the acts of Memory and Imagination; then by reason of their failure and disorders in their first spring or fount, (which are not enough taken notice of till they become uncureable) there is a necessity, that an impotency or an eclipse of the motive faculty, should succeed in the nervous appendix. But the Cure of these Distempers, as often as they are excited from such an occasion, is ever very difficult, because the antecedent cause is hardly or scarce ever taken away.

The second History more rare and notable. A young man, of a Sanguine temper, ingenious, and for the most part healthy, sitting in a Chair after a large supper, and immoderate drinking of Wine, was so distemper'd with a numness or stupidity in his right hand, that his Gloves which he held in it, fell of themselves out of his hand; then getting up, and endeavouring to walk, he felt a resolution or loosening in his Thigh and Leg of the same side, and

a little

Of the Palsie.

a little afterwards falling into a certain hebetude or dulness of mind, and stupefaction, yet without an *Apoplexy*; for he was still himself, answering aptly to questions asked him, though but slowly and with difficulty, and doing those things that were bid him. Presently a skilful *Physician* being sent for, *Phlebotomy*, Vomiting, and Purging, were celebrated in order, Cupping-Glasses, Scarification, Oyntments, Frictions, and other fit administrations were carefully applied: Nevertheless the *Palsie* increased, that besides the motion of his members on the right side being taken away, he also lost the sight of that eye; yet still being stupefied and sleepy, he was *compos mentis*, and knew his Friends, and being conscious of his infirmity, and solicitous for the recovering his health, he took all remedies were given him, but notwithstanding all this, the animal functions daily more and more languished, and at length by their consent the vital; so that about the seventh or the eighth day, from thence, falling sometimes into a Delirium, and sometimes into Convulsions, or other distractions of the Animal Spirits, his strength being at length quite lost, he yielded to Death.

His Head being opened, the anterior cavity of the Brain was filled, partly with *An Anatomick Observation, which the Cafe is explained.* ichorous Blood, partly concreted and in clodders or gobbets, with plenty of Serum; Hence, as it is easie to conceive, from this deluge, pressing upon one of the Streaked bodies, and binding up its Pores and Passages, the flowing of the Spirits into the nervous appendix of that side was hindred, and for that reason, the resolution in the respective members was excited; and because of the *optick* chamber, where it is inserted into the Streaked Body, being also pressed together, the Eye of that side lost its sight; further, because the *Callous* Body, chambring that den, was somewhat pressed by the heaped matter, from thence the hebetude and stupefaction of the chief functions of the soul were excited, yet without their subversion or inordination. By reason of the evil being fixed on the substance of the Brain, and the Spirits inhabiting it, these sorts of Distempers do proceed, and not from the impletion of the Ventricle, as appears clear enough by this instance, and by what we have elsewhere mentioned.

A Servant to a certain Nobleman, being about forty years of Age, indued with *The third History.* a sharp Blood, and Cholerick temperament, and for some time obnoxious to the *Vertigo*, whilst he was riding in the Country to a certain Village, being taken suddenly with a dizziness in the Head, he fell upon the ground headlong, and being instantly taken up by the inhabitants, and put to bed, he lay for many hours insensible, and as if dead. But afterward being awakened, he felt an universal *Palsie*, and all his members loosened on both sides. Visiting this Man the day after, I took from him presently about twelve ounces of Blood, and prescribed forthwith some other Remedies, both outward administrations and also inward Medicines to be carefully given him, and indeed with good success; for after five or six days, he began to bend and stretch forth his hands, and feet, yea, though slowly, to move them about hither and thither; then by the constant use of Remedies, within two months, he was able to rise up, to stand on his feet, and to walk a little with the help of Crutches; then using at home for some time daily a temperate artificial Bath, he got strength and motion by degrees in his members; at length as soon as the season of the year served, going to the *Bath*, within a fortnights time, by the use of the Baths, he grew perfectly well, and leaving his Crutches behind him returned whole.

In this case, the *Apoplectick* matter falling down out of the middle of the Brain, be- *The Reason of this.* ing divided and largely poured forth, entered both the Streaked Bodies, and so caused the universal *Palsie*; but forasmuch as being more stretched abroad, the same was the less thickly impacted in the Marrowy Pores, therefore being more moveable, and apt to be shaken off, it did admit so easie and quick a Cure. To this man the more hot Remedies were not agreeable, so that I was compelled sometimes to iterate *Phlebotomy*, and to give him only temperate Medicines. That the *Palsie* doth sometimes succeed, not only *Cephalick* Distempers, but also the *Colick*, and *Scurvey*, (as we have already hinted) the following History, (of which we have somewhere made mention as to its *Scorbutick* reason,) will manifestly declare.

A young and handsome Woman, after being brought to bed, fell into a Tertian *The fourth History.* Feavour, this coming at length daily upon her, and protracted, brought in a most cruel and continual *Colick*. The pains at first tormented her only in her Belly, with vomiting and most sharp torments. Being a long while vexed with these, and almost worn out; at length she began to be molested with a stupefaction, and a sense of tingling, such as comes upon a member laid upon. Nor was it long after that but a *Palsie* (which this other Distemper very often foreruns) follow'd in her whole Body. In this condition being brought to *Oxford*, she was committed to our Cure (the noted *Physician* Dr. *Lydell* being also called to our assistance.) In this sick Gentlewoman, not only all her greater Members, as her Arms and Legs, but almost every lesser

lesser joynt or limb, was almost wholly loosened, that she could not move hand nor foot, or the fingers or toes of either, Further, she was so distemper'd with a wasting away, that she was nothing but skin and bones, however (and from which only we had any hopes) she had a good Pulse, and a lively aspect.

The Cure expoposed. After we had administer'd to her for many weeks, most choice Medicines, both *Antiparalytick* and *Antiscorbutick*, almost of every kind, and according to the various methods, without any success; at length we proposed to her, and to her Friends, *Salivation*, as the most powerful, though also most dangerous of all other Remedies; they not long deliberating upon it, resolve to try a Medicine rather doubtful than none, and though the same should be wholly inefficacious. Therefore by God's help, we gave her in a small Dose, precipitate of *Mercury cum sole*, and the next day repeated it. On the third day, a moderate and easie Salivation beginning, gently succeeded for a week, without any malignant *symptom*; but then the sick complaining of a grievous Headach, and *Vertigo*, began to be afflicted with Convulsive motions; so that there was a necessity to let her lye down, and depress the Salivation, and as soon as we could, to break off this course, by the Serous Flux of water being called away from the Head, to the other parts; which indeed Clysters, frequently given, *Epispatick* or drawing and revulsive Plasters, applied to several places, together with Cordials and Opiates inwardly given her, did quickly effect; and then presently this Gentlewoman finding her self a little better, began to stretch forth and bend her fingers and toes, and sometimes to move her members from one place to another. Her spitting ceasing, being gently purged, she took for many days a Decoction of *China, Sarsa, Saunders, Ivory*, &c. with the addition of the dried leaves of Betony, Sage, female Betony, &c. and between whiles with that, Spirits of Hartshorn, or of Sut, *Cephalick* and *Cardiack* Confections, also Powders and proper *Juleps*. Within a months space, being held up by her Servants, she could stand on her feet, and walk a little in her Chamber; moreover, sleeping and eating moderately, she every day got flesh and strength, and at length by the use of the temperate Bathes at the *Bath*, she grew well.

The Reason of it. The reason of the aforesaid case seems to be after this manner: First, the vitious blood had contracted an intermitting Feavour, then by reason of the long stay of that Feavour, the same being made more vitious, did also impart its evil to the Brain and nervous Stock; the matter being poured forth from the blood on them, together with the nervous juice, being only at first *Spasmodick* or Convulsive, and entering much into the *Intercostal* Nerves, excited the *Colick*; but then, that being more largely poured forth into the Nerves of the *spinal* Marrow, brought on painful contractions in the nervous Fibres, in almost the whole habit of the Body; and when from the assiduous and plentiful incourse of the Convulsive matter, the passages of the Brain and Nerves being very much unlock'd, became very open; at length the more thick and *vitriolick* Particles entering with them, disseminated the *Paralytick* Distemper thorow the whole Body. Concerning its Cure, the Remedies used before Salivation did not profit, because they urging this Morbifick matter still forward, drove it more deeply and closely into the nervous passages; but the *mercurial* Particles, because they dissolved the matter so compacted, first opened the way of Cure, which afterwards being much helped daily by *Cephalick* Medicines, it was at length consummated by the use of the Baths.

The fifth History, shewing when the Baths are hurtful. But that Baths are not profitable to all *Paralyticks*, yea (as we said above) very hurtful to some, this following History (whose mournful *catastrophe* happened whilst we were writing these) will manifestly declare. A Merchant of *London* having put his foot out of joint, became upon it lame in that part, but as to all things else he was sound and strong enough; when he had tried for some time several kinds of *Topick* Remedies, and they effecting nothing; at length, by the counsel of a *Physician*, going to the *Bath*, he began to try the temperate Baths, by the use of which growing presently worse, and beginning immediately to have a Palsie in his other Members, he had abstained from them, but that the *Physician*, then present, promising him that he should afterwards be better, exhorted him to persist; wherefore he again enter'd into the Bath, for about thirty days, until at length all his lower members, to wit, from the *Os sacrum* to his Feet, being wholly loosened, withered away; besides in his Breast was excited a very great difficulty of breathing, and as it were *Asthmatical*: For that his breast was not able to be dilated sufficiently, by introducing the breath deeply, the Muscles dedicated to respiration being as it seems also affected with the *Palsie*; wherefore growing short-winded, he laboured with a continual endeavour of those parts, and with an agitation of the whole *Thorax*. In this condition leaving the *Bath*, he was bid by his *Physician*, to abstain for a whole month from any Remedies taken

from

Of the Palsie.

from Medicine; which when he had strictly observed, out of hope to grow well again, that time being elapsed, it was then too late to deliberate on the use of any Medicines; for besides his *Paralytick* and withered members, his belly swell'd, his breathing was yet more hard and troublesome, that he could now scarely draw breath: His Pulse was very weak, and upon any motion of his Body, he had frequent swoonings away, and loss of Spirits: Hence, as there was scarce any place left for purging, Cordials and Antiparalytick Remedies were only to be insisted on, but notwithstanding the use of which, this sick man, within a fortnights time, labouring for many hours under a *Dyspnoe* or want of breath, at length expired. The immediate cause of whose Death I suspect to have been the manifold concretions of the blood in the Heart; for when the motion of the *Præcordia* for a long time was very much hindred, there seems nothing more probable, than that these kind of gobbets as it were fleshy, should increase within the Ventricles of the Heart.

For the illustrating of the *Theory* of the *Palsie*, a little more, and also of the *Lethargy* and *Carus*, I shall add this other example, with *Anatomical* observations; which happened whilst the former were in the Press.

A little one a little above three years old, of a moist or humid Brain, as appeared by most grievous sore Eyes, and the watry whelks or pustles of the face, to which it was sometimes obnoxious; falling ill about the beginning of *Autumn*, with a slow Feavour, and lost Appetite, it became very torpid and sleepy, so that it would sleep almost continually day and night; but being awake, he knew those standing about him, and answered very aptly to their Questions. To this Child, fit Remedies being presently and diligently given, *viz.* Clysters, Blistering Plasters, Purges, also Juleps, Spirits of Harts-horn, Powders, with many others used in these cases, they prevailed so much, that within six or seven days the sick Child being free from its Feavour, waking enough, and desiring Food, seemed to grow well, and to have scarce any more need of a *Physician*: But in a short time after (by what occasion uncertain) falling into a relapse, and again sleepy, was presently seised with a most grievous stupefaction, so that it was hardly to be awakened, and scarce knew any one, or what it did it self; the next day being plainly stupid, though being strongly pulled, it did open its Eyes, it would roll them about hither and thither, and saw nothing; but within a day or two, a *Palsie* follow'd in its whole right side. The former Remedies were repeated, and besides sneezing Medicines, chawing Medicines to draw down Rheum by the mouth, a taking away of Blood, with Poultisses applied to the Feet, and all its Head being shaven, drawing Plasters were put all over its Head, with other Medicines, and ways of administrations prescribed in order, nothing profited, but that this sick Child, after its lying so insensible for four or five days, at length its breath and Pulse failing, dyed.

An Example of the Palsie from a Lethargy.

Its dead Body being opened, we found almost all things sound enough in the lower and middle bellies, (*i. e.* in the Belly and Breast) unless that in the right Kidney, a whitish mattery Humor, or as it were a thin Corruption, had begun to be heaped together, which plentifully flowed forth out of some parts of the Kidney being dissected and squeezed together: This did seem to have been the beginning, or a certain rudiment of a future Imposthum, and perhaps by reason of the Serum not sufficiently separated here, its greater plenty had flowed to the Brain.

For the top of the Skull being taken away, the anterior region of the Head, almost to the insertion of the fourth bosom, swelled up, being covered with clear water, shining thorow the Membranes, which presently flowed forth, when the *Meninges* were dissected: Further, in this place, portions of the Brain being by pieces cut off, appeared too wet, and without any red or bloody pricks: but in the hinder border of the Brain the Vessels were red with blood, and the *Cortical* substance appeared without tumor, or deluge of water, more close and firm: From these (as we have affirmed before) it manifestly appeared, that the cause of the *Lethargy* did depend upon the watry flood, or as it were *Anasarca* or Dropsie of the outward part of the Brain.

The Brain being cut piece-meal, and an hole made in the anterior cavity, distended by the water, the clear water being before as it were penned up, within a more narrow space, leaped forth, a great plenty of which had filled all the Ventricles to the top, and (as it seems) by compressing the *Optick* chambers, (as in the other case above described) brought in blindness, and by entring or pressing together one of the Streaked Bodies, or its Pores, caused the *Palsie*.

The *Choroeidal* Infoldings appeared as it were half boiled, whitish, and almost without blood. It is probable, that the water did flow forth of these Vessels, by which the Ventricles of the Brain were overflown, all, or at least the greatest part

A a of it;

of it; although in this case, if (as some think) the watry *Latex* or Humor sliding down lower from the shelly part of the Brain, the Brain being at length thorowly passed thorow, did rain down into these bosoms, we may from thence aptly fetch a reason, wherefore the *Lethargy* at first thought to be cured, returned afterwards more cruel, accompanied with blindness and the *Palsie*; to wit, because at first the stock of the sleepy matter falling down, from the shelly part of the Brain, into its cavity, the animal function was a little cleared; but afterwards, when new matter sprung up in the *Cortex* of the Brain, and this sliding forward into its bosom, was heaped up to a fulness, for that reason happened the relapse of the former Disease, with those companions of blindness and the *Palsie*.

But although the Dropsie of the interior Brain, or the inundation of its Ventricles, by compressing either the Streaked Bodies, or the *optick* chambers, raised up the *Palsie* or blindness, or by pulling the beginnings of the Nerves, the Convulsive Distempers; yet it appears most evidently by our late *Anatomical* observation, that the *Lethargy* did not arise from any such cause, but only from the exterior part of the Brain being overflowed, or pressed together.

A certain Gentleman a long time unhealthy, after he had laboured almost for five months with the *Colick*, or rather with a wandring *Scorbutical* Gout, in which not only the Viscera and Loins were troubled with great torments; but moreover the Membranes and Muscles of the whole Body, were almost continually tormented; and at length he suffered sometimes most horrid Convulsions in his Members, sometimes resolutions, and sometimes a Phrensie in his Head, and sometimes as it were *Apoplectical* fits, or a darkness in his Eyes, so that being worn out, his strength and spirits wholly exhausted, he dyed. Almost seven days (except the last but one) before he dyed, being more strong as to his Sense and Intellect, he lived almost perpetually without sleep; though gentle or the more strong *Opiates* were given him, yet he could not sleep at all. A little before this waking, from a *Vesicatory* applied to the hinder part of his Neck, an immense quantity of water flowed; and from that time even till he dyed, it still flowed forth; hence, as I suspect, he became so waking by reason of the watry humor being so greatly drawn away from the Brain.

The head of this dead Man being opened, the interior cavities of the Brain, or all the Ventricles being filled to the top with clear water, appeared as if they were distended; yea the medullary cord it self, about the top of the Back-bone, seemed to be drowned and compassed about with water laid up there. Without doubt, for this reason, the Pains and Convulsions so cruelly tormented him in his Loins, Members, and all over his Body; and by reason of the deluge in the Ventricles, he became obnoxious to blindness of his sight, and to frequent loosenings of his limbs: Nevertheless, hence no *Lethargy*, but a waking was induced, by reason of the waters being so much derived from the compass of the Brain by the Blistering Plasters. He had also a Dropsie in his Breast, by reason of his Lungs being much vitiated. His Liver appeared of a mighty bulk, besprinkled every where with white spots, and almost without blood: so that to these faults of the *Viscera*, the vices of the Blood and nervous juice ought in some measure to be ascribed.

CHAP.

CHAP. X.

Of the Delirium and Phrenſie.

THUS much concerning *Cephalick* Diſeaſes, by which the Animal Functions by *The Diſtempers* themſelves, and as they are Corporeal, without any reſpect to the Animal *of the Brain* Soul, are wont to be hindred or perverted: In ſome of which, *viz.* the *Ver-* *follow, in which* *tigo* and *Palſie*, the Intellect for the moſt part remains clear and lively, and in the *Reaſon is hurt* reſt, like the eye placed in an obſcure place, it beholds the ſpecies, either not at all, *as will as the* or a few objects only of a more rude appearance, but is not eaſily ſnatched into any *other Animal* great error or fury; which kind of *ſymptoms* are ordinarily induced by reaſon of other *Faculties.* Diſtempers of the Head, and of the Spirits inhabiting it, of which we are now about to treat. For if at any time the Imagination is ſo diſturbed, or perverted, that it falſly conceives, or evilly compoſes or divides, the ſpecies and notions brought from the Senſe or Memory; preſently for that reaſon the intellect beholds or forms con- *Who are ſaid to* ceptions and thoughts only deformed, diſtracted one from another, and very confu- *be Fooliſh, or* ſed: Which indeed are repreſented to it from the Brain evilly affected, and as it were *to talk idly.* monſters from a multiplying or diſtorted Glaſs. As there are many ways, by which *This is either* the Imagination, and by conſequence the mind and will, and the other powers of the *ſhorter, as the* ſuperior ſoul, are wont to be perverted or depraved, all of them are noted by the *Delirium;* common word Fooliſhneſs, or talking idly. But this Diſtemper is diſtinguiſhed into *or longer, and* ſhorter, which is called a *Delirium*; and into a longer or continual; which is either *with a Feavour,* conjoined with a Feavour, and termed *Phrenſie*; or it happens without a Feavour, and *& called Phren-* then their is joyned with it, either raving, ſadneſs, or ſtupidity, and ſo it is divided in- *ſie; or without* to madneſs, melancholy, and moroſity or fooliſhneſs: we ſhall ſpeak of each of theſe *a Feavour, as* in order; and firſt of the *Delirium* and *Phrenſie*. *melancholy, madneſs, ſtupidity.*

Although the *Delirium* is not a Diſeaſe of it ſelf, but only a *ſymptom* proceeding from other Diſtempers, yet becauſe it happens in ſome of them, that for the moſt part it is cured by Remedies appropriate to it, therefore it will not be amiſs for us to inquire a little more ſtrictly into the cauſes and nature of it. This word taken after an eſpecial manner, is the ſame with παραφροσύνη, or a going crooked, or out of the *What the Deli-* right or ſtraight way, and denotes an hurt of the ſame Animal Function ſuch as ariſeth *rium is.* in fits of the Feavour, Drunkenneſs, and ſometimes in the paſſions called *Hyſterical*, and induces men for a ſhort time to think, ſpeak, or do abſurd things, either ſome of theſe, or all of them together.

The *Delirium* is excited, foraſmuch as the Animal Spirits being either too much *Its formal Rea-* irritated, or acted into confuſion, are carried tumultuouſly into diſorders hither and *ſon.* thither, within the globous compaſs of the Brain, where the *Phantaſie* and *Memory* have their ſeats; and ſo whilſt the various images of the imagination and the memory being excited at once, are confounded together, they object only incongruous and abſurd *phantaſies* to the rational Soul, and ſo both the acts of the intellect and the will, are only inordinately choſen or drawn forth. In like manner it happens, by rea- ſon that the Animal Spirits being moved, within the middle of the Brain or the *Callous* Body, that incongruous conceptions, and confuſed thoughts, are objected to the rati- onal Soul; as in a long circumgyration or turning about of the body, the images of viſible things are carried to the common ſenſe, whence all things ſeem to be turn- ed about, and ſometimes to be lifted up, and ſometimes to be depreſſed to the ground; that nothing is beheld ſtable or ſtanding in its due place, and poſition. In a Brain rightly diſpoſed, the motion of the Animal Spirits are performed, as it were in certain numbers, ways and meaſures; whilſt ſome Spirits are raiſed up in theſe tracts, others lye ſtill in thoſe, and ſo they ſucceed one another in their motions; and the ſeveral acts of e- very faculty are made diſtinct, like ſo many wavings of water in a River; but in the *Deli- rium*, all the Spirits leap forth at once, and meeting one another tumultuouſly, or vari- ouſly laying hold on one another, are agitated like mad *Bacchanals*. Further, even as theſe being ſtruck with ſuch a fury within the compaſs of the Brain, do ſtir up manifold and ve- ry much diſturbed cogitations; ſo whilſt they are carried without its confines into the ner- vous original, they produce incongruous ſpeeches, abſurd geſtures of the body, and mem- bers, and not rarely Convulſive motions. But for that ſuch a rage of the ſpirits, (other- ways than in the *Phrenſie* or *Madneſs*) preſently grows cool, and their tumult being over, none of their wandring tracts are imprinted in the Brain, the *Delirium* ſoon paſſes

over,

Of the Delirium and Phrensie.

over, and the distemper'd come immediately to themselves again, without any marks left of their foolishness or idle raving.

The Causes of the Delirium.
If it be demanded, from whence this short fury is impressed on the spirits, inhabiting the Brain, that the Reins of the mind being shaken off, they turn thus all things upside down in their government; we say, that they conceive this kind of inordination, from a twofold reason; to wit, this rage or madness is brought immediately to

1. Either from the Blood: Or
them, from the blood washing the frame of the Brain; or some Animal Spirits, outwardly dwelling in the nervous Stock, enter first of all into some disorder; then the same being communicated by the nervous passages, affecting in like manner the

2. From exterior Spirits planted in the nervous Stock.
spirits there inhabiting, stirs them into a *Delirium*. There are various causes and kinds of either of these: the chief of which we shall here touch upon; and first shall be shewed, how, and for what occasions, the Blood, being either swelled up with too much heat, or being pregnant with an invenomed matter, is the parent of the *Delirium*; forasmuch as it insinuates into the Pores and passages of the Brain, either fierce and untameable particles, or such as are malignant and deadly to the Animal regiment.

By what, and how many ways the Delirium is caused by the Blood:
1. By reason of its too great heat.
First, As to the first, in the fits of intermitting and in the height of continual Feavours, the blood growing hot, by an immoderate burning, sometimes stirs up the *Delirium*, by the mere force of its Ebullition or boiling up; to wit, for that it swelling up very much, whilst it passes thorow the small shoots of the Arteries, every where diffused thorow the outward compass of the Brain, it very much blows them up and distends them; and so pressing together the substance of the Brain, variously drives in the Spirits, and as it were compells them into very confused troops: Moreover, from the blood so swelling up, with a frothy rarefaction, the Effluvia's of heat, and with them heterogeneous particles, entring into the Pores and passages of the Brain, agitate the Spirits, and tumultuously snatch them hither and thither.

2. By reason of untameable Particles carried from it into the Brain.
Secondly, Almost for the like reason Drunkenness, a deep Sleep, or a *Delirium*, is brought in; to wit, forasmuch as the bloody mass doth insinuate the spirituous particles of the Wine, (by which it grows hot) into the Pores and passages of the Brain, by which the Spirits dwelling in them, are either plainly overturned, or are moved into inordinate and confused motions. For that the untameable little Bodies of Wine or Beer plentifully drunk, open the shut places of any Brain, how sound and firm soever it be, and penetrating deeply into the Marrowy passages, disturb and plainly overturn the Acts both of reason and of the imagination.

3. By reason of malignant Particles suffused from it.
Thirdly, The blood suggesting not only feavourish and turgid, or vinous and untameable particles, but sometimes malignant, and as it were venomous to the Animal regiment, stirs up a *Delirium*, either with or without a Feavour. As to the former, in the Plague, Small Pox, malignant Feavours (although the heat be but moderate) the malignant matter being translated to the Brain, because it dissipates a great company of Spirits (rather than that it drives them into tumults) brings forth abrupt, incoherent, and at length distracted notions.

4. By reason of Effluvias, or venomous Particles, obtruded also on the Brain.
For the like reason also, some intoxicating and venomous things taken inwardly, and (as some affirm) outwardly applied, quickly cause a *Delirium*: This is commonly reported of the furious night-shade, *Mandrakes*, and some other plants; as for the roots of wild Parsnips, the thing is very well known. A certain intimate friend of mine told me, and he was a Man that might be credited, and also very learned, That he entring into the House of a certain Gentleman, found the Mistress of the Family, her Daughters, and all her Maids (excepting one) become all at once Delirious, and speaking absurd and incongruous speeches, run up and down and leaped about the House; and for that he plainly thought them all mad; he learnt of the sober Maid, who had her reason, and was her self, that all that had happened from their eating of Parsnips, which she had not tasted: Which indeed the event shewed to be true; for after they had tired themselves, and fallen to sleep, they all at length awakned sober. We have not here leasure to examine, whether this or other kinds of intoxicating things, infestous rather to the animal government, than the vital, do communicate to the Brain their evil, by the passage only of the Blood, or also in some measure, by a contact of the spirits residing in the Ventricle.

5. By reason of its afflux being denied to the Brain.
But moreover, we advertise you, that sometimes a *Delirium* is excited from a want, and great dissipation of the Animal Spirits; because their series or orders being broken off, and drawn one from another, like as if they were tumultuarily heaped together, cause confused and incongruous notions. Hence it is observed, that some have become Delirious by great *Hæmorrhagies*, or long watchings, and excessive want of Food; for this reason, many are wont to die delirious, and talking idly.

Of the Delirium and Phrenſie.

There remains the other kind of *Delirium*, in which the Blood being faultleſs, the *Animal Spirits* flowing ſome where in the nervous ſtock, firſt enter into diſorder; then the ſame affection creeping thorow the nervous paſſages to the Brain, ſtirs up the Spirits inhabiting its middle part into a *Delirium*. This is ſufficiently obvious in the paſſions that are called *Hyſterical*; to wit, after a ſwelling up of the Belly, and an oppreſſion of the Heart, doth ſucceed ſometimes a lying ſpeechleſs, ſometimes a talking idly, with weeping and laughing. In like manner I have obſerved in a moſt cruel *Colick*, that ſometimes after great torments obout the Bowels and the Loins, they have fallen into a *Delirium*, then a little after this ceaſing, the torments have returned. I knew a young Maid (as we have ſomewhere elſe mentioned) from the taking of an *Emetick* Potion, whilſt it worked, was wont conſtantly to fall into a *Delirium*. I have alſo often noted, that a *Gangrene* beginning in ſome external member, has cauſed a *Delirium*. And this in a Wound or Ulcer, is ordinarily noted for a mortal ſign; becauſe it denotes the Animal Spirits in the diſtemper'd part to be ſlain.

How a Deliriūm proceeds from the irregularities of the exterior Spirits.

Nor doth this *ſymptom* coming upon thoſe who are long ſick and almoſt worn out, give any better *prognoſtick*; in the fits of intermitting Feavours, it is almoſt ever ſafe; but in continual Feavours dubious, and of ſomething a ſuſpected event; in malignant it more often fore-ſpeaks evil; in Convulſive Diſeaſes, the firſt aſſaults of a *Delirium* for the moſt part are free from danger, but yet its frequent coming, frequently turns that diſpoſition into a *Carus, Apoplexy*, or *Palſie*.

The Prognoſtick of a Delirium.

This Diſtemper, as often as it is ſeen to be ſafe enough, requires not a Cure; for the fit quickly and eaſily paſſes over: yet, becauſe ſome, who have a looſe and weak Brain, and the Animal Spirits too eaſily diſſipable, and apt to flight and confuſion; being diſturbed by any light occaſion, are wont preſently to grow Deliriors and to talk idly; therefore there is need of Medicine for theſe, not only of *Hellebore*, but alſo *Cephalick* Remedies, which may ſtrengthen the Brain, and fortifie it againſt the incurſions of the Morbifick matter; alſo which may ſortifie the Animal Spirits, and render them more fixt and ſtrong for reſiſting. We have above deſcribed the forms of theſe kind of Medicines, and their manner of adminiſtration, which are profitable for the taking away the foregoing cauſe of any other *Cephalick* Diſeaſe.

Its Cure.

A *Delirium* coming upon continual and malignant Feavours, requires a peculiar way of healing: for in the firſt place, it ſhews the morbifick matter dangerouſly tranſlated towards the Head, and therefore ought to he called back from thence, by any means; for which end may be laid Plaſters that draw bliſters to the hinder part of the Neck, other Plaſters or Pultiſſes, or the fleſh of living Creatures, or their warm bowels to the feet; inwardly may be taken temperate *Cephalicks*, as Powder of Coral and Pearl, black Cherry Water, or Water of Cowſlip Flowers, or Poppy Water, and others ſweetning and cheriſhing the ſpirits.

Theſe being thus premiſed, concerning the firſt and moſt light manner of fooliſhneſs or talking idly, we will proceed to its higher degree, *viz.* the *Phrenſie*, which is far longer, and more durable, than the former Diſtemper. In the *Delirium*, a perturbation of the Spirits, inhabiting of the Brain, being excited, is like a waving of waters, from a ſtone flung into a River; but in a *Phrenſie*, their commotion ſeems as it were the ſtorm of waters, raging in a tempeſt.

The *Phrenſie* is defined, to be a continual dotage, or deprivation of the principal faculties of the Brain, ariſing from an Inflammation of the *Meninges*, with a continual Feavour. To this Diſeaſe there is another of kin, *viz.* the *Paraphrenſie*, commonly called, or additional *Phrenſie*, whoſe cauſe is not an inflammation of the Membranes which cover the Head, but as they affirm of the *Diaphragma*. Further, in either Diſtemper (as alſo in the *Pleuriſie* but falſly) it is affirmed, that the Feavour doth ariſe as it were only ſymptomatical, from the ſame conjunct cauſe, *viz.* from the Inflammation of ſome part. But indeed, that the *Phrenſie* doth rather ſucceed the *Feavour*, and is produced, becauſe the boiling blood doth transfer its aduſt or burnt recrements to the Head; *Hippocrates* long ſince, and now every common body, obſerves: to wit, for that the Urine of one ſick of a Feavour, being changed from a troubled and thick, into a thin and wateriſh Urine, ſhews a *Phrenſie* at hand: Wherefore, from hence, the cauſe of this Diſtemper is concluded to be a tranſlation of the Feavouriſh matter into the Brain.

Of the Phrenſie, what it is.

The Paraphrenſie.

But as to the conjunct cauſes of the *Phrenſie*, and *Paraphreneſis*, we may eaſily ſhew, that the former doth not always proceed from the Inflammation of the *Meninges*, nor this latter from the Inflammation of the Midriff. I have often ſeen in Anatomical Diſſections, the *Meninges*, yea ſometimes alſo the exterior compaſs of the Brain,

Their Conjunct Cauſes.

The Phrensie not from the Inflammation of the Meninges.

Brain, beset with an inflamed tumor, and the sick not distemper'd with a *Phrensie*, but on the contrary with a stupidity, and have dyed with a *Carus*, or some other sleepy Diseases. And truly, that it is so, reason plainly declares; for the *Meninges* being inflamed, and by that made more tumid, press together the Brain very much, and about its compass shut up the ways and passages of the Spirits; so that the functions of waking and memory being hindred, the *Lethargy* (as it appears de *facto*) necessarily follows: Notwithstanding, far otherways in the *Phrensie*, all the passages and Pores of the Brain, for the excursions of the Spirits, seem to be too largely open; because the Images hidden or laid up, are raised all at once, out of the utmost, and all the places of the memory, which together with others, suggested from the Phantasie to the common sensory, tumultuously, bring forth such manifold and highly confused notions. There is only wanting to the sensitive soul, for its expansion to be straitned or loosened, within the Head (which certainly the inflammation of the *Meninges* would effect) rather than that it should be dilated above measure, and that all the Pores of the Brain should be unlocked and carried beyond its wonted compass. Perhaps it may happen, from a long continuance of this Disease, that the Blood being greatly heaped up within the Vessels of the *Meninges*, and there stagnating, that it may at length bring forth an Inflammation in them; and then for that reason, we may suspect, (because it often so falls out) that the *Phrensie* doth pass into the *Carus*, or *Lethargy*, of which *phrensical* persons often dye.

The Paraphrenesis not from the Inflammation of the Diaphragme.

No less do we reject the Inflammation of the *Diaphragma*, which cause of the *Paraphrenesis*, *Galen* in times past, and moved by his authority, most *Physicians* in every age since, asserted: *Anatomical* observations plainly prove the contrary. Some time since, dissecting the dead Carcase of a Maid, dying of a sudden *Leipothymy* or swooning away, we found in the fleshy part of the *Diaphragma* a great Imposthume, with a bag full of filthy matter, and watery little bladders; yet she was not troubled ever with a *Delirium* or *Phrensie*. Some time since also when we had made an *Anatomical* Inspection of a Gentleman of the University, (of whom we have made mention in a late Tract) who dyed of a long spurious *Pleurisie*, it manifestly appeared, that a great Imposthume being ripened in the *Pleura*, and the intercostal Muscles, and broke inwardly, that a vast plenty of matter had flowed forth into the cavity of the *Thorax*, which gnawing the *Diaphragma* lying under, had made a great hole in it; nor was this man however in all his sickness *Delirious*, or Frantick. Wherefore, I think this Distemper scarce ever to be produced from such a cause: but that opinion seems to arise from hence, because oftentimes in a true *Phrensie*, together with a continual raving, the motion of the *Diaphragma* is wont to be hindred or perverted; as is gathered from the unequal and difficult breathing, to wit, sometimes anhelous or breathing short, and as it were suspended, sometimes short and swiftly repeated, *wherefore breathing is hurt in this Disease.* with sometimes a double breathing; which kind of *symptoms*, and also at the same time the alienation of the mind, are said to proceed from the Midriff being inflamed, and for that reason convulsed; wherefore the Ancients called the Diphragma *Phrenes*: But there was no need for this, if they had consider'd, that the whole action of the *Diaphragma*, doth depend upon the flowing forth of the Animal Spirits from the *Cerebel*, and therefore there is a necessity, if the *Phrenetick* matter invading the Brain, some part of it should with it rush into the *Cerebel*, that besides the raving, the motion also of the Midriff, though of it self innocent, should be altered; as we have shewed elsewhere more largely.

The formal Reason of the Phrensie.

Therefore the formal reason of the *Phrensie* seems to consist in this, that the Animal Spirits being at first very much irritated in the whole Brain, are driven into inordinate, very confused, and also impetuous motions; so that the acts of every Animal Function are depraved, and variously perverted; and at the same time, very many Ideas of things being raised up out of the memory, the old are confounded with the new, and some evilly joined, or wonderfully divided, are confounded with others, the imagination suggests manifold *Phantasms*, and almost innumerable, and all of them only incongruous; and the common sensory represents the images of sensible things distorted, double, or incoherent; that hence the mind and the will, choose or pick out nothing but ridiculous and impertinent conceptions and passions; and cause the actions of the body to become almost only irregular. Moreover, the spirits being struck as it were with madness, tumultuate not only in the Brain, but also in the *Cerebel*, and every where in the nervous Stock; wherefore, *Frantick* people not only talk idly, but breath unequally, speak aloud, strike with their fists, fling about their hands and feet, yea and stretch forth all their members with a mighty strength, and a most strong force, that indeed the whole Soul seems to grow hot and furious in the whole body, to be mad, or rather as it were to be inflamed

Of the Delirium and Phrenſie.

inflamed with a ſudden burning. And truly a *Phrenſie* cannot be more aptly defined, than that it is a burning or inflammation of the whole ſenſitive ſoul, or animal ſpirits, as to their whole *Hypoſtaſis* or Conſtitution. This burning always beginning from the ſpirits inhabiting the Brain, and wandring from thence into the other parts of the ſenſitive ſoul, ſeems to receive from the Blood, firſt growing hot and raging with a Feavouriſh fire, both the firſt incentive matter, and then the conſtant food of the burning. For indeed it is probable, that the blood burning Feavouriſhly, doth pour forth on the Brain ſometimes ſulphureous Particles, together with the ſpirituous, which being half inflamed, and after a ſort burning forth, penetrate together with the others, and from thence immediately entring into all the murrowy and nervous paſſages, adhere every where to the ſpirits, and ſo render them being inflamed, highly rageing and implacable. Certainly it is more likely, that the *Phrenſie* is rather excited after this manner, by an inflammation of the Spirits, than from that of the *Meninges* or of the Brain, which more ſurely cauſes an Headach or *Lethargy*, than a Fury, as we have frequently found by *Anatomy*. *This Diſeaſe proceeds from the burning of the Animal Spirits, the Inflammation of the Meninges ſtirs up rather the inveterate Headach, or the Lethargy, than the Phrenſie.*

And indeed, that it is ſo, is not only ours, or any new opinion, but that great follower and beſt interpreter of *Hippocrates*, *Proſper Martianus*, who hath affirmed the ſame thing, almoſt in expreſs words, *viz.* Comment on his Book *De Morbis* 3. *verſ.* 99. *pag.* 151. he ſays, "That *Hippocrates* doth call the *Phrenſie* a *Delirium* with a Feavour, "which is continual, and depends upon a firm and ſtable Diſtemper: to wit, from "an inflammation of thoſe parts, which ſerve to inſtitute Nature, Reaſon, and the "Mind; For ſo the Animal Spirits, whoſe viciouſneſs cauſe the *Delirium*, do not "grow hot as it were by a ſimple quality, but are altered as to their ſubſtance. This Man manifeſtly diſtinguiſhes between heat and flame, and affirming that to be in reſpect of quality, and this an alteration in reſpect of ſubſtance, plainly aſcribes the cauſe of the *Phrenſie* to the inflammation of the Spirits. He has in the ſame place more things appoſite to our matter, to wit, that the containing cauſe of the *Phrenſie* was not the inflammation of the *Meninges*, but of the Spirits, whoſe ſubſtance is indeed altered, that is, foraſmuch as it is become fiery, ſuch a continual *Delirium* is excited. *Proſper Martianus alſo aſſerts this.*

I have oftentimes compared the production of the Spirits from the Blood into the Brain, to a Chymical Diſtillation; of which it is obſerved, if the ſpirituous ſulphureous liquor be provoked with too ſtrong a fire, that in Diſtilling it ſometimes takes fire, and aſcends in the *Alembick* with a very great flame. This is known of Oyl of *Turpentine*, of it ſelf, or with the Flowers of *Sulphur*, to the great loſs of ſome. In like manner we may believe, that the blood growing more ſtrongly hot, doth often communicate alſo a burning to the Spirits diſtilled out of it, *viz.* that ſome half burnt Particles, do inſinuate themſelves into the Pores of the Brain, which ruſhing into all the paſſages of the Spirits, both there and in its appendix, every where inkindle the Spirits, and compel them into moſt ſwift motions, almoſt like Lightning. *Chymical Spirits in their diſtilling are ſometimes inflamed. So the Animal Spirits.*

But becauſe the *Phrenſie* doth not come upon all Feavours, but only on thoſe highly burning, the reaſon is plain by what follows; to wit, the cloſure of the Brain ought to be ſo ſhut up, that not only any extraneous thing might not be poured into them, but that the more intenſe flame of the Blood, however burning it be, and though planted round about, might not be able to break thorow; wherefore, ſome diſtemper'd with a burning Feavour, although the Blood grows hot thorow the whole, the Bowels burn, the Marrow rages, the Tongue and Jaws roſted like a coal, yet the Brain being ſtill firmly ſhut up, all the Animal Functions remain whole and ſound. But on the contrary, others who have a weak and too looſe a Brain, and their Blood more ſulphureous than it ought, become *Phrenſical* not only from a burning Feavour, but ſometimes from a more gentle viſit. By reaſon of what foregoing cauſe, and for what occaſions, or evident cauſes, this is wont to happen, is the next thing we ſhall inquire into. *What the Indiſpoſition of the Brain is to the Phrenſy.*

Hitherto hath been ſhown that the immediate ſubject of the *Phrenſie* is the ſenſitive Soul, or the *Hypoſtaſis* of the Animal Spirits, and that the formal reaſon of the Diſeaſe doth conſiſt in their Inflammation, and that the conjunct cauſe is the ſulphureous particles poured forth from the Blood into the incloſures of the Brain, and there continually inkindling the Spirits; and now it is no difficult matter to aſſign its *procatartick* or foregoing cauſes, which we find partly in the Blood, and partly in the Brain and its inhabitants *The Procatartick Cauſes of the Phrenſy,*

The previous diſpoſition of the Blood, diſpoſing to the *Phrenſie*, is ſometimes ſimple, ſometimes twofold; the former is an hot, ſharp, or bilous conſtitution of it, to wit, that contains very many ſulphureous Particles in it ſelf, which are apt to inflame the *which are partly in the Blood, and* the Blood in a Feavour more than ought to be, and to infinuate its burning into the Brain. This difpofition, when it is very potent and active, often produces this Difeafe of it felf; but for the moft part, there is another difpofition of the Blood, which helps that former, and renders it more efficacious, to wit, that, befides the fulphureous and inflameable Particles, there are others fharp and penetrative, which enter into the Pores, and open them, fo that the former more eafily enter in, or are introduced: This the faline little Bodies, conjoined with the fulphureous, do in a manner effect; hence Cholerick and Melancholick perfons growing Feavourifh, are more prone to become furious; but much more do the *Heterogeneous* Particles, implanted in the Blood, and moved by a Feavour, open the doors of the Brain, and intromit all that are inflameable: wherefore a *Phrenfie* frequently comes upon the Small-Pox, and malignant, and Peftilential Feavours.

Partly in the Brain.   The other provifion to a *Phrenfie*, which is of the Brain, confifts partly in its temper and conformation, and partly in the difpofition of the Spirits inhabiting it: As to the former, thofe indued with an hot and dry Brain, are found to be moft prone to a *Phrenfie*; not becaufe that conftitution is more obnoxious to an inflammation or burning, (for to this it is lefs apt) but becaufe in fuch a Brain, otherwife than in an hot and moift, or cold and dry, the Pores and paffages are more open, and too much gaping, and fo give an entrance to the incentive matter, fuggefted from the Feavour: which befides, they much more eafily admit, if the Spirits being very fugacious or apt to flight, or *pathetick*, or paffionate, are upon every light occafion ready to fall into paffions of fadnefs, fear, anger, or hatred; fo that they refift not the incurfions of the extraneous matter, and more readily conceive a burning themfelves.

The evident caufes of the Phrenfie.   The evident caufes of the *Phrenfie* are either more remote, *viz.* whatever things are wont to excite a Feavourifh intemperance; as Surfeits. Drunkennefs, a very vehement difturbance of either body or mind, ufual evacuations being fuppreffed, with many others; or more near, as a Feavour, and its dependences and adjuncts; to wit, if it be peftilential, malignant, or after an evil manner; if it arifes by reafon of a Surfeit taken from very incongruous Meats or Drink, or if it fucceeds violent paffions, as of Love, hatred, envie, indignation, or fadnefs; or immoderate ftudies: for thefe kind of occafions render the Blood and Animal Spirits, growing Feavourifhly hot, very propenfe to the frantick Diftemper.

The differences of it.   Since that this Difeafe depends rather and more immediately upon the Soul than upon the Humors or folid parts being diftemper'd, its kinds and differences are neither various nor manifold: In refpect of magnitude, the *Phrenfie* is either great or moderate, alfo continual or intermitting; to wit, according as the Animal Spirits are more or lefs inflamed, and as they receive the food of their burning continually from the Blood, or by turns. Secondly, As the burning begins only in the Brain, or together with it in the Cerebel, it is commonly diftinguifhed into the *Phrenfie*, or the *Paraphrenefis*; which is as much as to fay, that either the fpontaneous Animal Functions are only or chiefly hurt, or elfe together with them the vital alfo. But this Difeafe as to the Feavour, on which it depends, hath its nature and manner malignant, or free from malignity; alfo according to the temper of the fick, the *Phrenfie* is diftinguifhed into Sanguineous, Cholerick, Phlegmatick, or Melancholick; and this not improperly, for the Animal Spirits are wont to grow hot and burning, after a diverfe manner, in this Difeafe, according to their various difpofitions.

The Prognoftick.   The *Prognoftick* in this Difeafe is always doubtful, and the event is to be inftituted with an evil fufpicion: For the Phrenfie of it felf (as *Trallianus* fays) *is a moft acute and moft dangerous Difeafe*; then, if it comes upon a Peftilential, or malignant Feavour, or of fome other evil kind, we cannot but expect the end of it to be mortal.

If a *Phrenfie* happens in a found body, well habited, of a Sanguine temperament, and young, there is greater hopes of health, than if it were fickly, aged, lean, or Cholerick, and obnoxious to violent Paffions.

If the *Phrenfie* remitting by frequent turns, have lucid intervals, it is better than if the fury fhould be undifcontinued: But if the fick fometimes feem to be better, yet after moderate fleep to awake always furious, it is a fign that the Difeafe is pertinacious, and for that reafon dangerous; for that a new ftock of incentive matter is from thence carried to the Brain; which indeed we have elfewhere fhewn to be made far more plentifully in fleep than waking.

A *Phrenfie* is in a fhort time terminated with the Feavour, either in health or death; or elfe it is protracted, and remains after the Feavour; or at length it is healed, or paffes into other Difeafes, to wit, the *Lethargy*, or *Madnefs*, or *Melancholy*.

If the *Feavour* having a laudable *Crifis*, either by Sweat or great quantity of Urine, is

Of the Delirium and Phrensie.

is fully cured, for the most part the *Phrensie* also ceases; but if the Feavour be not cured and carries still the Morbifick matter to the Head, so that besides the Animal Functions being depraved, the vital begin to fail (which appears by the Pulse and breathing being altered for the worse) if the Urine be pale, if that frequent bleeding at the Nose, if Vomiting, and Convulsion happen, the *Physician* concludes death to be at hand.

Sometimes a *Feavour*, though it be not at once or fully Cured, yet passing away afterwards slowly and by degrees, leaves a *Phrensie*, or a talking idly behind it; which, if it doth not by its stay obliterate the former tracts of the Spirits in the Brain, either will end by little and little of its own accord, or is to be healed by the help of Remedies.

If that by reason of the *Phrensie* being long protracted, the *Meninges*, or the *Cortex* of the Brain, be possessed from the Blood; or *Serum*, there heaped up, and stagnating; with an inflamed tumor, or a serous deluge, the *Lethargy*, or sleepy Diseases follow; the Cure of which is often very difficult, or not at all. But if from a long *Phrensie*, either the Animal Spirits (though their burning should cease) contract a vicious nature, or that the passages and Pores of the Brain are perverted, a perpetual raving oftentimes succeeds, the former Disease passing into Madness, or Melancholy, or foolishness or stupidity. Wherefore it is vulgarly said of those that are *Frantick*, and not soon Cured, that their Brains are crack'd or broken, so that after that, they are always Mad or raving.

In the Cure of the *Phrensie*, we ought to respect at once the Feavour and the Fury. The Feavourish burning of the Blood, or its immoderate growing hot (which for the most part is the antecedent cause of the other effect) ought in the first place to be appeased and allayed, and the Animal Spirits to be cherished, and freed from any great burning. If the *Phrensie* happens about the beginning of the Feavour, or the middle of it, the same Remedies in a manner, and the same method of curing conduce to either end: But if this Distemper comes upon this, whilst it is at a stand, or at its height, the means of Curing are oftentimes repugnant to either, and there is need of great caution, lest whilst we endeavour to help one Disease, we do not increase the other; in this case, the vital indication concerning the preserving of strength, obtains the first place; and the taking away of blood, or purging, is not to be rashly and copiously celebrated.

The Cure of the Phrensie.

In the former case, when the Feavour and the *Phrensie* are almost both of an age, *Phlebotomy* rarely or never is to be omitted, but is presently to be performed, and if strength will bear it, let it be afterwards repeated. For nothing depresses and diminishes the immoderate flame of the blood, like to this Remedy, and nothing more averts or recals its burning from the Animal regiment: Wherefore, if the matter requires it, let a vein be opened, sometimes in the Arm or Hand, sometimes in the Leg or Foot, and sometimes in the Neck or forehead: perhaps sometimes it may be expedient to open the temporal Artery: yea also to take away blood in other places by Leeches, and sometimes by Cupping-Glasses. For this gives the chiefest help, and according to *Galen*, is the *most powerful and principal Remedy*, and is wont to fulfil very many indications in a *Phrensie*.

Phlebotomy.

But for the prevention of the Feavourish matter being carried from the Bowels into the Head, Clysters are of chief use; with which, if need be, let the Belly be continually kept slippery. Vomiting Medicines, and Purging, unless very gentle, have very rarely any place here. *Cataplasms* of Rue, Chamomel, Vervine, Bryony Roots, red Poppies, with Sope, may be laid all over the Feet; or instead of them, may be applied Pigeons or Chickens, cut up and laid warm: In the mean time, as you see occasion, there ought to be prescribed *Juleps, Apozems, Powders,* and *Confections,* by which the rage of the Blood, and the burning of the Animal Spirits may be allayed.

Clysters.

Take of *Pipin Water, Black Cherry Water,* and *Cowslip Water, each four ounces; Water of the whole Citrons two ounces, of Pearl powder'd one dram, of Syrup of the juice of Citron one ounce; mingle them and make a Julep. let three ounces be taken three or four times in a day.*

A Julep.

Take of *Grass Roots, of the Leaves of Wood-Sorrel, and Pimpernel, each one handful; of Barly half an ounce, of Apples cut, of Currans, or Strawberries, or Rasberries, one handful; let them be boiled in four pints of spring-water, till a third part be consumed; clarifie it, and strain it; then add to it of the Syrup of Violets one ounce, and of Sal Prunella a dram and a half.*

An Apozem.

B b

Of the Delirium and Phrensie.

A Drink. Take of the Leaves of Borage fresh gathered and young, four handfuls, of Wood-Sorrel two handfuls, two Apples sliced, of Sal Prunella two drams, the pulp of one Orange, of white Sugar one ounce; let them be bruised together, and pour to them of Spring-water two or three pints; let them be strongly squeezed forth, and kept in a Glass, and cleared from its setling; let six or seven ounces be taken of this often in a day, when they will. For the quenching of thirst, let the excellent drink of Palmerius, viz. Spring-water with Sugar, and the juice of Lemons, or Water, or Posset-drink with Elm leaves, or Pimpernel infused or boiled in it, be drunk: Emulsions of the Decoction of the roots and flowers of Water-Lilies, with Melon-seeds; or else Spring-water distilled with the pulp of boiled Apples dissolved in it.

Hypnoticks. Hypnoticks or Medicines causing rest, are often very necessary in this Disease; but yet the stronger are not convenient in the beginning, nor let them be frequently used; because sleep caused by Opiates, carries more morbifick matter to the Brain, and fixes it more deeply there.

Take of the Water of Cowslip flowers four ounces, of the Syrup of Poppies half an ounce, of Pearl one scruple; make a drink to be taken at night late.
Take of the Seeds of white Poppy two drams, of Sugar-Candy a dram and a half; bruise them together, and pour to them of white Poppy Water six ounces; make an expression, to be taken after the same manner.

Narcoticks or Stupefying Medicines, which are made of things meerly cold, are cautiously to be exhibited; because they agree not with some, who have the Fibres of their Stomach very tender and sensible. I have often observed these kind of Hypnoticks, to have stirred up a great oppression in the Ventricle, and then presently an Inflation or blowing of it up; and a little after distractions and inordinations of Spirits use to follow in the Brain, yea in the whole Body; so that there was not only a frustration of sleep, but great disquietness was stirred up.

Take of liquid Laudanum, prepared with the Salt of Tartar, or the juice of Quinces, Let a Dose of it be taken in a convenient liquor.

External Medicines causing Sleep. Things inviting Sleep, as Epithems or moist Medicines applied to the Temples and Forehead, are often used with success; of which sort are Rose-cakes dipt in Vinegar, Rose-water, and grated Nutmeg, an Embrocation or washing with Water or Milk, Oyntments of Oyl of Nutmeg by expression, Oyntment of Poplar, to which sometimes may be added of Opium five or six grains; or a Cake of Poppy flowers, with Vinegar and Nutmeg, &c. Further, for this end, rather than for the taking away the inflammation of the Meninges, the hot Lungs of a Lamb or Weather, as also Pigeons or *Epithems.* Chickins slit in two, do often give notable help. Also for this use Housleek bruised, and mixt with a Womans Milk, and applied to the hinder part of the Head being shaved, is wonderfully praised; Also the Epithem of Penotus, of twelve grains of Nutmeg, of Camphir half a scruple, and the Tincture of Rose-water impregnated with red Sanders twenty ounces, is commended by some.

Further, they are wont to apply Epithems not only to the Head, but also to the Heart, Liver, and other parts: A little bag of silk may be applied to the Præcordia, with Cardiac Species being sewed or quilted in it, with silk, and sprinkled with Rose-water, or Vinegar of Roses; also rags wet in Rose Vinegar, may be laid to the Testicles: The Feet way be bathed with a Decoction of Willow leaves, Lettice, or the heads of white Poppy. But these kind of cooling Topicks only, and cherishers are to be used in the beginning of the Disease; but in its height, resolvers and softners, are to be added, as the Flowers of Chamomel, Melilot, Elder, &c. also the leaves of Mallows, Orage, Marjoram, Hysop, and such like: In the declining of the Disease, resolvers only, and those sparingly are to be administred.

The means for the preserving of strength. In the mean time, there ought to be great means used, for keeping up of strength, for that too much failing, all hopes of Cure is lost. For strength is quickly worn out, by reason of great watchings, the perpetual agitations both of the body and mind, a thin Dyet, and Phlebotomy sometimes often requisite. Wherefore, great care must be had, lest whilst we endeavour to root out the Disease, by Purging or frequent letting of Blood, we should suddenly debilitate the Vital Function: If this begins to fail, the Phrensie being let alone, a better dyet may be granted, and especially Cordials are to be used.

Take

Of the Delirium and Phrensie. 187

Take *of the Tincture of Coral half an ounce, take of it twenty drops, twice or thrice in* Cordials. *a day, with a Dose of a Cephalick or a Cordial Julep; or let it be given with Coral dissolved in Milk, made with the juice of Oranges, one spoonful often in a day.*

Take *of the Rob or Conserves of Rasberries, and Barberies one ounce, of prepared Pearl, of Magistery of Coral, each one dram; of Confection of Hyacintha two drams, Syrup of the juice of Alchermes, what will suffice; make a Confection, and let the quantity of a Nutmeg be taken three or four times a day, drinking after it of the following Julep three ounces.*

Take *of the Water of the Flowers of Water-Lilies, red Roses, and of Elm leaves, each three ounces; of the Syrup of Coral two ounces, of the Cordial Water of Saxony one dram; mingle them.*

Take *of the Conserves of the Flowers of Water-Lilies, and of Violets, each one ounce; the Stalks of Lettice candied or preserved half an ounce, of the Powder of red Coral, bruised in a morter with the juice of Orange and dryed, two drams; of the Species of Diamarg. frigid. one dram, of white Poppy seeds one dram and a half, with what will suffice of the Syrup of the juice of Wood-Sorrel; make an Electuary; let the quantity of a Nutmeg be taken often in a day.*

In the *Phrensie*, not only the Belly, but also the Bladder, and their offices, ought to be thought on, and often solicited or provoked.

Wherefore, the sick are to be warmed, and the Urinal given them, and asked to make water; but if they will not, or cannot, let the region of the yard below the belly be bathed *with a Decoction of Pellitory of the wall, Elder Flowers, and of the Seeds of Parsley, and wild Carrot Seeds, or daucus; with a Sponge; and after the Fomentation, anoint it with Oyl of Scorpions, and Oyntment of Dialthea: In a long suppression of Urine, you may put up to the bladder a piece of Wax Candle.*

The Histories and cases of *Frantick* people are so many, and so diversly described, *The Histories of* and so accurately by *Hippocrates* in his Books *De Epidem.* that there seems little need *sick persons in* here to add others; especially, because it would be an immense work and tedious, to *Hippocrates* relate the various manner and cases of Mad-men: In the mean time, as to the event of *Lib. Epidem.* the Disease, there is great diversity; for that for the most part the Feavour being cured, the *Phrensie* ceases by little and little; or else, that having no, or an evil, *Crisis*; either death, or a long raving follows. But that our *Hypothesis*, of the Inflammation of the Spirits, may be illustrated, I shall propose here one more rare instance.

I was one time sent for to Cure a Maid, that was strong, and having a Feavour, *A notable History.* was highly raging, being continually bound in her Bed. I took from her a great quantity of Blood, and caused it to be again iterated; I often took down her Belly with Clysters; yea I ordered all the other administrations in order, usual in this case; in the mean time she took *Juleps, Emulsions* and *Hypnoticks*: But these little or nothing availing, she continued still for seven or eight days without sleep, and furious, perpetually calling and bauling for cold drink; wherefore an *Hydropick* being granted her at her pleasure, yea to satiety; she was nevertheless not any thing less quiet, or thirsty. I therefore bid them (for that it was Summer time) that in the middle of the Night she should be carried by Women forth of doors, and put into a Boat, and her Cloths being pull'd off, and she tyed fast with a Cord, should be drenched into the depth of a River, the Rope being tyed only about her middle, that she might not be stifled in the Water; but there was no need of that, for the Maid of her own accord, fell to swimming, that scarce any Man could do it better, who had learned the art: After about a quarter of an hour, she came forth of the Water sound, and sober, and then being had to Bed, she slept, and sweat very much, and afterwards, without any other Remedy she grew well. This Cure succeeded so happily and so suddenly, forasmuch as the excess both of the Vital and the Animal flame, being together immensly increased, was taken away by a proper Remedy for the more intense Fire; to wit, by the moistning, and cooling of the Water.

Bb 2   CHAP.

CHAP. XI.

Of Melancholy.

The Distemper of the Animal Spirits, being after a diverse manner, as it is the cause of the Phrensie, so it is of Melancholy, Madness, and Stupidity.

AS the *Phrensie* arises from the burning of the Animal Spirits, (as we have elsewhere shewn) or as *Prosper Mart.* seems to affirm, from their substance being inflamed; so indeed other Distempers of raving arise from their substance being altered by other ways, and from their genuine nature being changed, from a *spirituous-saline*, into an acetous or sharp disposition, like to *Stygian* Water, or else into a liveless; which therefore are either *Melancholy*, or *Madness*, or *Foolishness* or *Stupidity*: of which we shall now speak in order, and first of all of *Melancholy*.

The definition of Melancholy. That it is a Distemper of the Brain and Heart.

Melancholy is commonly defined to be, a raving without a Feavour or fury, joined with fear and sadness. From whence follows, that it is a complicated Distemper of the Brain and Heart: For as *Melancholick* people talk idly, it proceeds from the vice or fault of the Brain, and the inordination of the Animal Spirits dwelling in it; but as they become very sad and fearful, this is deservedly attributed to the Passion of the Heart.

Its Examples or Types various, and almost infinite.

It would be a prodigious work, and almost an endless task to rehearse the diverse manner of ravings of *Melancholy* persons; and there are great Volumes already of Histories and examples of this sort; and more new and admirable observations and examples daily happen. Fabulous antiquity scarce ever thought of so many *metamorphoses* of men, which some have not believed really of themselves; whilst some have believed themselves to be Dogs or Wolves, and have imitated their ways and kind by barking or howling; others have thought themselves dead, desiring presently to be buried; others imagining that their bodies were made of glass, were afraid to be touched lest they should be broke to pieces. There are extant manifold and various kinds of the Imagination so depraved, concerning which may be commonly observed; That the distemper'd are *Delirious* as to all things, or at least as to most; so that they judge truly almost of no subject; or else they imagine amiss in one or two particular cases, but for the most part in other things, they have their notions not very incongruous. We shall first inquire into this more universal Distemper, for that the Imagination is prevaricated concerning very many things; to wit, by what causes, and with what difference of Symptoms, this is wont to come to pass; afterwards we shall speak of the special raving or idle talking.

Melancholy is either, 1. Universal, or

2. Particular.

The primary Phænomena of a Melancholick Delirium.

Although the universal Distemper of *Melancholy* contains manifold Delirious *Symptoms*, yet they chiefly consist in these three; 1. That the distemper'd are almost continually busied in thinking, that their *Phantasie* is scarce ever idle or at quiet. 2. In their thinking they comprehend in their mind fewer things than before they were wont, that oftentimes they roll about in their mind day and night the same thing, never thinking of other things that are sometimes of far greater moment. 3. The *Ideas* of objects or conceptions appear often deformed, and like hobgoblins, but are still represented in a larger kind or form; so that all small things seem to them great and difficult.

After this manner the *Phantasms* in the Brain evilly affected, are objected to the Intellect, almost after the same manner as the visible images are shewed to the Eye, by the interposition of some Optick Glass; to wit, where every object appears an horrid and huge monster, and for that reason a small portion only of the visible matter or thing, being increased to that immensity, is received by the aspect; then by reason of its horrid and unusual appearance, the image being once conceived, is not easily or suddenly let go: we will now consider by what affection of the Brain and Spirits, these appearances happen.

From what disposition of the Spirits they proceed.

Here we shall first of all inquire into the disposition or preternatural Constitution of the Animal Spirits: For inasmuch as they are after an irregular manner, they always or for a long time continue in their irregularities; and when the *Palsie*, *Apoplexy*, *Vertigo*, or *Convulsion*, are not joined to this Distemper of theirs, which argue obstructions of the Brain, it may be inferred, that the Animal Spirits, not fetching their force elsewhere, are driven into such inordinations; nor do chiefly conceive their disorders, by reason of the Pores and passages of the Brain being obstructed; but rather, in this case, they cause these aforesaid *Symptoms* in the sick from the default of their own Nature.

Such

Of Melancholy.

Such an indisposition of the Animal Spirits is wont to be described after this manner; to wit, that they, when as they ought to be transparent, subtle, and lucid, become in *Melancholy* obscure, thick, and dark, so that they represent the Images of things, as it were in a shadow, or covered with darkness: The explication of which does not seem incongruous; forasmuch as we have already shewed, that the Animal Spirits flowing forth from the inkindled Blood, go forth after a manner, as the rays of light from a flame. And it sufficiently appears, that the light shews and illustrates it self diversly, according as it proceeds from the burning of bodies, flaming forth after a various manner; as of Spirits of Wine, Oyl, Fat, Mineral Sulphur, Nitre, and others: in like manner the Animal Spirits, forasmuch as stilled forth from the Blood, having got this or that, or some other disposition, they are either subtil, clear, or dull, thick, and as it were sooty, they variously pass thorow and irradiate the organs of the Animal Functions, and so for that reason, diversly pervert their actions. *As they are compared to Light, they are called opacous, or full of darkness.*

But further, when as the Animal Spirits are not wholly loose and free as the little bodies of light, but mutually cohere or stick together, and lest the continuity of the soul should be broken off, they ought to be contained in a certain *Latex*; therefore these, with the Vehicle to which they cleave, may be very aptly compared to some *Chymical* Liquors, drawn forth by distillation from natural mixtures. Which *Analogy* indeed seems fittest for the unfolding the mad distempers. *This kind of Spirits in Melancholy compared to those in Chymical Liquors.*

1. Liquors *Chymically* Distilled, are, according to the active Elements after a various manner combined in them, of a diverse kind: the chiefest of these, by the consent of all, are said to be such, as in which the Spirit being united with the Salt, doth volatise it, and on the other side is sharpned by it, and after a sort fixed or kept. Of this sort they conceive the great *Elixir* and the Liquor *Alcahest* to be; and indeed in a manner are the Spirits of Blood, of Harts-horn, of Soot, and such like, very subtil, volatil, and penetrating, yet not apt to be inflamed, or suddenly to be dissipated. And indeed, the Animal Spirits seem to be after a manner, having obtained a sound and legitimate disposition, like a spirituous liquor stuffed with a volatile Salt, which is distilled from Blood; besides, to this there is given from the fire an high Acrimony and *Empyreuma*, or smatch of burning, which are wholly absent from the liquor watering the Brain and Nerves. *1. They are not like the Spirit of blood, as they should be.*

2. Other *Chymical* Liquors are sulphureous and burning, as the Spirits of Wine and Turpentine, which consisting of Spirit and Sulphur combined together, are easily inflamed, and depart one from another of their own accord, and fly hither and thither what way they can find; the Animal Spirits of this nature, as we shewed in the former Chapter, seem to be in the *Phrensie*. *2. Nor like the Spirit of Wine: Such rather in the Phrensie.*

3. Some Liquors or Spirits are produced by *Chymical* operation, in which the fixed Salt being carried forth to a Flux, hath obtained the dominion; of which sort are such as are distilled from Vinegar, ponderous Woods, and some Minerals, with a gentle fire; whose particles are very moveable, and unquiet, but of a short activity, so that Effluvia's do not long flow from them, that if they should be distilled *in Balneo*, nothing but an insipid Phlegm would be carried into the *Alembick*. And indeed, the Animal Spirits in *Melancholick* Distempers, are to be suspected to be of this kind of acetous nature, with the dominion of a fluid salt, as shall hereafter be more largely shewed. *3. But these are like acid Spirits, distilled out of Salt, Vinegar, Box, and such like.*

4. Some *Stagmas* drawn forth by *Spagyrick* art, are sometimes most sharp, to wit, in which the untamed Particles of a fluid Salt, and also *Sulphureous*, and *Arsenical*, being combined together, are exalted; as are the *Stygian* Waters distilled out of *Nitre*, *Vitriol*, *Antimony*, *Arsnick*, *Verdigriece*, and the like, all which are of a fierce nature, very penetrating and not to be broken, so that their *Effluvia's* are agitated with a perpetual motion, penetrate every thing, and are also diffused far and wide. And these kind of Liquors, may be aptly likened to the disposition of the Animal Spirits, acquired in *Madness*, as shall be anon declared. *4. Stygian Waters are like the Nature of the Animal Spirits in Madness.*

But for the present, that we may deliver the formal reason and causes of *Melancholy*, let us suppose, that the liquor instilled into the Brain from the Blood (which filling all the Pores and passages of the Head, and nervous *Appendix*, and watring them, is the Vehicle and bond of the Animal Spirits) hath degenerated from its mild, benign, and subtil nature, into an Acetous, and Corrosive, like to those liquors drawn out of Vinegar, Box, and *Vitriol*; and that the Animal Spirits, which from the middle part of the Brain, irradiating both its globous substance, as also the nervous *System*, and do produce all the Functions of the Senses and Motions, both interior and exterior, have such like Effluvia's, as fall away from those Acetous *Chymical* Liquors. Concerning which there may be observed these three things, 1. Their *The formal Reason of Melancholy aptly represented by acetous Chymical Liquors.*

being

There are three chief affections of these, which agree with the Animal Spirits in Melancholy.

being in perpetual motion: 2. Not long able to flow forth: 3. not only to be carried in open ways, but to cut new Porosities in the neighbouring bodies, and to infinuate themselves into them. From the *Analogy* of these conditions, concerning the Animal Spirits, it comes to pass, that *Melancholick* persons are ever thoughtful, that they only comprehend a few things, and that they falsly raise, or institute their notions of them. We shall consider of each of these a little more largely.

1. Effluvias falling away from these Liquors are perpetually in motion.

1. Therefore we shall take notice, that the Effluvia's falling away from these distilled Acetous Liquors, are perpetually in motion: for the Spirits of Vitriol, or of Vinegar, or Sea Salt continually evaporate: the reason of which is, because those Particles of the fluid Salt do scarcely agree with any others, but where ever they are stopped, being apt immediately to leave their subjects, seem to endeavour to get new consorts. And hence some have thought nothing more like to perpetual motion, than the Acid Spirits of Minerals, shut up and *Hermetically* seal'd in a Phial; for so the Vapours or Effluvia's will creep about the sides of the Glass, with a continual Circulation.

In like manner also the Spirits in the Phantasie of a Melancholick person.

In like manner we may suppose, That the nervous Acetous Liquor is instilled from the Blood, sometimes stuffed with a fixed Salt, or with Vitriolick Particles, or other heterogeneous, into the Brain, for the matter and Vehicle of the Animal Spirits; and so these being admitted within the middle part of the Brain, for the acts of the Animal Functions, do not quickly pass thorow and irradiate all the Pores and Passages, but like little acid Atoms, creep about here and there, slowly, but incessantly, and as it were with a certain unquiet motion of tingling or creeping, diffuse themselves by little and little thorow the whole neighbourhood: Hence a storm of thoughts is perpetually stirred up, by which the Brain is wont to be busied without intermission; so that *Melancholic* persons have continually, day and night, disturbed Phantasies; for that their Animal Spirits consist of a continually moveable matter; Hence also they look with eyes turned inwards, or fixed, or obliquely, and sullen or clogged, and exercise the other faculties both sensitive and loco-motive inadvertently; because the Spirits being worn out and distracted by continual motion, do not well actuate or beam into the nervous *System*.

2. Effluvias from actous Chymical Liquors do not proceed far.

2. Though the Effluvia's continually fall away from an Acetous Spirit, prepared by *Chymical* Art, yet they do not go far, but gather together on an heap thickly, near the superficies of the liquor, and penetrate only the neighbouring bodies, not touching those that are at a distance: Hence the Spirits of *Vitriol*, Salt, or Vinegar, will not ascend out of the *Cucurbit* into the *Alembick* unless urged with a very strong heat; but being included in a low *Phial*, they shall corrode and pierce thorow the stopple.

In like manner the imagination of a Melancholick Person, though always employ'd, comprehends only a few things.

It is after the same manner, concerning the *Phantasie* of *Melancholick* persons; for inasmuch as the Animal Spirits being degenerate into an acid nature, do not irradiate or quickly pass thorow the whole compass of the Brain, as before, but flowing in the middle part, are carried with its force only into the nearest Pores and Passages; therefore cogitations raised up from thence, though they be continual, yet they comprehend but a few things: and so, as when many bands of Spirits are thrust together in strait bounds, every small object, and of very little moment, seems to them very great and of notable weight;

And therefore every thing is conceived with a greater Image than it should be.

certainly after the same manner, and for the same reason, as when the visible images passing thorow a *Microscoptick* Glass are carried to the Eye; for, because many beams of the same thing are concenter'd, its magnitude seems to be increased into an immense greatness; so when as every intentional Species or Image, by the conflux of very many spirits together, is formed in the Brain, it appears to the soul greater and of more weight than usual. Every one may experiment this truth in himself: For when as we become thoughtful, from eating gross or melancholick meats, or by reason of the passion of sorrow (the reason of which affection is, because the Animal Spirits are unfit for a more free expansion) then we are very solicitous and fearful, concerning every little thing, as if then our health or fortune were for ever in danger. Hence also, because the Animal Spirits, though almost ever in motion, are notwithstanding still limited within the same short bounds, *Melancholick* persons persist a long while in thinking and revolving in their mind often the same thing.

3. Effluvias from acetous Liquors do not evaporat so much from open Pores, as they make new.

3. But there yet remains another similitude of the Animal Spirits, with those distilled from *Vitriol*, and other saline bodies, to wit, that as the Effluvia's sent away from these kind of Acetous Spirits, do not evaporate so much from open spaces and tracts, before made, as they cut out Pores and Passages that are new, for themselves, in an objected body; so that they easily pass thorow, and render friable or crumbling, the Cork or stopple to the Vessel where they are; which happens not from the Spirit of Wine, to any thing that stops up the Phial; so indeed in *Melancholick* persons, it is usually wont to be. For because the Animal Spirits, being as it were pointed with saline

saline Particles, whilst they flow from the middle of the Brain, they observe not their former tracts and ways of their expansion, but they thickly make for themselves new and unwonted little spaces, within the globous substance of the Brain: Hence cogitations are brought before the Soul, not such as they were wont to be, but new and incongruous, and for the most part absurd. But indeed, because the *Phantasie* is prevaricated, about the Conceptions of things, and by reason that the acts of judgment and reason are falsly framed, the only cause is, for that the Animal Spirits leaving their former walks, and going backward and forward in their ways in the Brain, being carried hither and thither obliquely and transverse, affect altogether unaccustomed and bye ways, which indeed is proper for them to do, out of the Acetous disposition, with which they labour; to wit, forasmuch as the Effluvia of those kind of Liquors expand themselves not in a direct or free emanation, as the rays of light; but by a bending motion, and as it were creeping, they craul on every side into the neighbouring part. *And in like manner the Animal Spirits, whilst they form in the Brain new Tracts, produce unwonted and incongruous Notions.*

Thus much for the primary *Melancholick* Distemper, to wit, a *Delirium* or Raving, being excited by reason of the vices of the Spirits inhabiting the Brain: The beginnings of which, although they proceed chiefly, and oftentimes, almost only from the Acetous disposition of the Spirits; yet afterwards, the conformation of the Brain it self is often brought to be a part of the cause; to wit, forasmuch as the Recrements of the *Melancholick* Blood, being perpetually poured forth, renders its substance more thick and dark, and the primary tracts or paths of the Animal Function being near blotted out, new, oblique, and by-paths are made; insomuch, that the Spirits, though better should be begotten, could not easily irradiate the Brain, or presently recover their former passages. *In Melancholy, after the Animal Spirits being for some time vitiated, the Conformation of the Brain is also hurt.*

Melancholy is not only a Distemper of the Brain and Spirits dwelling in it, but also of the *Pracordia*, and of the Blood therein inkindled, from thence sent into the whole Body: and as it produces there a *Delirium* or idle talking, so here fear and sadness; but by what means we shall now see. *The Affection of the Præcordia in this Disease, as to fear and sadness, is delivered.*

First, in Sadness, the flamy or vital part of the Soul is straitned, as to its compass; and driven into a more narrow compass; then consequently, the animal or lucid part contracts its sphere, and is less vigorous; but in Fear both are suddenly repressed and compelled as it were to shake, and contain themselves within a very small spaces; in either passion, the Blood is not circulated, and burns not forth lively, and with a full burning, but being apt to be heaped up and to stagnate about the *Præcordia*, stirs up there a weight or a fainting; and in the mean time, the Head and Members being destitute of its more plentiful flux, languishes. The formal reasons of these Distempers, and their causes, we have before exposed. *After what manner the Corporeal Soul is affected in these two passions.*

But because these are habitual in *Melancholick* persons, the cause is partly in the Blood, and partly in the Animal Action of the heart. For the Blood, because of the saline particles being exalted, becomes less inflamable; from whence it is neither sufficiently inkindled in the Lungs, or doth it burn with a plentiful and enough clear flame within the passages of the Heart and its vessels; but is apt to be repressed, and almost blown out with every blast of wind: Hence, when that the vital flame is so small and languishing, that it shakes and trembles at every motion, it is no wonder if that the *Melancholick* person is as it were with a sinking and half overthrown mind always sad and fearful. By reason of this kind of saltish *Dyscrasie* of the Blood, *Melancholicks* rarely have a Feavour; yet being taken with it, by reason of the irregular burning of the Blood, they are more in danger. *The cause of these depends partly on the blood;*

No less doth it come to pass, by the fault of the Heart, that *Melancholick* persons become sad and fearful, by reason of the course of the Blood being retarded, and called back from thence: for, because that Muscle is actuated but with an inflowing of weak and enormous Spirits, it cannot perform its contractions strongly enough, and constantly, whereby the Blood may be driven forward into the whole body, without stop or leaping back: So the Blood and the Animal Spirits affect one another mutually, with a reciprocal evil, and bring hurt one to the other. That is, the *Melancholick* Blood consisting of *Saline* Particles, carried forth together with *Sulphureous*, begets Animal Spirits, indued with an Acetous nature, as hath been shown; and these Spirits wrongly performing the offices of the Vital Function, cause such an evil disposition of the Blood to be increased. *and partly on the Animal Action of the Heart.*

Thus much of *Melancholy* in general, *viz.* of its Essence, Conjunct Causes, and chief *Symptoms*, together with the reasons of them. Before we proceed to the kinds and differences of this Disease, we ought to explain, from what kind of causes, both *Procatartick* and Evident, it is wont to arise, and to be cherished; and first, from whence either part of the Soul, *viz.* both Animal and Vital, doth acquire their morbid dispositions. *The procatartick Causes of Melancholy, &c.*

First

Partly the acetous Nature of the Spirits, and partly the Melancholy Dyscrasie of the Blood: The Distemper begins sometimes from this, sometimes from that.

First we say, the former of these to be Acetous, like to the Spirit of *Vitriol* or Vinegar, and this to be *Salino sulphureous*, or Atrabilary or Melancholick; further, as the one doth cherish the other, so they at first beget one another. For sometimes *Melancholy* beginning, and for a long time persisting, from the Animal Spirits being disturbed, and driven into a certain confusion, causes the *Melancholick* disposition of the Blood; and sometimes also the Blood, at first contracting this evil disposition, perverts the nature of the Spirits.

How it begins from the Spirits and the Animal Government.

That *Melancholy* doth very often arise from the Animal Government, every common body doth sufficiently note; to wit, forasmuch as the Animal Spirits conceive inordinations from violent passions of the mind, in which, when they remain long, they bend the whole Soul, yea and the Body, from their due temper and constitution: So especially destroying Love, vehement sadness, panick fears, envy, shame, care, and immoderate study, are wont oftentimes to excite this Distemper. For by reason of these kinds of occasions, the Animal Spirits being thrust down, beyond their wonted paths of expansion, and remaining in their error, by reason of the assiduity of Passion, at last they go into these deviating tracts, which afterwards observing, they are hardly reduced into their former due ways. Then, forasmuch as for that reason, the motion and vigoration of the Heart (as hath been shewed) is lessened; therefore the Blood is defective in its due temper, and sanguification, and is from thence made more fixed and *Salino-sulphureous*, and the Animal Spirits coming from it, are but degenerate into a sourness; and so the Blood being depraved by the latter, encreases to the *Melancholick* disposition, begun from the Spirits.

By what means this Disease arises from the Blood.

No less often doth it come to pass, that the seeds of *Melancholy*, being at first laid in the Blood, do at length impart their evil to the Spirits: For this reason, some are made obnoxious to this Disease from their Parents. But an inordinate living, long intermission of wonted exercise, usual evacuations, as of the Menstrual Blood, or the Piles, or bleeding at the *Hæmorrhoidal* Veins, also the Seed, or the Serous Matter, being suddenly suppressed, and many other occasions, easily infect, and foul the Blood, and render it *Melancholick*; whose depraved disposition is of necessity communicated to the Spirits.

Melancholy doth not arise from an atrabilary humour heaped up in some place or mine.

But we cannot here yield to what some *Physicians* affirm, that *Melancholy* doth arise from a *Melancholick* humor, somewhere primarily and of it self begotten, and they assign for its birth, several places, to wit, the Brain, Spleen, Womb, and the whole habit of the Body; for besides, for that no such mines of such an humor appear, unless perhaps some be planted in the Spleen; moreover the Blood it self is it, which conceives at first the *Melancholick* intemperance, or any other by it self, and then deposes the Recrements of the same nature, in proper emunctories or receptacles. For neither is the yellow Bile or Choler laid up in the Gall-Bladder, or the black Bile so called, or *Melancholick* humor in the *Spleen*, unless the bloody Mass begets those humors before hand: If at any time these, or other Recrements, being any where laid up, are received of the Blood, they produce its effervescency or growing hot, but not presently or easily its intemperature.

By what means according to the Antients, it is said to arise from the Head.

Therefore, because sometimes the original of *Melancholy* is ascribed to the Head, and the intemperature of the Brain from these, to wit, too hot, and accused to be from those, too cold, I rather think it ought to be affirmed, that this Distemper doth sometimes at first begin from the Brain, and the Soul dwelling in it: because *Hippocrates* also plainly asserts it, 6 *Epidem*. Sect. 8. T. 58. For distinguishing *Epileptical* and *Melancholick* persons, being made so together, or else successively, as to the formal reasons of the Diseases, he saith, *The defluxion which floweth from the Brain, from the ill affection, state, or temperament thereof, if it flows into the Body causeth the Falling-sickness; if into the cogitation or the mind,* *Melancholy*. So in *Melancholy* he grants, the Soul distinctly, and as it were apart from the Body, or Brain, to be affected.

How from the Womb.

Secondly, Because sometimes the original of this Disease is deduced from the Womb, it is not to be thought, that the *Melancholick* humor is there at first generated, but the occasion of *Melancholy* doth proceed from thence; either because the whole Blood being infected, and made degenerate by reason of a stoppage of the *Menstrua*, strives to go into a *Melancholy Dyscrasie* or intemperature; or because, by reason of the provocations of *Venus* or Lust, being restrained, not without great reluctancy of the Corporeal Soul, the Animal Spirits being for a long time forced, and restrained, become at length more fixed and *Melancholick*.

How from the Spleen.

Thirdly, It is a common opinion, and also ours, that sometimes *Melancholy* is either primarily excited, or very much cherished from the Spleen, being evilly affected, and so from thence is called by a peculiar word, *Hypochondriack*; as we have shewed at large in another Tract of Convulsive Diseases. But the Blood is first in fault, begetting

Of Melancholy.

ting in it self from the beginning *Melancholick* foulnesses, deposes them in the Spleen, which receiving again, after their being exalted into the nature of an evil Ferment, is more vitiated in its disposition, by their foulness.

Fourthly, But besides, it is said, there is another kind of *Melancholy*, distinct from the *Hypochondriack*, and the former, that is begotten in the whole Body together; this is nothing else, than the Mass of Blood being degenerated from its true nature, by reason of errors in the six non-naturals, and for many other occasions, doth acquire an *Atrabilary* or *Melancholick* disposition; that is, where the Spirit being depressed, the *Sulphureous* Particles, together with the *Saline*, and also with some *Earthy*, are carried forth; for the *Melancholick* disposition of the Blood is very much a-kin to this *Sulphureous-saline*, which we have shewed oftentimes to excel in some kind of *Scurvy*. For what causes, and upon what occasions, this is wont to be produced, may be sufficiently known from the *Ætiology* of that Disease, being at large explained. *How from the whole Body.*

The differences of this Disease may be easily gathered from what hath been said: for in respect of its first subject, which is sometimes the Soul, sometimes the Body, or rather the Blood, it is called either Animal or humeral *Melancholy*. Again, it is impressed according to that, with various powers, to wit, it is first impressed either on the Rational Will, or the sensitive, concupiscible, or irascible Appetite; also it is divided into very many kinds, as it is employed about diverse things, to wit, either Sacred, or Magical, or Humane, the huge cense or bead-roll of which is almost infinite; the chief of which, that are wont to come within the Cure of Medicine, are Religious, Amorous, and Jealous *Melancholy*. *The Differences of the Disease. 1. In respect of its first Subject.*

2. By reason of the temperament of the sick, according to which, the Particles of the *Melancholick* blood, being made sometimes *Sulphureous*, sometimes Saline or Earthy, the Spirituous being depressed, are exalted more or less, a *Delirium*, or sadness, fury, or stupidity, are more or less variously joined to *Melancholy*. *2. By reason of the Temperament of the Sick.*

3. The Disease is either continual or intermitting, according to the conjunct cause, either stronger, both the *Hypostasis* of the Spirits, and also the bloody Mass, being both together vitiated; or else lighter, and less deeply fixed; so that the Distemper'd sometimes are well enough for many days or months, yet apt to relapse upon any great occasion. *In respect of the next Cause, as it is singular, or conjunct.*

4. In respect of the hurt Imagination, there are very many types of *Melancholicks* to be met with, yea almost innumerable; yet the chief difference of which is, that some are delirious in all things, and others in one thing only. *In respect of the Imagination diversly hurt.*

The *Prognostick* of this Disease, though as to health or death, it is for the most part safe; yet by reason of the event, it is very uncertain: For some quickly grow well, others not of a long time, and others are never cured. *The Prognostick of this Disease.*

This Distemper suddenly excited, from a solitary evident cause, as a vehement Passion, is far safer than by leasure invading, after a long *Procatarxis* or foregoing cause. For the former, if the evident cause be presently removed, often ceases of its own accord, or with a little help; but in this latter, for that the Mass of Blood, and the whole heap of Animal Spirits, are departed from their due disposition, and not rarely the conformation of the Brain, as to the tracts of the Spirits, is altered; The Cure very difficultly, and not under a long time succeeds.

Melancholy being a long time protracted, passes oftentimes into Stupidity, or Foolishness, and sometimes also into Madness; further, sometimes it brings on Convulsive Distempers, or the *Palsie*, or *Apoplexy*, yea sometimes a violent Death.

As to the Cure, there is little or no hopes, if the Distemper'd being very contumacious and refractory, reject all Medicines, and every method of Physick. Further, there is scarce any better thing to be expected from them, who lying sick with only imaginary Diseases, take all Remedies, and require still more, and of diverse kinds, to be given them.

As the Cure of *Melancholy*, as it is always difficult and long, so it is wont to be mighty intricate and perplexed; for that it ought to be diversly and variously instituted, in respect of the evident, *Procatartick*, and Conjunct causes of its kind, also by reason of the *Symptoms* daily arising. Neither is it only behoveful oftentimes to change the Remedies, and Method of healing, but also variously to make use of between whiles, warnings, deceits, flatteries, intreaties, and punishments. *The Cure of the Disease.*

But first of all, the Evident Cause of this Disease, if any noted thing went before, should be inquired into; and if it may be, either presently removed, or else its removal to be in some sort feigned. Further, the affections of the mind being vehement, and stirred up from thence, are either to be appeased, or subdued by others opposite. Wherefore, to desperate Love ought to be applied or shewed indignation and hatred; Sadness is to be opposed with the flatteries of Pleasure, Musick, a desire of vain glory, *The evident Cause first to be removed.*

Cc or

Of Melancholy.

or also a *pannick* terror. In like manner, as to the rest of the Passions, you must proceed to quiet, or elude them.

Three primary Indications.
The *Curatory* Method, accommodated for the healing of *Melancholy*, suggests many other Indications, the chief of which, and to which the rest may be the better placed, are these three, commonly noted, *viz. Curatory*, which respects immediately the Disease, and its Conjunct Cause; *Preservatory*, which cuts off the *Procatartick*, and Evident Causes; and *Vital*, which is imployed about conserving of strength.

1. Curatory.
As to the first Indication, the intention of the *Physician* is so much to lift up, make volatile, and corroborate the more fixed or dejected Animal Spirits, that being also apt to go backwards, or out of the way, that afterwards they may irradiate more freely, being stretched forth, the whole Brain, with a full and not broken beam, for the Acts of the Imagination, Judgment, and other principal faculties; and so lively actuate the *Pracordia*, and make them to vibrate or beat strongly, that the Blood being more plentifully inkindled, it may be projected from thence, without stop or stagnating, into the whole Body.

The healing of the Spirits, is best performed by admonitions and artificial inventions, concerning the business of Life.
Therefore, for the healing of the Spirits, first of all it is to be procured, that the Soul should be withdrawn from all troublesome and restraining passion, *viz.* from mad Love, Jealousie, Sorrow, Pity, Hatred, Fear, and the like, and composed to chearfulness or joy: pleasant talk, or jesting, Singing, Musick, Pictures, Dancing, Hunting, Fishing, and other pleasant Exercises are to be used. They who care not for Sports or Pleasures (for to some *Melancholicks* they are always ingrateful) are to be roused up by imploying them in more light businesses; sometimes *Mathematical* or *Chymical* Studies, also Travelling, do very much help; moreover, it is often expedient to change the places of habitation, in their native soil. Those who will still stay at home, are to be warned, that they take care of their Houshold affairs, and that they should govern their Family; that they should build Houses, plant and order Gardens, Orchards, or Till the Ground. For the mind being busied with necessary cares or duties puts aside, and at last deserts more easily, vain and mad cogitations. *Melancholy* persons are seldom to be left alone, for that then they indulge their airy phantasies and speculations, and suffer them to continue longer. The Soul sinks down inwardly, and leaving the body, enters into a certain *Metamorphosis*, and puts on a new shape, and oftentimes different from humane manners. Wherefore, the Distemper'd ought to be disturbed almost always with the discourses of their familiar Friends; to wit, that the Animal Spirits, being called outwards, may be solicited from their diversions, into their former and accustomed tracts. But if the sick be seduced with phantastical illusions, and imagine some prodigious things of themselves, and firmly believe them; their mind is to be drawn from them, by artificial inventions; very many causes and examples of this sort of Cure are to be found in Books, and a discreet Physician may institute the like as occasion serves.

Yet oftentimes there is need of Medicine besides.
Although a fresh *Melancholy* may be cured sometimes by the mere discipline and institution of the mind and Animal Spirits, yet in a long or inveterate, where the Spirits have contracted an acetous nature, and the Blood an *Atrabilary* or Melancholick disposition, and that the Brain is hurt, as to its Pores and passages: other Indications called

The Preservatory indication, concerning the Procatartick Causes of the Disease.
Preservatory are required, for the taking away of the *Procatartick* causes. Concerning this thing, the Medical intentions are first, that the Blood be reduced to a better temper, and genuine, to wit, a spirituous saline; then to enliven the Brain, and to render it bright and clear, its Pores being unlocked; and also to corroborate the Animal Spirits, and to excite them into a lively flowing forth. For which ends, the following method I think good to propose, which notwithstanding ought to be varied, according to the various constitutions of the sick.

Phlebotomy.
The taking away of Blood has place almost in all *Melancholicks*, and sometimes it is often to be iterated. For the adust and liveless Blood, being at times drawn away, a new and more spirituous comes in its place. Concerning the quantity, place, and manner of celebrating this Remedy, Authors have various opinions; but the motion and the affections of the Blood, being truly weighed, it will at first suffice to take a moderate quantity out of the Arm, and afterwards if need be, a lesser, or to draw it from the Sedal Veins by Leeches. How the *Salvatella* Veins being opened (as is said) should bring such notable help to *Melancholicks*, I confess I cannot understand: perhaps it may help them, if the *Melancholick* persons be firmly perswaded, that this *Phlebotomy* will cure them before any others: the frequent opening the *Hemorrhoidal* Veins, invites Nature to an indeavouring afterwards for that evacuation, which succeeding of its own accord (as *Hippocrates* says) does not seldom Cure this Disease.

Purging.
Purging, for that it draws back the nourishment of the Disease, from the firsts ways, and removes the impediments of other Remedies, ought to be celebrated at the beginning,

ning, and repeated at intervals. But that some think, for the sooner rooting out of this Disease, *Hellebore* or *Elaterium* are chiefly to be used, and cite *Hippocrates* for their Author; we apprehend, if the success be minded, those things do not ordinarily agree with, yea more often do hurt to the sick: For indeed, more strong Purgers do not take away the cause of the Disease, to wit, the *Dyscrasie* of the Blood, but rather encrease it; besides, they more debilitate and strike down the Animal Spirits, before dejected. But *Hellebore* was so often prescribed by *Hippocrates*, because in his Age other *Catharticks* were scarcely known, or at least they were not in frequent use: But now it is thought much better, gently to draw forth the receptacles of the humors, by more gentle and easie Purgers, and to cleanse only the Viscera and the first ways, without any great commotions of the Blood and Spirits.

Vomiting Medicines (as in most *Cephalick* Diseases free from a Feavour) are wont to help after a peculiar manner in all mad Distempers. The reason of this partly consists in this, because the viscous load of the Ventricle, which (as we have elsewhere shewn) doth very much burthen the Soul, being purged forth, the Spirits by that means being more free, expand themselves more lively and chearfully. Further, forasmuch as Vomiting presses together and evacuates the neighbouring receptacles of the humors, to wit, the *Gall-Bag*, the passage of the *Pancreas*, and the *Glandulæ* of the *Mesentery*, procures that their contents be not transferred into the Head. *Vomiting.*

Take *Oxymel of Squills one ounce and a half, of Wine of Squills one ounce, of the Syrup* *Vomitories.*
de Peto two drams; mix them, and make a Vomit: if it doth not work, or but slowly provoke Vomiting with a great deal of Carduus Posset-drink.
Take *of the Decoction of the middle bark of Elder four ounces, of the Salt of Vitriol one scruple to two scruples, of Oxymel simple three drams; mix them, and take it after the same manner.*
To robust and well set persons may be given *of the Infusion of Crocus Metallorum, or of Mercurius Vitæ*, also *the Emetick Tartar of Mynsicht, or the Sulphur of Antimony.*
Take *of the Root of Polypodium of the Oak half an ounce, of Epithimum three drams, of* *Purgers.*
Sena half an ounce, of Tamarinds six drams, of the seeds of Coriander three drams, of yellow Saunders two drams; let them be boiled in fourteen ounces of Spring-water, till it comes to ten ounces; adding to the Colature, or when it is strained, of Agarick two drams, of Rhubarb one dram and a half, being clarified, add of the Syrup of purging Apples two ounces; let six ounces be taken, and repeated within three or four days.
Take *of the best Sena three drams, Epithym, Rhubarb, each one dram and a half; of Yellow Saunders half a dram, of Coriander seed two scruples, of the Salt of Wormwood half a dram, of Celtick Spike a scruple; put these into white Wine, and the Water of Pipins, of each four ounces, kept close all night; to the liquor being strained five ounces, add of the Syrup of Epithimum six drams, of Aqua Mirabilis two drams; mix them and make a Potion. In strong bodies or hard to work on, may be added to these, of the strings of black Hellebore macerated in Vinegar one dram or two.*

For those who had rather make use of Pills, Boluses, Powders, or Syrups, take the following.

Take *of Pil. Tartar of Quercitan, or of Amber of Crato half a dram, of the Resine of* *Pills.*
Jalap or of Scammony six or eight grains, of Tartar vitriolated half a scruple, of Ammoniacum dissolved in Aqua Mirabilis, what will suffice to make a Pill: let four be taken going to sleep, and unless they work first, one in the morning following.
Take *of Calamelanos, of the extract of black Hellebore, each one scruple; of the Resine of Jalap six grains, of Ammoniacum solut. what will suffice; make four Pills, let them be taken with Government.*
The Powder of Haly, the Powder of *Valesco de Tarenta*, of *Peueda* and others, are very *Powders.*
much commended. And indeed in Country bodies, or robust, this Cathartick may seem convenient. Take *of Epithimum half an ounce, of Agarick, Lapis Lazuli, each three drams, Scammony one dram, Cloves thirty; make a Powder: the Dose is from half a dram to a dram.*
Take *of the Powder Diasenna, of Diaturbith with Rhubarb, each half a dram; make a Powder: let it be taken in a draught of Posset-drink, in a Decoction of Epithimum simple four or five scruples.*
Take *of the best Senna two ounces, of the Roots of Polypodia of the Oak two ounces, of* *Syrups.*
Epithimum one ounce and a half, of yellow Citrons half an ounce, of Tamarinds one ounce, of Coriander seeds six drams, boil them in Barnet water four pints, till half be consumed,
strain,

strain it, and let it be evaporated in a warm Bath, to the consistence of a Syrup, adding towards the end, of pure Manna, and of white Sugar, each four ounces; make a Syrup: the Dose is two spoonfuls or three, in three ounces of some convenient distilled-water, or in any other liquor. Or,

Take *of the same liquor evaporated to the consistence of Honey six ounces, of fresh Cassia four ounces, of the jelly of Currans two ounces, of Cream of Tartar, of the Salt of Wormwood, each one dram and a half; of the Powder of Diasen. two drams, of yellow Sanders powder'd two drams; mix them and make an Electuary: Dose three drams to half an ounce.*

Altering Medicines are of the greatest moment;

Purging is not to be used continually, nor too frequently, yea it suffices that it be administred within six or seven days space, and at other times, let the belly be taken down by Clysters, if it be bound. As to other Medicines, which are not evacuators, though the Ancients relied not much upon them, we put our greatest confidence of Cure in them. For they (to whom also many moderns consent) thought there was nothing more to be done for the curing of *Melancholy*, than to Purge forth the *Melancholick* humor; wherefore, making Purges their chiefest business, they instituted the other Medicines called Preparatory, only for the sake of this, to wit, making it their scope, that as soon as the humor being reduced to a fit consistency, by altering Medicines, and that the ways for its excretion were open enough, then that it should be *and not purging Medicines, as the Antients thought.* carried forth of doors by Purgers. Which kind of *Hypothesis* seems not agreeable, neither to reason, nor to Medical experience; because *Melancholick* people rather receive hurt than help by often Purging, how methodically soever it be instituted. Therefore, we, placing the cause of this Disease in the Dyscrasie of the Blood and Spirits, and in the weakness or evil conformation of the *Viscera* and the Brain, esteem altering and corroborating Medicines to be in the first rank for Remedies, and for the sake of these, that Purgers may be used sometimes between whiles. Therefore Purging being rightly prescribed at due intervals, for the removing impediments, as to the rest you may proceed according to these forms.

An Electuary.

Take *of the Conserves of the flowers of Gilliflowers, and of Borage, each two ounces and a half; of the rinds of Myrobalans preserved six drams, of Coral prepared, and of Pearl, each one dram and a half; of Ivory, and Crabs Eyes, each one dram; of Confection de Hyacintho two drams, of the Syrup of Coral and red Poppy what will suffice; make an Electuary: take two drams Morning and Evening, drinking after it three ounces of the following Julep, or the distilled Water.*

A Julep.

Take *of the water of the Flowers of Cowslips, and of black Cherries, each six ounces; of Balm four ounces, of Dr.* Stephens *his Water two ounces, of Sugar six drams; mingle it and make a Julep.*

A Distilled Water.

Take *of the leaves of Balm, Borrage, Bugloss, Fumitory, Water-Cresses, and Brooklime, each four handfuls; of the flowers of Pinks, Marigolds, Borrage, and Cowslips, each three handfuls; the outer rinds of six Oranges and six Lemons, being all cut and bruised, pour to them Whey made of Cyder eight pints; distil it in a common Still, and mix all the liquor together.*

Lozenges.

Take *of the Powder of Pearl, of Ivory, of Coral prepared, each two drams; of the Species Latificant (or making merry) of Diarrhod. Abbatis, each one dram; of the Oyl of the rind of Citrons half a scruple, of white Sugar, dissolved and boiled to the consistence of Lozenges, in what will suffice of Balm Water, six ounces; make Lozenges according to art, weighing a dram: take two or three at nine of the Clock in the Morning, and at five in the Afternoon, drinking after it a draught of the distilled Water or of Tea.* Or,

An Apozem;

Take *of the Roots of Chervil, of Polypodium of the Oak, each one ounce and a half; of the leaves of Harts Tongue, Ceterach, Scolopendria, Germander, each one handful; of Tamarisk half a handful, of the bark of the same half an ounce, of Raisins of the Sun stoned two ounces, one Apple cut; let them be cut and bruised, and boiled in four pints of Spring-water, to the consumption of a third part; about the end add of the leaves of Water Cresses one handful, let it be strained and clarified: take of it six ounces twice or thrice in a day; sweeten it with Syrup of Fumitory.*

Spaw-Waters.

*Spaw-*Waters coming from Iron, are wont oftentimes to give great benefit for the Curing of *Melancholicks,* to wit, because they being plentifully drunk, wash out *salino-sulphureous* Tincture of the Blood, and destroy its evil ferment. Moreover, they wipe clean the filthiness of the *Viscera,* unlock obstructions, and what is of great benefit, they corroborate, by their astriction, both the weak and too loose *Viscera,* and also shut up the little mouths of the gaping Vessels of the Brain, by which a passage lay open

into

into it for the extraneous matter, together with the nervous juice. And for this reason, to wit, by corroborating the Viscera, and by locking up the passages of the Head, *Vitriolicks* prepared of Iron are wont to be given profitably in *Melancholy*, and also in the *Vertigo*.

> Take of our Steel prepared three drams, put it into a quart of the Water above described, take of it three or four ounces twice in a day, by it self, or with any other solid Medicine. *Chalybeates.*
>
> Take of the filings of Iron one ounce, put it into a glass with the juice of Oranges two ounces; let it stand for a day, shaking it sometimes, then pour to it of the Water of Pipins, and of White Wine, each one pint; or of the more thin and sweet Cyder one quart: take of it three ounces, twice in a day, after the same manner. *Steeled Medicines.*
>
> Take of the Vitriol of Steel, of the Cream of Tartar, of Crabs Eyes, each one dram; mix them; make a Powder, and let it be divided into nine parts: Take one part every Morning in a draught of the distilled Water, or the Decoction, or in a proper Broth.
>
> Take of the Syrup of Steel four ounces: take of it one spoonful twice in a day, in a proper Vehicle.
>
> Take of the Extract of Steel, of our Steel prepared with a proper Decoction three drams, of the Powder of Ivory, of yellow Saunders, of Lignum Aloes, each half a dram; of the Salt of Tartar two scruples, of Ammoniacum dissolved in the Water of Worms what will suffice to make a mass; let it be made into small Pills; let three or four be taken every Evening, drinking after it three ounces of the water of Apples, or of Cowslip flowers.

Whey, if it agrees with the stomach, being drunk very plentifully, for many days, for the same reason as Spaw waters, viz. by washing out the Salt, and Sulphureous particles of the Melancholick blood, is often given with success. Whey with Epithimum infused in it, or boiled in it, is highly praised by some. *Whey.*

Let Broths be made of a boiled Pullet, with the roots of Polypodium, Chervil, Fenil, Butchers Broom, and the leaves of Ceterach, Harts Tongue, Scolopendria, &c. take a draught of it in the Morning, and at five of the Clock in the Afternoon, in which dissolve of the Vitriol of Steel six grains, to ten of the Salt of Wormwood, and of the Cream of Tartar, each a scruple. *Broths.*

The Juices of Herbs and their expressions bring sometimes not at all: help to the taking away the Discrasie of the Blood. Take of the leaves of Borage, of Water-Cresses, each six handfuls; two Apples pared, the Pulp of two Oranges, and of white Sugar one ounce; let them be all bruised together, and pour to them of the best Cyder a pint and an half; make an expression very strongly, and let it be kept in a glass. The Dose is four ounces twice or thrice in a day. *Juices of Herbs.*

In the Summer time, a Bath of sweet water, for that it wipes away the filth impacted in the Pores of the skin, and moves transpiration insensibly, is very profitable to some. *A Bath.*

Because *Melancholick* persons sleep but badly, and from long and frequent waking become worse, therefore *Anodynes,* and sometimes the more gentle *Hypnoticks* (when there is need) may be prescribed to be taken late at night, for this end are convenient, a Decoction of Cowslip flowers, or of the leaves of Lettice, or the water of red Poppies, or the Syrup of the same: Further, Emulsions of the Seeds of the white Poppy, of the Syrup *de Meconio*, and others that are only agreeable and cherishing of the Spirits. *Hypnoticks.*

As there is an infinite Company of *Melancholicks,* as well as of *Fools,* therefore we shall illustrate our *Hypothesis* with two Examples only, in one of which the Disease begins from the sensitive part of the Soul, or the Animal Spirits; and the other from its Vital part, to wit, from the Blood.

Sometime since, a noted person about forty years of Age, of a florid countenance, chearful, and nimble about any business, being afflicted in his mind, by reason of a certain affair, and very much dejected, he became thereupon very sad, *Melancholick,* and with a dark and cast down countenance. When I went first to visit him, he complained of a manifold hurry and distraction of thoughts, which were so many, that he was busied in his Phantasie almost night and day continually, he lived without any sleep: Nor were these cares concerning the commonweal, or the proper business of his Family; nor about the health of his Soul, or of his Body, was he at all solicitous; but was rather troubled perpetually about small matters, and of no moment. He was so fearful of all things, that he presaged loss or death immediately to happen to him, upon every small accident. And lastly, he was so sad, as if he would contend in weeping with *Heraclitus*. Further, he laboured with such a straitness of Heart, and so great a constriction, that he seemed to feel all his *Præcordia* to be drawn together like a Purse, *The first History.* *An Example of Melancholy beginning from the Spirits.*

and

and he thought that there still lay there an immense burthen, and mighty weight, under which he imagined he could not go, unless stooping towards the Earth. Whilst he talked, and discoursed with his Friends, this constriction of the *Præcordia*, and the weight did somewhat remit; but then again, they were wont to be repeated more vehemently, shaking for fear at any unaccustomed object: Nor did he labour only in his *Præcordia*, but with a certain constriction in his whole Body besides, and as if a certain burthen lay on the region of his Loins, and also on his shoulders and arms.

The Cure.

The reasons of these *Symptoms* are clear enough from our *Hypothesis*. As to the Cure, after various Medicines being given, without any success, I at last perswaded, because it was then Summer time, that he should drink of our Artificial *Spaw* Waters, for a fortnight: Therefore, first two quarts of Spring-water being poured upon half a dram of our prepared Steel, for a night, and afterwards as much in four quarts of water; the sick man every morning drunk the clear liquor, and within four or five hours he rendered the greatest part of it by Urine: He took besides, going to sleep and early in the morning, a Dose of an appropriate *Electuary*, (such as is above described) with a *Cephalick Julep*; within two months he became much better, and afterwards by degrees returned to himself.

The second History. An Example of Melancholy arising from the Blood.

Whilst I was writing these, a young Noble-man, being lately returned from his Travels beyond Sea, and becoming unhealthy, put himself upon our care. This person being formerly indued with a Sanguine and chearful temperament, splendid in his appearance, as also with an acute wit, and of a ready ingenuity, whilst he travelled in the Countries abroad; but one Summer living in *Spain*, he felt a great alteration in himself, from the great heats in that place: for first of all, from the frequent heatings of his Blood, he became obnoxious to an heat arising in the palms of his hands, and in the bottoms of his feet, with prickings over all his body, which in a short time vanished. Then he found himself very bad as to his Appetite and Sleep; moreover being dull and sad, he began not to mind, yea sometimes to avoid any pleasant business, or the converse of his Friends. At length his indisposition daily increasing, without any evident cause, or real trouble of mind, he became *Melancholick*, so that being ever thoughtful, fearful, and sad, nothing could delight him; for his studies, exercises, travelling, conversation with learned men, or any other thing which he before delighted in, now became to him a trouble and a terror. After this manner being distemper'd for two years, he was so changed from himself, as if he were another Man. For his Cure he had consulted the most skilful Physicians in *Spain, France*, and *Holland*, and lastly in *England*, and had tryed several methods of healing almost without any benefit. The *Melancholick* distemper of his blood, at first contracted by the intemperature of the Air, still remaining, and afforded to the Animal regiment, Spirits as it were acetous, that is such as we but now described. To this Noble-man, at the beginning, we thought good to recommend these following Remedies.

The Curatory Method proposed.

Take *of the Decoction of Senna Gerionis (with Tamarinds half an ounce) four ounces, of the Syrup of purging Apples one ounce, of Aqua Mirabilis two drams; mix them, and take it with government, repeating it within nine days. After Purging let Blood be taken away with Leeches, about four ounces.*

Take *of our Syrup of Steel six drams, take a spoonful in the morning, and at five of the Clock in the Afternoon, in the following liquor three ounces, walking after it for an hour or two.*

Take *of the leaves of Balm, Borrage, Buglofs, Pimpernel, Elm-tree, Harts Tongue, Water Cresses, each four handfuls; of the Roots of Borrage half a pound, of Pinks and Marigold flowers, each three handfuls; the outer peels of eight Oranges and four Lemons, of Mace half an ounce; these being cut and bruised, pour to them of Whey made of Cyder eight pints; let them be distilled in common Stills.*

Take *of the Conserves of Gilliflowers, Betony, Borrage, each one ounce and a half; of Pearl powdered two drams, of red Coral prepared one dram and a half, of the Species Confect. de Hyacintho two drams, of the Syrup of Coral, and red Poppies, each, what will suffice: make an Opiate to be taken going to sleep every night, the quantity of a Chesnut, drinking after it of Cowslip flower water two or three ounces.*

After sixteen or twenty days, changing the method of altering Medicines, the following things were used in their places.

Take *of the Powder of Ivory, Pearls, red Coral prepared, each two drams; of male Pæony roots one dram and a half, of the Wood-Aloes half a dram, Lozenges made out of Oranges four ounces, of the solution of Tragacanth made of Balm Water, what will suffice: make Troches weighing half a dram: let him eat four in the Morning, and at five in the Afternoon, drinking after them a draught of Tea.*

Take

Take *of the same Powder without the Lozenges half an ounce, of the flowers of Sal Armoniack, and of Salt of Coral, each one dram; with Turpentine of Chio six drams, make a Mass: take half a dram Evening and Morning, drinking after it of the distilled water three ounces.*

His food was only good and easily digested meats: he drank small Ale, with the leaves of Harts-tongue infused in it. He tasted sometimes a little Water and Wine, or Cyder, and he was almost continually employed, sometimes in some easie affairs, sometimes in moderate exercises, or in several sorts of recreations.

Thus much concerning universal *Melancholy*, by which the sick are affected almost indifferently by any object, so that they are intangled in every place, and by any accidents and circumstances, with a multitude of thoughts continually, with raving, fear, and sadness. We have largely enough handled the *symptoms* of this Disease being manifold, and the reasons of them, partly in this Chapter, and partly in another Tract. *Universal Melancholy. De Morbis Convulsivis, Cap. 2.*

It is called special *Melancholy*, when the sick respect a certain particular thing, or some kinds of things, of which they think almost without ceasing; and by reason all the powers and affections of the soul being continually imployed about this one thing, they live still careful and sad; moreover, they have absurd and incongruous notions, not only about that object, but also concerning many other accidents and subjects. In this Distemper, the Corporeal Soul, bending from its proper kind, assumes a certain new one, but not being conformable, either to the Rational Soul, or to the Body, or to it self, it enters into a certain *Metamorphosis*. *Particular Melancholy.*

This kind of Distemper, is produced by many ways, and on various occasions; for vehement passions, desire, fear, anger, pleasure, yea all other passions both of the *concupiscible* and *irascible* Appetite, being long continued, and carried forth to the height, are wont to excite the same. But there are two general occasions, from which special *Melancholy* chiefly and most frequently doth arise; to wit, first, when there lyes a most heavy pressure on the mind of some present evil, or an evil just at hand, whether it be true or imaginary: or secondly, if the loss or privation of some good before obtained, or desparing of something wished for or desired, happen. In these opposite cases, the Corporeal Soul being either drawn forth outwardly, omits all domestick care, either of it self, or of the Body, or of the Rational Soul: or being pressed inwardly, it relinquishes or perverts the offices of Reason, and of both the Vital and Animal Functions. It would be an huge work to enumerate the various cases in either kind, and their ways of affecting; out of the great plenty, which being of the greatest moment, seem to require the care of a Physician, are chiefly *furious Love, Jealousie, Superstition, despair of Eternal Salvation*, and lastly the *imaginary Metamorphosis* of the Body or its parts; and the good and evil phantasticks of fortune; of these, severally, we shall speak briefly. *is excited by reason of two sorts of Affections concerning Good or Evil.*

Concerning the power of Love, saying nothing here of some most noble Lord, or Heroick actions, (which appear chiefly on the stage of the *Theatre*, and on that of humane life) it is a most common observation, that if any one being taken with the aspect and conversation of any Woman, begins to desire her and to grow mad for her inwardly, and for his most devoted affection has nothing but loss and contempt allotted him, unless he be very much supported by a firm reason, or is averted as it were by other cross affections, there is great danger lest he falls into Melancholy, Stupidity, or Love-Madness; with which passion, if by chance he be distemper'd, he forthwith seems transformed from himself, as it were into an animated statue, he thinks on, nor speaks of any thing but his Love; he endeavours to get into her favour, with the danger of both the loss of his Life and Fortune; in the mean time, he not only neglects the care of his houshold affairs, or of the publick, yea his own health, but becoming desperate of his desires, he oftentimes lays violent hands of himself: But if he be content to live, yet growing lean, or withering away both in Soul and Body, he almost puts off man; for the right use of reason being lost, omitting food and sleep, and the necessary offices of Nature, he sets himself wholly to sighing and groaning, and gets a mournful habit and carriage of body. *Love-Madness.*

If we should inquire into the reason of this Distemper, it easily appears, that the Corporeal Soul of Man being obnoxious to violent affections, when it is wholly carried into the object most dear unto it self, viz. the beloved Woman, and cannot obtain and embrace her, there is nothing besides that can quiet or delight it; yea being refractory, it grows wholly deaf to the Rational Soul, and hears not its dictates, but carrying only tragical notions to the Imagination, darkens the sight of the intellect. Further, forasmuch as the *Præcordia* (the more plentiful afflux of the Spirits being *The Reasons of Symptoms in mad Love.*

ing denyed to them) do flacken of their motions, the blood heaped up in the bofoms of the heart, and apt to ſtand ſtill, ſtirs up a great weight and oppreſſion, and for that reaſon, ſighs and groans; in the mean time the face, and the outward members grow pale and languiſh, for that the affluence of the Blood and Spirits is withdrawn: Hence in our *Idiom* or Speech, the Heart of deſpairing Lovers is ſaid to be broken, to wit, becauſe this Muſcle is not lively enough actuated by the Animal Spirit, and ſo is ſhaken weakly and ſlowly, and doth not amply enough caſt forward the blood with vigor, into all parts. Indeed in Love, the Corporeal Soul intimately embracing the *Idea* of its moſt grateful object, endeavours all it can to be joyned, and fully united to the ſame; emitting toward her, the roots of the affections, with which it is moſt ſtrictly enfolded, ſeems from thence to draw its chiefeſt life and growth; ſo that the body being neglected, when as it inclines it ſelf wholly towards the thing beloved, if by chance being broken off from this union, it ſuffer a divorce, like a plant taken out of its natural ſoil, for that it does not receive any more, or aſſimilate food convenient for it ſelf, it ſoon withers: Hence the Animal Spirits leaving their accuſtomed offices, and wonted tracts of expanſion, do not actuate or irradiate either the Brain or the *Præcordia*, nor the nervous *Appendix*, after their due manner: wherefore, not only for the preſent an untrimmed, and a delirious diſpoſition of mind, with a mournful habit of body, are excited; but from thence the vitiated Blood, and the Spirits, having gotten an acetous nature, an habitual *Melancholy* is introduced.

Jealouſie. Such an inordination of the Animal Function as Mad-Love hath, about the acquiſition of its object, the ſame or very like hath *Jealouſie*, about the retention of the ſame, being gotten; ſo always (as well in the fruition as in the deſire) *Res eſt ſolliciti plena timoris Amor: Love is ever full of careful fear.* This Soul, if it be not ſecure of its moſt dear prey, it preſently grows hot, and pours forth darkneſs and clouds upon its own ſerenity: Then afterwards being infected by a *Choleric* tincture, it receives every object, as if it were imbued with a yellow colour: for indeed, as the ferment of the ſtomach being too much indued with a ſourneſs, perverts all things that is put into it, into its nature; ſo *Jealouſie* being once ariſen, changes all accidents and circumſtances, into the food of its poiſon; and when the ſenſitive Soul, being as it were bowed inward in this paſſion, becomes not conform to its Body, for that reaſon the Oeconomy of the Functions both Animal, Vital, and vegetative being depraved, *Jealouſie* makes rave, and to wither away.

Superſtition and Deſperation. Superſtition, and a deſpair of *Eternal Salvation*, are wont to impreſs on the *ſenſitive* Soul, the Blood, and the Body, almoſt the like Diſtempers of *Melancholy*, as *Love* and *Jealouſie*; but their way of affecting is ſomewhat different: for in thoſe the object, whoſe acquiſition or loſs is indanger'd, is wholly immaterial, and its affection being at firſt conceived by the Rational Soul, is impreſſed on the other Corporeal: In the proſecution of which, if ſhe eaſily obtains her deſires, then no perturbation of the humane mind ariſes; but if (as it often is wont to happen) the Corporeal Soul being oppugned or refuſed, it will not ſtand to the monitions of the Rational, but preſently growing hot, moves inordinately the Blood and Spirits, oppoſes the Corporeal goods and blandiſhments to the ſpiritual objects, from the intellect, and endeavours to draw the man to its ſide; and ſo whenas there is a continual skirmiſh between the two Souls, and that ſometimes the ſuperior Will, and ſometimes the ſenſitive Appetite prevails; at length the judgment ſeat of the Conſcience is erected by the mind, where *The reaſon of the Symptoms.* every ſeveral action is ſcrupulouſly examined. By reaſon of this more frequent ſtrife of the Souls, the Animal Spirits being too much and almoſt perpetually exerciſed, and often commanded, and as it were drawn hither and thither into contraries, at length they depart ſomething from their vigor and their nature, and at length being made more fixed and Melancholick, for that they are detained from their wonted expanſion, cut unaccuſtomed and by-tracts in the Brain, and ſo induce a *Delirium* or idle raving, with mighty fear and ſadneſs. In this ſort of Diſtempers, the Corporeal ſoul being ſnatched as it were violently, departs both from it ſelf, and from the Body, and according to the characters of the impreſſed *Idea* being modified, it is wont to aſſume a new image, either Angelical or Diabolical; in the mean time, the Intellect, becauſe the *Imagination* furniſhes it only with undecent and monſtrous notions, is wholly perverted from the uſe of right reaſon.

The imaginary Metamorphoſis of Melancholick Perſons. By the like means of affecting, it happens that ſome *Melancholick* perſons undergo imaginary *Metamorphoſes*, as to their fortunes, or as to their bodies, *viz.* whilſt one imagines himſelf, and plays the part of a Prince, and another a Beggar; another believes that he has a Body of Glaſs, and another that he is a Dog, or a Wolf,

or

or some other Monster; for after the Corporeal Soul's being distemper'd with a long *Melancholy* and the mind blinded, it wholly departs both from it self, and also from the Body, and affects, and as much as in it lyes, truly assumes a new image or condition.

CHAP. XII.

Of Madness.

After *Melancholy*, *Madness* is next to be treated of, both which are so much akin, that these Distempers often change, and pass from one into the other; for the *Melancholick* disposition growing worse, brings on *Fury*; and *Fury* or *Madness* growing less hot, oftentimes ends in a *Melancholick* disposition. These two, like smoke and flame, mutually receive and give place one to another. And indeed, if in *Melancholy* the Brain and Animal Spirits are said to be darkned with fume, and a thick obscurity; In *Madness*, they seem to be all as it were of an open burning or flame. But indeed, for that as we have already shewn, that the Animal Spirits being inkindled or inflamed do excite a *Phrensie* with a *Feavour*, which is wanting in *Madness*, their affection will be better illustrated in this Disease, as well as in *Melancholy*, by the *Analogy* of *Chymical* Liquors. *Madness and Madness are akin.*

Whenever therefore *Madness* without a *Feavour* being excited, with a remarkable hurt of the animal Function, is wont to be permanent, and continue long, its next and immediate subject are the Animal Spirits; which acting not by consent, nor from any force from another, but of themselves, are habitually distemper'd, and depart from their proper and genuine nature, to wit, a *Spiritual saline*, into a *Sulphureous-saline* disposition, like to *Stygian*-Water, as we have shewed above; therefore they perform only inordinate acts; and so persist a long while to act amiss or evilly. To this vice of theirs, perhaps the Brain, or the Blood, or other parts may contribute somewhat, but the Spirits themselves are first and chiefly in fault. *The Subject of Madness are the Animal Spirits.* *The disposition of which are like to Stygian Water.*

It is observed in *Mad men*, that these three things are almost common to all: *viz.* First, That their *Phantasies* or Imaginations are perpetually busied with a storm of impetuous thoughts, so that night and day they are muttering to themselves various things, or declare them by crying out, or by bauling out aloud. Secondly, That their notions or conceptions are either incongruous, or represented to them under a false or erroneous image. Thirdly, To their *Delirium* is most often joyned Audaciousness and Fury, contrary to *Melancholicks*, who are always infected with Fear and Sadness. These primary symptoms of *Madness* in the Animal Spirits, indued with the nature of *Stygian*-Water, may be thence most aptly deduced as appears clearly by what follows. *Three chief Accidents in Madness.* *Which are also to be found in Stygian Water.*

For first, the Particles of *Stygian*-Water are highly active and unquiet, and in perpetual motion; hence the Effluvia's falling from them continually strike the Nostrils, and the Liquor being poured forth from the Vessel, meeting with some other bodies grows very hot, and penetrates their Pores and Passages; the reason of which is, because the *Saline* Particles being conjoyned with the *Sulphureous*, shake one another, and will not cohere with any of another kind. In like manner we may suppose that the Animal Spirits being stilled forth from the Blood; filled as it were with a *Nitrous sulphur*, are indued with a notable mobility or unquietness; which, for that reason, being stretched forth from the middle of the Brain on every side, both in its compass and in the nervous *System*, and being from thence perpetually reflected, produce unbridled *Phantasies*, and almost never interrupted, and also great and perpetual inordinations, both of the sensitive and loco-motive function. *1. The Particles of this are always in motion.* *And in like manner the Animal Spirits in Mad-men.*

Secondly, the *Effluvia's* exhaling from *Nitrous* or *Stygian* Spirits, do not so much evaporate from open spaces, but being very penetrating, cut every where new ones, almost in every subject, where they are able to break thorow; yea most bodies containing these kind of Spirits, or the things laid upon the mouths of the Vessels, are so bored thorow by them, that they are presently rendred friable or brittle, and fall into small bits. In like manner we believe, that the Animal Spirits in the Distemper of *Madness*, becoming very moveable, and very much sharpned, out of their morbid nature, do so likewise leave their former tracts of going and returning to and fro, and do cut for themselves, every where in the Brain, new little spaces or walks, *2. The Effluvia's of Stygian Water, every where make new Pores and Passages.* *In like manner also the Animal Spirits in Mad-men.*

D d and

and plainly devious; in which, whilst they flow, they produce unaccustomed notions, and very absurd, whence there is a necessity, that the distemper'd do speak, and imagine for the most part incongruous and discomposed things; at once confounding things past with things present, or to come; and contrary or opposite things.

3. The Effluvia's of Stygian waters are diffused far.
Thirdly, It is observed, that the vaporous little bodies falling away from the *Nitro-sulphureous* Spirits of Minerals, do not only subsist in the neighbourhood, (as the breath exhaling from *acetous* Liquors) but are diffused very far, and on every side into remote places. I have often seen, when the Spirit of *Nitre* has been mixed with the Butter of *Antimony*, that the whole Chamber has been filled with a black smoke ascending from those *Stygian* Liquors: When *Aqua fortis* or the Spirit of *Nitre* being poured from the *Alembick*, or drawn forth by a gentle heat, a most sharp vapor has pierced the Nostrils and Lungs of those standing afar off; which certainly happens by reason of joyning together of the fluid *Salt*, and the raging *Sulphur*; the little bodies of either of which mutually incite one another, and so being combined together, are carried farther.

In like manner as the Animal Spirits in Madmen.
Indeed, after the same manner it seems to be concerning the Animal Spirits in Madmen, which, for that they are of the same nature as *Stygian* Water, quickly passing thorow both the frame of the Brain and its *Appendix*, cause the distemper'd not only to be furious, but as it were *Demoniacks* or possessed with the Devil; so that being free from any fear or languishing, they enter upon any thing boldly, and expose themselves fearless to sword or fire; also by reason of the prodigious putting forth of their Spirits, with a mighty strength, they often break asunder bonds and chains, and overthrow at once many strong men, resisting and going about to restrain them.

What the Conjunct Cause of Madness is.
The comparing of the Animal Spirits with *Stygian* Water, or the *Nitro-sulphureous* Spirit, clearly shews what is the conjunct or immediate cause of *Madness*; to wit, which seems to consist, not so much in an adust bile or humor, or black and sharp vapour, being suddenly suffused into the Brain, and inciting the Spirits inhabiting it into rage and fury; (for such a vapour or humor either exhales of its own accord, or may be soon removed by the help of Remedies; and so the madness thence excited, would pass away as quickly and as easily as the Fury or *Delirium* produced by the eating of wild Parsnips) but rather raging *Mad-men* are habitually so made, because their Animal Spirits degenerate from a gentle and benigne nature, as also a subtil and very active disposition, to wit, a *Spirituons-saline*, into another more sharp, to wit, partaking of a fluid *Salt*, an *Arsenical Sulphur*.

How the Animal Spirits acquire a disposition like to Stygian Water.
As to what belongs to the more remote or antecedent causes of *Madness, viz.* by reason of which the Animal Spirits acquire a most sharp disposition; before we come to these, we ought to shew how, and by what reason or means, a certain Corrosive *Latex* or water (such as we suppose the Animal Spirits with its Vehicle to be) is begotten, and is able to subsist in the humane body.

It is shewed in the first place that corrosive and as it were Stygian Particles, are begot in the humane Body.
Truly, that most sharp humors are sometimes begotten in our bodies, plainly appears by many observations. We have elsewhere made mention of a Noble Man, grievously obnoxious to distempers of the Brain and Nerves, whose sweat (when he was in a fit) presently eat thorow his shirt, or made it so crumbling or friable, as if it had been dipt in *Aqua fortis*. It is an usual thing for some to render by Vomit oftentimes as it were a *Vitriolick* water, corroding the coats of the *Oesophagus* and the Palat. Further, *Cancrous, Scrophulous*, and *Pestilential* Ulcers, shew a most sharp humor, by which the flesh and Membranes are eaten, as it were with *Aqua fortis*, with a blackness poured on them. Further it is observed, that Corrosive *Stigmas*, not chiefly brought forth in the Blood, are affixed to the musculous flesh, or to the *Parenchyma* of the *Viscera*; but more frequently being procreated in the nervous liquor, being laid up with its *Latex* in the nervous parts, or their *Emunctories*, do produce *Aposthums*, and *Pockey, Septick*, and other foul and filthy Ulcers. For these are most often excited in the *Glandulas*, or near the Tendons, or Membranes; and when as the humor falling away from them is first thin and watry, and afterwards becomes black very stinking, and corrosive; it is a sign indeed, that the nervous Liquor it self is changed into that sort of putrefaction.

Wherefore the nervous Liquor sometimes becomes corrosive. Because the volatile Salt most easily degenerates into an acid and most sharp, with the acquired Sulphur.
It easily occurs, if the reason of these be inquired into, that the *Latex* watering the Brain and nervous *Appendix*, doth contain in it self, together with a subtil Spirit, great plenty of volatile Salt. Therefore, when this is so depraved, that the Spirit being depressed, the Saline Particles degenerate into a flux, and acquire to themselves little *Sulphureous* bodies, it becomes plainly Corrosive and *Stygian*. Wherefore, malignant humors and Ulcers chiefly happen in the nervous parts, and their *Emunctories*, and there are excited upon any light occasion (as when a small hurt happens to the Breast of a Woman, a *Cancer* follows) because, indeed, the nervous humor being hindred somewhere in its passage, doth there stagnate, presently the Spirit being
depressed,

Of Madness. 203

depressed, or flying away, the Saline Particles degenerating from a volatile to a sour nature, get to themselves soon after strange companions, and snatching either Earthy or Sulphureous little bodies, or of some other kind, begin to congeal into *Scirrhous*, *Strumous*, or *Cancrous* Tumors. And when after this manner, by the stagnating of the nervous Liquor, and by its getting an heterogeneous concretion, the Mine of a Tumor is blown up in some part, and the supplements of the same liquor are continually perverted into the like nature of viciousness; to which also happen, the *Melancholick* impurities, poured forth from the Blood, and other humors, which with their joined forces encrease the rage (even as when diverse Salts and Sulphurs are distilled together) and constitute in the distemper'd part, a *Septick* matter, and like to the *Escharotick* or crusting up of *Stygian* Water. According to this reasoning or *Ætiology*, the irregularities of these kind of Tumors, as also the appearance of the Kings-Evil, are most aptly unfolded. If that the nervous Liquor so corrosive, and made degenerate, doth not grow into Tumors, flowing into the nervous Fibres, it is wont to cause here and there most cruel Pains and Cramps. *Hence the Reasons of Tumours and Ulcers in the Kings Evil and the Cancer, are given.*

But as this Liquor of the Nerves, being depraved after this manner, stirs up the aforesaid Distempers in the nervous parts; so it is not difficult to conceive, that the same water, for that it is for a Vehicle of the Animal Spirits, flowing in the Brain, doth acquire, together with those Spirits, a Corrosive and as it were a *Stygian* nature, and for that reason excites Madness. The depravation of the Animal Spirits, together with the juice watering the Brain, or the disposition of Madness, is wont to arise after various ways and for diverse causes; but truly, for the most part this Distemper (as we have observed of *Melancholy*) begins either from the Spirits themselves, or else from the Blood. *Hence also the Madness of the distempered Spirits.* *The Original of Madness either from the Spirits themselves, or from the Blood.*

First, *Madness* beginning from the Spirits, arises sometimes from an evident solitary cause, as a violent Passion; sometimes also it proceeds from a foregoing cause lying in the Brain, as when it comes upon *Melancholy* or a *Phrensie*. We shall a little weigh the reasons of either case, and the various manner of their being made. *It begins for two occasions from the Spirits.*

1. As to the former, when a vehement affection puts any one besides himself, that happens to be made thus; either because the Animal Spirits are too much overthrown, and hurried into confusion; or because they are elevated above measure, and endeavour to stretch themselves forth beyond their sphere. *1. By Reason of a violent Passion, by which*

First, The Spirits are wont to be cast down by a violent and terrible Passion; so it often happens, that some being struck with a panick fear, by seeing a true or an imaginary Spectre or Ghost, afterwards fall into a perpetual Madness. Further, some by reason of some notable disgrace or repulse, others by reason of their hopes of obtaining their Love being suddenly and unthought of frustrated, and others by reason of a rash breaking their oaths or vows, and violated Conscience, being first highly troubled in mind, anon become Mad. The reason of which is, because the Animal Spirits being driven beyond their orders and wonted passages, and put into confusion, do make for themselves new and devious ways, which entring into, immediately they bring forth delirious *Phantasms*; in the mean time, the *Saline* Particles of the nervous juice, the spirituous being depressed, depart from their volatileness; and suffering a flux, assume to themselves the *Sulphureous* little bodies poured forth from the Blood, into the then weak and open Brain; From whence this Liquor, being most sharp like *Stygian* Water, and the Animal Spirits becoming fierce and very much incited, become furious. *They are either too much cast down,*

Secondly, Sometimes the Animal Spirits, whilst they are too much elevated, almost after the same manner induce both to themselves, and the nervous juice, the mad disposition. Hence Ambition, Pride, and Emulation, have made some mad; the reason of which is, because whilst the Corporeal Soul swelling up with an opinion and pride of its own excellency, lifts up it self, and endeavours on every side to expand or stretch it self forth most amply, beyond the border or sphere of its body, the Animal Spirits being tumultuarily called into the Head, will not be contained within their wonted bounds, but being there broken and diversly reflected, by reason of their too much excretion, are compelled into new and plainly devious tracts; wherefore, both they being thrust forth from the course of their proper emanation, and also the nervous Liquor, do quickly acquire a sharp and incitative Disposition, as was said but now, for that reason *Madness* follows. *Or elevated above measure.*

Thus much concerning Madness, excited by reason of a solitary evident cause; but this Disease doth also arise from a *Procatartick* cause, preexisting in the Brain, and chiefly from *Melancholy* or the *Phrensie* going before; in that the Animal Spirits with the nervous juice being a little more exalted, and in this a little more depressed, acquire the disposition of Madness. As to the former, it is a vulgar observation, that sudden and great *Melancholy* is for the most part next to Madness: the reason of which is, because, when the *2. Madness beginning from the Spirits succeeds Melancholy, or the Phrensie.*

D d 2   Animal

Animal Spirits, together with the nervous liquor, degenerate into a sourness, are perverted, there only wants the accession of *Sulphur*, by which they afterwards getting a *Stygian* nature; may induce *Madness*; (as when an acid Liquor distilled out of *Vitriol* or Salt, by the addition of *Sal Nitrosus*, becomes *Aqua fortis*) but indeed, in a great passion of *Melancholy*, because the Spirits being disturbed, the passages of the Brain are too open, the *Sulphureous* Particles carried from the Bilous and Rancid Blood, find an easie entrance, and so the former sour or acid disposition, turns into a *Stygian* or Maddish. Hence it is observed, if any one of a more hot temperament, falls into a *Melancholick Delirium*, with fear and sadness, forasmuch as the *Sulphureous* Particles in its humors, are joyned to the Salts being depressed into a flux, that sadness and thinking at the beginning, very readily a short time after becomes madness. Secondly, for that also a *Phrensie* often ends in *Madness*, the reason is almost the same with the former, but inverted; to wit, because in a *Phrensie* the Spirits and the nervous Liquor becoming *Sulphureous*, and too much inflamed, afterwards burning forth, get to themselves *Saline* Particles, and so in like matter get a most sharp and as it were a *Stygian* nature; wherefore the *Feavour* then ceasing, the *Fury* becomes fixed and continual.

1. By what means it comes upon Melancholy.

2. How upon a Phrensie.

2. The disposition of *Madness*, hath no less frequently its roots in the bloody Mass, and is at length produced into act, to wit, when as the Blood being depraved, and becomes *Nitro-sulphureous*, it either perverts the nervous Liquor, as also the Animal Spirits, or supplies them but evilly. Which kind of taint of the Blood is either hereditary or acquired.

2. The Original of Madness sometimes from the Blood.

First, It is a common observation, that men born of Parents that use sometimes to be mad, are obnoxious to the same disease, and though they have lived above thirty or forty years prudent and sober; yet afterwards without any occasion or evident cause, they have fallen into Madness. The reason of which is, for that the Blood at that time bending from its due temper, by degrees into a *Nitro sulphureous*, affords to the Head Animal Spirits, and also the nervous juice, participating (as hath been said) of a most sharp nature. We have formerly shewn, that in our Complexion, Elementary Particles do persist during life, apart from the secondary, afforded by nutrition, and have their times of crudity, maturity, and defection; wherefore we suppose, the morbid seeds do ripen into fruit, according to the periods of Ages. Further, we take notice, that oftentimes the fruits of Diseases of this kind, do remain ripening for a long time, or perpetually as long as life; yet sometimes falling off as it were of their own accord, do wither away; then sometimes in another tract of time, from the infection being left, new fruits do spring up, and by little and little rise up to their height. Wherefore, *Hereditary Madness* is sometimes continual, and sometimes intermitting; Its fits are wont sometimes to come again after a shorter time, and sometimes after a longer interval.

1. It is either Hereditary,

The Reason of which is shewn.

Secondly, As the foregoing Cause of *Madness* sticking in the Blood, is oftentimes innate or original, so sometimes the same is by degrees begotten, either by an evil manner of diet, or by the suppression of usual evacuations, or by reason of a Feavour going before, or for some other causes, and at length being brought to maturity, breaks forth into *Madness*. It is an usual thing in great want of sustenance, that some poor people, being constrained to feed only on very disagreeing meats, and of ill digestion, become at first sad with an horrid aspect, louring and dark, and a little after Mad. The *Hemorrhoids*, and the after flowings of Women in Child-bed, being restrained in their flux, or some evil and foul running Ulcers being suppressed, dispose some towards this Disease. Further, those who originally, or by acquisition, are indued with a more sharp temper, and with fierce manners, and threatning countenance, by reason of the disposition of their Blood, being nigh to a *Nitro sulphur*, are in danger to fall into Madness, from some strong evident cause.

2. Or acquired, and so either,

By reason of errours in the six Non-naturals;

Thirdly, Venomous Ferments being insinuated to the Blood and nervous juice, as first of all from the biting of mad Animals, or by the taking of some poisons, are wont to stir up Madness. Concerning the reasons of the former, we have proposed our conjectures in another place. Of late a very Noble Lady, and to be credited, told me from her own knowledge, that a certain Gentleman, having eaten at dinner time the tender leaves of Wolfs-bane, in a Sallad with other herbs, in the Evening found himself ill, and complaining of a great unquietness and agitation of his Blood and Spirits, he desired his Friends to send for a Chirurgeon to let him blood, or that otherwise he should grow Mad; which indeed, as he said, came to pass; for before he could be let blood, he fell into Madness, and dyed in a nights space: This kind of deadly Distemper so suddenly happened, for that this poison had not only perverted the Blood and Animal Spirits, as to their temper, but had slain or beat them down immediately, with its malignant Ferment.

Or by reason of Poysons.

An History of a Mortal Madness, from eating the leaves of Wolfs Bane.

Thus

Of Madness.

Thus much for the formal Reason, and Causes of *Madness*. The *primary Symptoms* of it, we have mentioned to be a *Delirium* and a *Fury*; the reasons of which appear clear enough from what has been already said. To these we may moreover add Boldness, Strength, and that they are still unwearied with any labours, and suffer pains unhurt, of which we will speak briefly. *The Reasons of the symptoms of Madness explained.*

Mad men are not as *Melancholicks*, sad and fearful, but audacious and very confident, so that they shun almost no dangers, and attempt all the most difficult things that are. The reason of which is, because the Animal Spirits being very fierce and provoked, both fortifie the Imagination, that no object may seem greater or bigger than it is wont to be, and actuate also the *Pracordia* with vigor, so that they cast forth the Blood strongly and swiftly, and drive it forwards lively to the utmost borders of the Body. In this Distemper the Soul endeavours to be carried forth, and to leap beyond the compass or sphere of the Body, and so striving on every side, against the incursions of any exterior things, bears it self without fear. *1. Wherefore Mad-men are audacious.*

Secondly, *Mad men* are still strong and robust to a prodigy, so that they can break cords and chains, break down doors or walls, one easily overthrows many endeavouring to hold him. The certain cause of which is, because in the Blood and nervous juice of Mad people, are contained Particles as it were *Nitro sulphureous*, or otherways most sharp, and as it were *Stygian*; from whence the Animal Spirits are induced, or are strong with an *Elastick* or *Explosive* force, stupendous, great, and far beyond what's natural. *2. From whence their immense strength.*

Thirdly it is observed, that *Mad men* are almost never tired; for although by playing mad pranks, and striving many days and nights they strongly exercise their members, and live in the mean time without sleep or eating, yet they scarce languish at all, nor desist from their agonies for want of strength. Which without doubt comes to pass, for that the Animal Spirits, though very moveable and *Elastick*, are not however volatile and easily dissipable, but by reason of the *Saline* Particles being depressed from their volatileness into a flux, being joined with the *Sulphureous*, become firm and more fixed; and therefore continue longer in their activity. In like manner as we have observed in *Aqua fortis*, which though it be contained in a vessel that's open, perpetually sends forth very many Effluvia's, and yet still retains its substance unwasted, and its corrosive force, otherwise than the spirit of Wine or Blood, the virtue of which soon evaporates. *3. Wherefore they are never tired.*

In the fourth place, almost for the same reason, *Mad-men*, what ever they bear or suffer are not hurt; but they bear cold, heat, watching, fasting, strokes, and wounds, without any sensible hurt; to wit, because the spirits being strong and fixed, are neither daunted nor fly away. Further, the blood having gotten a *Nitro sulphureous Dyscrasie*, is incapable of any sudden mutation; wherefore, although insensible transpiration be hindred, and other usual evacuations suppressed, or the supplies of the nourishing juice degenerated, yet neither a *Catarrh*, nor *Feavour*, nor *Atrophy*, of evil digestion easily comes upon *Madness*. For in this Distemper, although the Particles of the Blood do greatly swell up, yet by reason of the abundance of Salt they do not conceive a Feavourish burning. Even as also *Aqua fortis*, though it grows very hot and burns other subjects, yet it self is not at all inflamed, but rather resists burning. *4. Wherefore they are not easily hurt.*

The differences of this Disease are easily gathered from what hath been before said; for first as to its beginning, it is either *occasional*, which sometimes quickly ceases, the evident cause being taken away presently; or *habitual*, depending upon a foregoing cause lying in the Blood, and that either *hereditary*, or *acquired*. *The Differences, 1. In respect of the Original.*

Secondly, by reason of the *magnitude*, *Madness* is either highly furious, that the distemper'd ought to be bound or lock'd up, lest they should attempt any mischief to themselves or others; or else it is more gentle, in which the sick, being conversant with others, abstain from any malice or hurt. Thirdly, In respect of time, *Madness* is wont to be long or short, continual or intermitting. Fourthly, As to the various kinds of *Deliriums*, the shapes or *types* of this Disease are almost innumerable; all which to run thorow, is neither possible, nor worth the while; but most commonly, the distemper'd are mad alike in all things, or else chiefly as to one particular thing, having their judgment concerning other matters for the most part right. *2. By reason of the Magnitude.* *3. In respect of Time.*

As to the *Prognostick* of *Madness*, if the distemper'd be not obnoxious to a *Feavour*, nor any other Diseases besides, nor easily hurt by external accidents the Disease is not mortal of it self; yet the Cure is very difficult, because there is made a great alteration in the Blood and Spirits, and the sick resist every method of healing, and are enemies to *Physicians* and to themselves. *The Prognostick.*

If *Madness* be inveterate or hereditary, or is caused by the biting of a Mad Dog, it is is hardly or not at all to be cured. What is excited upon some occasion, or from a solitary evident cause, or succeeds a Feavour, also upon which comes a Manginess, Whelks, the Hæmorrhoids, or spots in the skin, is easily cured.

Those who are obnoxious to this Disease at intervals, about *Midsummer*, or when the Dog Star arises, are in greatest danger; also those who are altered according to the changes of the Air, or when long cold and foul weather are opposite in the constitution of the Heaven.

The Cure.

As there are two kinds of *Madness*, to wit, Continual, and Intermitting; so the means of healing ought to be twofold.

What the indications are of continual Madness.

1. The *Curatory* method to be administer'd, as to continual *Madness*, suggests the commonly noted three primary Indications, *viz.* The first *Curatory*, which respecting the Disease it self, endeavours to correct or allay the furies and exorbitances of the Animal Spirits. Secondly, *Preservatory*, which being levelled against the causes of the Disease, endeavours to take away or amend the sharp and *Nitro-sulphureous Dyscrasies* of the nervous Juice and the Blood, as also the *Stygian* disposition of the Spirits. Thirdly, *Vital*, which directs such a means of dyet and restraint, which is only fit in this Disease, for the nutritive and vital function to have and be sustained with.

1. The Curatory Indication.
As to Discipline.

The first Indication, *viz.* *Curatory*, requires threatnings, bonds, or strokes, as well as *Physick*. For the *Mad-man* being placed in a House convenient for the business, must be so handled both by the *Physician*, and also by the Servants that are prudent, that he may be in some manner kept in, either by warnings, chiding, or punishments inflicted on him, to his duty, or his behaviour, or manners. And indeed for the curing of Mad people, there is nothing more effectual or necessary than their reverence or standing in awe of such as they think their Tormentors. For by this means, the Corporeal Soul being in some measure depressed and restrained, is compell'd to remit its pride and fierceness; and so afterwards by degrees grows more mild, and returns in order: Wherefore, Furious Mad-men are sooner, and more certainly cured by punishments, and hard usage, in a strait room, than by *Physick* or Medicines.

As to Medicine.

But yet a course of *Physick* ought to be instituted besides, which may suppress or cast down the Elation of the Corporeal Soul. Wherefore in this Disease, Blood-letting, Vomits, or very strong Purges, and boldly and rashly given, are most often convenient; which indeed appears manifest, because *Empericks* only with this kind of *Physick*, together with a more severe government and discipline do not seldom most happily cure Mad folks. But indeed, this more sharp handling is not convenient for all Mad people, but to the most furious. Others more remissly Mad, are healed often with Flatteries, and with more gentle Physick.

Phlebotomy.

In most Mad folks the taking away of Blood copiously ought to be in the beginning of the Disease, as it is the common practice and vogue of the people. And indeed, while there is strength, the opening a vein ought to be repeated, sometimes in the Arm, sometimes in the Neck Vein, Forehead, or Foot; and sometimes it is expedient for the *Hæmorrhoidal* Vessels to be opened by Leeches; for these evacuations being timely made, both the raging of the Spirits and the lifting up of the Soul, are best of all suppressed; then besides the *Dyscrasies* or evil habits of the Blood (for that what was sharp and Corrosive in it being drawn forth, a new and gentler comes in its place) are amended.

Vomiting Medicines.

That Vomiting Medicines are highly profitable for the curing of Mad people, it is almost a Proverb, so that the most part of *Hellebore*, yea almost all *Anticyra* is allotted to them. By what means *Emeticks* do often help in *Cephalick* Diseases, we have shown already. *Quack-salvers* in this case, give with success many times, though rashly and with danger, a large Dose of *Stibium*: But *Chymical* things are here more convenient, both because they move more strongly, and because also the sick may be more easily deceived by them.

Take *of the Sulphur of Antimony eight grains to ten, of the Cream of Tartar half a scruples; mix them together by pounding them; make a Powder: let it be given in a spoonful of grewel;* or if it be to be given deceitfully, to one not knowing of it, let it be put into a bit of white Bread, and so let it be taken in Milk or Broth. Let this Vomiting Medicine be often repeated, to wit, once in four days.

Take *six or seven grains of Mercurius Vitæ; let a Powder be made, and given after the same manner.* The *Emetick Tartar* of *Mynsicht*, and of *Hercules Bovius*, and other various preparations of *Mercury* may be given after the same manner. *Aurum vitæ* or the *Solar* Precipitate, also the *Lunar* Precipitate, are esteemed by *Chymists* for specifick Remedies against madness; and indeed, *Mercurial* Medicines, for that they operate not only by Vomit and Stool, but oftentimes by Sweat, Urine, or Salivation, do notably help. A long and plentiful spitting or flux at the mouth hath perfectly cured some Mad people.

3. The

3. The more strong Purging Medicines, (where strength and the constitution may *Purging Medi-* bear them) because they depress the raging of the Spirits, and of the Blood, and very *cines.* much evacuate the *Emunctories*, that are for the receiving the recrements of the Blood, and nervous Juice, do often bring help in this Disease. For this use preparations of black *Hellebore*, as chiefly its extract, and Wine of the Infusion of its strings, or the pulp of an Apple with the roots of it boiled together are much praised.

Take *of the Extract of black Hellebore, of Calamelanos of each one scruple: make a Bolus.*
Take *Calamelaros one scruple, of Diagridium from twelve to fifteen grains; make a Powder.*
Take *of Confectio Hamech, or of the Electuary of the juice of Roses half an ounce to six drams: let it be given in broth.*
Take *of the Decoction of Senna Gereonis, or of Epithimum (with the roots of black Hellebore two drams) six ounces; make a draught.*
Take *of the Powder of Diasenna two drams: let it be taken in Posset-drink.*

In the mean time, whilst these things are doing, let the Preservatory Indication re- *The preservatory* spect the cause of this Disease. Wherefore, with these frequent purgings and letting of *Indication.* Blood, between whiles let altering Medicines or Remedies be used, which may attem- *Altering Medi-* per the Blood and nervous juice, and reduce them to their due temper; if that the sick *cines.* be tractable and orderly enough, they will not refuse to take such things methodically.

Take *of Crystal Mineral, or of the best purified Nitre two ounces, of Pearls powdered two drams, of Sugar Candy two drams and a half, of Camphor half a scruple; let them be all beaten together to a moist fine Powder: let two drams of this be put into a glass vessel that will hold two quarts of Spring-water, or of clear small Ale, or Beer and mild; let it be given for ordinary drink at pleasure.*

Put to *Whey* being made hot the flowers of *Violets* or *Water-Lilies*, and after they have *Whey.* infused for two hours, let them drink it plentifully; also the *Spaw* Waters are convenient for Mad people to drink orderly, and plentifully.

Take *of the tops of green and the tenderest Borrage, and Bugloss, each four handfuls; An Expression.* *three Apples pared, of Sal Prunella two drams, of Sugar half an ounce; let them be bruised together, and pour to them of Spring-water three pints; make a strong Expression: take half a pint thrice in a day or oftener.*
Take *of the Conserves of Borrage flowers, and of Violets, each three drams; Confectio de An Electuary.* *Hyacintho, of Alchermis, each two drams; of Coral prepared a dram and an half, of the Powder of Pearls one dram, of the Salt of Coral one dram, of the Syrup of red Poppies what will suffice; make an Electuary, of which take two drams twice or thrice in a day, drinking after it of the following liquor four ounces.*
Take *of the waters of the flowers of the Water-Lilie, Borrage, Bugloss, and of black Cher- A Julep.* *ries, each four ounces; of red Poppies six ounces, of red Rose-water two ounces, of Camphor tyed in a rag and hang'd in the glass half a dram, of the Syrup of Coral one ounce and a half; mix them and make a Julep.*
Take *of the yellow flowers of the Willow-tree what will suffice, let them be distilled in a Distilled Wa-* *common Still, and let the Distillation be repeated, by putting to it fresh flowers for three ters.* *times: Give of it four ounces twice or thrice in a day, sweetning it with the Syrup of Water Lilies.*
Take *of the leaves of the Willow, Meadowsweet, Pimpernel, Borrage, Balm, each six handfuls; of the flowers of the Water-Lilie, of the tops of St. Johns-wort, each four handfuls; of Camphor powdered three drams, all being bruised together, pour to them eight pints of new Milk; let them be distilled in common Stills.*
Let the brains of Weathers be distilled with Milk, and give of the water three or four ounces thrice in a day.

Further there are to be used Specifick Remedies, so called, of which is famous, a *Specificks.* Decoction of *Pimpernel* with the purple flower, also the tops of *Hypericon* or St. *Johnswort*, and other Decoctions, Opiates, and Powders of *Antilyssi* are frequenly noted among all the famous *Empericks*.

Concerning the cure of *Madness*, excited from the biting of venomous or mad Ani- *A Decoction* mals, for that it is almost only *Emperical*, and commonly known, we shall not discourse *and Infusion of* of it in this place, and since we have elsewhere proposed our conjectures concerning it. *Apples.* But a Decoction or an Infusion of Apples, either raw or boil'd in Spring-water, the liquor

Of Madness.

quor of *Tea*, Emulsions, with many other things, whose forms we have shewn in the Cure of *Melancholy*, are convenient in this case.

Other Chirurgical Remedies. Moreover, from *Chirurgical* Remedies, besides opening of a Vein, many other helps are wont to be had for the curing of this Disease. *Cupping-glasses* with Scarification, often help. *Blisterings*, *Cauteries* both actual and potential are praised of many. Others commend cutting an *Artery*, others *Trepaning*, or opening the Skull, others *Salivation*. But these kind of administrations, besides that their effects are uncertain, can hardly be performed, or not at all safely, by reason of the intractability of the sick; wherefore, it were here superfluous to inquire into the reasons of help or cure to be expected from them: The hair being shaven off, sometimes it is expedient to apply to the forepart of the Head the hot Lungs of a Lamb or Weather, and other Fomentations, and so to change them. But these sorts of Remedies also are hardly to be applied and repeated methodically, because of the reluctancy of the sick, and so often afford more hurt than help.

3. The vital Indication. 3. The vital *Indication* institutes how mad people ought to be handled, concerning their government, dyet, and sleep. In this Disease there is no need of keeping up the flesh, as in most other Diseases: For the spirits ought not to be refreshed with Cordials, nor strength to be restored with Medicines; but on the contrary, both being too raging of themselves, things are to be administer'd as it were for the suppression or extinction of a flame raging above measure. Therefore let the diet be slender and not delicate, their cloathing course, their beds hard, and their handling severe and rigid. But sleep, for that it is very necessary, ought to be caused sometimes by *Anodynes*; for which end, *Hypnotick* Remedies or Medicines above prescribed for *Melancholy*, are also convenient in this Disease. In inveterate and habitual Madness, the sick seldom submit to any *Medical* Cure; but such being placed in *Bedlam*, or an *Hospital* for Mad people, by the ordinary discipline of the place, either at length return to themselves, or else they are there kept from doing hurt, either to themselves or to others.

Histories and Examples of mad people are to be sought in Bedlam, or Hospitals for mad people. There is no need to illustrate the nature of this Disease with Histories and Examples, or to describe the manifold Types of it; but rather let them go to the *Hospitals* of Mad people, where they may behold, not without a wonderful spectacle, as it were a new and monstrous nation of men, contrary to rational people, and as it were our *Antipodes*; all which, if they were gathered together in one place, and that all, Madmen and Fools were joyned to them; I know not whether this world would not be equally divided between them and the sober and prudent.

The Cure of Intermitting Madness. Thus much concerning the cure of continual *Madness*. The intermitting, either has perfect lucid intervals, in which the sick return to themselves, or the fury only ceases, the *Delirium* being still left, insomuch that the distemper'd become gentle and tractable, yet still they continue amiss, as to their imagination and judgment, and speak and do many absurd or incongruous things, and afterwards sometimes again become furious.

The Curatory Indication. The Cure of either of these Distempers, as to the Curatory Indication, is the same, as in continual *Madness*, so that there is no need to shew here any other Medicines, or method. But as to what respects the *Prophylaxis* or Preservatory Indication, by which the means of healing is instituted out of the fits, cautions and threatnings are to be given them; in whom only the Fury intermits, the *Delirium* remaining, the very same Remedies of Medicine, which we have prescribed for the taking away the foregoing cause of *Melancholy* are convenient.

Preservatory. In *Madness* which perfectly intermits, as to all its *Symptoms*, at the chiefest convenient times, to wit, Spring and Fall, they ought to enter into a solemn course of *Physick*; and besides, there is a continual need of looking to, or governing the sick, both as to diet and to their manner of living, that they may be always preserved in an equal and a moderate temper; and also, that as soon as the signs of the approaching fit appear, its coming may be hindred by Blood-letting, and by administring of Medicines.

Therefore, in the times of the *Æquinoxes*, let Blood be taken out of the Arm, and seven or eight days after out of the *Hemorrhoidal* Veins by Leeches. Let Purges and Vomits be given twice or thrice at due intervals. Moreover, between whiles, let them take in order altering Remedies, at *Physical* hours. The *Formulas* or *Recipes* of these are set down both in this Chapter and in the former for the cure of *Melancholy*. Let the dyet be slender and of good digestion; as concerning exercise or motion, sleep, and other *non naturals*, let them be all moderate. When the approach of *Madness* is seen to be at hand, and constantly before the Summer *Solstice*, let *Phlebotomy* be celebrated, with Vomiting, and a more slender or sparing diet.

CHAP.

CHAP. XIII.

Of Stupidity, or Foolishness.

Stupidity, or *Morosis*, or Foolishness, although it most chiefly belongs to the Rational Soul, and signifies a defect of the Intellect and Judgment, yet it is not improperly reckoned among the Diseases of the Head or Brain; forasmuch as this *Eclipse* of the superior soul, proceeds from the Imagination and the Memory being hurt, and the failing of these depends upon the faults of the Animal Spirits, and the Brain it self.

We have before clearly shewed, that the Rational Soul doth subsist in a sensitive or corporeal Soul, and that its principal seat is the Imagination: Further from *this*, and the *Memory*, either the notions themselves, or their occasions of all things are supplied, which the Mind beholds; wherefore, when it happens that these Corporeal Functions are defective or hindred, forthwith the eye of the Intellect, as if covered with a vail, is wont to be very much dulled, or wholly darkned. Therefore, that the reason of *Foolishness* and *Stupidity* may be rightly delivered, first we ought to inquire by what means, and from what causes, the *Imagination* and the *Memory* are often defective or fore-hindred. *Stupidity arises chiefly from the failing of the Imagination and Memory.*

That we may proceed methodically, concerning these, hither ought to be referred, what we have discoursed before concerning the Functions of the Corporeal Soul, and their subjects and instruments. we have at large declared that the *Callous Bodies*, or the middle of the Brain is the seat of the *Imagination*; and the Cortical Marrows of the Brain, the seat of the *Memory*; and further, that the Animal Spirits are the immediate organs of either. Wherefore, because their powers being hindred (which are the first or chief movers of any other Function, both rational and sensitive) the Imbecillity and dulness of the mind, the slowness of the ingenuity, stupidity and madness at length do often arise; the fault is either in the Brain it self, or the Animal Spirits, or both together, and at first now these, now that. *Wherefore the Organs of these Faculties labour in this Disease.*

1. As to the Animal Spirits, we have largely enough declared, of what sort they ought to be, of their proper and genuine nature, and what they are by reason of their preternatural disposition, in the *Phrensie*, *Melancholy*, and *Madness*. But besides (which we before mentioned) it may be suspected, that these Spirits being sometimes almost destitute of active Particles, become as it were liveless or vapid; to wit, when the spirituous Particles ought to excel, and to get to themselves volatile Salts; in *Stupidity*, both these, together with the Sulphureous, being too much depressed, they are almost drowned and overwhelmed with the watery and terrestrial. For indeed, Fools are not so dull or of such thick understanding, as their soul seems to be indued with, and their Animal Spirits are rather formed of clay than their Heart. There are many occasions or evident causes, by which the Animal Spirits acquire so deadish a texture, the chief of which we shall touch on by and by.

2. But it doth not frequently come to pass, that *Stupidity* is excited by the mere solitary fault of the Spirits, or of the Corporeal Soul it self, but more or rather the Brain it self is found to be first in fault: For as there are many things requisite, by which this exact subject or machine of the Animal Function is constituted, if by chance any thing of them be deficient or depraved, it easily follows, that such so distemper'd have little wit.

First, It is a vulgar observation, That the wit and ingenuity doth depend somewhat on the magnitude and figure of the Head, and consequently of its Brain; for as to its bulk, it is a Proverb, that it argues little of Brain or too much Foolishness. And although this does not always happen, yet it does for the most part. The reason of which is, because in a little Brain but a few Spirits are begotten and exercised; but in a greater, consisting for the most part of a vile or base texture or frame, it is less fitted for the quickness or sharpness of the mind. *1. As to Magnitude.*

Secondly, The genuine and best figure of the Brain ought to be globous; to wit, for the end that the Spirits may be poured forth with an equal efflux on every side, from its middle part to the whole compass, and may be from thence retorted every where by equal angles of reflections. But those who have a flat head, or too sharp, or otherways improportionate, are affected for the most part with some noted fault of the Animal Function; for these kind of Brains, like distorted Looking-Glasses, do not rightly *2. By Reason of the Figure.*

Of Stupidity or Foolishness.

rightly collect the Images of things, nor truly object them to the Rational Soul.

3. As to its Substance or Texture. Thirdly, The substance of the Brain should be well temper'd, and of a laudable frame; not only as to the qualities of heat and cold, of driness and moisture, but its *Systasis* or Constitution consisting of plenty of a volatile Salt and Spirit, with a moderate proportion of the rest should be thin and airy, that the Spirits may pass thorow the whole, and cut out to themselves paths; also it should be moderately firm and compacted, that the tracts and passages being made, may remain, and not be presently blotted out again, by the sinking of the too soft parts. But in *Stupidity*, it is to be suspected, that there is in the Brain an excess of some manifest quality, as of moisture or coldness, for which reason, Children and old people are wont to be affected with a dulness of their senses; or sometimes, the Texture is too thick, and Earthy; so that the spirits do not easily irradiate it, or cut tracts for themselves; to wit, they cannot penetrate an opacous or thick body, no more than rays of light. To this kind of deadish Texture of the Brain, those that are born of Plowmen and Rusticks, as if they were formed of a worser clay, are obnoxious; hence in some Families, reckoning many descents backward, there is scarce one witty or wise man found. In some places, the influences of the Heaven and Air incline, as it is thought, the Inhabitants to Stupidity; so, to be born in *Batavia*, is proverbially, as much as to say, a Fool.

4. The evil conformation of the Brain, as to its pores and passages. Fourthly, Besides these vices of the Brain, which are for the most part original and born with it, sometimes its evil conformation, as to its Pores and Passages, by reason of some acquired inordinations, is a cause that the Animal Function is not rightly performed. For first of all, as to what appertains to the smaller Passages and Pores of the Brain (which the spirits themselves frame every where thorow its whole substance, and perpetual flow into them for the exercise of the Animal Functions) it sometimes happens that these are either defective or perverted, and so bring on a dulness of mind, or *Foolishness*. These little spaces are defective, because the consistency of the Brain being either too obdurate or too fluid, it will not indure to be cut thorow after a due manner, or to remain or continue so bored thorow. But we suspect those Passages to be perverted, either because they are too loose or too strait, or else, for that their making is unequal. Too strait Pores do not sufficiently admit store of matter for a good plenty of Spirits: Those loose above measure, receive together with that matter, *Heterogeneous* Particles, and infesting the Animal Regiment. They seem to be unequally formed, where they are more open in one part of the Brain, and more strait in another. For this cause we think it to be, that some understand, or know things well enough, but still judge evilly; for that their notions and conceptions, like the visible Images, passing thorow a diverse Medium, become distorted. Further, perhaps for this reason it comes to pass, that some excel, or are strong in Imagination and Phantasie, yet are very deficient in Memory, and others on the contrary.

3. Stupidity sometimes proceeds from both of them being in fault together. 3. It sometimes happens, that both these conjunct causes do concur together to Foolishness, to wit, because both the Animal Spirits are dull and torpid, and also the Brain evilly conformed. And in truth, which part soever is first in fault, it quickly will make the other in like manner guilty. Because when the Spirits being blunt and sluggish do not freely pass thorow the Brain, the Pores and Passages in it are not either sufficiently cut thorow, or else they close again; and the Spirits if they cannot expand themselves, by reason of the evil texture of the Brain as they should do, they at length becoming slothful and idle, grow heavy, and acquire a vicious disposition.

What the Antecedent Causes of Foolishness, are. Thus much concerning the Conjunct Causes of *Foolishness*, as to its *Procatartick* and *Evident*, there belong more occasions, by reason of which the aforesaid evils are wont to be brought to the Brain, or the Spirits, or to both together.

1. An Hereditary Disposition. For in the first place, *Stupidity* (as we but now observed) is sometimes original or born with one, and so it is either *hereditary*, as when Fools beget Fools, the reason of which is clear enough, to wit, the same weak Particles flowing for the constituting the Animal Organs in the Son, which were in the Father: or *Stupidity* being born with one, is as it were accidental, to wit, it frequently happens, that wife men and highly ingeni-

Why strong or wise men are not always begotten of strong and wise Men. ous, do beget Fools and Changelings, or heavy witted: which we suppose so to come to pass sometimes for this cause, for that the Parents being too much given to study, reading, and meditation, the Animal Spirits that inhabit the Brain, are so much wasted, that for the supply of them, the most generous Particles of the Blood are still carried to the Head, and but few only, and small, are permitted to descend to the *Spermatick* Bodies.

The first Reason. When the rational Soul becomes greatly solicitous in bringing forth its child (which are the works of the Intellect) then the Corporeal Soul (the Spirits being called away to wait on the other) becomes not at all, or very weakly prolifick.

A Second Reason. Besides this reason, there is another frequently to be met with, wherefore the first implanted sagacity of men, as well as of *Brutes*, is not often propagated from the Parents

Of Stupidity or Foolishness. 211

Parents to the Children. For when as we presume certainly, the Colt of a generous Horse, or of a delicate strain, or the Chickens of a Game-Cock, that they will *patrisfare*, or be like their Sires, so that they are sold at a great rate, and the virtues of these, if not broken by inordinate and preternatural feeding or bringing up, descend by a long series to their young from age to age: This often happens otherwise to men, to wit, because the Parents do so enervate and weaken their bodies by intemperance, luxury, and evil manners, that they beget only languishing and unhealthy Children. Hence it is, that for the most part, those who are born of Parents broken with old age, or of such as are not yet ripe or too young, or of drunkards, soft, and effeminate men, want a great and liberal ingenuity or wit. Nor does there happen a less detriment to them of the Animal Faculty, whose sires are obnoxious to evil affections of the Brain, as the *Palsie*, *Epilepsie*, *Carus*, *Convulsions*, and the like; so that to be born of Parents who *have a sound mind in a sound body,* is far beyond a large patrimony.

Secondly, There are more evident causes, by which *Stupidity* is wont to be induced, to some originally whole. Some at first crafty and ingenious, become by degrees dull, and at length foolish, by the mere declining of age, without any great errors in living; to wit, because the nervous liquor, and the blood, (whose evil dispositions the Animal Spirits partake of) like some Wines, and other fermented liquors, depart from their vigor after a perfect Fermentation; and by little and little degenerate into a dead and pallid substance. For it is observed, the wits of some people do receive a various increase and decrease, according to the periods of their Ages. I have known many in their childhood very sagacious, and extreamly docil or apt to learn, that by their literature and discourse have caused admiration, who afterwards becoming young men, were dull and heavy: and those who at first were very beautiful, were afterwards not at all handsome, or beautiful in their aspect. In like manner, it often happens on the contrary, that many at first indocil or unapt to learn, and wholly unfit for literature, and seeming of an ill favour'd countenance, when they have become young men, or have put off their childhood, have had both an excellent wit, and become beautiful. The reason of the former is, that some ripe wit, or ingenuity, like garden fruit, does not remain long in the same condition, but soon declining, quickly withers. For in every mixture or concretion rightly made, there is required, that a progression from crudity to maturity be made gently and by little and little, that is, the active elements do not at first arise above the rest, and shew themselves above measure, but being involved with the others, rise up and put forth themselves by little and little; for otherwise, being too free in the beginning, and made loose, they easily fly away, leaving their subject almost dead or taste less. Wherefore, Boys who are seen to be dull in their first Age, may be hoped afterwards, when the temper of the Brain (the superfluous moisture being evaporated) is come to maturity, to become ingenious enough.

2. Ripeness and the Declination of Age dispose some to Foolishness.

Thirdly, Sometimes great strokes or bruising of the Head, especially such as happen from a fall from some high place, do bring hurt or debility to the Animal faculties. I have known some very learned, and men of great wit and judgment, who outliving some of these falls by chance, afterwards were of a heavy and dull ingenuity. It is commonly said of such so distemper'd, that their Brain is turned; and indeed a vehement Convulsion or shaking of the Brain, greatly perverts, and not seldom presses together, or shuts up the accustomed tracts and paths of the Spirits, so that they perform the acts of the Memory and the Imagination for ever after, hardly, and amiss; so as some by some great wound inflicted on the Head, have become sottish, and afterwards mad.

3. Great hurts of the Head sometimes cause Doting, or want of Ingenuity.

Fourthly, Frequent Drunkenness and Surfeiting, especially if they sleep in their Cups, and lie as it were buried in Wine and Sleep, do very much decay the wits of some, and make infirm the use of their Reason; to wit, because by them, *Heterogeneous* little Bodies, and infesting very much the Animal Regiment, are introduced. Almost for the same reason, the frequent use of *Opiates* very much troubles the sharpness of the mind.

4. Frequent Drunkenness.

Fiftly, Violent and sudden passions, as in the first place, an unexpected and very great affright, or terror or vehement sadness, have caused Sottishness or Foolishness in some, so that they have been scarce able to express the sense of their mind in words, or to perform the familiar actions of life. Which certainly comes to pass, forasmuch as the spirits inhabiting the Brain upon such an occasion, are very much dissipated and drawn asunder one from another, and afterwards, are not able to repeat the the former footsteps of their motions; in like manner as Souldiers, being put to flight by a sudden and violent attack of the enemy, recover not easily their orders and stations.

5. Vehement Affictions.

Sixthly, It is observed, that some men have contracted also *Foolishness*, by reason of cruel Diseases of the Head. This frequently happens in a great and long *Epilepsie*, for that this Distemper, possessing the middle part of the Brain, perverts, and so fills and stuffs

6. The more grievous Diseases of the Head, oftentimes excite Foolishness.

Ee 2

stuffs up with feculencies, all the Pores and paſſages, the Spirits being thereby frequently and vehemently thruſt forth, that the tracts of the Spirits being ſhut up; the acts of the internal Senſes and Motions are hindred. I knew a young maid, at firſt of an acute wit, and lively ingenuity, who after ſhe had long laboured with the Falling-ſickneſs, became ſottiſh and fooliſh, like a changeling. Further, I have taken notice in many, that *Stupidity* hath accompanied the *Palſie*, or has gone before it (as we mentioned in the Chapter of the *Palſie*) to wit, the ſame matter which brings a reſolution or looſning, being in the Streaked Body, being heaped up in the *Callous*, cauſes often, if not an *Appoplexy*, or *Carus*, a *Fooliſhneſs*.

The Differences of this Diſeaſe. Many differences of this Diſeaſe are to be met with; and firſt, there is commonly wont to be a diſtinction between *Stupidity* and *Fooliſhneſs*, for thoſe affected with this latter, apprehend ſimple things well enough, dextrouſly and ſwiftly, and retain them firm in their memory, but by reaſon of a defect of judgment, they compoſe or divide their notions evilly, and very badly inferr one thing from another; moreover, by their folly, and acting ſiniſtrouſly and ridiculouſly, they move laughter in the by ſtanders.

How fooliſhneſs and ſtupidity differ. On the contrary, thoſe who are *Stupid*, by reaſon of the defect of the Imagination and Memory, as well as of the Judgment, do neither apprehend well, or quickly, nor argue well; beſides they behave themſelves not as the others by toying and geſticulation, but ſottiſhly, fooliſhly, or like a dull Aſs; ſo that the *ſimplicity* of theſe is the more miſerable, who ſhew ſo the Diſeaſe in their countenance and behaviour. In *Fooliſhneſs*, it ſeems, that the Animal Spirits being ſomewhat active, though leſs firm, do paſs thorow only more ſhort and oblique tracts, and do not beam thorow the Brain, with an equal and conſtant irradiation, but leaping forth, or running out deſultorily or after a leaping manner, ſometimes here ſometimes there perform the acts of the Animal Functions, perfunctorily only, or ridiculouſly. But in *Stupidity*, the Spirits being obtuſe and dull of their own proper nature, and flowing, very little pervious in the more thick Brain, cannot exerciſe themſelves rightly, for the performing the offices of the Animal Regiment.

Degrees of Stupidity. Stupidity (whoſe *Pathology* we here chiefly deliver) hath many degrees; for ſome are accounted unfit or incapable, as to all things, and others as to ſome things only. Some being wholly fools in the learning of letters, or the liberal Sciences, are yet able enough for *Mechanical* Arts. Others of either of theſe incapable, yet eaſily comprehend *Agriculture*, or Husbandry and Country buſineſs. Others unfit almoſt for all affairs, are only able to learn what belongs to eating or the common means of living: Others merely *Dolts* or drivling Fools, ſcarce underſtand any thing at all, or do any thing knowingly.

The Prognoſtick of the Diſeaſe. As to what belongs to the *Prognoſtick*, *Stupidity* being contracted from the birth or hereditary, or happening from unknown cauſes, if it ſtill perſiſts to ripe age, it is almoſt never healed: but when it happens that Children being at firſt dull and almoſt inſenſible, by reaſon of the complexions of both their Brain and Spirits being ripened, they are made ingenious and docil enough.

Evil if from an hurt of the Head. This Diſeaſe excited from an evident ſolitary cauſe, as from an hurt of the Head, or a violent paſſion, alſo coming upon an inveterate *Epilepſie*, if it continues for ſome time, it is afterwards incurable.

What is excited from a Lethargy admits a Cure. What ſucceeds a *Lethargy*, and any other ſleepy Diſeaſes, depends chiefly on the hurt of the Memory, and ſometimes vaniſhes of its own accord, thoſe Diſtempers being cured. Therefore, when in theſe caſes the cure of *Stupidity* is inſtituted, here are convenient almoſt the ſame method of healing and Remedies, which we have preſcribed in the Preſervatory *Indication* of the *Lethargy*; the chief intentions of which are, that the Animal Spirits being freed from any torpor or benummedneſs, cut forth or frame Pores and paſſages within the tranſlucid Brain, and may be expanded truly in them.

Sometimes it is cured by a Feavour. Sometimes a *Feavour* has cured ſome Fools, and ſtupid, and render'd them more acute. *Huartus* tells of a certain man that was a Fool in the Court of *Corduba*, that being diſtemper'd with a malignant Feavour, came ſo much to himſelf in the midſt of the Diſeaſe, and with that judgment and diſcretion, that the whole Court ſtood in admiration; and ſo remained his whole life afterwards, one of the moſt prudent men of his time. We our ſelves have known a certain man of a very blunt, *Bœotick* or dull wit, who talking idly in a Feavour, moſt ſuddenly brought forth moſt acute ſpeeches, and ſeaſoned with a great deal of ſalt or ingenious wit. Further, we before ſpoke of a generous old Gentleman, who having loſt his memory, and ſo the uſe of diſcourſe, received great help by the diſtemper of a Feavour happening afterwards; the reaſon of which ſeems to be, becauſe the feavouriſh burning ſometimes rarefies and diſpels the darkneſs covering the Brain.

As

Of Stupidity or Foolishness.

As to what respects the cure of this Disease, *Stupidity*, whether innate or acquired (if it be not plainly *Madness* or *Stolidity*, uncapable of all learning) though it may not be cured, yet is often wont to be amended. Wherefore it must be the work both of a *Physician* and a *Teacher*, that the wit of such that are so affected, may be somewhat trimmed, and they being at least brought to the use of reason in a little measure, may be accounted out of the number of *Brutes*. *The Cure requires both a Master and a Physician.*

For this end, because dull or senseless Beetles, or the more dull Loggerheads or Blockheads, do not readily learn the common notions of things, no more than Children the first elements of letters, therefore they are to be instituted in all things, by the frequent care of a Master, and the same things are again and again to be inculcated to them. For by this means, the Spirits, though slow and torpid, are a little sharpened by perpetual exercise, and they being continually excited in the Brain, how rude and crasse soever they be, do cut forth at length for their expansion, some tracts or passages, though more imperfect. But that this may the more happily and easily succeed, medical Remedies ought to be administred, which may purifie and volatize the Blood and nervous Liquor, together with the Animal Spirits; and also, that may clarifie the Brain, and render it as it were *Diaphanous*. *What the labour of the former ought to be.*

What the Medical intentions are.

For the purifying the Blood, let there be sometimes administer'd a gentle Purge, and Phlebotomy in a small quantity, if there be strength, several times; for that end also Issues are convenient, in the Arm or Leg, or both, for the driving the filthiness from the Brain: In fat folks, and such as are indowed with a moist Head, let them sometimes be made between the shoulders. Further, some in this case cry up with wonderful praises a *Trepaning*, by which the Brain may more freely breath forth, and evaporate. Let their diet be light and attenuating; their dwelling in a free air, and dry; their sleep moderate. *What kind of Remedies are shewn.* *1. Evacuating Remedies.*

After these have for some time been administred, in the ordinary and usual manner, if that in the left part of the breast *there is no beating of the heart in the Arcadian youth*, or if there be no sign of hopes, it will be in vain to spend labour and pains, and Medicines any further on them: but if by the use of these, any signs of help, or any hopes appear, sometimes it will be to the purpose to add to these, altering Remedies, to be daily taken at medical hours, for a long time. The *Recipes* or *Formula*'s of these are already delivered in our *Pharmaceutice* for the taking away the foregoing causes of most *Cephalick* Diseases; and thence may be taken: moreover what do besides respect this particular case, we think here good to add, being some magisterial Receipts. *2. Altering Medicines.*

Take of the Spirits of *Armoniacum*, succinated, or with Amber six drams; let it be given from fifteen to twenty drops Evening and Morning, in three spoonfuls of the following distilled water; drinking after it seven spoonfuls of the same. *Spirits.*

Take of the fresh leaves of *Misletoe* of the Apple tree six handfuls; of the lesser Sage, Rosemary, Savory, the greater Rocket, Mother of Thyme, Calaminths, Penyroyal, Marjoram, each four handfuls; of the roots of *Angelica*, of *Imperatoria*, each six ounces; of *Zedoary*, the lesser *Calingal*, of the *Aromatick Reed*, of *Winterans Bark*, each two ounces; of Cloves, Nutmegs, Mace, Cinnamon, Ginger, each one ounce; of *Cubebs*, *Cardamums*, Grains of Paradise, each six drams; all of these being cut and bruised small together, pour to them twelve pints of the best Canary; let them be digested cold, and close shut in a vessel for three days, then distilled according to art: let the whole liquor be mixed together, and sweetned with Sugar when it is taken: The Dose is two or three ounces. *A Distilled Water.*

After the use of the *Spirits of Armoniack* for fifteen or twenty days, other Medicines about that time may have their turns, such as *Spirits* of *Harts-horn*, of *Sut*, *Humane Skull*; *Tinctures* of *Coral*, *Antimony*, *Castor*, *Amber*; the *Elixir Vitæ Quercitani*, *Elixir Proprietatis*, Spirits of *Lavender*, &c. *Tinctures, Elixirs.*

Or Take of the Conserves of the flowers of the Lilie of the valley six ounces, of the roots of *Acori veri* preserved six drams, of Ginger preserved in India, of preserved Nutmeg, each half an ounce; of Species *Diambra* two drams, of Lignum *Aloes*, yellow Saunders, the picks roots of Zedoary, of Cubebs, of Jamaica Pepper, each one dram and a half; of Coral prepared two drams, of the Syrup of Candied Ginger what will suffice; make an Electuary. The Dose two drams Morning and Evening, drinking after it of the distilled Water three ounces. *An Electuary.*

For those whose Brain is too abounding with moisture, let them drink every Morning a draught of *Coffee*, with Sage leaves boiled in it: For those who have their Animal Spirits too poor and liveless; let them take *Chocalate*, as we have described it above, *Coffee.* *Chocalate.*

which

Physical Beer.   which seems most profitable. For ordinary drink let small Ale or Beer be prepared in a vessel containing three or four Gallons, and after it has work'd, put into it in a little bag, these following things. Take *of the leaves of Sage, the sharp leaved and dryed, four handfuls; of Cubebs one ounce, of Cloves and of Nutmegs bruised, &c.* Mix them according to art.

Outward Applications.   Outward Applications have also a place here; such are a quilted Cap, Plasters, and Liniments: and sometimes let these, sometimes those or others be administer'd.

A Cap or quilted thing for the Head.   Take *of the flowers of the Lily of the valley, Rosemary flowers, Stœchadoes, each one handful; of Celtick Spike two drams, of the roots of Cypress, the lesser Galingal, the Florentine Iris, each three drams; of Labdanum, Benzoin, of Toluvian Balsam, of Amber, each two drams; of Nutmegs, Cloves, Mace, Cinamon, each one dram and a half: make of them all a fine powder, quilting it in a Cap with silk between.*

A Plaster.   Take *of the Plaster of Floris unguent. so called, two ounces, of Tachamahac, of Carrane, of the Balsom of Tolu, each three drams; of the Powder of Amber, Myrrh, each two drams; of Cloves, Nutmeg, Mace, each one dram; being all liquefied or melted together, let them be made into a mass, of which make a Plaster, spread it on leather, and the head being shaved, put it to it.*

A Liniment.   Take *of the Oyl of Palms half an ounce, of Capive Balsom three drams, of the Balsom of Peru one dram, of the Oyl of Nutmeg, by expression two drams, Oyl of Amber half a dram; make an Ointment for the Head.*

I might here add many other Medicines, and ways of Administrations, but in this almost desperate case, where oftentimes no Remedies are wont to help, and the Cure never perfected, these may suffice.

CHAP. XIV.

Of the Gout.

The Distempers of the Gout and Colick are Distempers of the nervous Stock.   AMong the Diseases of the Head and the nervous stock, we may refer hither some Distempers that are chiefly wont to infest the Feet and the Belly, to wit, the *Gout* and the *Colick,* That the seat of either is in the nervous parts, we may very well conclude from the primary *Symptom,* to wit, pain. The cause of this latter, *Charles Piso* has affirmed to exist within the Head, and *Fernelius* affims the same of the other. Wherefore we shall endeavour to deliver the *Pathologie* of either, together with the apposite means of healing them; and first we shall speak of the *Gout.*

The Subject of the Gout.   The name of the *Gout* denotes plainly its subject; because that it is almost only *Articulate,* or is in the space where the heads of two or more Bones meet together. This Disease is wont to be excited more frequently about the *Internodia* or knittings of the Bones of the Feet; because this part being greatly declining, and remote from the *Præcordia,* and the fountain of Heat, receives readily the Morbifick matter, and does not easily overcome it, or quickly put it off. Yet the *Gout* often happens in the jointings of the Hip or huckle bone, the knee, the bending of the arm, the shoulder, the wrist, the ancle, and of other parts.

Its appearances rehearsed.   The fits of this Disease (which are almost ever intermitting) invade either wandringly, or periodically; which being finished, sometimes sooner, sometime more slowly, the intervals happen lucid or quiet enough; presently after the first assault of it, for the most part pains arise without any tumor; though afterwards, about the height of the Disease, the distemper'd part often swells up; the pains in the beginning yield to no Remedies, but are made more cruel by *Catharticks,* and are not presently put to flight by *Topicks,* or wont to be allayed. The Fit most often falls upon one without any previous distemper, but suddenly; yet sometimes there will be an heat of the blood, or a little feavourish distemper going before. The disposition to this Disease is sometimes hereditary, and sometimes acquired, by reason of an evil manner of living. The occasions or causes, which being wont to move this disposition, stir up the *Gouty* pains, are all violent alterations or passions, inflicted on the humors or spirits. Hence Surfeiting immoderate drinking, especially of sharp and thin Wines, transpiration being hindred, wrath or indignation, immoderate Venus or Lust, sadness, also the changes of the air, and of the year, and any great mutations ordinarily induce fits of this Disease. Those obnoxious

Of the Gout.

to this disease, are sometimes in danger to be distemper'd also with the *Stone*, or *Gravel* in the *Reins*; and so on the contrary, those obnoxious to the Stone, are wont to be troubled with the *Gout*. Yea the *Gout* growing grievous, it every where heaps up about its nests, to wit, in the joynts, a calculous or stony matter, and there excites a stony or hard bulk.

The distemper'd parts, whose pains are stirred up in the hauled Fibres, for the most *The parts affect-* part are the *Periostea*, or the heads clothing the Membrane of the Bones, and perhaps *ed.* the *Tendons* and Ligaments there planted about. But sometimes the pain in these parts, wholly depends upon a breach of the unity, and this proceeds from a certain matter being impacted in those Bodies, or lying upon them; first of all we shall inquire, what sort of morbific matter this is; secondly, from whence it comes; and thirdly, by what means it so stirs up periodical *Gouty* Fits, by breaking the unity in them.

As to the *Morbifick* Matter it seems, first that it is not the Blood or nervous juice of *The Morbifick* it self; nor is it one only simple humor laid up a part from the others. We deserved- *Matter.* ly excuse the Blood from this censure, because these pains only infest Bodies for the most part without Blood; yea, and almost them only. For although in the neighbouring parts, by reason of the course of the Blood being hindred, sometimes a tumor happens with an inflammation; yet this is not the Disease, but a *Symptom*, and for the most part comes upon the *Gout*. Further it appears, that the nervous juice (how ever sharp, or biteing, or pricking, or pulling it is supposed to be) does not excite of it self the pains of the *Gout*; because then the Distemper would cause pains also, or as much in some other passages of the nervous parts, and also in the *Internodia* or knittings of the Bones.

It is improbable, for the same reason, that any singular, excrementitious, or super- *It is not any* fluous Humor or Matter deposited from the Blood or nervous juice, to cause the pains *simple or singu-* of the *Gout*. For if such were only carried thorow the Nerves, it would excite pains *lar Humour sug-* by order, and a continual tract, not first in the feet or extream joints, but by irritating *gested from any* the nervous Stock in its whole journey. If that according to the opinions of *Hollerius*, *of them.* *Sennertus*, and other Moderns, it be affirmed, that some impurities falling off from the heated Blood, and received by the joints, is the material cause of the *Goutish* pain; then it should follow, that all who are greatly obnoxious to the *Goutish* Distempers, are also most prone to Feavourish burnings or heats; and that a Feavourish heat should precede every assault of this Disease; neither of which to be true, common observation doth witness. For those troubled with the Gout, as it were with a priviledge (to wit, by reason of the *Saline* dispositions of the Humors) are free from a *Feavourish* Distemper. Further, the Fits of the *Gout* most often arise of a sudden, without any great swelling up or ebullition of the Blood, and presently at the beginning become very cruel; which also argues, that the Morbifick Matter is not by degrees laid up in the distemper'd part, as in a Mine, and then to excite pains by its fulness. For if it were so, the beginnings and the increase of the Disease, being always made *gradatim*, they would be longer and more durable; nor doth the distemper (as it often is wont) being presently vehement, by and by change its seat, and quickly vanishing in one place, anon arise up in another.

When therefore any singular humor (of which sort soever it be supposed) seems not *In the Mint of* efficacious enough, for the provision of the Fits of the *Gout*; we may affirm, That in *this Disease two* the nest or mine of this Disease, (whether it be one or many), that many fermentative *humours concur,* juices, and those not easily to be mixed, do meet together; then from the strife and *and mutually* growing hot of these, the painful Vellications or pullings of the nervous Fibres do a- *grow hot.* rise.

Formerly discoursing of the wandring *Scorbutick Gout*, and the *Rheumatism*, we plain- *In like manner,* ly shewed what was also the cause of this *Gout*, of which we now treat; *viz.* forasmuch *as when the* as it appears by a very vulgar experiment, that salts being put in a diverse state, to *Spirits of Vi-* wit, some of them being fixed or *Alchalizate*, and others having gotten a flux, or sharp, *triol are pour-* or acetosous things, being put together, do very much boil up and grow hot, and their *Tartar.* humidity causing a white and hardish *Coagulum* or curdling; as for instance well known, when the spirit of *Vitriol* is poured to oyl of *Tartar*, it manifestly appears; and why may ⟨ ⟩ ot think, that in the fits of the *Gout*, there is something like it? to wit, that from the fighting and mutual conflict of the Liquors, which are of a diverse *Saline* nature, the nervous Fibers are pricked and provoked, and at length, from the various *Coagulations* of either juice, that there is sometimes heaped together in the distemper'd places, a *Calculous* or stony matter.

That we may shew the genuine matter of the *Gout*, we ought to referr hither, what *A Vitriolick* we have elsewhere said, concerning the nourishment of the solid parts. For indeed, *Matter partly* we have shewed, that to that office both the Blood, and the nervous Liquor do bring *the Nervous Li-* their *quor.*

their tributes; to wit, when the nourishing juice is carried from the Blood, thorow the Arteries, to all the parts of the whole body, another liquor being deposited from the Brain, thorow the Nerves, and their dependences, doth actuate that former, as it were with an inspired spirit, so that it is made full and fertil, and so more easily insinuates into the Pores and passages of the part that is to be nourished, and is assimilated into its substance. There will be no need to repeat here what we have formerly discoursed at large; as to what respects the present matter, we shall take notice, that the nutritious humor, distributed from the blood, consists of a little Spirit, but of more plenty of Water, Earth, and Sulphur, and moderately of Salt, somewhat volatile; further, whilst the nutritious humor is distributed, for that its Particles, which are for the cherishing or nourishment of any part, ought to be proportionate, and to remain like it self; therefore, whilst the spirituous are destinated to the Brain, and the sulphureous to the flesh, the inwards and the fat, it is behoveful, that the most *Saline* and more fixed, should be laid up about the jointings of the Bones, and then growing full with the nervous liquor, to be assimilated with them.

Either Matter, growing degenerate or depraved, turns to the Gout.
1. From the Blood, for that it becomes full of a fixed Salt.
2. From the nervous Liquor, for that it is acetosous or sharp.

But if by reason of the vitious *Dyscrasie* of the Blood, it happens that Particles saltish above measure, and fixed, should be laid up in the joints, and by reason of their incongruity are not presently assimilated; they soon after grow together into an heap, or a certain Morbific mine. But the Fit of the *Gout* is not wont for that reason to be excited, but an heaviness only and languishing of the distemper'd member, which is oftentimes taken away by abstinence, or exercise, or Physick; the strange Particles being discussed, or supped back again into the Blood.

But if the Particles of the nervous liquor degenerate from a volatileness into an acetous Flux, a flowing arising from thence, they fall down in too great plenty into the little joints, and because they there grow hot, with the *Saline* or *Lixivial* Mine, there before laid up, they stir up the Fits of the *Gout*.

The former is, as it were, the feminine Seed of the Gout;
The other masculine.

The *Saline* or *Tartarous* Matter therefore being laid up from the Arterous Blood, about the jointings together of the Bones, is as it were the feminine seed of this Disease; which notwithstanding, though there be heaped together a great plenty of it, is of it self wholly unfruitful, like an Egg without a Cock; until the nervous liquor growing turgent, sends its acetosous Recrements falling from it, into the nest of the former; which immediately, as it were the masculine seed, renders the other prolifick. For inasmuch as those two Particles which are of a different state and original, do meet together, and mutually concur, they pull or haul the Fibres of the Membranes and Tendons, and so stir up the fit of the Gout; the allaying of which, wholly depends upon the mutual subaction or bringing under, and the difflation or blowing away of the most sharp Particles of either kind.

The Procatartick, or foregoing Causes of the Gout.

These things concerning the formal reason, and the conjunct cause of the *Gout*, being thus laid down, we will proceed to the further unfolding its *Procatartick* or foregoing causes: And we say, that these are a *Saline* matter, laid up from the Blood in the joints, and *acetous* or sharp Recrements, sent into the same nest, from the swelling up of the nervous liquor.

1. A Mine of fixed Salt laid up about the Internodia, or Knitting together of the Bones.
This Matter is not merely Excrementitious,

First therefore, that this sort of *Saline* Mine is laid up about the jointings or knitting of the Bones together, is plainly argued by the sudden and unlook'd for assault of this Disease, and from its difficult cure; for the matter doth not flow into the distemper'd part altogether, and at once, in such abundance, that it should excite a fit so grievous and tedious; besides, for that the pains are repeated still within the accustomed nest, it seems that their setation or hatching doth most certainly depend upon the Egg somewhere laid up before hand. But that this matter is not merely Excrementitious, but a portion of the nourishing juice, degenerate towards a fixed Salt, being destinated to the same bony parts, we may lawfully conjecture, because an humor merely Excrementitious, would cause in the distemper'd place, a continual trouble and tumor; moreover, this plainly convinces, from the cure of the *Gout*, by torture or cutting of the part: For *Authors* worthy to be believed, have told us in their writings, that the Member being cut off, in which the sickness uses to be, or greatly wounded, that the Disease has ceased without any relapse; in like manner as a most grievous Tooth-ack, and continual, is most often cured by pulling out the distemper'd Tooth.

nor a Bilous or Phlegmatick Humour.

If that the *Goutish* humor were (as it is commonly said) a *Cholerick*, or a *Phlegmatick* humour, or any other merely Excrementitious, it flowing afterwards to some other member, after the former distemper'd were cut off, would there excite a new Morbific Mine; but this happens only in some accustomed joints, for that this or that part is become more weak, and so admits into it self the more easily, all other filthy portions; and neither assimilating nor sending them away, suffers them to increase into a Morbific Mine. Further, the Recrements also of the nervous juice, that are sharp and acetous, fall down more readily into the same part by reason of its debility. But

Of the Gout. 217

But to the *Saline Procatarxis*, or foregoing cause of this Disease, lying in the Joints; not only the weakness of the distemper'd member, but much more and first of all, the evil disposition of the Blood doth help. We shall weigh a little the reasons, and the manner how it is done, of either.

To this previous procatarxis, to wit, a fixed Salt, the Disease of the blood, and the debility of the Distemper'd Member doth help.

1. And in the first place, the fault of the Blood is, that its elementary Particles, and chiefly the Saline, are not in a fit state or condition. For they ought to be within the mass of the Blood, in the middle betwixt a fixed and a volatile constitution: they are called fixed, so long as the Sulphur and Earth being combined, do pertinaciously adhere to them; as it is observed in fresh and raw Urine, from which you shall not easily draw by distillation, either Salt or Spirit: But the saline Particles are volatilised, when leaving the Sulphur and Earth, they adhere to the spirituous, and with them fly away; as it is seen in the spirit of Urine, being distilled after a long digestion. Then there is a middle constitution between these, when the Saline Particles are so loosned and dislocated from the Sulphureous and Earthy Particles, that upon occasion they may be easily laid hold on by the Spirituous, and ascend together with them; as it is in Urine putrefied by digestion, from which with a very little heat, you may force out Spirit and Salt. In like manner the Saline Particles in a living body, seem first of all to be in a degree of fixity, within the *Coyle*; from which, notwithstanding, through Concoction in the Bowels, being rightly made, they begin to come forth a little. Secondly, these are made volatile in the nervous juice: And, Thirdly, they are of a middle constitution in the bloody mass; to wit, which are exalted by a continual circulation or digestion, so that they are in some manner volatile, that being associated, partly with spirituous particles, and distilled forth with them into the Brain, they go into Animal Spirits; and partly going into the nutritious juice, together with the sulphureous and others, they increase in their nourishing the solid parts.

What the Saline Particles of the blood ought to be, to wit, in a middle state, between fixation and volatilisation.

But sometimes it happens, that the saline Particles (at least not all) are not rightly exalted within the bloody mass, but remaining in a state of fixity, give a beginning or cherishing to many Diseases. That we may say nothing of the *Scurvy*, *Dropsie*, and many others, we only say for the present, it may be suspected, that the first seeds of the *Goutish* distemper depend upon this cause; for when the nervous juice, being destinated to the heads of the bones (where it is chiefly received) ought to consist of very much Salt, there is a necessity, that its Particles, because they are too fixed and thick, cannot be admitted presently into the Pores and passages, should increase into a Morbifick Mine Besides, that more easily and more often happens, if the weak or broken Fibres of the bodies, planted near, cannot by wrinkling themselves, shake off what is troublesome or superfluous.

When, being too fixed, they become Morbifick. And so they bring forth the Scurvy, Dropsie, and other Diseases, and especially the Gout.

As to the secret leading or evident causes, from which the nutritious liquor being brought from the blood to the joints, is imbued too much with a fixed Salt, and by reason of which, these parts become too prompt and easie for the receiving what is improportionate to them, the chief of these, for that they are various and manifold, we will briefly touch upon.

The Saline fixed, or Arthritical Disposition of the Blood, proceeds from various Causes.

1. And first of all, an hereditary disposition is wont to produce either evil. For those troubled with the *Gout*, for the most part beget Gouty Children, and this Disease descending from the Parents to the Children, is wont not only to have the like fruits in both, and also to ripen about the periods of the same age; but for the most part, it hath its first roots in the same members, and observes every where the like progresses: concerning the reason of which, I think, we have already said enough, being the same as other Diseases propagated *ex traduce*, or from the Parent.

1. Sometimes it is Hereditary.

2. But indeed, the *Gouty* disposition is brought in oftentimes without any original fault, by reason of an evil manner of living, and errors in the six *non-naturals*. For those who are given to Surfeiting and drinking much, and indulge their appetites by an inordinate eating and drinking, and especially if they feed on salt and spiced meats, and guzle down great plenty of Wine, easily contract this Disease. For by this means, the *Coyle* is indigested, and indued with very unfit and untameable Particles, and so ill prepared in the Bowels; and then from a more liberal drinking of Wine, saltish settlements and heterogeneous feculences or dregs, which subsist somewhere in the first passages, being too much exalted, are carried into the Blood: to which enormities of living, if a sedentary life, idleness, or sleeping at noon be added, so that the superfluities neither exhale, nor the *Saline* impurities are dissipated by exercise, but left to settle about the jonts, certainly too much of this *Alchalisate* seed is sowed for a plentiful harvest of this Disease of the *Gout*.

2. Oftentimes acquired, by reason of an evil manner of living.

3. The debility of the little Joints, and *Goutish* disposition is not only hereditary, but excited frequently by reason of various occasions. The falling down of the Morbific matter often induces this: for if by chance it happens, that at first, the fit of the *Gout* comes

From what Causes the debility of the Joynts is excited.

F f

comes in this or that part, afterwards the peccant humor more easily falls down into the same member; and quickly constitutes, as it were, a nest, where the Eggs may be continually laid up. Besides, a solution or breach of continuity also, or some hurt inflicted on any joint, by wet, or cold, by a blow, or putting out of joint, oftentimes stirrs up the *Goutish* disposition.

2. The other foregoing Cause of the Gout, from the acetous part of the nervous humour.

Secondly, But indeed, as the Blood brings a *Saline* Mine for the Morbid seed, and the Joints receive and hide it readily; yet this provision, without the coming of the other seeds, is like an addle Egg, wholly barren and unfruitful; because, for the constituting of this Disease into act, it is required, that the nervous liquor, by chance swelling up or growing turgid, pours forth *Saline* impurities of another condition, to wit, acetous, falling away with a certain effervescency, or heat, and as it were a firing of the other Mine. Wherefore, we think good to set down this other foreleading cause of the *Gouty* Disease in the nervous humor, and its acetous or sharp affluxions, or flowing to the parts.

Such an acetous disposition does not come upon the whole Mass of the nervous humour, but only some portions or recrements of it.

And indeed, that the *Saline* Particles of this Liquor degenerating from a *volatilization* to a flux, do become acid, we have shewed by very many instances and reasons; both formerly, and also in this Tract. But for the provision of this Disease, it is not requisite that the whole Mass of the nervous juice should be acetous; but it is sufficient, that some portions of it in the Brain, or elsewhere in the nervous stock, being depraved, or that its Recrements laid up here and there, had contracted this kind of Nature, from which afterwards growing turgid, when as the acid Particles run together to the *Saline* Mine laid up in the Joints, they stir up the *Gouty* fit after the manner aforesaid.

It is shewn that acetous fluxions do proceed from the nervous humour.

But truly, it manifestly appears, that *acetous fluxions* being brought from the nervous humor, do frequently happen; by a notable instance or experiment, often cited by me; *viz.* I have often observed, That those obnoxious to the passions or pains of the Nerves, have suffered or felt a light rigor or stiffness in their whole Body (which is a corrugation or wrinkling of almost all the nervous parts) and then presently, the Convulsive Distemper would follow; at which time the Urine was rendred very copiously and clear, which being without any lixivial or nitrous savour (which otherwise it always has) was very sharp, like mere Vinegar: indeed by this most clear sign it appears, that the humor being risen up to a fulness in the nervous parts, and moved by its swelling up, doth bring in the Convulsive Distempers; and when a portion of the same sweating or dropping forth, is laid up in the *Glandulas,* immediately being reduced thence into the Blood, by the passage of the Veins and *Lympheducts,* it did excite the flood of the sharp Urine: Indeed in like manner, from the same humor swelling up in a lesser measure, and still remaining within the nervous passages, and setling in the Joints, we think the *Gouty* fits do arise.

And so part of the Gouty Mine is sent from the Brain and Nerves.

Indeed it is an argument, that part of the *Goutish* matter doth proceed from the Brain and Nerves, because for the most part, those obnoxious to this Disease, do complain a little before the fit, of an heaviness of the head, and of a dulness, with a *Vertigo,* and sleepiness; but as soon as they begin to suffer the pains of the *Gout,* as if the Clouds were blown away from the Brain, they enjoy a more free understanding, with a great and unwonted sharpness of wit. Besides, when as there are sometimes many *Saline* Mines of this inveterate Disease, deposited in diverse Members, it is observed, that the pains do very much invade, first the superior places, and then by degrees descend to the rest; wherefore, when perhaps at first the *Vertebræ* of the neck were troubled, a little while after the shoulders, or other members of the Arm were possessed, then the Disease reached to the Loins, or the Hips, and lastly the joints of the Legs, and so to the lowest joints, sometimes these, and sometimes those.

The evident Causes of the Goutish Fit.

The *Evident Causes,* which in respect of the nervous liquor stir up the *Gouty* Fits, do either pervert the Particles and portions into an Acetousness, or else stir them up before degenerated into Fluxions.

1. The drinking of sharp Liquors.

1. Acid liquors, as thin Wines, Cyder, stale Beer (experience being mistress, are to be shunned by *Gouty* persons, more than a Mad-Dog, or a Snake. For these kind of Drinks do not only bring into act the cause of this Disease, but contribute more Acetous Particles, (by carrying them to the Brain, and nervous Fibres) to its nest, and increase the Morbific matter.

2. Immoderate Exercise.

2. Immoderate or unseasonable exercises of the Body, violent passions, immoderate Venus, and a disorderly feeding, and whatsoever besides greatly disturbs the spirits and humors or shakes them, and by that means stir up the fluxions of the nervous juice or its recrements, induce the pains of the *Gout.*

3. Evacuations being suppressed.

3. Usual evacuations being suppressed, also taking of cold and wet, for that by this means the blood, and by consequence the nervous liquor, conceive effervescencies and fluxions, do bring on the fits of this Disease.

4. For

Of the Gout.

4. For the same reason, the changes of the Heaven and of the Air, as also the Tropicks of the year, are wont to bring on the pains of the *Gout*; so that it is become a Proverb, That *Gouty* persons carry their *Almanack* in their joints; and deduce most certain *Prognosticks* of the weather, from their pains: For as often as the humid constitution of the year, or the blowing of the Southern, or the Northern Winds, or Snow, are at hand, they are wont to predict these from the coming of their pains. Further, every Quarter of the Year, especially Spring and Fall, they are more grievously tormented. Wherefore the *Æquinoxes* are always religiously observed by them. The reason of these consists partly in this, forasmuch as insensible perspiration is variously altered, by reason of the mutations of the Air and Year; therefore the Effluvia's which are wont to transpire, being restrained, do ferment the Blood and the nervous Humor, and easily stir them up into *Goutish* Fluxions. Besides, the humors of our Bodies, even as the Sap of Vegetables, and other natural and artificial Liquors do diversly grow hot, about the changing of times, and enter various states or conditions of either fixation, or sometimes of volatileness, or of a flux.

4. The Circulations of the Heavens, Air and Year.

The chief differences of this Disease, are taken from the distemper'd places, and so there are ordained as it were distinct *species* of the same, to wit, the *Chiragra* or Hand *Gout*, the *Ischia* or Hip *Gout*, the *Gonagra* or Knee *Gout*, and the *Podagra* the Foot or Toe *Gout*; in the mean time, pains are wont to be excited in some other members, and are noted by the common name of the *Gout*. Whether the pains of the Teeth, or of the Loins, and pains of other parts ought to be referred hither, we have not now leasure to inquire.

The differences of the Gout.
1. As to the places affected.

This Distemper, as to its original, is said to be hereditary, or acquired; as to the temperament of the sick, it is Hot or Cold, or *Sanguine*, *Cholerick*, or *Phlegmatick*, to wit, because the Blood being hindred in its circuit, about the distemper'd places, sometimes an Inflammation, or a watry swelling come upon the pains.

2. As to its Original.

As to the relation of other Diseases, the Distemper of the *Gout* is either singular, or else complicated with other Diseases, and chiefly with the *Scurvey*, or the Stone. Of which kind of combinations, because they are intimate and frequent (as if they were of kin to this Disease) it will seem to the purpose, for us to inquire into the reasons.

3. In respect of other Diseases.

A long *Gout* oftentimes gets to it the *Scurvey*, and some *Scorbutick* Distempers are so like the *Gout*, that they are not easily distinguished. The reason of the former is, both the like *Dyscrasie* of the Blood in either Distemper, depending upon a fixed Salt, as also for that *Gouty* people, being for a long time fixed either to their Bed or Chair, the *Scorbutick* disposition easily comes upon them. Secondly, The *Scorbutick* Distempers which imitate the *Gout* are the *Rheumatism*, and the wandring *Scorbutick* Gout; the reasons and causes of which, and how they may be discerned from the *Gout*, we need not repeat here, having already delivered them in our tract of the *Scurvey*.

It is wont to be complicated with the Scurvey.

The *Gout* hath so near a relation to the *Stone*, or *Gravel* in the Reins, that either distemper, as if they had the same original, most often meet together; for scarce any is sick of the *Gout*, but is found to be also obnoxious to the other Disease. Further, an inveterate *Gout* is wont to excite stony Concretions in the Joints, such as the *Stone* doth in the Reins. Hence I think it is most likely, that the *Stone* or *Gravel* in the Reins, doth arise from a like, if not wholly the same cause, that we assigned for the *Gout*, to wit, the *Saline* fixed matter, being deposited from the Blood, in the Reins, doth grow hot with the acid humor, being there poured forth thorow the nervous passages, and by that means doth frequently induce *Nephritick* pains, or of the Reins; then, from either matter being coagulated, after growing hot, doth form the Stone. For the illustrating this *Pathology* farther, (here being no place for it) it shall be deferred to another time.

2. With the Stone.
The Reason of this is shewed.

Every Body is wont to give a *Prognostick* of the *Gout*, to wit, that it is safe enough, but most hard to be Cured. 1. As to the former, this Distemper is not only free of it self from danger, but on the contrary, preventeth most other Diseases. For *Gouty* people, by reason of the *Saline* fixed *Dyscrasie* of the Blood, are little obnoxious to *Feavours*; but for the most part live free from a Consumption, and other more grievous Distempers of the Bowels or Head; because the Recrements of the Blood and nervous Juice are continually laid up in the Joints. 2. But as to the latter, the so great difficulty of Cure, the reason is, that for the taking away the foregoing cause of this Disease, there is required a most perfect amendment, of a double Humor, *viz.* of the Blood and nervous Juice; to wit, that they may beget no *Saline* fixed or plainly acid Particles; and moreover, a restitution of the weakned Joints; neither of which can ever be easily obtained. And besides this, it happens, that the Conjunct Cause of this Disease subsists in places greatly at a distance, so that the virtues of no Medicine are able to reach them.

The Prognostick of this Disease.

Ff 2

Some-

The Gouty Matter being restrained, or any other way translated, oftentimes excites dangerous Distempers.

Sometimes it happens, by reason of the Fluxions of the *Gouty* Matter, being suppressed or beat back, that sometimes torments of the Ventricle, of the Bowels, and of the Belly, sometimes a straitness of breathing, an *Asthma*, or other Distempers of the Breast, and sometimes also an *Apoplexy*, and other sleepy, or Convulsive Diseases are excited; which being observed, it may be objected, that the Mine of the *Gout* is not the same as we but now described: because its *Saline* part, if it were the same which is destinated for the nourishing of the Joints, would not be from thence expelled or deferred, or laid up elsewhere; then as to the other part, to wit, the laying up of the acid seeds in the accustomed place, it seems that it should not be easily repercussed, or of it self suppressed in its way, or any where else translated, to be very hurtful to any part. But indeed, it is easie to reply to this, that an acetous portion of the *Gouty* Matter, may be repelled or suppressed, flowing thorow the nervous passages, and so it being poured into other parts, doth oftentimes excite most grievous evils. Indeed the nervous Liquor and its Recrements, for that they consist of very subtil and active Particles, upon every light stop or repulse, are driven into diverse deflections and flowings; moreover, when these grow turgid, or meet with the Particles of humors of another kind, and grow hot with them, they stir up various Distempers, or such as are painful and Convulsive; and not rarely, because the dissimilar Particles are mutually coagulated, sometimes *Strumous*, sometimes *Cancrous*, or otherways malignant Tumors arise. Instances very remarkable of these kind of effects, we have shewn in our Treatise of *Convulsive Diseases*; But especially concerning a Maid, who by reason of the *Inguinal Glandulas*, or the Kirnels about the Groin, being hardly pressed and hurt with a Truss for a Rupture, fell into a *Vertigo*, and Convulsive Distempers, and shortly after had great *Scropula's* or running Sores, growing on the same side, in the Neck. After the same manner, by reason of the *Goutish* Mine being restrained from its wonted place, and suppressed within the nervous Passages, or otherways translated sometimes most wicked Distempers arise.

The acetous recrements of the nervous Liquor do chiefly effect this.

The first Instance of such an Effect.

A second Instance.

Whilst I was writing these, I was sent for to a Noble Matron, who sometimes past being obnoxious to the *Gout*, and that very much, after about three months last past, she had laboured almost continually with a languishing of the Ventricle, with a queasiness, nauseousness, and vomiting; at length, I know not upon what occasion, falling into frequent swoonings or loss of spirits, a little after she was troubled with a *Vertigo*, with a loss of memory, and sometimes with a light *Delirium*; and when she had continued thus for some days, and free in the mean time from the *Gout*, and growing well in her stomach, she eat with an appetite broth twice or thrice in a day, and once a day flesh meat, and digested it without any trouble: by this manifest sign indeed it appears, that the Recrements of the nervous humor, which were wont before to fall down by the *Spinal* Nerves into the Feet, to the Mine of the *Gout*, afterwards being deposited in the Ventricle, thorow the Nerves of the wandring pair, and the *Intercostals*, did stir up the continual troubles in it; which at last partly restagnating in the Brain, and being partly translated into the *Cardiack* Nerves, (or those going to the Heart) those last Distempers of Swooning, of the *Vertigo*, and the *Delirium* succeeded.

The Cure.

The *Curatory* method suggests three primary *Indications*, the first of them *Curatory*, to be administer'd only in the Fits, for the allaying the pains, and for the sooner ending of them. Secondly, *Preservatory*, being destinated for the intervals of the fits, endeavours the taking away of the foregoing cause of the Disease, that the fits of the pains may more rarely, or less, or not at all be repeated. Thirdly, *Vital*, which institutes, by what kind of food, and by what Remedies, strength may be sustained in the cruel Torments, and life be prolonged, and also refreshed or cherished, notwithstanding the frequent and almost continual troubles of the Disease.

Three primary Indications.

1. Curatory, for the allaying the pains in the Fits.

1. The first *Indication*, to wit, the allaying of the pains, contains these two chief intentions, to wit, that the breach of the unity be taken away; and in the mean time, that the irritation, or the growing hot of the Fibres, or of the Spirits flowing in them, may be quieted or appeased.

1. For the taking away of the Breach of the Continuity.

1. For the taking away of the breach of the unity in the distemper'd places, both the flowings of the humors, which are apt to tend thither, ought to be hindred, and the Mine already impacted to be dissipated, and shaken off, and its Particles suppressed, from their mutual effervescencies or growing hot. For these ends are destinated, evacuating and altering Remedies, and of either both internal and external. We shall here add some forms of these, and the more select ways of administration, in their order.

Phlebotomy.

Phlebotomy or letting of Blood, in a fresh *Gout*, or not very inveterate, and especially in a more hot constitution, being used about the beginning of the Disease, doth often bring help; but in an habitual Disease, and in a frigid temperament, and old age, it is is wont to be more hurtful than profitable; becauſe it depreſſes the vigor of the Blood, and of the Spirits, not too much raging, without a leſſening of the Morbific matter.

The buſineſs is very much controverted concerning Purging about the beginning of *Purging.* the Diſeaſe, whilſt ſome *Phyſicians* moſt ſtrictly abſtain from all Purging, before the declination or end of the fit; others on the contrary, conſtantly give ſtrong Purges about the beginning of the Diſeaſe, and oftentimes with good ſucceſs. The reaſon of the difference ſeems to be placed chiefly in this, to wit, becauſe ſome *Gouty* perſons are yet firm in the conſtitution and tone of the humors, and the Veſſels containing them, and being not yet weakned in their joints, as often as the Blood and nervous Liquor are diſturbed by Medicines, their ſuperfluities and recrements are not preſently precipitated into the Mine of this Diſeaſe, yea theſe being provoked by the Medicine, and alſo obeying the incitement, are drawn forth by the mouths of the Arteries, into the cavities of the *Inteſtines*; and in the mean time, the Veſſels being emptied, they draw or ſup back a certain part of the Morbific Matter. But it is otherwiſe in tender and weak Conſtitutions, for from the leaſt commotion of the Medicine, the purgings of either humor fall down into the *Gouty* place. Therefore to whom Purging is convenient, it ought to be inſtituted with the more ſtrong Medicines, and *Elaterium*. For this matter, theſe are *Forms of Purges.* of known uſe. The Electuary *Caryocoſtinum*. The Purging Syrup *de Ramno*. Pills of *Hermodactyls*. The Compounded Pill *ex Duobus*. The Pill of *Rhaſis*; which if we may believe the Author, will quickly make the ſick to walk. Take *of the beſt Aloes half an ounce, of red Roſes two ſcruples, of Hermodactils barkt one dram and a half, of Diagridium one dram, of Honey of Roſes what will ſuffice; make a Pill.* Roderick of *Fonſeca*, wonderfully crys up the root of black Hellebore, and among other things, an Apple with its ſmall ſtrings put into it, to about half a dram, roaſted under the aſhes, and ſo eaten.

Take *of Calomelanos one ſcruple, of the Reſine of Jalap three grains, or of Scammony three grains, of the Oyl of Cloves one grain, of the Balſam of Peru what will ſuffice; make three or four Pills, for one Doſe.*

In the time of Purging, it will be of ſome moment, perhaps, as *Solenander* adviſes, to reſtrain the falling down of the humors into thoſe places, by a Plaſter, or other defenſive Medicine, laid upon the diſtemper'd places.

Vomiting, to whom it is wont to be ſafe and eaſie, may be alſo convenient in this *Vomiting.* Diſeaſe; for which end, the *Emetick Tartar* of *Mynſicht*, the *Sulphur of Antimony*, or its *Flowers, Mercurius Vitæ, Vinum Emeticum, Gambogia*, may be adminiſter'd.

But in the *Goutiſh* fit, the Powders of Stones, Bones, and Shells, as alſo of ſharp Ve- *Altering Medicines,* getables, do help; which being called the *Alexiteria* of this Diſeaſe, ſubjugate all the *or ſuch* Particles, and by growing hot with them, do as it were mortifie them, and at laſt they *as preſerve from* being overcome, they carry them forth either by Urine or Sweat. *the Gout.*

Take *of the Powder of Crabs claws compounded two drams, of Ivory, of the Root of Cre- Pills. tick Dittany, of the Root of male Pæony, each one dram; of the Wood of Aloes, of yellow Saunders, each half a dram; make a Powder, let it be taken half a dram or a dram, either by it ſelf, in a ſpoonful of red Poppy Water, drinking after it ſix ſpoonfuls of the ſame, or let it be reduced into a Bolus, or Pills, with Andromach Treacle, or Venice Turpentine what will ſuffice: the Doſe one dram twice a day, drinking after it of the diſtilled Water afterwards deſcribed two or three ounces.*

Or Take *of the ſame Powder ſix drams, of the Conſerves of Gilliflowers, and of Betony, An Electuary. each one ounce and a half; of Diaſcordium one dram, of the Syrup of Poppies what will ſuffice; make an Electuary: the Doſe one dram to two, Evening and Morning.*

In the mean time, while theſe things are doing, beſides, altering Medicines, and allaying, have their turns, for the calling away to ſome other place, the flowing of the Morbific matter into the places diſtemper'd, or for the carrying it forth; ſuch as may allay the ſwelling up of the Blood, and the nervous Juice, and ſtop the Fluxions of the Recrements falling from them; for this end a ſlender diet, and ſpoon meat (if it be convenient) being ordered; let *Emulſions, Juleps*, and *Apozems* made of gentle things, and *Anodynes*, be preſcribed.

As to what belongs to the other intentions of healing, *viz.* the Diſcuſſion of the im- 2. *The Spirits* pacted Mine, and for the allaying the burning or growing hot of the Fibres and the Spi- *ought to be al-* rits; this latter muſt be endeavoured, without which, being performed, the other in- *layed, or qui-* tention will not ſatisfie: for this end therefore it is expedient, to give both external *eted.* Medicines, *viz. Topicks* of a various kind; as alſo internal, *viz. Hypnoticks*.

For that there are an immenſe company of *Topicks*, theſe are only *Anodynes*, which re- 1. *By Topick* ſpect *Remedies.*

spect only the pain by it self, or are such as aim at this together, and the tumor; or they are repelling, or resolving, and discussing: There are various *Formula's* of every one of these, and ways of administrations: But the chief in use are *Fomentations, Pultesses,* and *Plasters*; of these we shall shew the most celebrious; and first of all, *Anodyne* Applications, which please the Fibres with a certain delight. For this use the most common

Pultesses. practice with the vulgar are, *Cataplasms* or Pukesses of Milk and crums of Bread, or of those with a *Muccage,* or jelly of the leaves and of the roots of Mallows, and Marshmallowes, and such like.

Others praise a Pultesse of the fresh dung of a Cow applied warm.

A Fomentation. Take of the *Water of Nightshade,* and of the *Sperm of Frogs,* each *six ounces*; mingle them: Lint being dipt in this, let it be applied warm.

Take of red Lead three ounces, of distilled Vinegar one quart; let them digest for several days; and use this liquor by it self, or else the water drawn off by distillation.

Also a *Water* distilled, made of a *Tincture* of *Verdigriese,* distilled in *Vinegar,* oftentimes allays the pains.

I had from a Gentleman, oftentimes heavily obnoxious to the *Gout,* that he in the most cruel torments of this Disease, had always present ease, from a Fomentation, of the water distilled from the contents in the stomach of an Ox fresh killed.

Outward Narcoticks. For the extream torments of the *Gout,* outward *Narcoticks* ought sometimes to be applied. Take *of the leaves of Henbane,* and of *Hemlock,* each three handfuls; let them be put into boiling water, and as soon as they grow tender let them be taken out: These being bruised, add to them, *of the Powder of Chamomel flowers about two drams, and the yoalk of one Egg*; make a Poultesse.

Or take of the Tincture of Saffron, made in the Spirit of Wine four ounces, of Camphor, of Opium, each one dram; let them digest close shut and warm, till they are dissolved; anoint the pained part with this liquor. There are to be found other innumerable Medicines of this sort in Medical Books, and are every where ordinary, and wont to be prescribed almost by every vulgar person; which also suffices for the fulfilling of the other Intention, to wit, the repercussion of the Humors, when it is seen necessary.

Resolving Topicks consisting chiefly of Saline Particles, even analogic, or correspondent to the Morbific Mine. As to what respects *Resolving* and *Discussing Topicks,* they are not required to be of the same kind, which open only the Pores, and evaporate the *Serum,* and make the Blood circulate, as in an Inflammation, or a white hard swelling; but whose *Saline* Particles, being destinated for the opposing those Salts of the *Goutish* Mine, may either by embracing them carry them forth of doors, or by precipitating them may suppress them from their painful heats. Wherefore in this Disease, when Fomentations or Pultesses of *Chamomel, Mallows, Marsh-mallows, Line* and *Fenegreek* seeds, bring little or no help; yea by loosning the nervous parts, do oftentimes much hurt; the Salt of *Armoniack,* or Sea Salt, or *Nitre,* or of *Vitriol,* quick Lime, and dissolutions of the like, or distilled Liquors, always troublesome to other humors or pains, are wont to give the greatest help.

Forms of these. These kind of Liquors in the *Goutish* Fits, to be applied to the grieved part, are variously prescribed, by *Quercitan, Crollius, Hartman,* and other *Chymists*; and as other famous *Physicians* have often found them by experience good, and approved of them, we may conclude that they are helpful for the aforesaid reason.

There will be no need here to repeat the forms of these, though I could easily set down many other preparations of this sort; yet I shall here give you one or two of them only.

Take of *Sal Tartari,* and *Armoniac* powdered, each *two ounces*; put them into rain or spring water two quarts, and with a linnen cloth dipt in it warm, apply it.

Take of the Spirits of Vitriol not rectified one pint, of Sea Salts calcined and powdered one pound; distill them in a Glass retort in sand; a very pure Spirit of Salt will come forth, which being expulsed from its lodging by a Vitriolick Stagma, leaving the possession, easily ascends: To the dead head pour two pints of the Spirit of Wine, digest it close and warm; adding of Camphor two drams; let it be applied warm to the grieved part with linnen rags.

Take of the Filings of Iron, of the Flowers of Sal Armoniack, each six ounces; mingle them well by pounding them together; let it be distilled in a Glass retort till the Flowers are sublimated; to the Caput Mortuum being pounded, pour the Spirits of Wine, digest it, and keep it for use.

I have

I have heard of some that for the allaying of the pains of the *Gout*, have inclosed the distempered foot in a little Bay, filled with Sea Salt calcined and powdered; from which they have still expected a certain and sudden help.

In the declination of the Fit, for the strengthening the part, and for the shaking off the reliques of the Morbific matter, Plasters are profitably applied; which however are not all convenient to all, but for some more, for others less hot; But the most efficacious to most people are those in which are *Red Lead*, *Ceruse*, and *Soap*, boiled with *Oyl*. Or Take *of the Plaster of Red Lead two parts, of Paracelsus one part, mix them, and spread them upon Leather*. *Plasters in the declination of the Fit.*

2. Internal Remedies for the pains of the *Gout*, that are made use of, are only *Narcoticks*, or such as stupefie, which ought to be administer'd in cruel and long torments. Of these we shall chiefly commend Preparations of *Opium*, with *Salt of Tartar* or its *Tincture*. Further, for this use, the *Laudanum* of *Paracelsus*, or that of *London*, Pills of *Styrax*, and *Cynogloss*, or Dogs Tongue, Syrup *de Mæconio*, or of Poppies, *Treacle Andromach*, and *Diascordium*, are wont to be helpful or give ease. *Opiates.*

The Indication *Preservatory*, or so called, respects the taking away of the foregoing causes of the *Gout*; wherefore, that the fits of pains may more rarely, or less or not at all infest them: For this end, *Evacuating*, *Altering*, and *Corroborating* Remedies, together with an exact dyet, are prescribed to be given out of the Fits. *2. The preservatory Indication, out of the Fit.*

1. *Gouty* people therefore ought constantly to be purged Spring and Fall; and then also it will be expedient to Vomit, if nothing gainsays it; and sometimes afterwards at intervals, to repeat them. Let those who are indued with a more strong stomach and *Præcordia*, take Emetick Minerals prepared out of *Antimony* or *Mercury*. Those who are of a more tender constitution, may take after the eating of slippery meats, Wine of *Squills*, or the Salt of *Vitriol* with Posset drink; and then the stomach being filled with warm water, or simple Posset-drink, or with the leaves of *Carduus* boiled in it, let Vomiting be twice or thrice or oftner provoked. For Purging to be often celebrated also at convenient times, between, the forms of purging Medicines already prescribed are convenient enough. Or Take *of the strings of black Hellebore cleansed one ounce, of Lignum Aloes and of Cloves, each two drams, bruise them, and pour to them of the Spirits of Wine, not rectified, one quart; let them digest warm and close shut, for several days.* The Dose two or three spoonfuls in the morning, twice or thrice in a week; and let Vomiting and Purging be always begun before the *Æquinoxes*, lest perhaps the Fit being first begun should pervert the course of the Medicine. *Usual Purging and Vomiting.*

Letting of Blood, or the opening of the *Hemorrhoidal* Vessels, are sometimes convenient Spring or Fall, in an hot temperament, and for such as are indued with a more sharp Blood. *Cauteries*, made in the Arms, and between the shoulders, are profitable to every one almost obnoxious to this Disease. *Phlebotomy.*

But besides, altering Medicines, *Antidotes* so called by the Ancients, against the *Gout*, are of known use; and in a long time, together with an exact method or Government concerning the six *non-naturals*, often bring great help; in this rank the chief are Medicines indued with a *Volatile Salt*, and *Balsamick Sulphur*, forasmuch as these exalt the fixed Salt, and reduce what is *Acetous*; besides, bitter and astringent things, as these Herbs, *Chamepitys*, *Centaury*, *Germander*, the Roots of *Gentian*, and *Aristolochia*, or *Birthwort*, &c. (as by experience has been approved of in this Disease) for this reason seem to be profitable; because they help the offices of *Concoction*, and *Chylification*, or making of *Chyle*; and restrain the *Saline fixed seculencies* or dregs, that they may not be carried into the Blood. We shall here set down some forms of each of them. *Altering Medicines called Antidotes of the Gout.*

Take *of the Powder of Chamæpitys six drams, of Crabs Eyes two drams, of Venice Turpentine what will suffice, make small Pills, take three or four Morning and Evening, for thirty or forty days, drinking after them of the following distilled water two or three ounces.* *Pills.*

Take *of the leaves of Cypress Tree, of the Ash, and of Misleto of the Apple tree, each six handfuls; of the roots of sweet smelling Avens, Burdock, each one pound, the outer rinds of ten Oranges, and of six Lemons, of Nutmegs, and Mace, each one ounce; let them be all cut and bruised, and pour to them seven pints of new Milk, and of Malaga one pint; let them be distilled according to art, and the whole liquor mixed together.* *A Distilled Water.*

Or *let there be a simple Water prepared of the leaves of Burdock, by pouring it twice or thrice upon fresh leaves.*

Take *of the Powder of the Seeds of Burdock six drams, of Crabs Eyes two drams, of Nutmeg half a dram, of Capivæ Balsom what will suffice to make a Mass, which form into small Pills: let four be taken Evening and Morning for many days.*

Take *of the Tincture of Antimony one ounce; the Dose twenty drops to twenty five, Evening and Morning, with three ounces of the water but now described.* *Tinctures.*

For

Of the Gout.

Powders.

For poor people I was wont to prescribe after this manner. Take *of the Powder of the leaves of Sage half a pound, of Crabs Eyes, and of the Sugar of Crystal, each two ounces; mix them; let it be kept in a Glass, and take one spoonful twice in a day, with a draught of a Decoction of the leaves of Sage, or of the roots of the Burdock.*

Or of the Powder of *Dorncrellius* prescribed to be taken after the same manner.

Take *of the Powder of the leaves of Germander, of Gout Ivy, of the lesser Centaury, of Marjoram, of Sage, of Betony, of the roots of Gentian, and of round Birthwort, each one ounce; of Sugar one pound; mix them and make a Powder.*

Or of the *Powder* of *John Anglicus*, called by himself *Saracenick.*

Take *of the Powder of the leaves of Chamæpitys, one ounce, the bones of a Mans foot burnt two drams, of Liquorish three drams, mix them.*

Medicated Beer.

For ordinary drink, let there be prepared a *Bochet* of *Sarsaparilla*, of *Saunders*, wood of *Rhodium*, shavings of *Ivory*, *Harts-horn*, &c. or let there be prepared *small Ale*, in a Vessel holding about four gallons, instead of *Hops* let their be boiled the leaves of *Germander* and *Chamæpitys*, and after it has work'd, put into it of the leaves of dry *Sage* four handfuls, of *Sassaphras* two ounces, of the roots of sweet smelling *Avens* eight ounces.

A Milk Diet.

Among *Altering* Medicines a *Milk dyet* has not the last place, that the Patient should use for three or four Months, no other food: let him drink Morning and Evening new Milk from the Cow; about noon, and at other times, let him eat white Bread boiled in Barly, or Water-gruel of Oatmeal: I have known some by this kind of dyet to have received notable help; but others, to have received much hurt or to grow worse, by the use of Milk, and the *Gout* being nothing cured, to have contracted great obstructions of the *Viscera*, and a *Cachochimical* disposition or fulness of evil humors. Therefore this method is not rashly to be entered upon, without the counsel of a prudent *Physician*, and by a sedulous observation, whether it be convenient or not.

Drinking of ones own Urine.

Of late it has been a common custom, for people having the *Gout*, to drink every Morning their own Urine; which I know has been beneficial to some. The reason of which help seems to be, because the *Saline Latex* of the *Urine*, passing thorow the Blood, doth carry with it to the Reins, the *Saline fixed* Particles that were before wont to be carried into the joints. Wherefore, this method, when it is helpful to the distemper of the *Gout*, for the most part encreases the *Stone*: which I think sufficiently appears from the following History.

A notable History of the Stone converted into the Gout, and on the contrary of the Gout into the Stone.

A very Learned and Pious Man of this Nation, and also the glory of Learned Men Dr. *H. H.* after he had lived for many years, grievously obnoxious to frequent fits of pains, of Vomiting, and a making of bloody Urine, at length by the constant use of the following Remedies, he lived above seven years almost free from the *Stone*, and without any grievous Fit. The method of Cure which had been taught him by a certain Gentleman, was after this manner, without any *Physick* or medicine, abstaining from Wine and Cyder, he drank for his ordinary drink small Ale, made of Oaten Malt; further, once in a week in the Morning, he took a draught of the same Ale, to about a pint, with the Powder of small old rotten Bones three spoonfuls dissolved in it. By the use of these, within a few months he seemed to be in health, and freed from the *Stone*, but shortly after he began to be sick of the *Gout*, and was infested with most grievous Fits of it, all the time he was free from the *Stone*; and at length upon every light occasion, was become so obnoxious to them, that presently after feeding, if he exercised either his body or mind, by walking or study, he most certainly expected the Fits of his pains. The reason of which was, because the Blood being filled to a plenitude with *Saline* fixed Particles, and the nervous Liquor still with *Acetous*, when being incited, and also poured forth on the fresh nutritious juice, they grew turgid, presently they deposed their superfluities, *viz.* the Morbifick matter of either kind, into the very weak Joints.

This venerable person therefore, being tyred out with so frequent and almost continual torture, by the counsel of a certain Friend, drank every morning of his own Urine, by the use of which, within a month or two, he was less tormented with the *goutish* Fits, but with an evil turn, the Distemper of the Stone began to grow again upon him, for he was from thence troubled with a pain about his Loins, with Vomiting, and a pain in making water, and a little after a total suppression of Urine followed, which being not to be helped by any Remedies, in about a fortnights time this Reverend Gentleman dyed.

The reason of this shewed by Anatomical Observation.

The Carcase being opened, all the *Viscera*, except the Reins appeared most sound and firm, but the right Kidney was almost consumed, a small heap of the *Glandula's* being only left, all the Vessels and the *Ureter* being joined together, and wholly shut up,

so

Of the Colick. 225

so that no Urine at all had passed there of a long time: The left Kidney being large enough, contained within the cavity and its passages, a great heap of Sand or Gravel, and little Stones; besides there was a round hard and whitish stone fallen into the *Ureter*, three inches deep, and there fixed, and had wholly shut out the passage of the water; the *Membrane* of the *Ureter*, where the Stone stuck, was become so thick and callous, and so free from pain, that here it could by no means be moved either upwards or downwards.

It seems in this case, that when the coagulated Particles of the Blood and nervous juice, to wit, the *Saline fixed* and the *Acetous*, meeting together at first in the Reins, did stir up for a while the Distemper of the *Stone*; afterwards, by the use of the abovesaid Powder, the *saline* Particles being still thrust forward into the habit of the Body, and not easily rendred, heaped together the *Goutish* seed plot in the Joints, the Reins being in the mean time free. But at length, when by the drinking of his own Urine, the *saline* Mine was brought back into the Reins, the Disease of the *Gout* was changed into the mortal Disease of the *Stone*.

CHAP. XV.

Of the Colick-Passion.

IT has been mentioned in the former Chapter, by what right we have referred this Disease among the Distempers of the Brain and nervous Stock, to wit, both in respect of the *Symptoms* urging, which are pain, and Convulsive motions, as also from the reason of the cause, by *Charles Piso* placed in the head, and truly not improbably. *Why the Colick is counted among the Distempers of the Brain, and the nervous Stock.*

Concerning the word *Colick*, from the *Intestine* called the *Colon*, we shall not strive, for that it is supposed, though wrongfully, to be chiefly affected in this Disease. The Distemper may be described, That it is an hauling or notable pulling of some parts of the *Abdomen* or the *Belly*; from whence a very acute pain arises, and with it for the most part, a Vomiting, as also Convulsions, and Contractions almost of the whole *Viscera* of the Belly, are wont to be joined. And for that the Navil, and its neighbouring parts, are sometimes as it were with a Perforation, or boring thorow, drawn inwards, and sometimes swell out, with an inflation or blowing up, and as it were with a great leaping forth; the *Intestines*, by an inverse motion of the Fibres, are oftentimes pulled together upwards: wherefore the Belly being extreamly bound together, renders little or nothing; yea although it be often provoked by Clysters, it doth not easily part with its contents: It appears clearly, that the Ventricle, with the *Duodenum*, and the bladder of *Gall*, are in like manner pulled, by Vomiting, and by the casting forth of great plenty of yellow or green *Choler*: Sometimes the *Ureters*, and the bladder of the Urine, are so contracted, that in all the fit, the Urine is wholly suppressed, or but very sparingly rendered: Besides, a *Vertiginous* Distemper of the Head, frequently preceeds, or follows the fits of this Disease: yea, the *Colick* growing worse, and inveterate, oftentimes causes pains in the outward members, and at length ends in the *Palsie*: Therefore, forasmuch as very many parts are wont to labour in this Disease, we shall inquire, which is primarily affected, and by what means the other suffer; then what is the conjunct cause of the Disease, in what place it subsists, and from whence it draws its original. *From whence the denomination. A description of the Disease.*

As to the part primarily or first of all distemper'd, though the Disease being urgent, the whole region of the Belly is wont to be disturbed, yet its primary seat ought to be placed, where the pain chiefly infests, and pertinaciously sticks: But this, by the consent of very many *Physicians*, is said to be some where in the Gut *Colon*. Wherefore *Celsus* saith, *That the Colick is a Distemper of the greater Intestine*; which also reason seems to perswade, something; for whether the *Morbific* Matter is supposed to be heaped up in the Cavities of the Intestines, or to be wholly fixed in their Membranes, certainly there are extant deep little Cells in the folds of the *Colon*, for its receptacles, and thick coats of this *Intestine*, in which the peccant humor may be deeply fastned. But indeed this opinion (to which we cannot easily assent) as also the denomination of the Distemper, seems to have grown in credit in the Schools of the *Physicians*, from this only, because we ordinarily observe, that the *Intestines* enter into pains and torments, being irritated by wind, medicines, *Choler*, and perhaps other humors, contained within their cavities; *The seat of the Disease is not always, or often in the Intestine, or Gut Colon. viz. neither in its Cavity or Coats.*

G g hence,

hence, as it is obvious, may be inferred, that the *Colick* pains do arise from the sharp and provocative contents of the *Intestines*, and especially of the *Colon*. But if it were so, without doubt, those things which loosen the Belly, and draw forth plentifully the wind, and the dregs or *Fæces*, should give certain ease; the contrary of which often happens, to wit, by some more violent, or often Purging, the Disease has grown worse.

Pains commonly taken for Colicks.
Wherefore, that the seat of this Disease, and the nature of it may be truly known, we ought first of all to distinguish here, concerning the torments of the Belly, or pains commonly esteemed for *Colicks*: to wit, these are either meerly occasional, arising from a solitary evident cause, and ordinarily happen without any previous disposition to some men, and especially to those who being of a tender constitution, have very sensible Fibres, and Spirits quickly dissipated; after this manner, disagreeable or unwonted eating or drinking, also medicines, taking of cold, and many other alterations about the six *non-naturals*, oftentimes excite great perturbations, with pains in the *Viscera* of the lower part of the Belly: which kind of Distemper, ought to be esteemed, not the Disease, but only *Symptoms* excited from a manifest cause.

These are meerly accidental or habitual.

These latter are properly the Disease.
But besides, the *Colick* properly so called, happens to some, not only produced by an accidental cause, but falling upon some men predisposed by a peculiar right, depends wholly upon a foregoing cause ripened by degrees. The more grievous fits of this Disease, for the most part, have their periods, and observe the changes of the Air and Year; further, being excited, they do not easily give place to any Remedies, nor quickly pass over; but notwithstanding the use of Fomentations, and though the Belly be taken down very much by *Cysters*, or Purging, there often times continue with great fierceness for many days, and sometimes weeks. The pains in every fit still repeat the same part, and are followed with a concourse, for the most part, of other the like *Symptoms*: But the pains of the *Colick*, though they have not the same seat in all, but sometimes exercise their cruelties under the *Ventricle*, sometimes about the *Navel*, or the *Hypochondria*, and sometimes in the lower part of the Belly, or about the Loins; yet as often as they are repeated in the same sick person they mostly observe the same nest.

The conjunct cause of the Disease are not the Contents of the Intestines.
For the unfolding the *Ætiology* of this Disease, it is not enough to affirm, that the Intestines are pulled, either by their sharp contents, or irritated by the Blood, and other humors poured into them, and breaking the continuity. For as to the former, it is extreamly improbable, that the *Bile*, or *Choler*, or *Phlegm*, or the *Pancreaick* Juice, or any other simple humor, or growing hot or fermenting with others, should be able to excite such fixed, cruel, and long continuing pains: Besides, because the *Intestines* being besmeared with their own dung, cannot be easily pricked by the Contents, though sharp; nor are they wont to be exasperated by them; insomuch that the sharpest stools, which oftentimes fetch off the skin at the Fundament, very little trouble, or not at all, the passages of the Guts; further, these being grievously provoked, whatever is troublesome, contained in their cavity, is easily shaken forth, and either by driving it forward, upwards, or downwards, is quickly thrust forth; as is plainly perceived in the Disease of the *Choler*, and other *Dysentrick* Distempers; nor indeed is there almost any loading of these provoking the Membranes, and stirring up pains, which may not be exterminated or carried forth of doors by one purge or other. Then, secondly, as to what respects the suffusions of the Blood, or *Serum*, within the coats of the *Intestines*, by which an Inflammation or painful Tumors are excited; Indeed we grant, that sometimes it may so come to pass, yea I have known it by ocular inspection; but from thence we have observed, not the *Colick*, but the *Iliack* passion to have been excited. For when I have opened several dying of the *Iliack* passion, I found almost in all, that the cause of the Disease, and of their Death, was an Inflammation or Ulcer of some Intestine; neither is this any wonder, because a *Solution* of the continuity, in a very tender and highly sensible Membrane, doth stir up Convulsions, and painful Corrugations or wrinklings together, and so continual and cruel; that therefore the *Peristaltick* motion of the distempered Intestine, whereby the dung or dregs of the Belly are carried forward toward the *Anum* or Arse-Gut, should be hindred and wholly inverted.

Not the humors impacted in the Membranes.

The nervous Liquor seems most of all to contribute to the cause of this Disease.
Therefore, that we may thorowly inquire out both the Matter and Mine, as also the seats, and the ways of flowing to them, of this Disease of the *Colick*, by some other means; it may deservedly be suspected, that it is the nervous Juice, and its Recrements; and that the rather, because this passion hath so intimate an agreement or consent with the other Distempers of the Brain and the nervous Stock, as we have already shewed. *Charles Piso* hath affirmed, That as most distempers of the whole Body, so also the pains of the *Colick*, are excited by a *Serous* heap or deluge gathered together in the head; and he contends, that the seat of this Disease, is neither in the coats nor cavities of the *Intestines*, but in the *Peritonæum* or inner rim of the Belly, and that

Of the Colick.

that the cause sticks wholly in the Brain, near the original of the Nerves. To wit, he supposes, (which he saith he hath found by *Anatomical* observation) "The serosities *Charles Piso's* "laid up in the hinder region of the Brain, to beset the little heads of the Nerves of *Opinion cited,* "the wandring pair, and so some of the utmost branches and shoots of them inserted in "to the *Peritonæum* or inner rim of the Belly by the Caul, to move into Convulsions; "and from the contraction or drawing together of this, most cruel pains, both in it, "and in the underlying *Viscera*, as it were breaking them to pieces, to be excited. For the proof of this opinion, he brings an example of a certain man dissected, being dead of a most grievous fit of the *Colick*, in whom *the hinder region of the head near the Cerebel, was so much drowned with a clear water, as also the nervous original of the wandring pair, that the marrowy substance appeared very much moistened, like wet Paper,* Sect. 4. Chap. 2

But indeed, though we should grant, that the *Colick* should arise from the humor of *and examined.* the Brain, and from the default of that watering the nervous parts; yet we think that this painful passion is excited, not after that manner as this *Author* has laid down. Because we think neither the seat of this Disease to subsist in the *Peritonæum*, nor its primary cause to be within the head. For as to this, although the *Morbisick* matter being heaped up in the head, near the origine of the Nerves, doth sometimes produce in the parts at a great distance, Numnesses, Cramps, and Convulsive motions, as we have elsewhere shewn, by many instances, with the reasons of the Distemper; yet it is much otherwise in a very cruel pain, such as the *Colick* is wont to be: For as to this being excited, which always proceeds from a breach of the continuity, it is required, that the dolorifick cause or improportionate object, should be fixed in the distemper'd member it self, or at least a certain part or portion of it: Neither is it sufficient to say, that the Convulsion proceeds from a remote cause, and so the pain from the Convulsions: For although pain oftentimes doth pro- *The seat of the* duce Convulsive motions, yet these do not produce pain of themselves, at least great *Morbisick Mat-* and continuing long. Wherefore in the pain of the *Colick*, the matter drawing asun- *ter not in the* der the sensitive Fibres, and pulling them one from another, and so provoking them into *Brain.* painful Corrugations or wrinklings, doth not still stay in the Brain; but descending from thence, thorow the nervous passages, towards the *Intestines*, seems to be heaped up somewhere in their neighbourhood, nigh to the pained parts, and there either growing turgid or swelling up, by reason of their fulness, or growing hot with some other humor, do bring in the fits of this Disease.

We indeed reject the Mine of the *Colick*, from the *Peritonæum*; because this Mem- *The part pri-* brane being very thin, and gifted but with very few and only small Vessels, is neither *marily affected* capable of any great affluxions of Humors, neither can it self, though pulled together, *in the Abdo-* be able to urge the *Viscera* lying under it, into pains, by compressing or drawing them *men, not in the* together. But the Morbifick matter being slid down from the Head, by the Nerves, into *Peritonæum.* the Belly, finds very convenient nests in the *Mesentery*; in which very many and great *ly it seems to be* Nerves have there their noted infoldings and distributions: Wherefore, as this part is *the Mesentery.* very sensible, and very much obnoxious to the flowings in of the humors of the nervous Stock, it may be deservedly affirmed to be the seat of this Disease of the *Colick.*

We have shewn formerly, the causes of some Convulsive motions in the *Abdomen, where the seat of* which are commonly called *Hysterical*, to lye hid in the *Mesenterick* Infoldings; more- *the Distempers* over, in the same places, we did then assert, That the *Colick* pains had sometimes their *called Hysteri-* nests, and confirmed it sufficiently by *Anatomical* observation. But the matter is some- *cal, often lyes* thing diverse, and not the same, that is wont to excite the so different Distempers of *hid.* either, under the same roof. In the Passions called *Hysterical*, we have largely declared in a former Treatise, That the Animal Spirits being burthened with an *Elastick Copula,* are let off, or as it were exploded one from another, and so the containing bodies are unwillingly forced into irregular or preternatural Motions. But in the pains of the *Colick*, the same Spirits, by reason of the matter troublesome to them, and improportionate, being provoked, and so pulled and distracted one from another, do put the sensible Fibres into very troublesome Corrugations, or wrinkling themselves together: By what means this comes to pass in the pains of the *Colick*, also what are the conjunct, and the foregoing causes of this Disease, and the reasons of the *Symptoms*, we shall a little further explain.

Therefore we shall suppose, that for a Seed-plot or Mine of the *Colick* Distemper, *The Colick-mine* some Recrements of the nervous humor being fallen from the Brain, thorow the Nerves, *is affirmed to be* and slid down into the *Mesentery*, and other infoldings of the *Abdomen*, are there heap- *within the ner-* ed up; which if they be thick, and very viscous, so that they cannot be received by the *vous, and other* Lymphaducts or water-carriers, and so sent away, or that they cannot sweat forth by *mesenterick in-* the small shoots of the Vessels into the cavities of the *Intestines*, stagnating in those *Abdomen.* parts, and being by degrees heaped together, do arise at length to a provocative fulness;

fullness; then this matter growing more degenerate by standing, and becoming more infestous, grows turgid occasionally, or of its own accord, or perhaps grows hot or ferments with a *Saline fixed* humor, poured forth thither, from the Blood, torments the shoots of the Nerves, and the nervous Fibres (of which the *Mesentery* hath an infinite number) with very troublesome and painful Corrugations; which kind of Distemper of these, doth not plainly cease, till the hot or Fermentative matter being shaken off, or pressed forth into the cavities of the *Intestines*, is at length overcome.

From which, planted thereabouts, the Colick Symptoms are excited.

Further, forasmuch as from the *Mesentery* and its Infoldings, nervous shoots and Fibres are most thickly put forth into the bottom of the Ventricle, the bladder of the Gall, the *Choledoch* passages, all the *Intestines*, and on every side almost into all the *Viscera* of the whole *Abdomen*; therefore whilst the *Colick* matter grows hot or ferments in its Mines, it there stirs up torments, and oftentimes most cruel pains; and together with them in many other Membranous parts Cramps, and Convulsive or painful Contractions, are every where excited. Hence, by reason of the *Mesentery* being primarily distemper'd, a most sharp pain under the Navil shews it self, like as if a stake were driven thorow it, or a wimble a boring it; then round about almost in the whole *Abdomen* or lower region of the Belly, by reason of the *Intestines* being variously drawn down, or backwards, in diverse places together, wandring pains run about hither and thither; and by reason of the motions of the Fibres being disturbed or inverted, both in these, and also in the urinary Vessels, the Belly is almost always bound up, and sometimes a suppression of the Urine, or a rendring but a very little succeeds: yea also the *Duodenum*, the *Gall*-Bladder, with its passages, and the bottom of the Ventricle, being distemper'd with a *Spasm* or Cramp, and their Fibres drawn upwards, from thence frequent Vomiting, with a copious casting forth of yellow or green Choler, doth infest during the fit.

The yellow or green Bile or Choler, that is cast forth by vomiting, in the Colick-Fits, is not the material cause of this disease.

But some do contend that this *Bile* or Choler (which is sometimes cast forth as green as a Leek) is the material Cause of the Disease; and that abundance of it dropping or distilling forth into the *Viscera*, doth excite the *Colick* pains in the *Intestines*. I say, that this humor about the beginning of the fit, is contained without any offence in the Bladder or bag of the Gall; but afterwards by reason of the Convulsions of the *Viscera*, being from thence pressed forth, and as it were drawn or stroked out into the Stomach, it is carried from the distemper'd Ventricle by Vomit; but there perhaps meeting with some other acid humor, it acquires a greenish colour, yea sometimes a blackish (as we have sometimes found by *Anatomical* observation.) And indeed, it appears clear from this, because those who are of a more cold temperament, and beget little Choler, when they are sick of the *Colick*, cast forth by Vomit little or nothing of the yellow or green *Bile*; and yet they are wont to be vexed with as cruel and sharp pains as others.

Why sore pains of the Loins often come upon the Colick pains.

In the fit of the *Colick*, to the pains of the Belly, most cruel pains, raging about the Loins, in the bottom of the back, are very often joined; which certainly cannot arise from the irritation of any *Intestine*. But it may be easily conceived, that these are excited from the Morbific cause implanted in the *Mesentery*; forasmuch as some most noted Nerves, belonging to the Loins, enter into the greatest nervous infolding of the *Mesentery*; hence not only painful Convulsions are delivered by consent from one part to another; but besides, it is probable, that some Recrements of the Back and Loins, are derived by this passage into the *Mesentery*; and in some measure, for this reason *Scorbutical* people are so very obnoxious to pains of the Belly, and to a Flux.

In what the foregoing cause of this Disease consists.

Thus much concerning the nature and seat of the *Colick*, as also of its conjunct cause, and of the *Symptoms* of the same coming into act: As to what belongs to the foregoing cause, it consists chiefly in these two things, to wit, first of all for that many Recrements are heaped together in the nervous Liquor; and secondly, because they being chiefly received from the Nerves, destinated to the *Viscera* of the lower Belly, and brought into the *Mesentery*, constitute the Morbid Mines there: 1. The former of these happens for the most part, from the fault and vice of the Brain; to wit, because this admits together with the nervous liquor, *Heterogeneous* Particles, and infestous to the Animal Regiment within its borders; besides also, for that it doth not send away presently these and other ordinary Recrements by convenient sinks: Wherefore, the incongruous matter, when it cannot be otherways carried from the Brain, it most easily rushes into the most open Nerves of the wandring pair. And for this Reason it is, that Women from every inordination of the Brain, frequently contract the disposition called *Hysterical*; to wit, because the Recrements of the nervous Liquor, whether they are *Spasmodick* or Convulsive, and *Elastick* or letting off, or painful, or provocative only, being more apt to be deposed into the wandring pair, so ordinarily excite Convulsive *Symptoms*, like to the *Colick*. 2. Because this matter running into the pair of the wandring Nerves, is laid up in the *Mesentery*, or in other Infoldings within the *Abdomen*; the reason is, that in these

1. The nervous Liquor is in fault, because the Morbifick Matter is gathered together in it.

2. The nerves of the wandring pair, and their mesenterick Infoldings, because they receive into themselves this matter.

these nervous Infoldings, many and large Nerves of the same conjugation are at last terminated: wherefore, if the Recrements of the nervous humor, subsiding here as it were upon its bottom, neither can be drawn back by any of the Vessels, nor pass into the cavities of the Intestines, there is a necessity that it must erect in this part its morbid nests.

The evident causes are of a double kind, to wit, first, those that do injury to the Brain and nervous stock, by causing a greater provision of the Morbific matter: or, secondly, those which by agitating or shaking the Blood and humors, stir up the Mines gathered together, and before quiet, and provoke them into painful heats or fermentings. It would be tedious here to examine the manifold, and diverse occasions, by which the *Colick* pains are brought upon those predisposed; for these often are caused by great inordinations in the six *non naturals*, and the mutations of the Air, and the Year; and moreover (by what help should be expected) by the untimely administring Medicines themselves. *The evident causes of this Disease.*

From what has been said, the differences of this Disease may be easily known. For, first, by means of the causes, we have shewn the *Colick* to be either accidental, which is caused by reason of the *Intestines* being provoked by sharp contents, such as we but now described it. Secondly, By reason of the place affected, the *Colick* is sometimes superior, sometimes inferior, sometimes *lateral* or of the side, as the Morbific matter is fixed, either sometimes in this part, sometimes in that part of the *Mesentery*, or in other infoldings of the *Abdomen*. Thirdly, By reason of the sickly condition and temperament of the sick, it is called a *Bilous*, or *Cholerick*, a *Phlegmatick*, or a *Melancholick Colick*; also either simple, or *Scorbutick*; nor that these imaginary humors excite of themselves the *Colick*, but according to the dispositions of the Body distemper'd, various *Symptoms* are made, or caused to vary. *The differences of this Disease.*

As to its *Prognostick*, it is commonly known, that the accidental *Colick*, to wit, excited from a solitary evident cause, is most often safe, and with an easie matter cured; but the habitual, as to its disposition, is very difficult to be rooted out, so that the fits may no more return; and its fits sometimes are pertinacious, notwithstanding Remedies, and sometimes continue many days, yea weeks, and months. *Its Prognostick.*

2. The *Colick* disposition frequently succeeds long intermitting Feavours, and continual, being evilly handled; for that the nervous Liquor being highly vitiated, gathers together many Recrements, which are deeply deposited into the Infoldings of the *Abdomen*, as it were the more open receptacles. Further, for this reason, an *Epidemical* Feavour rages some years, to which the *Colick* is joined, as its *Pathognomonick* or peculiar *Symptom*: hence in like manner, a long and grievous *Scurvy* causes also the *Colick*, because it perverts the nervous liquor.

3. After the *Colick* pains have raged for some time in the Belly, they fall oftentimes into the Loins, and then the Disease increasing or growng worse, they enter upon the members, and the muscles almost all in the whole Body, and at length oftentimes end in the *Palsie*; which certainly is a manifest sign, that the Morbific matter is not carried by the Arteries, but by the Nerves; and that its subject or seat, is not the cavities or the coats of the *Intestines*, but the nervous Infoldings of the *Mesentery*: For because the *Lumbary* pains, or those of the side, do come upon the torments of the Belly, besides that the Nerves of either place communicate, the cause is further, for that the Morbific matter being much increased in the Head, slides down, not only into the wandring pair, but also into the *Spinal* Marrow; and entring into it, and setling in its bottom, causes pains to arise in the Loins, and afterwards in many other Nerves, which proceed from the *Spine* or Back bone, and in other Members and Muscles distemper'd; lastly, it brings in the *Palsie* by the passages of the Nerves being stuffed by the Morbific Matter heaped up to a plentitude in them.

4. The more cruel *Colick*, and very much raging, whose cause is an Inflammation, or an Imposthum of some *Intestine*, for the most part induces the mortal *Iliack* Passion.

The *Curatory* method in the *Colick*, as in most intermitting Diseases, suggests three primary *Indications*: The first of which *Curatory*, to be administer'd in the fit, respects the allaying of the pains, and for the sooner and more easie taking away the coming of the Disease. Secondly, *Preservatory*, which shews the taking away the cause of the Disease without the fit, that the fits may not be often repeated, or more grievously infest. Thirdly, *Vital*, which supplies Remedies for the preserving of strength in the torments, and most cruel Cruciations, and for the cherishing of the Spirits. Concerning these we shall speak a little more fully in order. *The Cure.*

1. We almost only respect the *Curatory Indication* in the accidental *Colick*; for the evident cause, which is an irritation of the *Intestines* by sharp contents, being removed, the pains for the most part cease of their own accord, nor do they return without the *1. The first Indication Curatory.*

like

like occasion. Wherefore, for the quick curing of this Disease, the practice is well enough known to every common person, among the vulgar, to wit, presently to administer softning *Clysters*, *Topick Anodynes*, and *Narcoticks*; to which, if a Feavour be joined or feared, letting of blood is often used with success. We shall set down forms of these, and the order of using them in the Cure of the habitual *Colick*.

What the chief Medical intentions are in the Fit.

Therefore, for the healing of this Distemper, in the fit, there are two chief *Intentions*; to wit, both to take away the painful breach or solution of the unity, and to allay the burning or growing hot of the Fibres, and the Spirits in them. For the former, you must endeavour, both that the matter impacted in one or more Mines, may be shaken off or subdued; and also, that a flowing in of new matter may be hindred. The second *Intention*, which ought chiefly and continually to be insisted upon, is performed by *Anodynes* chiefly, and *Narcoticks*: After what manner, and by what Remedies, every one of these are methodically to be done, we shall now shew you.

For the most part Clysters are to be begun with,

Most often, the Cure of the pain of the *Colick*, and that rightly, is begun with a *Clyster*. Let this at first be gentle, and only emollient, by which the Corrugations or the wrinklings of the Fibres may be allayed, and the burning Spirits flattered or pleased. For this end, warm Milk with Sugar, or *Molossus*, or Syrup of Violets, is convenient; as also Emollient Decoctions of Mallows, Marsh mallows, Mercury, with the Flowers of Melilot, and Elder, with the Oyl of Almonds, or of Olives; also a Decoction of a Sheeps-head, or Calves-feet: sometimes a *Clyster* of mere Oyl of Olives, or of Linseed Oyl, is wont to help before any others.

Which are at first to be gentle;

afterwards more sharp Clysters.

But if the more gentle *Clysters* do not loosen the Belly, nor are easily ejected, there must be given such as will more provoke, and press, or as it were stroke forth the humors, by the little mouths of the Arteries: For which end, let there be prepared Carminative Decoctions, or such as expel wind, or bitter Decoctions; in which are dissolved *Electuary Diacatholicon*, *Diaphœnicon*, or of *Laurel berries*, or *Species Hiera*: Also to these Liquors it is usual to add the Infusion of *Crocus Metallorum* three or four ounces, or of the *Emollient* Decoction one pint: add of *Venice Treacle* dissolved with the yolk of an Egg one ounce or an ounce and a half; or Take *of sound Urine one pint, of Venice Turpentine dissolved one ounce and a half, of Molossus one ounce*, mix them, and make a Clyster. I have known this oftentimes to bring great help; the reason of which seems to be, for that the Balsamick Particles of the *Turpentine* comfort the *Intestines*; and besides, being received by the Blood in the Veins, and with it circulated thorow the whole Body, moves the Urine, so that by such a *Clyster*, plenty of water follows, and always is rendred with a smell like Violets. Perhaps also, the Particles of the *Turpentine* being every where diffused, either move the stagnating Morbifick matter, or incline the acetous, or otherways degenerate, to a better disposition.

Fomentations.

Whilst the *Intestines* are thus washed with *Clysters*, and are cherished within, Fomentations are likewise to be applied to the outer parts of the Belly. Take *of the leaves of both the Mallows, of Mercury, of Pellitory, each four handfuls; of the Flowers of Elder, Chamomil, and Melilot, each two handfuls: the head of a Sheep cut in pieces*. Let them be boiled in as much Spring-water as will suffice; strain it, and use it for a Fomentation, with hot linnen stuphes dipt in it, and wrung forth, and shifting them apply them by turns. Repeating them as often as the more strong pains do come upon them: In the intervals, *Pultesses* or *Oyntments* may be administer'd.

Pultesses.

Make *a Pultess of bruised Herbs, adding to it of oaten meal what will suffice; which may be laid to the belly, covering it with little square bags made for that purpose. Let one of these at a time be made hot in a pan set over hot coals, with the Oyl of Earth-worms, or of Frogs*; lay them on warm, shifting them as soon at one grows cold.

An Oyntment.

Or Take *of the Oyl of Earth-worms or of Frogs what will suffice; and anoint the pained part, after the Fomentation, and lay upon it a thin sheet of fine brown paper dipt in it*.

The Caul of a Lamb, or the Lungs, or the Inwards of any other Beast, being laid warm to the Belly, and so shifted, sometimes wonderfully eases the pain.

Cold Fomentations.

I have observed in some Constitutions and temperaments, that *Fomentations* or Bathings made of hot things, and applied hot, have rather made the pains worse than eased them: wherefore in these cases, it will seem good to prescribe Fomentations of the solutions of *Nitre*, or of *Sal Armoniack*, or other *Chymical* Liquors, as in the pains of the Gout, and sometimes (as *Septalius* says) of pure cold water.

But if the torments of the Belly do not remit by the use of these, *Hypnoticks* must be used; which being given in a just Dose, oftentimes give great truces: In the mean time, that the tired Spirits may be refreshed, and strength preserved, there must be yet instituted a farther provision against the Disease.

Take

Take of liquid *Laudanum Tartarisated*, from sixteen drops to twenty, let it be given going *Opiates.* to sleep, in a spoonful of the water of Chamomil flowers, drinking after it six spoonfuls of the same water: Let it be repeated every other, or every third night, if the pains be very great. In a more hot Constitution, Take *of the water of Chamomil flowers three ounces, of the Syrup of Poppies half an ounce, of Aqua mirabilis two drams; make a draught, to be taken at the hour of Sleep.*

In the mean time, whilst these things are doing, for the allaying the pains, evacu- *Evacuating* ating Remedies have their turns, for the discussing, or at least for the loosning the mat- *Medicines.* ter impacted in the morbid nests; to wit, that both the *Colick* Mine may be wholly extirpated; and also that the supplements or its cherishment be cut off, that they may not more increase. For these ends a *Vomit* (where it is convenient) and a gentle purg- *Vomiting Me-* ing, ought to be ordered; and also in an hot temperament, where there is a Feavour, *dicines.* or where it is feared, letting of Blood.

Take *of the Sulphur of Antimony, from five grains to seven or eight, of the Conserves of Borrage one Dram*; let it be given in the Morning with government. In this case may be given, according to the judgment of the *Physician* present, either an Infusion of *Crocus Metallorum*, or of *Mercurius Vitæ*: The *Emetick Tartar* of *Mynsicht*, the expression of the leaves of *Asarum*: and in more tender Constitutions, Salt of *Vitriol*, and Wine and *Oxymel* of *Squills*.

Purges must be given only in a small Dose, and such as are choice, lest they move a *Purges.* nauseousness in the stomach of the sick.

Take *of the Resine of Jalap, of Scammony, each five grains, of the Cream of Tartar one scruple, of Cinnamon powdered four grains; make a Powder, or let it be reduced into Pills, or into a Bolus, with the Conserves of the Flowers of Borrage, or Damask Roses.*
Take *of Scammony sulphurated half a scruple, of the Cream of Tartar fifteen grains, of Diaphoretick Antimony one scruple; make a Powder, and let it be given after the same manner.*

If there be not a Feavour, a Dose of Stomach *Pills cum Gummi* may be given, or of *Amber* by it self, or with the *Resine* of *Jalap*.

Take *of Pill. Rudii twenty five Grains, or half a dram, of Laudanum one grain; make four Pills,* let them be taken at the hour of rest: These at first cause sleep, and Purge in the morning. Or, Take *of Calomelanos one scruple, of the Resine of Jalap six grains, of* *Salivation.* *Scammony four grains, of Ammoniacum what will suffice; make four Pills to be taken go- ing to rest.*

In a long and tedious *Colick*, when all other Remedies help little or nothing, I have often known this Medicine, being once or twice given, to have moved *Salivation*, with the greatest ease to the sick. For when the morbifick matter, being heaped together, and thorowly impacted in the nervous Infoldings, and other places about the *Abdomen*, could not be moved by any other Medicines; the *Mercurial* Particles every way unfold- ing themselves, easily dissolve it, and divide it into small bits, and drive it up and down hither and thither, and at length wholly dissipate it. Wherefore in a long and pertinacious *Colick*, a gentle *Salivation* sometimes may be very happily administer'd.

Baths, and *Sweating* Medicines, are ordinarily wont to be prescribed in the pains of *Baths.* the *Colick*; but as to our observation, very rarely with success: For that these, by sha- king the Blood and nervous humor, cause them to lay up still more matter into the *Colick* Mine, yea and that matter there deposited, to grow more hot and raging, and very rare- ly wholly shake it off.

Diureticks are wont much more profitably to be given, by which when the Blood is *Diureticks.* poured forth, and its serosities plentifully precipitated, the nourishment of the Disease is cut off, and the bloody Mass being emptied, receives part of the Morbifick matter, so that its reliques are more easily shaken off. For this end,

Take *of the best Spirit of Tartar rectified half an ounce; let half a dram be given twice or thrice in a day, in a spoonful or two of the following Julep, drinking after it five spoonfuls of the same.*
Take *of the Water of the leaves of Burdock, or of Aron, or of Arsmart, one pint; of the Water of the flowers of Elder and of Chamomil, each four ounces; of the compound water of Gentian, of the compound Water of Raddishes, each two ounces, of Sugar six drams; mix them together.*

After

After the same manner as the *Spirit* of *Tartar*, may be given in a just Dose, sometimes the *Tincture* of the *Salt* of *Tartar*, sometimes the simple mixture, or the Spirit of *Sal Armoniack* succinated, or impregnated with *Amber*.

Take of *Millepedes* prepared two drams, of the flowers of Sal Armoniack Tartarized one dram, of the Oyl of Nutmegs half a scruple, of Turpentine what will suffice; make a Mass, and let it be made into Pills; take three or four once or twice in a day, drinking after it a Dose of the Julep, or of the following distilled water five or six spoonfuls.

Take of fresh Millepedes or Hog-Lice cleansed one pint and a half, the outer rind of six Oranges, and of four Lemons, six Nutmegs; let them be cut small, and add to them one pound of the crumbs of stale white Bread: all being bruised together and well mixed, pour to them four pints of new Milk, and of Sack one quart; let them be distilled according to art, and the whole liquor mixed together; you may sweeten it with Sugar, or the Syrup of Violets as you please.

Mineral Purging Waters. In a long and pertinacious *Colick*, to those who are of a more cold temperament and *Viscera*, Purging *Spaw* Waters, or Whey with the Syrup of Violets, are wont to be given oftentimes with great help; for both liquors, where they are agreeable, being plentifully drunk, refrigerate the stomach and the hot Intestines, and presently loosen and help them in their painful Cramps and wrinklings, or from the Convulsive winds or blasts that extend them; besides, they chiefly help (as I suppose) for that they tame and subdue the *Saline* Particles of another nature, insinuating themselves into the Morbific Mine, and other *Saline* and irritative Particles inhabiting it, and oftentimes carry them forth by Purging.

In this Disease, as all things are not convenient for all men, yea neither the same thing always for the same person, there is dayly need of the careful observation of a prudent *Physician*, that by the co-indications from things taken, that hurt or help, a right method of healing may be instituted, and varied as occasion serves.

2. The Vital Indication suggests Remedies. 2. The *Vital Indication* ought to be joyned to the *Curatory*, and that between whiles. For when the sick, being afflicted with torture, watching, Vomiting, and abstinence almost continual, often fall into languishment, and sometimes in danger of their lives; Remedies which sustein strength, refresh the Spirits, and procure some truces against the fierceness of the Disease, to wit, *Cardiacks* or *Cordials*, and *Hypnoticks* or such as cause rest, have here their turns.

Cardiack. Take of the Water of the flowers of Chamomil, and of Elder, each four ounces; of Barlyed Cinnamon, and of the whole Citron, each two ounces; of Pearl powdered one dram, of Sugar three drams; make a Julep, take of it five or six spoonfuls.

Take of the Powder of *Pearl*, and of *Crabs Eyes*, each one dram; let it be divided into four parts; let one part be given twice or thrice in a day, with the Julep, or with a Decoction of the roots of Contrayerva.

Take of the Conserve of *Clove-Gilliflowers* one ounce, of the Confection de Hyacintho, of Alchermes, each two drams, of Pearl powdered half a dram, of the Syrup of the juice of Citrons what will suffice; make a Confection, give of it the quantity of a Nutmeg, three or four times in a day with the Julep.

In less hot Constitutions, *Spirits* of *Harts-horn*, of *Sut*, of *Sal Armoniack* impregnated with *Amber*, also the *Tincture* of *Antimony*, or of *Coral*, do oftentimes give notable help.

Hypnoticks. *Opiates* are of necessary use in the Disease of the *Colick*, without which, the sick cannot live, nor the *Physicians*, nor those who attend them be at quiet, or have any leasure time. Take of the water of Cowslip flowers three ounces, of the Syrup of Poppies half an ounce, of Aqua Mirabilis two drams; mix them and make a draught to be given going to sleep.

If the pains be very strong, and yield to no such Remedy, prepared *Opium* and its compositions ought to be given. The *Laudanum* of *Paracelsus*, or the *London Laudanum*, Pills of *Styrax*, or of *Hounds tongue* are convenient; a Solution of *Tartarisated Opium* from sixteen to twenty grains is much used by me. Which Medicine indeed I have given with very good success, to some, that for a long time have been miserably vexed with this Disease, sometimes a great while every night or every other night.

3 The Preservatory Indication, by which art indicated. 3. The *Preservatory Indication* hath only place in the intervals of the fits, and endeavours the taking away the present foregoing cause of the Disease, and hindring it for the future, so that the fits of the pains may seldom or never afterwards return: For which end, the Blood and the nervous liquor ought to be purified, lest they should beget the morbific matter, and conserved in its due temper, and the Brain and the nervous Infoldings

Of the Colick. 233

foldings of the *Abdomen* corroborated, left they should too readily receive it. For these ends, a strict dyet being ordered, let them enter into a course of *Physick* Spring and Fall; such as we prescribed for the prevention of the *Gout*.

Vomiting in this case is never to be omitted, if it be agreeable, to wit, by which the *Vomiting*. Emunctories of the *Viscera* being emptied, the Recrements of the Blood, and the nervous Liquor, which otherwise would augment the morbific matter, may be received more plentifully; besides the nervous Infoldings, and all the parts are so shaken, that nothing of that which is about to go into the Mine of the Disease, is suffered to stagnate or to be heaped up there.

Let Purging for three or four times, with due intervals, and also in a hot Constitution, *Purging,* *Phlebotomy* be celebrated; moreover, let altering Remedies, and especially *Chalybeats*, or such as are made out of Steel, when they do not Purge, be daily taken at medical hours.

But before all other Remedies whatsoever, the drinking of Mineral Waters, such as *Altering Reme-* come from Iron, for a month, in the Summer time, is wont to give the greatest help: *dies.* But when these are drunk, you must take heed, that they be rendred well and quickly by Urine or Stool, lest if they should chance to stay long in the body, by running into the Head or Feet, (as they often do) they should cause a *Vertigo* or the *Gout*.

Take *of our Tincture of Steel one ounce, and let fifteen to twenty drops be taken twice in a day in seven spoonfuls of the following Julep.*
Take *of the Waters of the leaves of Aron, and of Burdock, each half a pound; of the Magisterial of Earth Worms, of Gentian compound, of Paeony compound, each two ounces; of Sugar half an ounce; mix them.*

After the same manner, here deservedly have place the Tincture of *Antimony*, and of *Amber*, yea and many other altering Remedies above prescribed for the Distempers of the Head, may also be used for the preservation from the *Colick*, whose foregoing cause proceeds from the Brain.

As to *Charles Piso*'s Observation, by which he endeavours to prove, that the cause of *The Objection of* the pain of the *Colick* remains wholly in the Brain, because he had found a *Serous* de- *Charles Piso* luge in the Head of a certain person dead of that Disease: I say, that this *Serum* being *solved.* heaped up in the head, was the remote and antecedent cause of this Disease, and not the conjunct cause. But indeed it is probable, that from this first spring a certain portion of this superfluous and sharp Serum did descend, by the nervous passage, into the nervous Infoldings of the *Abdomen*, and there constitute the Mines of the *Colick* Distemper. Further, although the Morbific matter there sliden down, because of the tenuity of the parts, and the smallness of the nests, can rarely be seen with the eyes, yet I have plainly seen and handled such a Mine of this Disease become inveterate and very cruel, not long since, in the *Mesentery*, opening the dead body of a certain Gentlewoman, of whom I have elsewhere made mention.

Being sometimes since consulted with, concerning the curing of a Reverend old Man, *The first History.* grievously obnoxious for many years to the Disease of the Colick; I administer'd to him the same method of healing, and the Remedies I but now described; by the use of which, he found himself much better after a month or two, and within half a year he seem'd to be perfectly well, so that he lived afterwards wholly freed from any fits of the pains: But the *Colick* disposition had not long ceased, and he had omitted the usual course of Medicine, but he suffer'd about his throat a resolution or loosning in the Muscles serving for swallowing, which troubled him oftentimes, so that he was in danger to be choaked by Food, and chiefly by liquid things sticking in that place. Against this evil receiving help by *Antiparalytick* Remedies, he continued from thence six or seven years in moderate health; at last, being taken, the first time in the midst of a journey with an *Apoplexy*, he dyed. It is obvious enough in this case, that the Recre- *The Reason of it.* ments of the nervous liquor, that were wont to be deposed about the nervous Infoldings of the *Abdomen*, did at first stir up the Distemper of the *Colick*; then the same being shut forth from that part, getting another nest for themselves about the *Ganglioform* nervous Infoldings of the Throat, brought in the resolution or short Palsie of the *Oesophagus*; and lastly, by reason of the same matter restagnating in too great a plenty in the middle part of the Brain, that deadly senslesness followed.

A certain cunning and crafty little Lawyer, about fifty years of Age, was wont to *The second Hi-* be troubled for many years with a periodical Headach, and with a stupor or numness *story.* of his Senses, and a great weight of his head; about the middle of Summer labouring very much with the aforesaid Distempers, he perceived a sudden ease from the applying of Topical Remedies; but a little after, he was taken with a very cruel *Colick*, then
H h being

being the first time; whose fit fell upon him with so much cruelty, that his strength suddenly failing, he fell into frequent swooning fits, with a cold sweat, which fit notwithstanding by leasure vanished within twenty four hours, without any breaking of wind, or going to Stool. But after that, he suffer'd frequent fits, and became obnoxious to the Disease; all which (as I was carefully informed) for the most part were usher'd in with a pain of the Head, with a *Vertigo*, and amazedness, or stupidity, and from hence he was wont to presage the pains of the *Colick* would very suddenly follow. In a certain fit, which lasted for twelve days with great cruelty, the sick person himself observed, and told me, that whilst the distemper troubled him in his Belly, he felt no trouble in his head, but the *Colick* pains remitting, presently the *Vertigo* returned, with the

The Reason of it. Headach: from which reciprocal translation of these *Symptoms*, from the Head into the Belly, and so on the contrary from the Belly to the Head, we may lawfully argue, that the same Morbific matter, flowing in the nervous Passages, falling down sometimes below, brought in the *Colick* Passion, and sometimes above; and restagnating, caused those distempers of the Head. Hither may be referred, what *Charles Piso* hath accurately observed concerning himself, being wont to be affected with *Cepha'ick* distempers, and the *Colick* pains by turns, and with a mutual dependency, *Sect.* 4. *C.* 2. *p.* 355.

The third History. Not long since, a certain studious young Gentleman, and living a sedentary life, began to complain of a great stupidity of his senses, and a dulness, as also of a great weight of his Head, and almost continual sleepiness; further, his Ventricle or Stomach was become so slothful and stupid, that he wanted all manner of Appetite, whilst a Cure was instituted against this evil disposition, by Remedies which roused up the Spirits, and shook off their burthens, this Gentleman fell into a most cruel *Colick* Passion (which he was never obnoxious to before) from which a most cruel pain, like the boreing of an Auger, possessed the middle of the *Abdomen*, his Navil being drawn inwards, and notwithstanding the daily use of all kind of Remedies, it continued for three weeks, with great cruelty; that in the time he could take no rest, but what he received from *Narcoticks,*

The Reason of it shew'd. nor could he receive any ease from his pains, unless by an hot fomentation. Certainly in this case it is plain enough to every one, that the impurities of the nervous liquor being gathered to a certain fullness, was the immediate or conjunct cause of the whole sickness; which matter subsisting first in the Head, brought in the notable stupidity of the Brain and the oppression of the Animal Function; then being fallen down, by the passage of the Nerves, into the nervous Infoldings of the *Abdomen*, caused that cruel and daily *Colick*.

FINIS.

A TABLE.

A.

Affections, how wont to be iterated, and how allayed or obliterated, 49. they are more than eleven, 54. the two primary affections or gestures of the Soul, are pleasure and grief 48

Altering Medicines are of the greatest moment, in the cure of melancholy Diseases, and not purging Medicines as the Antients thought 196

Anatomy of an Oyster, 9. of a Lobster 11

Anger, its character, 54. 'tis of kin to boldness ibid.

Animals reduced into classes, 7. as Fire and Light are chiefly energetical in mechanical things, so in Animals. In perfect ones there ought to be many senses 56

Animal spirits, what they are, 23. to what compared, ibid. they abound in an objective, and an active virtue, 24. they are the efficient cause of sense and motion, 56. a most swift communication of them implanted within all the parts, ibid. an opposite tendency of them effect both sense and motion, ibid. they pass through the sensible species; and not the effluvia of the object, penetrate even to the head, 59. they actuate the Rainbow of the Eye very much, 85. they are the immediate subject of sleep, 87. and the immediate subject of the Vertigo, 147. their distemper being after a diverse manner, as it is the cause of the phrensy, so it is of Melancholy, Madness and Stupidity, 188. from what disposition of them the primary Phænomena of a melancholick Delirium proceed, ibid. as they are compared to light, they are call'd opacous or full of darkness, 189. these kind of spirits in melancholy compar'd to those in Chymical Liquors, ibid. they are not like the spirit of Blood as they should be, nor like the spirit of Wine, for such is rather in the Phrensy, ibid. they are like acid spirits distill'd out of Salt, Vinegar, Box, and such like, ibid. Stygian Waters are like the nature of the Animal Spirits in madness, ibid. three chief affections of acetous Chymical Liquors, which agree with them in Melancholy; first the effluvias falling away from these Liquors are perpetually in motion; in like manner also the Spirits in the Phantasy of a Melancholick Person; thence the effluvias from acetous Chymical Liquors do not proceed far; in like manner the imagination of a Melancholick Person, though always imployed, comprehends only a few things, and therefore every thing is conceived with a greater Image than it should be: Lastly, effluvias from acetous Liquors do not evaporate so much from open Pores as they make new; and in like manner, whilst the Animal Spirits form new tracts in the Brain, produce unwonted and incongruous notions, 190, 191. after they have for some time been vitiated in melancholy, the conformation of the Brain is also hurt, 191. how they acquire a disposition like to Stygian Water, 202. they are the subject of Madness 201

Antiscorbutick Medicines good for pains in the head 116

Apoplexy, its seat, 153. a description of the disease, ibid. its subject, ibid. the spontaneous functions only deficient in it, ibid. the opinions of others concerning this disease, ibid. the theory of this disease is best shown by Webster, 154. a reason added by the Author, ibid. a twofold Apoplexy, 155. The Theory of the former delivered, ibid. this disease either accidental or habitual, ibid. the cause of the former, 156. an extinction of the Spirits comes from opiates or immoderate drinking of hot Waters, ibid. the formal reason of the habitual Apoplexy, ibid. what its conjunct cause is, 157. it consists in the Pores of the Callous Body, being suddenly stopp'd, and the spirits being driven away by the contact of malignant matter, ibid. what the nature, or disposition of the morbifick matter, ibid. the procatartick cause of the habitual Apoplexy, ibid. the differences of this disease, 158. its prognosticks, ibid. the curatory method, ibid. what is to be done in the fit, and in what position the sick ought to be kept, ibid. Phlebotomy and other administrations noted, as Vomiting-medicines, Comforters, Cupping-glasses, hot or glowing Iron, 159. the preservatory method, ibid. purging and bleeding Spring and Fall, ibid. Cephalick remedies, ibid. Spirits and Tinctures, Lozenges, Tea, Coffee, and Chocalet prepared,

pared, how to be made and taken, 160 *a medical Ale*, ibid. *Examples and Histories of Apoplectical Persons*, ibid. *an Anatomical observation* 161
Appetite, *it stirs up local motion*, 36. *the Appetite, Imagination and Phantasy in the callous Body of the Brain* 25
Approach *of the sensible object is made either by contact or effluvias sent forth, or by reflected or repercussed particles of the Air, Breath or Light* 56
Arguments *and Reasons of very many Authors, perswade that the Soul of Brutes is not only Corporeal but Fiery* 5
Artery *cutting, what it may profit in the head-ach* 120, 121
Authors *for two distinct Souls in man* 40

B.

Baths, *when their use is hurtful to the Palsy* 173
Bewailing, *wherefore oftentimes joined with weeping* 80
Blasting, *or withering of Trees like the Palsy* 164
Blood *animated, but hardly sensible*, 55. *its disorders allayed by sleep*, 92. *it performs its offices (which are the generation of the Animal Spirits, and nourishing the parts) better in sleep*, ibid. *how it excites the head ach*, 108. *the Blood and its contents are sometimes the means of the conjunct, sometimes of the evident cause in head-achs*, 109. *for what causes it is wont to be moved and bring hurt to the distempered head*, ibid. *it delivers to the head the morbifick matter received from any other part*, 110. *its inordinations, how they may be taken away and prevented*, 114. *its exclusion from the Brain does not easily happen, because all the Arteries communicate one with another, and some of them supply the defects of others*, 154. *its total exclusion from the Brain sometimes happening, causes a terrible Syncope*, 155. *which depends oftnest on the motion of the heart being hindred, and so either by reason of the Cardiack Nerves being bound together, or by reason of the Spirits in the Cerebel being hindred from their flowing into the Nerves*, ibid. *the original of madness either from the Blood, or the Spirits themselves* 203
Bloody *Brutes, why some more hot, some more cold* 13
Bloodless *Creatures, whether they have Fiery Souls* ibid.
Brain *and Cerebel*, 2. *Roots of the sensitive Soul*, 23. *a twofold action in the Brain and its Appendix, of begetting and dispensation, and of Exercise and Government*, 24. *the reason and manner of the former*, ibid. *an exact anatomy of the Brain through its corticated or shelly part*, 25. *the Brain and Præcordia the two Roots of the Soul*, 48. *vices of the Brain noted*, 148. *its distempers, wherein the reason is hurt, as well as the other Animal functions*, 179. *what its indisposition is to the Phrensy*, 183. *the Procatartick cause of the Phrensy partly in the Brain*, 184. *Melancholy a distemper of it and the Heart*, 188. *its conformation is hurt after the Animal Spirits being for some time vitiated in melancholy Diseases*, 191. *the Brain labours in stupidity as to its magnitude and figure*, 209. *as to its substance or texture*, 210. *and in its evil conformation as to its pores and passages* ibid.
Bridges *passing over them, looking down from on high places, and drunkenness, how they cause a turning round of the head* 146
Brutes, *their various kinds with their Souls described*, 7. *all their Souls after the manner of Fire want a twofold Food, viz. a Sulphurous and Nitrous*, 6. *the more perfect Brutes are indued with knowledge, either inbred or acquired*, 34. *what natural instinct brings to them*, ibid. *some examples and instances of it*, ibid. *Brutes in some things are taught by the impressions of sensible things*, 35. *the direct sensible Species creates in them the Phantasy and memory*, ibid. *the reflected the Appetite*, 36. *by example, imitation and institution also*, 37. *how far 'tis they are able to know*, ibid. *their Syllogisms*, 38. *their raciocination what, and how vile* 39
A Burning-Glass *placed before a dark Chamber declares how light is made* 77

C.

Caros, *how it differs from the Lethargy and Apoplexy*, 136. *its seat a little deeper in the Brain than that of the Lethargy*, ibid. *its conjunct cause*, ibid. *'tis either a primary Disease, or comes upon other distempers*, ibid. *its prognosticks*, 137. *its cure the same with the Lethargy and Apoplexy*, ibid. *its Histories* ibid.
Cartesius *and others, their opinions concerning the Souls of Brutes* 3
Coma *waking its description*, 141. *its causes shown*, ibid. *more often a Symptom than a Disease*, ibid. *V.* Caros
Colick, *whence its denomination*, 225. *why counted among the Diseases of the Nervous stock*, ibid. *its description*, ibid. *its seat not always or often in the Gut Colon, neither in its Cavity or Coats*, ibid. *its conjunct cause are not the contents of the intestines, nor the humour impacted in the Membranes*, 226. *the Nervous Liquor seems most of all to contribute to its cause*, ibid. *its seat and part affected*, 227, 228. *why pains of the Loins often come upon Colick pains*, ibid. *in what the foregoing cause consists*, ibid.

the

the evident cause, 229 *the differences of this disease,* ibid. *its prognosticks,* ibid. *its cure,* ibid. *to* 233. *its Histories* 233. 234
Corporeal Soul the subject of the rational, 41. *after what manner 'tis affected in melancholy and madness* 191
Custome, *its force,* 89. *a notable example thereof* ibid.

D.

Deafness *sometimes proceeds from the loosness of the Drum* 73
Declination *of age disposes some to foolishness* 211
Delirium, *what it is,* 179, *its formal reason,* ibid. *its causes either from the blood, or exteriour Spirits planted in the Nervous Stock,* 180. *by what and how many ways it is caused by the blood,* ibid: *how it proceeds from the irregularities of the exteriour spirits,* 181. *its prognosticks,* ibid. *its cure,* ibid. *the primary Phenomena of a melancholick Delirium, and from what dispositions of the Spirits they proceed* 188
Desire *and aversion chiefly imploy the Soul,* 51. *how excited, &c.* ibid. *to* 53
Digby *and others their opinion of the Souls of Brutes* 3
Dreams, *what they are,* 93. *sometimes excited by the Spirits inhabiting the Brain, sometimes inhabiting other parts, viz. the Stomach, &c.* 94. *they sometimes stir up local motions* ibid.
Drunkenness *and looking down from high places, &c. how they cause a Vertigo* 146

E.

EAr, *and its uses* 71, 72
Eating *is a certain solution* 62
Epicurus *and his late followers opinion that the Soul is made of Atoms* 2, 3
Epilepsy, *its seat the middle of the Brain, which is the seat of the Apoplexy also* 161.
Eye, *its description and reason of its diverse conformation inquired into a p.* 78 *to* 86

F.

FEar, *its character, &c.* 53, 54
Feeling, *more thick, but most ample of all the senses,* 60. *its kinds, &c. from* 60 *to* 62. *what its proper organ* 168
Fire, *its definition agrees, by its causes and essences, with the Soul of Brutes* 5
Fishes, *why they rejoice rather in the Water than Air* ibid. *they breath by the Gills* ibid.
Flame *V.* Fire, *part of the Soul,* 22, 31, 33. *its difference from light* 76
Foolishness, *V.* Stupidity.

G.

GAssendus *his assertion of the Soul,* 4 *according to him every body is either lucid or illustrated* 77
Gometius *and* Pereira *deny the Souls of Brutes to have sense and perception* 2
Gout, *a distemper of the Nervous Stock,* 214. *its subject, its appearances rehearsed,* ibid. *parts affected,* 215. *morbifick matter, not any simple humour,* ibid. *in its mixe two humours concur and mutually grow hot, exemplifyed how,* ibid. *the Blood full of a fixed Salt, as it were its feminine, the Nervous Liquor being sharp, the masculine seed,* 216. *its foregoing causes,* ibid. *&* 217, 218. *the evident causes of the goutish fit,* 218. *whence the debility of the Joints,* 217. *differences of the Gout,* 219 *wont to be complicated with the Scurvy and Stone, and the reason of that shewed,* ibid. *its prognostick,* ibid. *cure,* ib. *a notable history of the Stone converted into the Gout, and of the Gout into the Stone* 224

H.

HEad-ach *the most common, and chiefest affection among diseases,* 105. *its causes so manifold that they can hardly be methodically recited,* ibid. *hence its cure often instituted empirically,* ibid. *what things belong to its pathology,* ibid. *its subject,* ibid. *its formal reason, differences and kinds,* 106. *either within or without the Soul, universal or particular,* ibid. *many other differences noted,* ibid. *an habitual one hath always a more remote cause besides the evident,* ibid. *its causes, a p.* 107 *ad* 110. *arising from the Nervous Liquor it chiefly infests in the morning,* 108. *how stirred up by many humours meeting together and growing hot,* ibid. *the habitual one chiefly depends on the fault of the Nervous humour,* 109. *its kinds noted at large,* 112, 113. *how it seems to arise from the Spleen, mesentery or womb,* ibid. *its prognosticks,* 113. *cure, from* 114 *to* 125. *Histories,* ibid. *a continual head-ach not to be accounted incurable* 123
Hearing, *its excellency as to use and activity, performed at a distance, &c.* 69. *its organ described* 71
Heart *hardned, what it is* 47
Histories *of head-achs, from* 121 *to* 125. *of one killed presently by taking too large a dose of Opium,* 128. *of Lethargicks,* 232, *&c. of continual sleepiness,* 135, 137. *of long waking,* 140. *of the Vertigo,* 151, 152. *of the Apoplexy,* 162. *of the Palsie,* 174, 175, 176, 177. *of the delirium or Phrensy,* 187. *of Melancholy,* 197, 198. *Histories of mad people are to be sought in Hospitals for mad people,* 208. *A notable History of the*

A TABLE.

the Stone converted into the Gout, and the Gout into the Stone, 224. *of the Colick,* 233, 234. *of a mortal madness from eating the leaves of Wolfs-bane* 204
Hope, 53, 54

I.

Images, *light, and colour are of the same substance* 75
Imaginary *Metamorphosis of melancholick persons* 200
Imagination, *V. Phantasy.*
Incubus, *or Night-mare its seat in the cerebel,* 142. *its description,* ibid. *it most often proceeds from natural causes,* ibid. *its seat falsely placed in the Brain,* ibid. *the Præcordia truly labour in this Disease,* ibid. *its cause doth not stick partly in the Brain, and partly in the Breast,* ibid. *its next cause is the hindrance of the inflowing of the Spirits to the Præcordia,* 143. *this not in the parts affected, nor Nerves themselves, but in the cerebel, where the first spring of the spirits is,* ibid. *from whence the sense of the weight and loss of motion proceeds,* ibid. *why the fit being so grievous is so often ended without leaving any evil,* ibid. *whence the trembling of the Heart and Præcordia after the fit,* ibid. *the Incubus of it self rarely dangerous,* ibid. *its prognosticks,* 144. *its Cure,* ibid. *how infants and boys obnoxious to this Disease ought to be handled,* ibid.
Insects *appear to have fiery Souls, because they want sulphureous and nitrous food* 8
Instances *of passion merely Physical* 46
Instinct *natural, what it is,* 34. *what it brings to Brutes,* ibid. *examples of it,* ibid. *it dictates to them what's wholesome, what not,* 35. *leads not only to simple actions, but to very complicate ones,* ibid. *yet those always, and in all, of one kind only,* ibid. *how 'tis wont to be compared with acquired notions,* 37. *and with the impressions of sensible things,* ibid. *with habits learned from example or institution,* ibid. *with notions learned from experience and imitation* ibid.
Intellect *in man presides o're the imagination, &c.* 38. *and discerns its errors, sublimates its notions, and divests them from matter, and contemplates immaterial substances, judges and directs its propositions, deduces from these others more sublime thoughts, beholds it self by a reflected action, and contemplates other things remote from sense, as God, &c.* 39. *it depends upon the Phantasy,* 41. *by reason of the various constitution of this and the Brain, Souls seems unequal* 42
Issues *made upon or near the distemper'd place help little* 119

K.

ALL Knowledge *from sense* 57

L.

Lethargy, *its seat the same with that of Sleep and Memory,* 125. *its Fits are call'd by this name,* ibid. *and the soporiferous disposition also,* 126. *of which are various kinds,* ibid. *its causes,* ibid. *to* 128. *what things belong to its theory,* 129. *the chiefest of its symptoms,* ibid. *by what means the other faculties of the Soul, as the knowing, desiring and locomotive are affected* ibid. *its evil reaches also to the cerebel,* ibid. *hence breathing often hurt or altered,* ibid. *which proceeds not from the inflammation of the midriff,* ibid. *its Fever from whence,* ibid. *and* 130. *none dyes without one,* ibid. *its prognosticks,* ibid. *its cure,* 131 *to* 133. *Histories,* ibid. *its ends or limits as to the places distempered are constituted,* ibid. *some sleepy distempers lesser than it, the Caros greater* ibid.
Light, *Colours and Images the same substance,* 75. *Light and Flame their differences,* 76. *wherefore Light either reflected or refracted goes forward only in streight lines,* ib. *it can pass through a Chamber, in the mean time not to be perceiv'd,* ibid. *'tis primary or secundary,* ibid. *the differences of these,* 77
Lobster, *its Anatomy* 11, 12
Local *motion stir'd up by the appetite* 36
Love, *how excited,* 50. *it and hatred transitory passions,* 51. *its object set up like an Idol in the Phantasy and worshipped* 50
Love-madness, 199. *reasons of its symptoms* ibid.
Lucid *part of the Soul,* 22. *shines diversly,* 31. *alteration of the flamy part impressed by it* 32
Lungs, *how differ in Birds and four footed Beasts,* 17. *for what end perforated in Birds* ibid.

M.

Madness *and Melancholy are a-kin,* 201. *the subject of Madness are the Animal Spirits, the disposition of which are like to Stygian Water,* ibid. *three chief accidents in Madness, which are also to be found in Stygian Water,* 201, 202. *the conjunct cause of Madness what it is,* ibid. *the original of Madness, either from the Spirits themselves, or from the Blood,* 203. *it begins from the Spirits from two occasions,* ibid. *by what means it comes upon Melancholy,* 204. *how upon a Phrensy,* ibid. *the original*

A TABLE.

ginal of Madness sometimes from the Blood, ibid. it is either hereditary, the reason of which is shown, 204. or acquired, and so either by reason of errors in the six non-naturals, or by reason of Poysons, ibid. History of a mortal Madness from eating the leaves of Wolfs-bane, ibid. the reasons of the symptoms of Madness explained, 205. wherefore mad men are audacious, ibid. from whence their immense strength, ibid. wherefore they are never tired, ibid. wherefore they are not easily hurt, ibid. the differences in respect of the original magnitude and time, ibid. the prognosticks, ibid. the cure from the indications of continual Madness, 206. the curatory indication as to discipline, ibid. as to Medicines, ibid. the preservatory indication consists in altering Medicines, as whey, &c. Specificks, &c. ibid. the vital and curatory indications 208

Melancholy, its definition, 188. 'tis a distemper of the Brain and Heart, ibid. its Examples or Types various and almost infinite, ibid. 'tis either universal or particular, ibid. the primary Phænomena of a melancholick Delirium, and from what disposition of the Spirits they proceed, ibid. as they are compared to light they are call'd opacous or full of darkness, 189. these kind of Spirits in Melancholy compared to those in Chymical Liquors, ibid. they are not like the Spirit of Blood as they should be, nor like the Spirit of Wine, for such is rather in the Phrensy, ibid. but these are like acid Spirits distill'd out of Salt, Vinegar, Box, and such like, ibid. the formal reason of Melancholy aptly represented by acetous Chymical Liquors, ibid. there are three chief affections of these which agree with the Animal Spirits in Melancholy, 190, 191. in Melancholy after the Spirits being for some time vitiated, the conformation of the Brain becomes also hurt, 191. in this Disease the affection of the Præcordia, as to fear and sadness is delivered, ibid. after what manner the corporeal Soul is affected in Melancholy and Madness, ibid. the cause of either depends partly on the Blood, and partly on the Animal action of the Heart, ibid. the Procatartick causes of Melancholy are partly the acetous nature of the Spirits, and partly the Melancholy discrasie of the Blood; and the distemper begins sometimes from this, sometimes from that, 191, 192. how it begins from the Spirits and the Animal Government, 192. by what means it arises from the Blood, ibid. Melancholy doth not arise from any atrabiliary humour heaped up in some place or vein, ibid. by what means, according to the Ancients 'tis said to arise from the Head, ibid. how from the Womb, ibid. how from the Spleen, ibid. how from the whole Body, 193. the differences of this Disease, in respect of its first subject, and by reason of the temperament of the Sick, and in respect of its next cause, as it is singular or conjunct, and in respect of the imagination being diversly hurt, ibid. its prognosticks, ibid. in the Cure the evident cause is first to be removed, ibid. and herein are three primary indications, first Curatory, &c. 193, 194. secondly Preservatory, &c. 149, altering Medicines are here of greatest moment, and not purging as the Ancients thought, 196. Histories of this Disease, 197. particular Melancholy is excited by reason of two sorts of affections concerning good or evil 199

Melancholick persons their imaginary Metamorphosis 200
Metamorphosis imaginary of melancholick Persons 200
Millepedes notably help in the cure of the head-ach 118

N.

Nemesius attributes sense and perception to corporeal Souls, and farther the use of an inferiour reason 3
Nervous Liquor how a cause of the head-ach, 108. the habitual head-ach depends chiefly upon its fault, &c. 109, wherefore it oftimes becomes corrosive, &c. 202
Nutritious juice, how it excites the head-ach, 108. 110, 111

O.

Opiats, how they cause sleep, 128. how they operate in the Ventricle or Brain, how as assigned by Webfer 156

P.

Palace or seat of the humane mind in the Phantasy 41
Palsie, what it is, 161. its seat, ibid. its conjunct causes, 162. in the Palsie either motion or sense only, or both together is hurt, ibid. spontaneous motion is abolished by reason of the ways being obstructed, either in the beginnings or middle passages, or about the ends, ibid. the ways are obstructed by impletion or compression, or by a breaking of the unity, ibid. an obstruction in the streaked Bodies causes the universal Palsie, or the Palsie of one side, ibid. why sense is not hindered as well as motion in every Palsie, 163. why all Muscles of the Eyes and Face are not loosened in an universal Palsie, ibid. a compression of the streaked Body sometimes stirs up the Palsie, ibid. a paralytick obstruction doth sometimes happen in the oblong and spinal Marrow, ibid. a Palsie often succeeds Stupidity, ibid. a Palsie sometimes from the pressing together of the Marrowy chord,

chord, ibid. *sometimes from the unity being broke,* 164. *the seat of the Palsie sometimes in the Nerves themselves, which are either obstructed, or compressed, or the unity broken,* ibid. *an obstruction sometime in the beginning of the Nerves, sometimes in the middle, or in their utmost processes,* ibid. *the other conjunct cause of the Palsie,* ibid. *in every Palsie the matter is not so thick or cold, as it is vitriolick and other ways infestious to the Spirits,* ibid. *the blasting or withering of Trees like the Palsie,* ibid. *the more remote foregoing causes of the Palsie,* ibid. *the Palsie is either a primary Distemper, and a Disease of it self, or secondary, coming upon or succeeding other Diseases,* ibid. *why the Palsie often succeeds convulsive Diseases,* ibid. *why the distemper of the Colick,* 166. *why the Gout,* ibid. *the evident causes of the habitual Palsie,* ibid. *want or paucity of Spirits oftentimes the cause of the spurious Palsie,* ibid. *for which reason old men are obnoxious to this Disease,* 167. *also scorbutical Persons, and such as are full of ill humours,* ibid. *also others long sick,* ibid. *hence some dare not venture on local motion, others endeavouring cannot bear it long,* ibid *the second kind of Palsie in which motion and sense are hurt at once,* ibid. *the third kind in which sense only is affected,* 168. *why feeling is sometimes lost and motion safe,* ibid. *the Prognostick,* ibid. *the Cure,* 171. *Histories and Examples of Paralyticks* 174
Paraphrensis, *what it is,* 181. *its conjunct causes,* 181, 182. *wherefore breathing is hurt in this Disease,* ibid. *its Prognosticks,* 184. *Cure* 185
Parts *of the corporeal Soul,* 22. *parts serving for hearing, how they differ in man and some four-footed Beasts* 74
Passions, *their History, from* 45 *to* 55
Phantasy, *or imagination the power thereof in Brutes,* 38. *'tis often deceived,* ibid. *in man 'tis the intellect presiding over the imagination,* V. Intellect, *the seat or palace of the humane mind in it,* 41. *the pleasing of it and the senses cause sleep* 90
Phantastick *desires are immense* 52
Phrensy, V. Delirium.
Platonists *and* Pythagoreans *affirm'd the Soul of Brutes to be an incorporeal substance* 2
Pleasure *and* Grief *the two primary affections of the Soul,* 48. *they affect the two roots of the Soul, viz. the Brain and Præcordia* ibid *and* 49
Præcordia, *wherefore and how esteemed the seat of holy affections,* 47. *why call'd the seat of Prudence and Wisdom,* ibid. *they and the Brain the two roots of the Soul,* 48 *they truly labour in the Incubus* 142
Prototype *of a sound by and by stirs up innumerable Ectypes* 70
Pupil *of the Eye in some round, in others longish, the reason inquired into,* 83. *its colour in some black, in others grey, reddish or otherwise colour'd, the reason shewn.* ibid.

R.

Reasons *of very many Authors perswade that the Soul of Brutes is not only corporeal but fiery,* 5. *the reason of good and evil either concerns the corporeal Soul by it self, or united to the Body, or subjected to the rational,* 45. *reasons of Colours and Images unfolded,* 77. *reasons of the symptoms in Love-madness explained,* 199. *of Tumors and Ulcers in the Kings Evil, &c.* 202, 203. *of symptoms in Madness,* 205. *why wise and strong men are not always begot of strong and wise men* 210

S.

Salivation *in inveterate head-achs, without suspicion of the Venereal Disease, whether it ought to be administred,* 119. *the means and manner of salivating by Mercury unfolded* 119, 120
Sense, *what it is* 56, 57 to 60
Serum, *how it excites the head-ach,* 108. *its evacuation through its right way being suppressed, brings its Flux to the head* 110
Sight, *the most noble Sense* 75, 77, 78
Sleep *unknown, or greatly controverted, what it is,* 86. Schneiderus's *opinion that it is an inorganical faculty of the Soul,* ibid. *its subject not the whole Body,* 87. *the Animal Spirits its immediate subject,* ibid. *all the Spirits injoy rest but not in sleep, &c.* ibid. *its immediate subject is the knowing part of the sensitive Soul,* ibid. *the mediate are the Bodies contemning it,* 88. *its formal reason and beginning,* ibid. *and causes,* 89. *'tis either natural, not natural or preternatural,* ibid. *by what and how many ways it begins from the Brain first affected,* 90. *not from fumes,* ibid. *its matter conveyed only by the Arteries,* 91. *why raw and indigested meats induce sleepiness,* ibid. *how it seems to begin in the Eyes,* ibid. *the effects thereof,* 92. *why those that sleep are apt to be cold outwardly,* ibid. *the Blood performs its offices better in sleep,* ibid. *what it affords to the lucid part of the Soul,* ibid. *benefits of sleep noted* ibid.
Soul, *the contemplation thereof whereto it conduces,* 1. *divers opinions of the Soul,* 2, 3. *three things to be considered in the Soul of Brutes,* 6. *various kinds of Brutes Souls described, &c.* 7. *Insects have fiery Souls, &c.* 8. *whether fiery Souls in Bloodless Creatures,* 13. *the corporeal Soul in man subject to the rational,* 18. *a double subject of the Brutal Soul,* 22. *whence two parts thereof, &c.* ibid. *the sensible part divisible,* 23. *the Animal Spirits constitute its Hypostasis,* ibid. *its beginning,* 29. *frames it self before*

A TABLE.

fore the Body, and increases with it, ibid. *the Bodies duration depends upon it,* ibid. *like flame it has its trepidations, &c.* 31. *as strong in sense and motion as a machine,* 32. *if immaterial, also rational,* ibid. *the common sensory not the whole Soul,* 33. *'tis like a self-moving musical Organ,* 34. *the rational far exceeds the Brutal, how both joyn'd in man, and how they frequently disagree,* 38. *the rational Souls priority,* ibid. *the first act of either is simple apprehension,* ibid. *the second enunciation,* 39 *how little the Brutes Soul can do in respect of man,* 40. *Authors for two distinct Souls in man,* ibid. *which reason also dictates,* 41. *the rational does not exercise the Animal faculties, nor obliterate the sensitive by its coming, nor transmute it into a mere power,* ibid. *by what bond united to the Body,* ibid. *the corporeal its subject,* ibid. *created and poured into the formed Body, not propagated ex traduce,* 42. *plurality of Son's in man manifested by their differences,* ibid. *the rational of it self without affections, and how it governs and orders them and the Phantasy,* 43. *in things to be known the corporeal obeys it, but not in things to be done, and inclining it self to the flesh fights against it,* ibid. *how 'tis reduc'd to obedience,* ibid. *it oft seduces the mind,* ibid. *its twofold state,* 45. *its lucid part feels or perceives the impulse of all objects, and is moved by them,* 56. *after what manner the corporeal Soul is affected in Melancholy and Madness* 191

Spirits, *their distinct offices in various provinces, &c.* 24, 25. *how they receive sensible species so very divers,* 57. *the Animal the immediate subject of Sleep,* 87. *for what causes they lye down of their own accord,* 89. *compell'd into sleep by Narcoticks,* 90. *their penury perswades to sleep,* ibid. *the distemper of the Animal Spirits being after a diverse manner, as it is the cause of the Phrensy, so it is of Melancholy, Madness and Stupidity,* 188, *compared to light they are opacous or full of darkness,* 189 *these kind of Spirits in Melancholy compared to those in Chymical Liquors, for they are not like the Spirits of Blood as they should be, nor the Spirits of Wine, for such are rather in the Phrensy, but like acid Spirits distill'd out of Salt, Vinegar, &c.* ibid. *Stygian Waters like the Animal Spirits in Madness,* ibid. *three chief affections of acetous Chymical Liquors which agree with the Animal Spirits in Melancholy,* 191. *after the Animal Spirits in Melancholy being for some time vitiated, the conformation of the Brain is also hurt,* ibid. *how the Animal Spirits acquire a disposition like to Stygian Water,* 202. *the original of Madness either from the Spirits themselves, or from the Blood,* 203. *it begins from the Spirits for two occasions* ibid.

Squinting, *whence it comes* 82
Stupidity *arises chiefly from the failing of the imagination and memory,* 209. *wherefore the Organs of these faculties labour in this Disease,* ibid. *chiefly the Brain, first as to magnitude, and by reason of figure,* ibid. *as to substance or texture,* 210. *its evil conformation as to its pores and passages, whence Stupidity sometimes proceeds from both of them being in fault together,* ibid. *what the antecedent causes of foolishness are,* ibid. *ripeness and the declination of Age dispose some to foolishness,* 211, *great hurts of the head sometimes cause doting or want of ingenuity,* ibid. *and frequent Drunkenness,* ibid. *and vehement affections,* ibid. *and the more grievous Diseases of the head,* ibid. *the differences of this Disease,* 212. *how Foolishness and Stupidity differ,* ibid. *Stupidity its degrees,* ibid. *the prognostick,* ibid. *if from an hurt of the head evil,* ibid. *if excited from a Lethargy it admits of Cure,* ibid. *sometimes 'tis cur'd by a Fever,* ibid. *the Cure requires both a Master and a Physician,* 213. *what the labour of the former ought to be,* ibid. *what the Medical intentions are* ibid. *what kinds of remedies are shown* ibid.

T.

Tangible *species immediately carried either to the cerebel, or to the streaked Bodies,* 61. *and from thence go forward sometimes to the other faculties* ibid.
Taste *of kin to feeling, &c.* 62, 63
Tears, *their matter* 80
Touch, *the same Nerves are observ'd to serve for its sense and motion* 63

V.

Venus *an enemy to the Brain and Nerves,* 55. *necessary to the preserving of the individual* 62
Vertigo, *its seat,* 145. *a description of it,* ibid. *the causes and manner of an unnatural one,* ibid. *why looking down from on high, and passing over Bridges cause it,* 146. *how Drunkenness causes it,* ibid. *from what causes the preternatural one is wont to be excited,* ibid. *sometimes 'tis a symptome of other cephalick Diseases; sometimes 'tis excited by reason of the distemper of other distant parts, viz. from the Stomach, Spleen, &c,* 146, 147. *not by reason of Vapors elevated from these parts,* 147. *its immediate subject is the Animal Spirits,* ibid. *its formal reason,* ibid. *its conjunct cause,* 148. *is seen by things helpful and hurtful,* ibid. *the more remote foregoing cause,* ibid. *the differences of this Disease,* ibid. *its prognosticks,* 149. *the Cure,* ibid. *the curatory method shown,* 150. *why vomiting Medicines are so much*

A TABLE.

noted in this and other Diseases of the head, ibid. *what is to be done out of the Fit for prevention sake,* ibid. *cases and examples of the sick in three Histories, and the reason of the case of the second History described,* 151, 152

Vices *of the Brain noted* 148

W.

IN Waking *the Spirits inhabiting the cerebel are disturbed with the Spirits of the other Regiment,* 93. *why those being disturb'd perform their offices better whilst these lye quiet in sleep,* ibid. *a double consideration of waking* 95

Long Waking, *of two sorts, 'tis either the symptom of other Diseases, or a Disease it self,* 138. *how many ways the unquiet or elastick Spirits stir it up,* 139. *its causes assign'd,* ibid. *its Cure and History* ibid.

Natural Waking *its cause consists in the restlesness of the Spirits and the openness of the cortical part of the Brain* 138

Want *or paucity of the Spirits oftentimes the cause of the spurious Palsie* 166

Watching *preternatural depends either upon the restlesness of the Spirits, or the openness of the cortical part of the Brain* 139

Weeping, *its causes, and the manner of its being made, described,* 80. *wherefore a bewailing is oftentimes joyned with weeping,* ibid. *wherefore it comes from sudden joy,* 81. *why mankind only or chiefly weep* ibid.

Wise *and strong men, why not always begotten of wise and strong men* 210

Withering *or blasting of Trees like the Palsie* 164

FINIS.

Advertisement.

DOctor *Willis*'s Practice of Physick, being all the Medical Works of that Renowned and Famous Physician, Containing these Ten Treatises following, *viz.* I. Of Fermentation. II. Of Feavers. III. Of Urines. IV. Of the Accension of the Blood. V. Of Musculary Motion. VI. Of the Anatomy of the Brain. VII. Of the Description and Use of the Nerves. VIII. Of Convulsive Diseases. IX. Pharmaceutice Rationalis, the first and second Part. X. Of the Scurvey. Wherein most of the Diseases belonging to the Body of Man are treated of, with excellent Methods and Receipts for the Cure of the same. Fitted to the meanest Capacity, by an Index for the explaining of all the hard and unusual Words and Terms of Art, derived from the Greek, Latin, or other Languages, for the benefit of the English Reader. With a large Alphabetical Table to the whole. With Thirty Copper Plates. Done into English by *S. Pordage* Student in Physick. Printed for *T. Dring,* and *C. Harper* in *Fleetstreet,* and *J. Leigh* at *Stationers Hall.* Price Thirty Shillings.

There is now Published the second Volume of Dr. *Nalson*'s Impartial Collections of the Great Affairs of State, from the beginning of the Scotch Rebellion, in the Year 1639. to the Murther of King *Charles* the First; wherein the first occasions, and the whole series of the late Troubles in *England, Scotland,* and *Ireland,* are faithfully represented, taken from Authentick Records, and methodically digested, with a Table. Published by his Majesties special Command. Sold by *Thomas Dring* at the *Harrow,* at the Corner of *Chancery Lane* in *Fleetstreet.*